Neurosurgery of complex tumors and vascular lesions

For Churchill Livingstone

Senior Medical Editor: Miranda Bromage
Project Editor: Deborah Russell
Project Controller: Mark Sanderson

Freelance

Copy Editor: Graham Wild
Proof Reader: Gillian Landsberger
Cover Design: Andrew Jones
Indexer: Anne McCarthy

Neurosurgery of complex tumors and vascular lesions

EDITED BY

Shigeaki Kobayashi, MD PhD
Professor and Chairman,
Department of Neurosurgery,
Shinshu University School of Medicine,
Matsumoto, Japan

Atul Goel, MCh
Associate Professor,
Department of Neurosurgery,
Seth G. S. Medical College and
King Edward Memorial Hospital,
Parel, Bombay, India;
Honorary Visiting Professor,
Department of Neurosurgery,
Shinshu University School of Medicine,
Matsumoto, Japan

Kazuhiro Hongo, MD PhD
Associate Professor,
Department of Neurological Surgery,
Aichi Medical University,
Aichi, Japan

Illustrations by

Junpei Nitta, MD
Staff Neurosurgeon,
Department of Neurosurgery,
Shinshu University School of Medicine,
Matsumoto, Japan

NEW YORK EDINBURGH LONDON MADRID MELBOURNE SAN FRANCISCO TOKYO 1997

CHURCHILL LIVINGSTONE
Medical Division of Pearson Professional Limited

Distributed in the United States of America by Churchill Livingstone Inc.,
650 Avenue of the Americas, New York,
N.Y. 10011, and by associated companies, branches and representatives throughout the world.

First published 1997

ISBN 0 443 07870 X

British Library Cataloguing in Publication Data
A catalogue record for this book is available from the British Library.

Library of Congress Cataloging in Publication Data
A catalog record for this book is available from the Library of Congress.

Medical knowledge is constantly changing. As new information becomes available,
changes in treatment, procedures, equipment and the use of drugs become necessary.
The editors/authors/contributors and the publishers have, as far as it is possible,
taken care to ensure that the information given in this text is accurate and up-to-date.
However, readers are strongly advised to confirm that the information,
especially with regard to drug usage, complies with
latest legislation and standards of practice.

The
publisher's
policy is to use
**paper manufactured
from sustainable forest**

Printed in Great Britain

Contents

List of contributors and commenting experts

Ossama Al-Mefty, MD FACS
Professor and Chairman, Department of Neurosurgery,
College of Medicine, University of Arkansas, USA

Ahmed Ammar MB, ChB DMSc
Chairman, Department of Neurosurgery, King Faisal
University Hospital, King Faisal University, Al Khobar,
Saudi Arabia

James I. Ausman MD PhD
Professor and Chairman, Department of Neurosurgery
(M/C 799), The University of Illinois at Chicago,
Neuropsychiatric Institute, Chicago, Illinois, USA

Issam A. Awad MD MSc FACS MA (Hon)
Professor of Surgery (Neurosurgery) and Program Head,
Neurovascular Surgery Program, Section of
Neurosurgery, Yale University School of Medicine,
New Haven, Connecticut, USA

H. Hunt Batjer MD
Professor and Chairman, Division of Neurological
Surgery, Northwestern University Medical School,
Chicago, Illinois, USA

Jacques Brotchi MD
Professor and Chairman, Service de Neurochirurgie,
Erasme Hospital, Free University of Brussels, Belgium

Vinko V. Dolenc MD PhD
Professor and Chairman, Department of Neurosurgery,
University Hospital Centre, Zaloska, Ljubljana, Slovenia

Fred Epstein MD
Professor and Director, Fred J. Epstein Division of
Paediatric Neurosurgery, New York University Medical
Center, New York, USA

Georg Fries MD
Department of Neurosurgery, Johannes Gutenberg
University, Medical School, Mainz, Germany

Steven L. Giannotta MD
Professor of Neurosurgery, University of Southern
California, Los Angeles, California, USA

Bernard George MD
Professor, Service de Neurochirurgie, Hospital
Lariboisere, Paris, France

Akira Hakuba MD DMSc
Professor and Chairman, Department of Neurosurgery,
Osaka City University Medical School, Osaka, Japan

Dae Hee Han MD
Professor and Chairman, Department of Neurosurgery,
Seoul National University College of Medicine, Seoul,
Korea

Kazuo Hashi MD
Professor and Chairman, Department of Neurosurgery,
Sapporo Medical University, Sapporo, Japan

Nobuo Hashimoto MD
Chairman, Department of Cerebrovascular Center,
Suita, Osaka, Japan

Harold J. Hoffman MD
Chief, Division of Neurosurgery, The Hospital for Sick
Children; Professor, Department of Surgery, University of
Toronto, Toronto, Ontario, Canada

Anil P. Karapurkar MS MCh
Professor, Department of Neurosurgery, Seth G.S.
Medical College and King Edward Medical Hospital,
Bombay, India

Takeshi Kawase, MD
Professor and Chairman, Department of Surgery
(Neurosurgery), Keio University, School of Medicine,
Tokyo, Japan

Andrew H. Kaye MBBS MD FRACS
Professor of Neurosurgery, The University of Melbourne,
Director of Neurosurgery, The Royal Melbourne Hospital
and The Melbourne Neuroscience Center, Melbourne,
Australia

Phyo Kim MD PhD DMSc
Associate Professor, Department of Neurosurgery,
Dokkyo University School of Medicine, Tochigi, Japan

Kazuhiko Kyoshima, MD
Associate Professor, Department of Neurosurgery,
Shinshu University School of Medicine, Matsumoto,
Japan

Manu Kothari MS
Professor Emeritus, Department of Anatomy, Seth G. S.
Medical College and King Edward Medical Hospital,
Bombay, India

Edward R. Laws Jr MD FACS
Professor of Neurosurgery, Professor of Medicine,
University of Virginia, Health Sciences Center,
Department of Neurological Surgery, Charlottesville,
Virginia, USA

Michael T. Lawton MD
Division of Neurological Surgery, Barrow Neurological
Institute, University of Arizona, St Josephs Hospital and
Medical Center, Phoenix, Arizona, USA

Arnold H. Menezes MD FACS FAAP
Professor and Vice Chairman, Division of Neurosurgery,
University of Iowa Hospitals and Clinics, Iowa City,
Iowa, USA

Williams T. Monacci MD
The George Washington University Medical Center,
Medical Faculty Associates, Washington DC, USA

Trimurti Nadkarni MS MCh
Lecturer, Department of Neurosurgery, Seth G. S.
Medical College and
King Edward Medical Hospital, Bombay, India

Tatsuya Nagashima MD
Department of Neurosurgery, Kobe University School of
Medicine, Kobe, Japan

Hiroshi Nakagawa MD
Professor and Chairman, Department of Neurological
Surgery, Aichi Medical University, Aichi, Japan

Junpei Nitta MD
Staff Neurosurgeon, Department of Neurosurgery,
Shinshu University School of Medicine, Matsumoto,
Japan

Stephen Nutik MD PhD
Consultant Neurosurgeon, The Permanente Medical
Group, Inc., Redwood City, California, USA

Akira Ogawa MD
Professor and Chair, Department of Neurosurgery, Iwate
Medical University, School of Medicine, Morioka, Japan

Chang-Wan Oh MD
Instructor, Department of Neurosurgery, Seoul National
University College of Medicine, Seoul, Korea

Kenji Ohata MD
Assistant Professor, Department of Neurosurgery, Osaka
City University Medical School, Osaka, Japan

Hideyuki Ohnishi MD
Assistant Professor, Department of Neurosurgery, Nara
Prefectural Medical University, Kashihara, Nara, Japan

Evandro de Oliveira MD
Director, Sao Paulo Neurological Institute; Chief,
Vascular and Tumors Groups, Neurosurgery Division,
Sao Paulo University School of Medicine, Sao Paulo,
Brazil

S. J. Peerless MD FRCS
Director, Clinical Professor of Neurosurgery, Mercy
Neuroscience Institute, University of Miami, Miami,
Florida, USA

Azel Perneczky MD PhD
Professor and Director, Department of Neurosurgery,
Johannes Gutenberg University, Medical School, Mainz,
Germany

Prem Pillay MD FRCS
Director, Brain Center, Singapore General Hospital and
Postgraduate Institute, Singapore

Elen Piontek MSc
Department of Neurosurgery, Hadassah University
Hospital, Jerusalem, Israel

Vendatam Rajshekhar MS Mch (Neuro)
Associate Professor, Department of Neurological
Sciences, Christian Medical College and Hospital,
Vellore, India

Albert L. Rhoton, Jr MD
R. D. Keene Family Professor and
Chairman of Neurological Surgery, Department of
Neurological Surgery, College of Medicine, University of
Florida, Gainesville, Florida, USA

Madjid Samii MD
Professor of Neurosurgery, Hannover Medical School;
(Chair), Director of Neurosurgical Clinic, Nordstadt
Hospital Hannover, Hannover, Germany

Hirotoshi Sano MD
Associate Professor, Department of Neurosurgery, Fujita
Health University School of Medicine, Toyoake, Aichi,
Japan

Laigam N. Sekhar MD
Professor and Chairman, Department of Neurological
Surgery, George Washington University Medical Center,
Medical Faculty Associates, Washington DC, USA

Chandranath Sen MD
Professor and Vice-Chairman, Department of
Neurosurgery, The Mount Sinai Medical Center, Mount
Sinai School of Medicine, New York, USA

Mr R. P. Sengupa Msc FRCS FRCS (Ed)
Senior Consultant Neurosurgeon, and Lecturer in
Neurosurgery, Regional Neurosciences Centre, Newcastle
General Hospital, Newcastle upon Tyne, UK

Masato Shibuya MD
Associate Professor, Department of Neurosurgery,
Nagoya University, School of Medicine, Nagoya, Japan

Hiroaki Shigeta MD
Staff Neurosurgeon, Department of Neurosurgery,
Shinshu University School of Medicine, Matsumoto,
Japan

Sergei Spektor MD
Department of Neurosurgery, Hadassah University
Hospital, Jerusalem, Israel

Robert F. Spetzler MD
Director, Barrow Neurological Institute; Professor,
Division of Neurological Surgery, University of Arizona,
St Joseph's Hospital and Medical Center, Phoenix,
Arizona, USA

Toshiki Takemae MD
Lecturer, Department of Neurosurgery, Shinshu
University School of Medicine, Matsumoto, Japan

Norihiko Tamaki MD
Professor and Chairman, Department of Neurosurgery,
Kobe University School of Medicine, Kobe, Japan

Yuichiro Tanaka MD
Assistant Professor, Department of Neurosurgery,
Shinshu University School of Medicine, Matsumoto,
Japan

Mamoru Taneda, MD
Professor and Chairman, Department of Neurosurgery,
Kinki University School of Medicine, Sayama, Osaka,
Japan

Michael J, Torrens BSc MBBS MPhil ChM FRCS
Chairman of the Division of Neurosurgery and
Consultant Neurosurgeon to Ygeia Hospital, Athens,
Greece; Honorary Consultant Neurosurgeon, Frenchay
Hospital, Bristol, UK

Felix Umansky MD
Professor and Chairman, Department of Neurosurgery,
Hadassah University Hospital, Jerusalem, Israel

Yukitaka Ushio, MD
Professor and Chairman, Department of Neurosurgery,
Kumamoto University School of Medicine, Kumamoto,
Japan

Alberto Valarezo, MD
Department of Neurosurgery, Hadassah University
Hospital, Jerusalem, Israel

U. S. Vengsarka MS Mch (neuro)
Consultant Neurosurgeon, Sir Hukissonda Hospital,
Bombay, India

Eiju Watanabe MD
Department of Neurosurgery, Tokyo Metropolitan Police
Hospital, Tokyo, Japan

Preface

The improvements in neurosurgical techniques are primarily a result of revolutionary advances in the technological aids that facilitiate diagnosis and surgery. We have selected in this volume a group of complex vascular lesions and tumors for discussion. The list of complex lesions obviously cannot be complete as none of the lesions involving the brain can be considered easy. The issues discussed are those which are of particular interest to the authors. The book comprises chapters written primarily by Shigeaki Kobayashi, Atul Goel and Kazuhiro Hongo. The cases and clinical data are collected from records of Shinshu University (Matsumoto) and King Edward Memorial Hospital (bombay). Each chapter is followed by a technical discussion on the subject by experts in that particular field. With this format we have made an attempt to introduce to the reader our perspectives and ideas of dealing with a particular problem and have complemented it with current opinion. As far as possible we have tried to exclude discussion on non-technical issues. Line drawings by Junpei Nitta and operative sketches by Shigeaki Kobayashi are an attempt to depict the surgical technique in a step-wise fashion and to show the operative scenario in which these techniques were used.

The book has been inspired by late Professors Kenichiro Sugita and Thoralf M. Sundt Jr.

Shigeaki Kobayashi, Atul Goel, Kazuhiro Hongo

Foreword

Professor Kenchiro Sugita and Thoralf M. Sundt, Jr., whose work provided the inspiration for this text, and whose careers focused on complex neurosurgical problems would be proud of the high standards embodied in this text. Dr. Sugita, in whose department Dr. Kobayashi worked, would be extremely proud of Dr. Kobayashi's beautiful drawings in which one can see a reflection of the eye and hand of a gifted artist and master surgeon like Dr. Sugita. In addition, Dr. Sundt, one of Dr. Kobayashi's teachers, would be excited by Dr. Kobayashi's mastery of the complex lesions with which Dr. Sundt so expertly dealt and which are the subject of this text. The text has a high level of continuity and quality which can be achieved only by having a small core of authors write all the chapters, and yet provides the broad perspective of having the world leaders on each subject comment on each topic following the core authors' presentations. The combination of the chapters written by the core authors in addition to the comments by other leaders from throughout the world provides an unusual breadth of perspective which spans the globe. Complex anatomy and technical detail have been dissected and refined into understandable concepts using simplified line drawings and carefully crafted text. They have de-mystified and simplified the management of numerous complex lesions. It is a great honor to have been asked to write the foreword to this text, which brings order to some of the most complex lesions with which the neurosurgeon will deal. I had the good fortune of being one of Dr. Kobayashi's teachers and am pleased to see him and his co-authors emerge as respected colleagues and international leaders in neurosurgery. These authors have prepared a text which will be of value and will enhance the work of their neurosurgical colleagues from around the world. Drs. Sundt and Sugita, whose work and aspirations will live on in the artistry and writing of these authors, would be extremely proud of this text which reflects their high standards and aspirations for neurosurgery.

Albert L. Rhoton, Jr., M.D.
R. D. Keene Family Professor and Chairman, Department of Neurological Surgery, University of Florida College of Medicine, Gainesville, FL 32610, USA

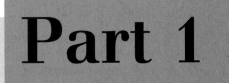

Vascular
lesions

Carotid cave aneurysm of the internal carotid artery

Shigeaki Kobayashi   Kazuhiro Hongo   Junpei Nitta
Kazuhiko Kyoshima

1

Carotid cave aneurysms were first described by Kobayashi et al (1989). The carotid cave is a dural fossa at the medial ventral side of the carotid dural ring at the site of entry of the internal carotid artery (ICA) in the intradural space (Fig. 1.1). This type of aneurysm is ventrally protruding and in general is not in relationship to the ophthalmic or any other branching artery.

PATHOGENESIS

As regards the pathogenesis of the aneurysm, there is an opinion that the superior hypophyseal artery junction could probably be the site of the origin of these aneurysms (Day 1991). However, it is difficult to conceive that all aneurysms can originate at the junction of the superior hypophyseal artery, which is such a small artery. It appears to us that hemodynamic stress with the curving internal carotid artery in the region of the carotid siphon plays a more important role in the formation of an aneurysm in this region. As we describe in a separate chapter, what we call dorsal ICA aneurysm is also typical of an aneurysm without branching arteries associated at its neck (Nakagawa et al 1986). While the dorsal ICA aneurysm is

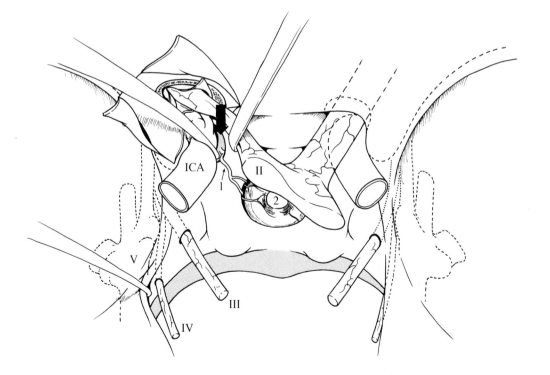

Fig. 1.1 Location of the carotid cave (arrow). It is a dural fossa on the medial ventral side of the carotid dural ring at the site of entry of the ICA in the intradural space. (II, optic nerve; III, oculomotor nerve; IV, trochlear nerve; V, trigeminal nerve; ICA, internal carotid artery; 1, superior hypophyseal artery; 2, pituitary stalk.)

occasionally considered as a dissecting aneurysm, the ventrally protruding aneurysm is not considered as such.

HISTORICAL PERSPECTIVE

The ventrally protruding aneurysm of the ICA in its proximal intradural segment, namely between the dural ring and the origin of the posterior communicating artery, was first described by Drake et al (1968). Yasargil & Fox (1975) called these aneurysms ventral aneurysms, while Nutik (1978) described them as paraclinoid aneurysms. Nutik's description of the aneurysm was that the neck was located on the ICA opposite the origin of the ophthalmic artery. He was the first to describe the aneurysms in this location as a category distinct from carotid–ophthalmic aneurysms. He experienced difficulty in dissection of the aneurysm in his initial cases and the outcome was not a great success. Kobayashi et al (1989) recognized a group of aneurysms similar to that described by Nutik. These aneurysms arose intradurally in the carotid cave and the origin of some even extended into the cavernous segment of the artery. These aneurysms require special varieties of clips and surgical techniques. Of the 24 carotid cave aneurysms in our series, four patients presented with subarachnoid hemorrhage. Direct surgical occlusion of the aneurysm is indicated in a suitable patient.

TECHNICAL CONSIDERATIONS

The neck of the carotid cave aneurysm is not seen with the usual pterional approach unless the anterior clinoid process is removed and the optic canal unroofed. Usually an ipsilateral pterional approach is employed. With the patient in the supine position and the head turned to the opposite side by about 45°, a frontotemporal craniotomy is performed. Extradurally the lesser wing of the sphenoid bone is removed substantially. The anterior clinoid process is not removed completely extradurally; this procedure could be dangerous as the aneurysm lies in close proximity or may even be buried within it. The dura is then opened and the sylvian fissure is opened widely. The intradural situation is observed around the region of the dural ring, optic nerve and carotid artery. Such information helps in orienting the surgeon for further intradural removal of the anterior clinoid process. If the aneurysm is not visible prior to removal of the anterior clinoid process, the ICA or the optic nerve may be retracted slightly. More often the aneurysm is not seen or only a small portion of the aneurysm may be visualized in the carotid cave.

The next step is to remove the anterior clinoid process. This may be done with the dura over the sphenoidal ridge cut open along the ridge so that both the intradural and extradural anatomy may be seen well. Removal of the anterior clinoid process requires appropriate skill in drilling. We observed that some technical alterations could help in drilling the anterior clinoid process. In order to remove the anterior clinoid process, the patient's head is rotated back to about 30°, as the tip of the anterior clinoid process now lies vertically in the field. Raising the head by tilting the operating table is helpful in visualizing the sphenoidal ridge and anterior clinoid process. Using a 3 mm diamond burr, the cortical bone of the lateral aspect of the clinoid process is drilled, after which one enters the diploic portion of the anterior clinoid process. Drilling is then continued towards the medial (deeper) side of the cortical bone. The deeper cortical bone is drilled in such a way as to detach the tip of the anterior clinoid process. The last part of the removal is usually done either with the assistant or the surgeon holding the bone with a mosquito forceps, needle-holder or a specially made punch, and the residual tip is dissected out with the help of a silver dissector. Because the aneurysm may be lying just under the periosteum, or the cavernous sinus may be opened, dissection here should be carried out with meticulous care. During or after removal of the anterior clinoid process, the optic canal is unroofed using a 3 mm diamond burr and then a 1 mm burr to drill the medial border of the optic canal. The drilling may be continued medial to the optic nerve to facilitate its mobilization (Fig. 1.2).

After removing the anterior clinoid process, the head of the patient is rotated contralaterally by about 60° so that the optic nerve and the carotid artery lie more or less parallel. This facilitates the removal of the optic strut which lies between them (Fig. 1.3). While drilling the optic strut one should be careful in avoiding damage to the adjoining dura as the ophthalmic artery often courses very close to it and is likely to be damaged. The optic canal may be unroofed up to the annulus of Zinn. The bone between the optic canal and the superior orbital fissure can be removed. Although it is not always necessary to remove the bone between the optic strut and the superior orbital fissure, this procedure may be helpful when the ICA is taking an unusual course or when one wishes to widen the field by dissecting the dura from the structures going through the superior orbital fissure. In the event of opening up the cavernous sinus during removal of the anterior clinoid process, small pieces of Oxycel may be packed into the space. If the ethmoidal or sphenoidal air sinuses are opened, whenever intact the mucosa should not be damaged but may be pushed away with the help of a small piece of temporalis muscle. If the mucosa is damaged the opening in the sinus should be firmly plugged with the muscle piece and fibrin glue.

After removal of the anterior clinoid process, the local anatomy is inspected. The oculomotor nerve is observed by following it distally from its intradural course towards

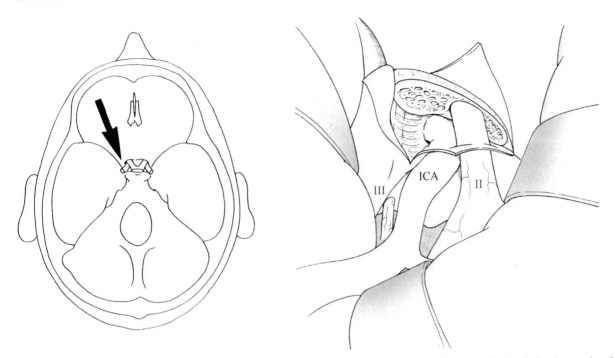

Fig. 1.2   The anterior clinoid process is drilled off. Drilling is continued medial to the optic nerve. The dural sheath covering the optic nerve is opened to facilitate its retraction if necessary. These maneuvers expose a larger area of the carotid cave. (II, optic nerve; III, oculomotor nerve; ICA, internal carotid artery.)

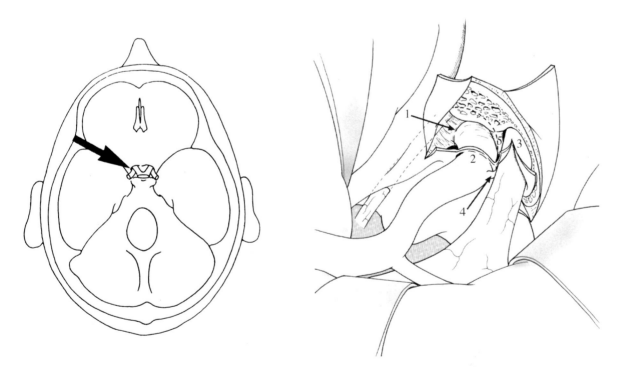

Fig. 1.3   After removal of the anterior clinoid process, the head of the patient is rotated contralaterally by about 60° so that the optic nerve and carotid artery lie more or less parallel. This procedure facilitates the removal of the optic strut. (1, proximal ring; 2, distal ring; 3, optic sheath; 4, ophthalmic artery; 5, optic strut.)

the superior orbital fissure; its extradural part is covered with periosteal membrane. The clinoidal segment of the artery may make an acute turn or may be stretched towards the superior orbital fissure. Usually one cannot see the origin of the ophthalmic artery unless the optic sheath is cut. Observation of the space created along the clinoid segment of the ICA is interesting. What Dolenc called the distal ring is certainly dural, but we have noticed that his nomenclature of medial ring is not a dural structure (Dolenc 1989). The medial ring covering the clinoidal segment of the ICA is a membrane coming off from the third nerve and traversing around the clinoidal segment of the ICA. Inoue et al (1990) called this the carotid oculomotor membrane. But it does appear to be forming a ring around the carotid artery. This is actually periosteum of the anterior clinoid process conjoined with the anteromedial border of the cavernous sinus. When this membrane is perforated, venous bleeding is likely to occur. This can be controlled by packing with a small piece of Oxycel or Surgicel (we prefer the former). The carotid oculomotor membrane extends halfway or all the way up to the distal ring. This means that the cavernous sinus may extend anteromedially either halfway along the clinoidal ICA or all the way to

the distal carotid dural ring. In any case, in order to prepare for clipping of the carotid cave aneurysm, the proximal membrane has to be opened around the carotid artery.

As the proximal ring membrane is opened, Oxycel is packed around the carotid artery to control the bleeding from the cavernous sinus. Packing should be delicate, and overpacking should be avoided to prevent injury to the oculomotor nerve. After opening up of the proximal ring one can identify the 'axilla' or 'genu' of the carotid artery (Kobayashi et al 1989) (Fig. 1.4). The carotid axilla is a space created by curving ICA from C3 to C4. The genu is the medial side of the carotid, but this cannot be fully exposed until the optic sheath is dissected and the distal ring is removed.

The optic sheath is sectioned longitudinally along the lateral border of the optic canal: if it is cut medially, the optic nerve can be damaged during retraction by the edge of the drilled bone.

Because the ophthalmic artery varies greatly in its origin and in its course through the optic canal, one cannot carry out the subsequent procedure without a clear knowledge of the local anatomy. Also, unless a few millimetres of the ophthalmic artery is dissected, it is difficult to perform the

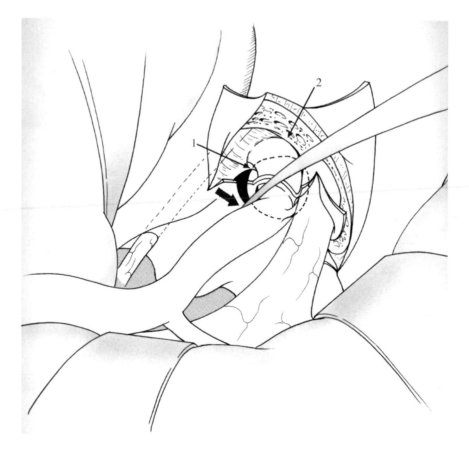

Fig. 1.4   The axilla and genu of the clinoidal segment of the ICA are shown. The lateral side of the dural ring is dissected from the axilla. (1, axilla; 2, genu.)

clipping with a ring clip. The dural ring over the carotid artery is sectioned close to the adventitia, so that it does not interfere with placement of the clip.

With this preparation one may be able to see by retracting the ICA or optic nerve a part of the aneurysm in the carotid cave. The next step will be to dissect the carotid laterally. This should be done prior to dissection around the dural ring on the medial side, as the aneurysm is in close proximity. Lateral dissection of the dural ring is initiated by first confirming the position of the carotid axilla and from here the dural ring is cut laterally (Fig. 1.4) in a stepwise fashion using a bipolar coagulator and scissors. When the cavernous sinus and the medial triangle (Hakuba et al 1987) are entered, it is packed with small pieces of Oxycel to stop venous bleeding. After the carotid dural ring is sectioned laterally about halfway round the circumference of the artery, dissection is then started in the region of the cave. The purpose of the dissection is to mobilize the ICA and free the ophthalmic artery in its first segment. After the origin of the ophthalmic artery is exposed, it is dissected from the optic sheath and also from the medial side of the dural ring. This procedure has to be done carefully as the

wall of the ophthalmic artery is thin when compared with the adjoining dura and the carotid wall. After freeing the ophthalmic artery for some millimeters, the dural ring is cut medially along the carotid cave (Fig. 1.5). One should not enter the cave where the aneurysm is located; instead the dura is cut just outside the cave along the bone which is actually the lateral wall of the pituitary fossa. This dissection is carried around the carotid artery so as to connect with the dural dissection which has been made laterally. During this course one may enter the cavernous sinus anteriorly. At this point we have dissected the medial border for the carotid artery all around and the genu for the carotid artery is freed. In the region of the genu some venous bleeding from the cavernous sinus may occur. Dissection of the genu is relatively easy as it has only periosteal border. However, occasionally one sees fibrous adhesions in this region. After this preparation, we reach the stage of clipping the aneurysm. The proximal ICA in its C3 portion is exposed for possible temporary clipping. Temporary clip occlusion of the carotid could be performed here but it is difficult to place the permanent clip to the aneurysm, with the temporary clip in place as the heads of the two clips

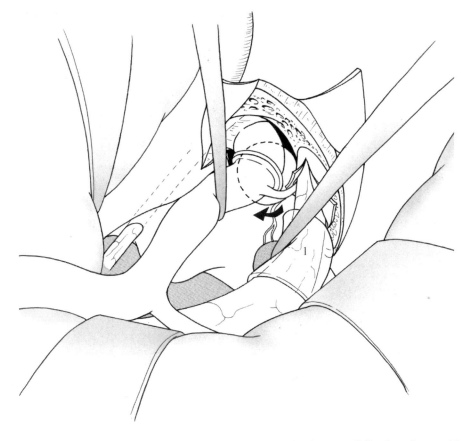

Fig. 1.5 After freeing the ophthalmic artery for some millimeters, the dural ring is cut medially along the carotid cave (arrow). The carotid cave is not entered but the dura is cut just outside the cave along the bone which is the lateral wall of the pituitary fossa. The dural dissection is carried around the carotid artery. (1, silastic sheet covering optic nerve.)

collide with each other, making it difficult to form a good alignment when applying the final clip. Exposure of the carotid artery in the neck may preferably be obtained for the purpose of temporary clipping. Usually one does not have to resort to temporary occlusion of the carotid artery. Temporary occlusion of the artery resulted in thromboembolism of the parent artery in one of our early cases. The clip preferred by us for this variety of aneurysm is a ring clip with curved blades. Depending upon the side of surgery, a clip of adequate curvature and length is chosen (Fig. 1.6). Placing a clip needs special maneuvering, as the clip is right angled and is to be used in a narrow space. A multi-jointed clip applier (Sano) is helpful in placing the clip, and if necessary the clip is adjusted to a proper position by a regular straight clip holder. When placing a clip

the axilla of the carotid artery is secured with one blade and the other blade goes under the ophthalmic artery; we then rotate this clip clockwise toward C3–4 if it is in the right side, or counterclockwise if it is in the left side. When closing the clip one should observe the tips of the blades clamping the proximal neck and also the angle of the clip clamping the distal neck. One can occlude and then readjust (Fig. 1.7). In our experience this procedure can be done safely.

After placing the clip, the parent artery and the ophthalmic artery are checked for patency by visual confirmation, as well as by Doppler flowmeter study, if available. It is important to see the tip of the blades crossing the proximal neck and also, in the genu, the clip occluding the distal neck of the aneurysm without causing stenosis. In closing the clip, the superior hypophyseal artery(s) is likely to be included in the clip but we have not found this particularly harmful for the outcome of vision or pituitary function.

Repair of the region is done with pieces of Oxycel and temporalis muscle; the opened dura is closed over the sphenoidal ridge as much as possible and the dural defect in the region of the parasellar area is filled with pieces of temporalis muscle and fibrin glue.

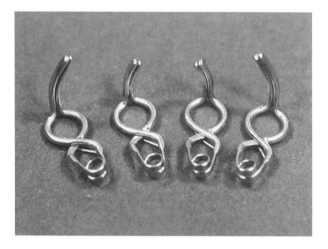

Fig. 1.6   Some varieties of clips suitable for carotid cave aneurysm.

CASE 1   Carotid Cave Aneurysm, Left

This 67-year-old male had undergone left middle cerebral artery aneurysm clipping when he was admitted in Grade 3 2 months earlier. The bone flap was left out for decompression. The patient recovered well after the surgery to near normalcy. The present surgery was undertaken to clip the incidental left carotid cave aneurysm and for cranioplasty (Fig. 1.8). The patient was also developing a normal-pressure hydrocephalus.

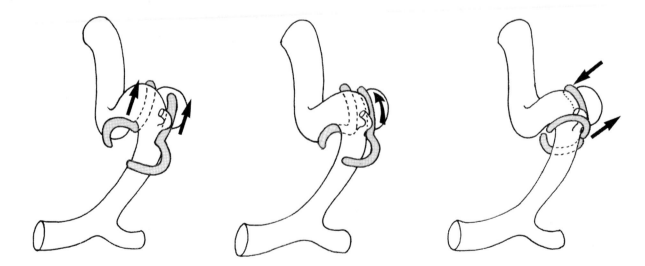

Fig. 1.7   Stepwise application of the angled fenestrated clip with curved blades.

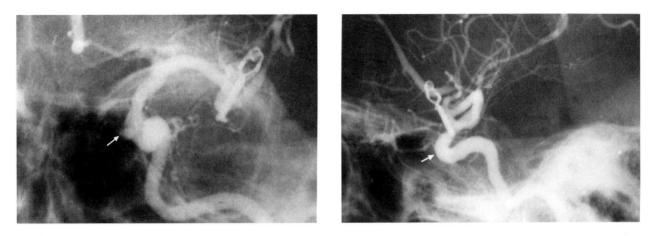

Fig. 1.8 Preoperative angiograms of the incidental left carotid cave aneurysm.

The patient was placed in the lateral position. The carotid artery was exposed in the neck. The previously performed frontotemporal craniectomy was reopened. After durotomy, the sylvian fissure was opened, draining cerebrospinal fluid (CSF) from the sylvian and carotid chiasmatic cisterns. The clinoid process was drilled intradurally and the optic foramen was unroofed, the bone being extremely porotic. The carotid (distal) dural ring was sectioned and the genu and the axilla of the carotid artery were exposed. The patient had an extremely tough distal dural ring just medial to the course of the oculomotor nerve. By raising the head of the patient the cavernous sinus venous pressure was maintained low. The dural ring on the lateral side was cut almost circumferentially. On the medial side of the carotid ring, dissection of the ophthalmic artery was difficult, as usual. The dura over the optic nerve was sectioned vertically to the edge of the bone. The ophthalmic artery appeared to be actually embedded in the medial part of the carotid ring; or it may be that its origin was slightly inside the carotid ring, but it became incorporated in the medial side of the carotid ring, where tracing the artery was difficult as the ring here was unusually tough. During dissection of the ophthalmic artery bleeding occurred from the wall of the artery which was easily controlled with a small piece of Bemsheet. The carotid cave was identified. Although the superior hypothalamic artery could be seen emerging from the cave, the aneurysm could not be seen until a thin membrane was opened here. The base of the aneurysm was then visualized. Lateral to the carotid the proximal part of the neck could be seen just proximal to the

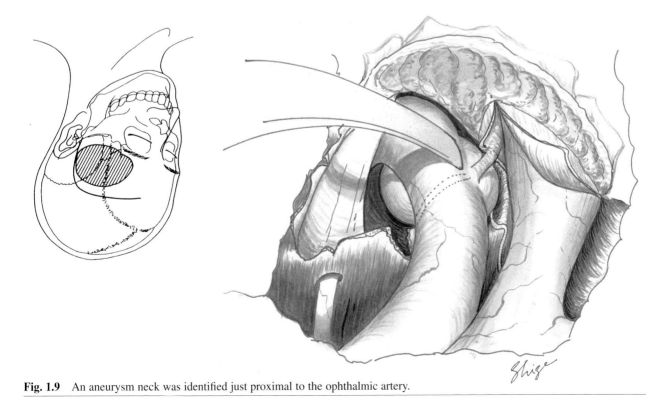

Fig. 1.9 An aneurysm neck was identified just proximal to the ophthalmic artery.

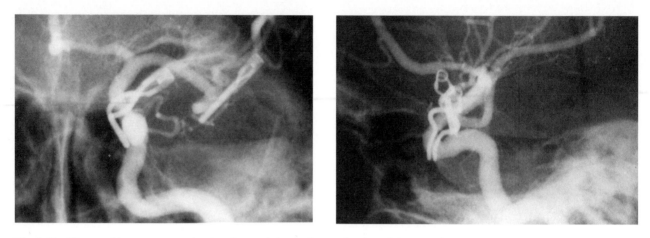

Fig. 1.10   The carotid artery appeared to be of normal shape after application of the curved-bladed ring clip.

carotid axilla. A curved-bladed ring clip was applied without temporary occlusion of the parent artery. The carotid artery appeared to be of a normal shape after the clip was applied (Figs. 1.9, 1.10). As the ethmoid and sphenoid sinuses were opened medial to the optic nerve and the carotid artery, packing of the region was performed meticulously using temporalis muscle pieces and fibrin glue. Cranioplasty was then performed using the previously removed bone flap which was kept frozen. The postoperative course was uneventful.

Comments

1. Circumferential section of the carotid ring and adequate dissection of the ophthalmic artery appeared to the chief reasons for success in this case.

2. The ophthalmic artery seemed to be embedded in the medial part of the tough carotid ring. In such a situation, dissection of the ophthalmic artery can be very difficult.

3. There was no need in this case for temporary occlusion of the carotid artery, although it was exposed in the neck. It appears that it is possible to expose the artery for the purpose of temporary occlusion in Hakuba's triangle instead of exposing it in the neck.

CASE 2   Carotid Cave Aneurysm, Right

A 56-year-old male with incidental right carotid cave aneurysm, detected during the investigation of an episode of sudden occipital headache, vertigo and vomiting which occurred 4 months earlier. He was on anticoagulant therapy. The angiogram showed a typical carotid cave aneurysm on the right side (Fig. 1.11, arrow shows the aneurysm).

The patient was placed in the supine position and the head was tilted by 45° to the other side (Figs. 1.12a,b). Cervical carotid arteries were exposed for proximal control. A right frontotemporal craniotomy was performed and the sphenoid ridge was removed substantially extradurally. After durotomy, the sylvian fissure was opened. The optic nerve, carotid artery and oculomotor nerves were identified. CSF was drained from basal cisterns. Inspection around the anterior clinoid process revealed that there was a carotid cave aneurysm with two superior hypophyseal arteries emerging from the cave. Whether these arteries were located proximal or distal to the aneurysm was not clear as further dissection around the region at this point was considered hazardous. The intradural arteries were very sclerotic, which was compatible with the fact that the patient had previously had an ischemic episode. In order to remove the anterior clinoid process, a dural flap was made and reflected over medially for later sealing the cavernous sinus. The anterior clinoid process was well pneumatized with extension into the sphenoid air sinus. After the anterior clinoid process was removed, the dural ring was sectioned, initially on the lateral and then on the medial side. On the lateral side, the ring was dissected as far down as the anterior margin of Hakuba's triangle and toward the carotid cave. During this procedure, the proximal ring was opened in the axilla, whereby bleeding from the cavernous sinus was controlled with pieces of Oxycel. The optic sheath was then opened along the course of the optic nerve laterally and the ophthalmic artery was exposed. The origin of the artery was identified and it was separated from the optic nerve. Efforts were not made to free the artery from the optic sheath distally as there was a risk of injury to the artery. The distal dural ring was sectioned medially toward the carotid cave, care being taken not to cause rupture of the aneurysm. In order to expose the carotid genu, the optic strut was further drilled with a 1 mm diamond head. After the carotid genu was exposed, the dissection was extended distally toward the carotid cave under the ophthalmic artery. Bleeding from the cavernous sinus was controlled with Oxycel. The course of the carotid artery proximal to the genu (C2–3) could not be ascertained despite the opening of the proximal dural ring. The axilla of the carotid was exposed laterally. Clipping of the neck of the aneurysm was performed using a ring clip with curved blades (no. 75), with initially a multi-joint applier (Sano) and later a straight clip applier being used. However, the position of the tips of the blades could not be ascertained (Fig. 1.12c). The flow through the carotid seemed to have significantly diminished when checked by Doppler flowmeter. In order to see the tips of both the blades, the axilla of the carotid was further dissected. The no. 75 clip was removed and a regular L-shaped

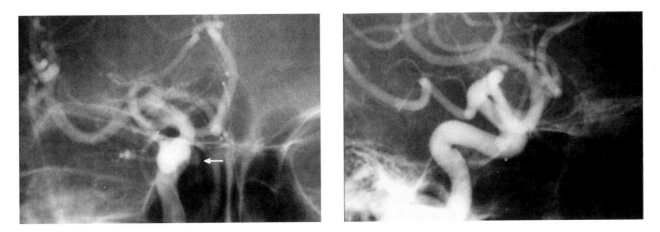

Fig. 1.11   Angiograms showing a typical carotid cave aneurysm on the right side (arrow).

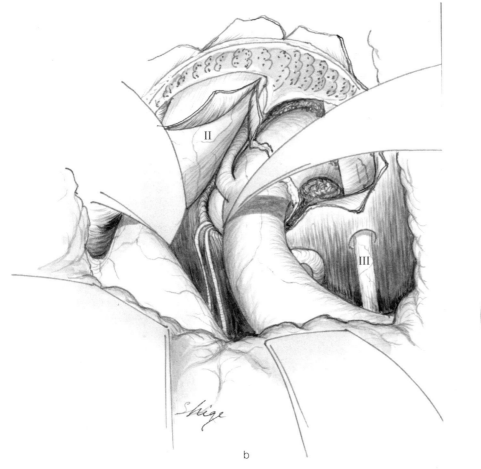

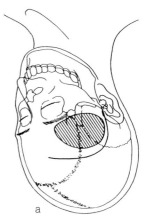

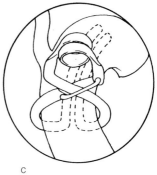

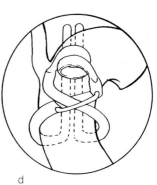

Fig. 1.12   **a** Head tilted by 45°. (II, optic nerve; III, oculomotor nerve.) **b** The optic nerve, carotid artery and occulomotor nerves were identified. **c** Clipping of the neck of the aneurysm using a ring clip with curved blades (the position of the tips of the blades could not be ascertained). **d** Application of a regular L-shaped ring clip.

ring clip (no. 43) was applied (Fig. 1.12d). As a curved blade clip was not used, the parent artery appeared straightened at the end of the clipping procedure. However, the adequacy of clipping was reasonably certain. The patient tolerated the procedure well. The postoperative course was uneventful except for rhinorrhea which disappeared with spinal drainage. The postoperative angiogram showed satisfactory clipping (Fig. 1.13).

Comments

1. Since the patient had had cardiac ischemic symptoms, efforts were made not to temporarily occlude the internal carotid in the neck. No induced hypotension was carried out during surgery.

2. In this case, figuring out the course of the intracavernous ICA was difficult, so that identifying the tips of the blades was important. For this purpose, using a regular L-shaped clip was found to be better than a curved blade because the tips could be seen more easily on the medial side of the ICA in the carotid groove (Fig. 1.12d). In 90% of cases in our series of carotid cave aneurysms, ring clips with curved blades were used.

CASE 3   Large Carotid Cave Aneurysm, Left

A 74-year-old female was incidentally detected to have a large unruptured left carotid cave aneurysm, while she was being investigated for ruptured anterior communicating, clipped 5 weeks previously. At the time of clipping of the aneurysm, a small aneurysmal dilatation was noticed at the dural ring ventromedially, but most of the aneurysm was hidden under the anterior clinoid process; therefore a direct attack to this aneurysm was deferred at that stage. After surgery, the patient developed an increasing hydrocephalus and became a little drowsy. Because of the fear of rupture of the cave aneurysm following shunt operation, it was decided to clip this aneurysm and follow it up with shunt surgery. The preoperative grading this time was 3 (Hunt and Kosnik). The angiogram showed that the cave aneurysm was larger than 1 cm in diameter, projecting ventromedially (Fig. 1.14). Due to this feature it was difficult to confirm whether it was a Nutik type or a carotid cave aneurysm.

With the patient in the supine position, the previous left frontotemporal craniotomy was reopened (Fig. 1.15). Prior to this the cervical carotid arteries were exposed for proximal control. The dura was first opened to confirm the cave aneurysm partially appearing under the ICA ventrally at the site of the exit of the artery from the distal dural ring. Extradural removal of the sphenoid ridge and the floor of the temporal fossa was done as far as the superior orbital fissure. The dura was then divided vertically to the tip of the anterior clinoid process, thereby exposing both intra- and extradural structures in the same field. Drilling of the sphenoid bone and orbital roof was further advanced to expose the infraclinoid structures. This dural opening was very effective and both intradural internal carotid and optic nerve and the extradural bone structures could be seen directly. The anterior clinoid process was removed as usual and then the bone over the optic nerve and part of the orbit, as well as the bone under the superior orbital fissure, was removed. The optic strut was then removed as much as was safely possible down to the carotid groove, taking care not to injure the ophthalmic artery underlying the optic sheath.

We first tried to identify and delineate the proximal neck of the aneurysm in the carotid axilla, which was done without much difficulty. Then, the distal dural ring was sectioned toward the optic sheath, whereby the origin of the ophthalmic artery was identified and followed distally in the optic sheath. The dural ring around the medial side of the carotid artery was carefully exposed, initially by dissecting the origin of the ophthalmic artery in the dural fold and then sectioning the dura outlining the medial bulge of the aneurysm. On the lateral side of the carotid artery, it was difficult to dissect the dura from the aneurysm body because of the fear of possible rupture of the aneurysm in doing so. Because the lateral side of the carotid artery could not be dissected, we had to further dissect the medial side of the carotid artery in order to allow the clip to close without causing stenosis of the parent artery. Finally the ICA proximal to the aneurysm was mobilized. At the end of the dissection, the medial wall of the aneurysm and ICA were freed

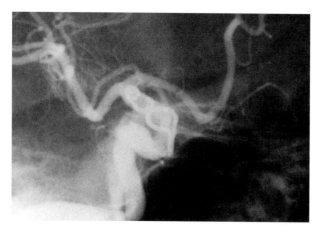 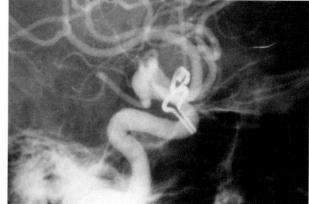

Fig. 1.13 Postoperative angiograms showing satisfactory clipping.

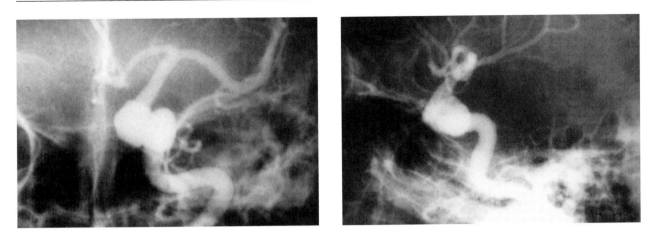

Fig. 1.14 Angiograms showing cave aneurysm (>1 cm diameter) projecting ventromedially.

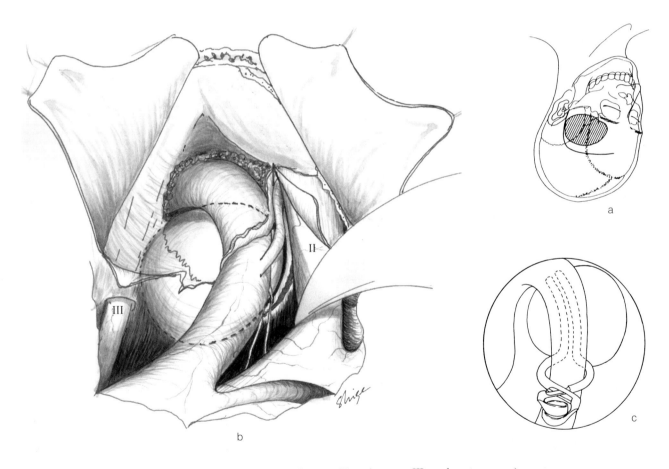

Fig. 1.15 Reopening of previous left frontotemporal craniotomy. (II, optic nerve; III, oculomotor nerve.)

from the bony carotid groove of the sphenoid bone. A no. 79 Sugita clip, a ring clip with curved blades 1.5 cm, was chosen for clipping. While making a trial clipping attempt, the ICA proximal to the neck (C4 segment) was injured by the tip of the clip blades, causing arterial bleeding. The carotid artery was occluded in the neck for about 15 minutes. Under the temporary occlusion the injured portion of the artery was pressed with Oxycel and a spatula which controlled the bleeding. Initially with a Sano clip applicator held in a reverse manner, a no. 79 clip was applied tentatively to the aneurysm, which caused stenosis of the parent artery. This was because the initial dissection was not sufficient. With this tentative clipping, the medial margin of the dura along the aneurysm was further dissected to allow complete clipping. The straight clip applicator was now used, and the clip was adjusted so that there was no stenosis of the parent artery (the straight clip applicator allowed pressing of the jaw portion of the clip down to the bone ventrally at the distral dural ring).

On inspection the parent artery was of normal size and the aneurysm was completely occluded; the tips of the clip blades were not compromising the parent artery (Fig. 1.16). The injured portion of C4 was sealed off with pieces of Oxycel and thin pieces of Bemsheet treated with fibrin glue. After confirming hemostasis, the dura over the cavernous sinus was closed as tightly as possible, supplemented with a piece of temporalis muscle. The wounds were closed after setting up an external drainage from the left lateral ventricle. The operative procedure around the aneurysm took about 3 hours. The postoperative course was uneventful.

Comments

1. This aneurysm can be categorized as a carotid cave aneurysm but was larger than the usual aneurysms in this site. The aneurysm may have originated as a carotid cave aneurysm and become large. It was difficult to determine whether this was a carotid cave aneurysm or Nutik type aneurysm preoperatively. At surgery, however, it was seen that the aneurysm was mostly covered by dura and was located in the enlarged carotid cave; a very small portion of the aneurysm had erupted through the dura under the ventral side of the ICA at the dural ring.

2. For a large cave aneruysm like the present one with firm adhesions to the surrounding dura, dissection of the medial side of the carotid over a substantial length around the medial border of the aneurysm was helpful when combined with mobilization of the parent artery in the carotid groove, where usually the adhesions are minimal.

3. A ring clip with curved blades was helpful in this case.

4. Sectioning the dura vertically along the sphenoid ridge facilitated removal of bone under direct visualization of the important intradural structures. It was very helpful in carrying out exact extension of bone removal necessary for clipping of a particular aneurysm.

5. The carotid artery was vulnerable in this elderly patient with sclerotic arteries as just touching with the tip of the clip blades resulted in arterial tear.

6. Bony removal extended to the superior orbital fissure, which was adequate for this large carotid cave aneurysm.

7. Several superior hyphophyseal arteries were found in this case. The most proximal two of these were coagulated and sectioned, while the distal three were preserved.

8. Circumferential section of the proximal ring was effective in exposing the C4 portion of the ICA.,

9. The entire procedure was performed medial to the course of the oculomotor nerve.

References

Day A L 1991 Aneurysms of the ophthalmic segment: a clinical and anatomical analysis. Journal of Neurosurgery 72: 677–691

Dolenc V V 1989 Anatomy and surgery of the cavernous sinus. Springer-Verlag, Vienna, pp 4–35

Drake C G, Vanderlinden R G, Amacher A L 1968 Carotid–ophthalmic aneurysms. Journal of Neurosurgery 29: 24–31

Hakuba A, Matsuoka Y, Suzuki T, et al 1987 Direct approaches to vascular lesions in the cavernous sinus via the medial triangle. In: Dolenc V V (ed) The cavernous sinus. Springer-Verlag, Vienna

Inoue T, Rhoton A L Jr, Theele D, Barry M E 1990 Surgical approaches to the cavernous sinus: a microsurgical study. Neurosurgery 26: 903–932

Kobayashi S, Kyoshima K, Gibo H, et al 1989 Carotid cave aneurysms of the internal carotid artery. Journal of Neurosurgery 70: 216–221

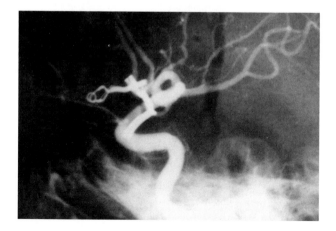

Fig. 1.16 Angiograms showing fully occluded aneurysm (the tips of the clip blades are not compromising the parent artery).

Nakagawa F, Kobayashi S, Takemae T, Sugita K 1986 Aneurysms protruding from the dorsal wall of the internal carotid artery. Journal of Neurosurgery 70: 841–846

Nutik S 1978 Carotid paraclinoid aneurysms with intradural origin and intracavernous location. Journal of Neurosurgery 48: 526–533

Yasargil M B, Fox J L 1975 The microsurgical approach to intracranial aneurysms. Surgical Neurology 3: 7–14

Surgery of Paraclinoid Aneurysms
Stephen Nutik

The preoperative evaluation of the surgical anatomy and the surgical treatment of aneurysms at the carotid dural ring are often difficult. Angiographic characteristics of these aneurysms include a neck on the distal turn of the anterior loop of the cavernous carotid artery near the origin of the ophthalmic artery and projection of the aneurysm over the anterior clinoid process. Those aneurysms which project either medially or towards the cavernous sinus often have a large component of their fundus below the dural ring. Nevertheless, most of them are accessible to clipping by an intracranial approach. Although the following remarks are applicable to most aneurysms in this region, the details refer to my experience with ventral paraclinoid aneurysms.

The key to the surgical exposure of dural ring aneurysms is the removal of the anterior clinoid process and unroofing of the optic canal. This dissection allows mobilization of the optic nerve and exposure of the carotid artery from its proximal ring to that area distal to the dural ring which is covered by overhanging clinoid. The ophthalmic artery and most aneurysms which project below the dural ring are hidden prior to this maneuver. Removal of the anterior clinoid can be done extradurally, but an intradural approach is preferred for these cases. This technique allows opening of the sylvian fissure which facilitates easy retraction of the brain and the simultaneous visualization of the carotid artery and optic nerve which are used as guides to the clinoid dissection. The cervical carotid artery is exposed for proximal control only in cases of large aneurysms where trapping and deflating the fundus may be essential for clipping or in the rare cases where the aneurysm projects laterally against the anterior clinoid process, increasing the risk of rupture during clinoid removal. In the case of unexpected need, direct compression of the artery exposed by the clinoid removal will give proximal control of the aneurysm.

Removal of the anterior clinoid process is not technically difficult. The dura is removed from the floor of the anterior fossa over the superior orbital fissure, anterior clinoid process and optic canal except for the falciform fold at its posterior end. Although it is possible to elevate and save this dura as a flap, there is a risk that this tissue will become entangled in the drill during bone removal. Next, as much as possible of the remaining dura attached to the anterior clinoid on its hidden posterior and medial surfaces is elevated with a small angled sharp dissector starting at the cut dural edge. Pledgets of gelfoam are packed between the posteroinferior surface of the bone and dura if there is venous bleeding. Most of the bone dissection is done with diamond burrs, but cutting burrs may be used along the sphenoid wing anteriorly. Bleeding from the diploic space of the sphenoid wing is easily stopped with small balls of bone wax packed into place with the suction tip over a cottonoid. If an air cell is opened, it is packed with gelfoam. After the aneurysm is clipped, a watertight closure of the opening is achieved by wedging temporalis fascia tightly into it. The drilling is started over the optic canal using the intradural optic nerve as a guide. Approximately 5 mm of the canal roof at its posterior end is removed. Bone removal is then carried from the anterolateral extent of the optic canal dissection to the posterolateral edge of the lesser sphenoid wing. Drilling is continued posteromedially along the posterior canal wall towards the clinoid and deepened below the level of the canal floor into the optic strut. This maneuver isolates the anterior clinoid process and exposes the cavernous carotid artery where the distal part of its anterior loop touches the strut. The loose bone is steadied with forceps and a small curette is used to dissect it free from any remaining soft tissue attachments. Venous bleeding from the clinoid bed is easily stopped with a gelfoam pack. However, this pack should be replaced with small gelfoam pledgets packed directly into the bleeding hole, which take up less space and are less likely to be removed by accident.

Dissection of the soft tissue exposed by clinoid removal is necessary to complete the carotid artery exposure. The dural sleeve over the optic nerve is opened longitudinally from posterior to anterior, forming a posterolateral and anteromedial flap of dura. The posterolateral flap of the canal dura and the dura which covered the medial intradural clinoid surface is removed. The dural incision for this removal is started at the anterior end of the optic sheath incision, carried posterolaterally to the drilled posterior edge of the canal floor, extended posteromedially along this edge to its carotid attachment at the dural ring, continued posteriorly around the lateral half of the ring and finished by carrying it to the site of the removed clinoid tip. Removal of the dural ring and the clinoid periosteum which covers the carotid artery proximal to the ring completes the dissection. The dural ring may be sectioned down to the carotid wall with a knife and then used as a handle to dissect the soft tissue away from the proximal carotid artery. Bleeding here can be controlled with bipolar coagulation or gelfoam.

The removal of the anterior clinoid process and dissection of the dural ring exposes the neck of a ventral paraclinoid aneurysm. The proximal neck of the aneurysm often extends medial to the carotid artery where the artery starts to curve posteriorly. This curve is really the lateral turn of the vessel on the sphenoid bone at the level of the anterior clinoid process which can be seen on an anteroposterior angiogram. The plane between the proximal aneurysm neck and the overlying artery is developed with blunt dissection to allow the passage of the lateral clip blade. On the medial surface of the aneurysm, the dural ring is loosely attached. Gentle retraction of the aneurysm wall develops the plane along which the medial clip blade will be placed. The aneurysm should be freed as much as possible to avoid narrowing of the carotid artery with the clip. If more mobilization is necessary, it is possible to free the medial surface of the carotid artery from the carotid sulcus after cutting the dura on the tuberculum sella just medial to the dural ring. However, this dissection is dangerous posteromedially where visibility is poor, and the dura may overlie aneurysm rather than bone and it has not been used to treat a ventral paraclinoid aneurysm. The blades of the aneurysm clip are passed from distal to proximal and placed parallel to the artery. Right-angle aperture clips allow the blades to be placed on the aneurysm neck situated on the far surface of the artery. The Sugita clips designed for carotid cave aneurysms are also useful here because the gently curved blades conform to the curve of the artery. If possible, the aneurysm is aspirated with a small needle after clipping to confirm its obliteration. However, postoperative angiography is also recommended because the clip tips and aneurysm fundus are usually hidden. Reoperation to advance the clip in the case of an incomplete clipping is an option.

Operative Management of Paraclinoidal Aneurysms

Georg Fries   Axel Perneczky

Introduction: The unique anatomical and clinical features of paraclinoidal aneurysms arising from the proximal internal carotid artery (ICA) between the distal dural ring at the roof of the cavernous sinus and the origin of the posterior communicating artery require a special operative management of these lesions. Because of the close topographical vicinity of these so-called ophthalmic aneurysms to osseous, fibrous, nervous and vascular structures of the skull base, they less frequently than other aneurysms become symptomatic with subarachnoid hemorrhage. While the most frequent clinical symptoms related to paraclinoidal aneurysms is visual deficit, quite a large number of them are only identified incidentally in the course of magnetic resonance imaging (MRI) and cerebral angiography for other intracranial lesions. The anatomical structures of the paraclinoid area not only provide a limited space for expanding vascular lesions of the carotid ophthalmic segment themselves but also for the neurosurgeon during the operation. Nevertheless, sufficient proximal arterial control and minimal traumatization of the optic nerve and chiasm are of utmost importance for the postoperative outcome of patients with paraclinoidal aneurysms.

The following paragraphs are a description of our current operative management of paraclinoidal aneurysms, with special regard to the surgical anatomy and its impact on surgical strategies.

Achievement of Proximal Arterial Control: There are several techniques to achieve safe proximal control of the ophthalmic segment of the ICA. One is to resect the distal dural ring of the ICA at its emergence from the roof of the cavernous sinus (Knosp et al 1988); another is to use ICA balloon occlusion via femoral artery catheters with the additional option of intraoperative angiography; a third and fourth would be the exposure of the cervical ICA (Batjer et al 1994) or the petrous segment of the internal carotid artery.

1. Resection of the Distal Dural Ring of the Internal Carotid Artery: We routinely open the distal dural ring of the ICA (Knosp et al 1988). This is a collagenous ligament easily identified during surgery of aneurysms arising from the C3 and the C4 segment.

The first step in this procedure is to drill the osseous structures which partially cover the superior transversal plate of the cavernous sinus, that is, the anterior clinoid process including the optic strut in ipsilateral approaches and the medial part of the tuberculum sellae in contralateral approaches. For that purpose we use a high-speed air drill with a 2–3 mm diamond burr.

It has been shown that, in a second step, after it has been carefully exposed, the distal dural ring of the ICA can be resected without causing major bleeding from the cavernous sinus. Using this technique, it is possible to expose an additional proximal ICA segment about 3–10 mm in length sufficient to apply temporary clips and thus to gain an excellent proximal arterial control of the ophthalmic segment.

In addition, it is important to note that, quite frequently, aneurysms of the ophthalmic segment extending into the subarachnoid space arise even proximally or at the level of the distal dural arterial ring. Especially with such aneurysms it is important to resect the distal dural ring in order to be able to safely identify the complete neck of the lesion.

2. Intraoperative Angiography and Balloon occlusion: Balloon occlusion of the ICA can easily be applied during surgery of paraclinoid aneurysms provided that intraoperative angiography is feasible. Our current technique, in the presence of an experienced neuroradiologist, is to insert an angiography balloon catheter in the petrous segment of the ICA. The inflation of the balloon provides an excellent proximal control and is extremely useful for pre-clipping decompression of the aneurysms or during premature intraoperative rupture of the aneurysms. To further increase the safety of this technique we recommend performing a preoperative balloon test occlusion of the ICA in the awake patients, including neurological examination and determination of collateral flow capacity by transcranial Doppler sonography. Usually the results of this preoperative test allow for a reliable estimation of the tolerance of temporary or even permanent ICA occlusion.

3. Cervical Exposure of the Internal Carotid Artery: We currently only use the first two techniques, as there are no advantages of the operative ligation of the extracranial or petrous ICA over ICA balloon occlusion. However, in neurosurgical departments that do not possess intraoperative angiography equipment the cervical or petrous exposure of the ICA should be a good alternative to intraoperative balloon occlusion.

Preservation of Visual Function: In the operative treatment of paraclinoidal aneurysms it should always be taken into consideration that the very close topographical vicinity of the optic nerve and the chiasm to the aneurysm and the intraoperative retraction of these structures influence the postoperative neurological outcome of the patients. The surgical preservation of the visual function is not only achieved by reducing the size of a space-occupying paraclinoidal aneurysm but by minimizing intraoperative retraction of the optic structures as well.

1. Preoperative Planning of the Approach: To preserve the optic structures and to apply as little retraction to the optic nerve and the chiasm as possible, we perform a very careful preoperative planning of the surgical procedure, taking into account the precise relation of the aneurysm to the optic structures, the displacement of these by the aneurysm, the microanatomy of the ophthalmic artery and the superior hypophyseal artery, the length of the optic nerve, the position of the chiasm, the precise identification of the neck of the aneurysm, and the displacement of the carotid ophthalmic segment. The summary of all this information gives us important hints for the correct choice of one of five different craniotomies to safely close the aneurysms and to take care of the optic structures.

To approach the paraclinoid area and the ophthalmic segment of the ICA we determine in each case the best individual craniotomy, whether ipsilateral supraorbital, ipsilateral frontolaterobasal, ipsilateral pterional, contralateral supraorbital or contralateral frontolaterobasal. The common feature to all these

approaches is the unroofing of the optic channel and the untethering of the optic nerve at an early stage of the procedure. The supraorbital approaches are keyhole craniotomies via eyebrow skin incision with diameters of 2–3 cm.

2. Ipsilateral Approaches to the Paraclinoid Area: All giant paraclinoidal aneurysms as well as all aneurysms which arise from the lateral wall of the ophthalmic segment of the ICA and displace the optic nerve or the chiasm medially should be treated via ipsilateral craniotomies. With the optic structures displaced medially by the aneurysm there is no need for the surgeon to retract these structures to prepare the neck of the aneurysm. The precise type of ipsilateral craniotomy is chosen individually depending on the diagnosed or estimated position of the aneurysm neck. Superior hypophyseal aneurysms and ophthalmic artery aneurysms expanding superomedially or inferomedially can best be approached via ipsilateral supraorbital or frontolaterobasal craniotomies, provided they displace the optic structures medially or superomedially. Aneurysms of the proximal posterior wall of the ICA can best be approached via ipsilateral pterional craniotomies.

At a very early stage of these procedures care is taken to untether the optic nerve. This important step is achieved by resection of the falciform ligament, which is first incised in the middle of its circumference in a longitudinal fashion with a hook knife or a diamond knife. Then both flaps of the ligament including the adjacent dura are mobilized laterally and medially. Hereafter, unroofing of the optic nerve is completed by drilling the superolateral aspect of the osseous optic canal including the anterior clinoid process. This usually gives a good access to the ophthalmic segment of the ICA and prevents impinging on the optic nerve in its canal during aneurysm dissection.

3. Contralateral Approaches to the Paraclinoid Area: In most patients the ophthalmic and the superior hypophyseal artery, which are the most important branches of the carotid ophthalmic segment, arise medially. Thus the origin of these vessels at the ICA cannot be seen from a lateral aspect, that is, through an ipsilateral craniotomy. According to their respective branches originating medially, ophthalmic artery aneurysms as well as superior hypophyseal artery aneurysms quite frequently arise medially and tend to displace the optic nerve superolaterally and the chiasm superiorly. In these situations the best approach to paraclinoidal aneurysms is from the contralateral side. The contralateral approach makes use of the retracting effect of the aneurysms on the optic nerve, and in most instances the necks of small aneurysms arising medially or superiorly and/or large aneurysms arising superomedially, superiorly or superolaterally can be nicely exposed, an experience also reported by others (Day 1990).

One of the first aims of the contralateral approach, as

ICA–posterior communicating or ICA–anterior choroidal artery aneurysms.

TECHNICAL CONSIDERATIONS

Technical differences between large to giant aneurysms and small aneurysms of the ICA artery are as follows:

1. Neck occlusion is difficult with a single clip; therefore multiple clips are usually necessary to occlude the neck completely.
2. In order to dissect the aneurysm for clipping, temporary occlusion of the ICA is usually necessary.
3. Important surrounding structures such as the optic nerve, oculomotor nerve, and branching vessels (ophthalmic artery, posterior communicating artery, anterior choroidal artery) are located close by and distorted, and often are difficult to spare and preserve.

In planning the surgical strategy, it is important to perform elaborate preoperative radiological studies and analyze the data carefully. The angiographic study of the location of the neck and projection of the aneurysm is important and this can be done with pictures taken from multiple projections. Recently we have found cineangiotomography helpful (Shigeta et al 1994). It is important to know prior to surgery whether the patient can tolerate the temporary occlusion of the ICA. This can be done by a balloon occlusion test, observing the clinical symptoms and, if possible, using xenon cerebral blood flow or single-photon emission computed tomography (SPECT). Although this test is not foolproof, a reasonable idea regarding the dominance of the artery can be had on the basis of this test. Some transitional aneurysms arising in the region of entry of the carotid artery intradurally or from the site of its exit from the cavernous sinus can be difficult to analyze on the basis of the angiogram. One would like to know precisely whether the aneurysm is originating intradurally or in the cavernous segment of the artery. If the aneurysm is proximally located, one could plan a skull basal approach, removing the anterior clinoid process and unroofing the optical canal. If it is located distally, these procedures are not likely to be necessary. Proximal control of the parent artery is very important in giant aneurysms. In the case of giant aneurysm closer to the anterior clinoid process, this is done most safely by securing the ICA in the neck. In the distal variety of giant aneurysm, proximal control of the artery can be obtained in its supraclinoid segment.

APPROACH

The aneurysm is usually approached by an ipsilateral frontotemporal craniotomy. The craniotomy is preferably larger than that used for the usual ICA aneurysms. As discussed earlier, preliminary exposure of the ICA in the neck is done in the proximal type of aneurysms prior to craniotomy. Whenever necessary, removal of the anterior clinoid process and unroofing of the optic canal can be done extradurally. However, because the aneurysm is close to the anterior clinoid process or may have even eroded it, extradural drilling of the bone could be dangerous as it is essentially a blind procedure. Drilling of the bone could be performed intradurally after directly exposing the aneurysm complex. The ICA is secured in the paraclinoid space and the dural ring is cut circumferentially as necessary. The sylvian fissure is widely opened to obtain larger exposure and to reduce retraction of the brain. Cerebrospinal fluid (CSF) is drained from all the available cisterns. The ICA is exposed from proximal to distal and also A1 and M1 are exposed for possible temporary occlusion. Proximal type aneurysms have a close relationship with the ophthalmic and posterior communicating arteries, while distal aneurysms are closely related to the posterior communicating and anterior choroidal arteries. All the branching arteries in the vicinity of the aneurysm are exposed.

When an aneurysm is of a proximal ventral type, it is important to recognize its technical difficulties as described. It is essential to know the anatomical interrelationship between the anterior clinoid process and the proximal aneurysmal neck for planning the surgical strategy to the proximal type of aneurysm (Sengupta et al 1976). However, the upper and lower limits of the orifice of the giant ICA aneurysm are often difficult to define, because the parent artery is usually overshadowed on the angiogram. Therefore, angiography with a double-lumen balloon catheter is very helpful to obtain precise information about the level of the proximal neck (Berenstein et al 1984, Mikabe et al 1991).

CLIPPING TECHNIQUES

Large (15–25 mm) and giant (>25 mm) aneurysms often require special clipping techniques compared to those used in aneurysms of a smaller size (Tanaka et al 1994). The parent artery frequently must be reconstructed with part of the aneurysmal wall itself (Sugita et al 1981, 1982) (Fig. 2.2). Application of multiple clips with short blades is valuable to obtain a satisfactory configuration of the parent artery and also to obtain the optimum closing pressure (Drake 1979, Drake et al 1984, Sugita et al 1981, 1982, Sundt & Piepgras 1979).

In our series, the number of clips utilized was considered to correlate more with the size of the aneurysmal neck than the volume of the aneurysm itself. Although the size

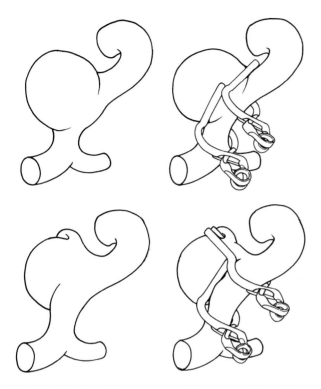

Fig. 2.2 Clipping of the aneurysm with reconstruction of the parent artery using part of the aneurysmal wall.

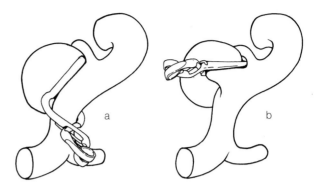

Fig. 2.3 Parallel clipping of the aneurysm (**a**) is more suitable than the perpendicular clipping (**b**), which may result in a dog-ear formation.

of the neck of the aneurysm generally correlates with the volume of the aneurysm, in some cases we observed that the neck of the aneurysm was disproportionately small when compared to the size of the aneurysm. Technical difficulty in reconstructing the parent artery is basically dependent on the projection of the dome, the location of the neck, and the size of the neck.

Application of the clip

Parallel application was more suitable to restore the original configuration of the parent artery than perpendicular application because a dog-ear formation was a frequent problem in aneurysms with wide necks where perpendicular clip application had been used (Fig. 2.3). A parallel method of clip application was also possible even in aneurysms protruding ventrally in the operative field (Sugita et al 1981, 1982). For ventrolaterally or ventromedially protruding aneurysms, an angled fenestrated clip with laterally located blades could be useful (Fujita 1986), although for most of these aneurysms standard fenestrated clips can be applied with widening of the operative field by retracting further the frontal and/or temporal lobe.

When using multiple ring angled clips in parallel fashion three combinations are available according to the direction of the blades. Tandem clipping involves a combination of fenestrated clips applied with the tip of the clip blades in the same direction. Another combination technique described is the counter-clipping method, in which the tips of the slip blades are placed in opposite directions. This method includes two variations: the facing fashion, in which the tips of the blades of the opposing clips are approximated, and the crosswise fashion, where the blades of one clip are located inside the fenestration of another clip (Fig. 2.4). Crosswise clip application was found to be good to avoid shifting of the clip blade, as the strongest pressure is applied at the center portion of the aneurysmal neck. Another advantage of the crosswise clip application is that less space is required for manipulation of the clip than in tandem clipping (Fig. 2.5).

In one of our cases the ICA was occluded when the blade of one of the four obliquely angled fenestrated clips applied in a tandem fashion shifted. This case showed that the closing pressure created by four clips was not enough to obliterate the large neck. The closing pressure of the angled fenestrated clip has a linear pressure gradient along the blade like a regular straight clip, such that the pressure at the tip of the blade is weaker than that at the other end of the blade close to the fenestration (Sugita 1985). Therefore, the blades of the second clip should be placed outside the fenestration of the first clip to prevent the inward shift of the blades (Fig. 2.6).

Duplication clipping is an alternative method to reinforce the closing pressure. Use of booster clips seems to be effective in preventing the slippage of the clips (Sugita 1985, Sundt & Piepgras 1979) (Fig. 2.7).

Straightening of the ICA

It is possible that sometimes straightening of the ICA following clipping of the giant aneurysm occurs, producing kinking of the middle cerebral artery (MCA). In some of our cases, we observed a low-density area in the territory

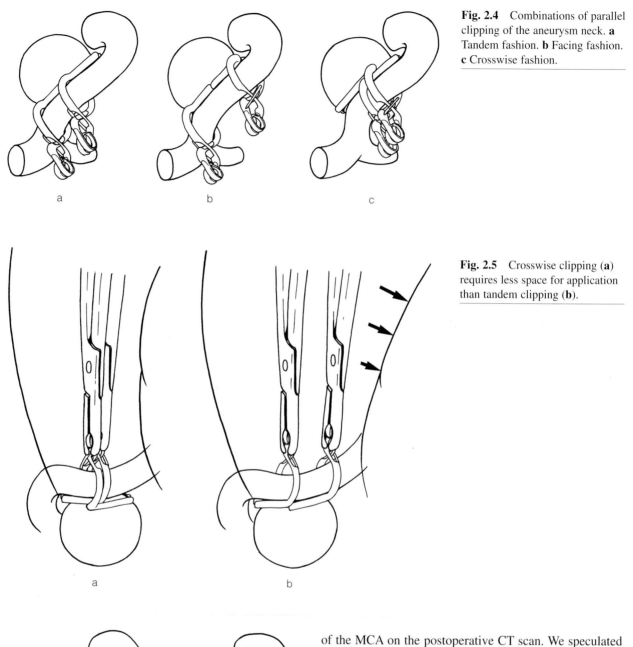

Fig. 2.4 Combinations of parallel clipping of the aneurysm neck. **a** Tandem fashion. **b** Facing fashion. **c** Crosswise fashion.

Fig. 2.5 Crosswise clipping (**a**) requires less space for application than tandem clipping (**b**).

Fig. 2.6 Tandem clipping. The blades of the second clip are placed outside the fenestration of the first clip to avoid slipping and causing stenosis of the parent artery.

of the MCA on the postoperative CT scan. We speculated that the lesions were caused by hemodynamic changes due to the kinking. Straightening of the ICA is more likely to occur with the proximal ventral type of aneurysm (Fig. 2.8) (Tanaka et al 1994).

When the aneurysm is classified as a proximal ventral type from preoperative angiogram, reconstruction of the carotid siphon in its original configuration appears to be important to minimize the risk of hemodynamic change. The proximal portion of the MCA should be observed after clipping, because kinking of the artery usually occurs preferentially at this portion. When kinking is observed, alternative methods that include relocation of the clip, replacement of the clip with one with shorter blades, and changing of the combination of clips may be tried. Freeing the

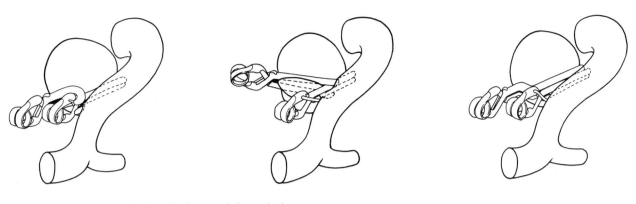

Fig. 2.7   Varieties of duplication clipping to reinforce closing pressure.

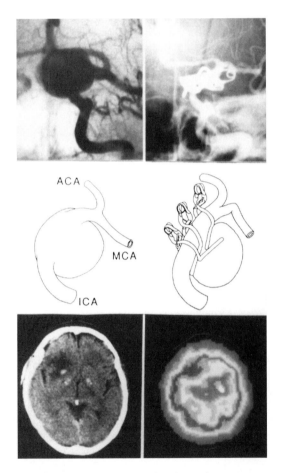

Fig. 2.8   Upper left: angiogram showing a giant aneurysm (maximum diameter 29 mm) of the proximal ventral type. Upper right: two fenestrated clips have been applied in crosswise fashion with an additional clip, showing straightening of the ICA artery and kinking of the middle cerebral artery. Center: schematic drawings of the pre- and postoperative (right) condition. (ACA, anterior cerebral artery.) Lower: postoperative CT scans showing a low-density area in the watershed area between the ACA and MCA (left) that corresponded to the hyperperfusion area revealed by ^{133}Xe inhalation SPECT scan (right). (From Tanaka et al 1994, with permission.)

MCA around the kinked portion by further opening the anteromedian sylvian fissure may help relax the kinking. Extensive removal of the anterior clinoid process to increase the flexibility of the carotid siphon also appears to be effective in reducing the incidence of complications, because straightening of the artery usually occurs in the proximal–ventral type aneurysm where the neck is located close to the knee of the siphon at the point where the ICA describes a major curve (Kobayashi et al 1989, Nutik 1988b, Punt 1979). Using an angled fenestrated clip with curved blades (Fig. 2.9) (see also Fig. 1.6) also appears to be a good method for reducing the degree of straightening (Kobayashi et al 1989). At the time of clipping, suction decompression of the aneurysm can help to provide enough space for clipping and makes it possible to design the configuration of the parent artery (Batjer et al 1988, Flamm 1981, Kyoshima et al 1992, Sekhar & Nelson 1983, Tamaki et al 1991).

After the clipping technique is completed, to relieve the mass effect the aneurysm is decompressed. It is not wise to peel off the aneurysm from the surrounding brain because it may injure the perforating arteries or important neural structures. Care is taken particularly not to retract or manipulate the optic and oculomotor nerves. The optic

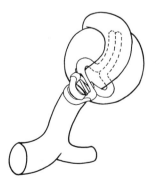

Fig. 2.9   The use of an angled fenestrated clip with curved blades.

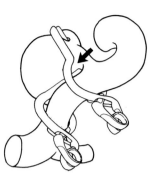

Fig. 2.10 Bleeding can occur through the point where two clips meet (arrow).

nerve can be retracted by about 5 mm when it is normal (Hongo et al 1987), but the stretched and thinned nerve with the giant aneurysm cannot tolerate even a minor retraction. After clipping, one should be certain that all branching arteries and perforators are spared and the major branches are not kinked. When performing multiple clipping, especially, ample caliber of the parent artery should be formed even if a part of the neck is left, because the thick wall of the aneurysm is likely to narrow the lumen of the parent artery. One should be careful not to cause leakage by applying multiple clips because junctional leakage may occur at the point where the blades of two clips meet (Kobayashi & Tanaka 1993) (Fig. 2.10). It is best to see a good alignment of the parent artery, and adequate designing of multiple clips is necessary before the final application. When designing multiple clips one should keep in mind the three-dimensional picture of the aneurysm and the parent artery. Angiography films, being two-dimensional images, may sometimes confuse the surgeon. One must remember that struggling to find the right combi-

nation of clips to occlude the aneurysm adequately is a usual feature and one should not get disturbed about it during the surgery. One should not hesitate to perform clip readjustment or clip removal and reapplication until a satisfactory result can be obtained. To confirm satisfactory clipping of a giant aneurysm, intraoperative angiography is useful.

CASE 1   Giant ICA Aneurysm, Multiple Clipping

A 40-year-old female was diagnosed as having an unruptured right ICA giant aneurysm of the proximal–ventral variety. The aneurysm was detected while she was being investigated for worsening vision. The aneurysm was located between the origin of the ophthalmic artery and the posterior communicating artery and measured 25 mm in its maximum diameter (Fig. 2.11). Visual acuity in the right eye just prior to the surgery was 14/20. The balloon occlusion test of the ipsilateral ICA indicated that there was no change in EEG and neurological status during the test occlusion time of 5 minutes. With the patient in the supine position, the carotid artery was first exposed in the neck. A frontotemporal craniotomy was performed (Fig. 2.12a). The sylvian fissure was widely opened. The dura over the sphenoid ridge was vertically sectioned in an open-door fashion, taking care to preserve the sphenoparietal sinus. The sphenoid ridge was then drilled under vision and the superior orbital fissure was exposed and protected. The anterior clinoid process was then drilled. The optic canal was unroofed and the optic strut was removed to expose the genu of the ICA. While protecting the aneurysm with a silastic sheet, the carotid ring was circumferentially sectioned and the genu and axilla of the clinoidal ICA were further dissected. The proximal dural ring was sectioned and the bleeding from the cavernous sinus was controlled with pill-rolled pieces of Oxycel around the ring. After mobilization of the clinoidal segment of the carotid,

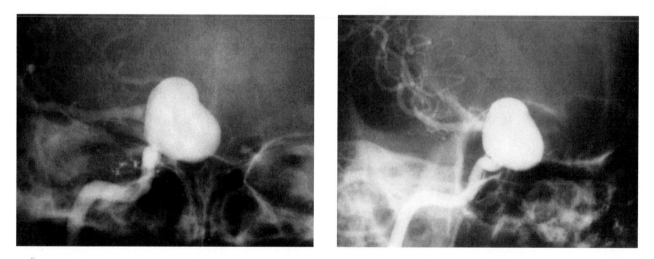

Fig. 2.11 Angiograms showing aneurysm (maximum diameter 25 mm) located between the origin of the ophthalmic artery and the posterior communicating artery.

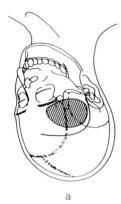

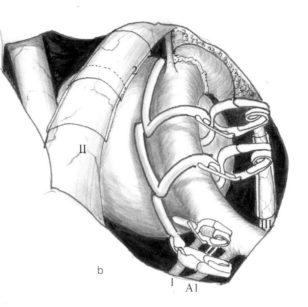

Fig. 2.12 **a** Frontotemporal craniotomy. **b** A curved regular no. 63 clip was applied distally to the aneurysm. (1, posterior communicating artery; 2, silastic sheet protecting the nerve; II, optic nerve; III, oculomotor nerve; A1, A1 portion of the anterior cerebral artery.)

dissection was carried out between the optic nerve and the aneurysm. Here a few superior hypophyseal arteries had to be coagulated and sectioned. The wall of the aneurysm in the lateral side seemed thick, whereas its distal portion under the optic tract seemed thin. The optic and oculomotor nerves were protected by silastic tubes of different sizes. This helped to protect the nerves from mechanical injury and also kept the nerves moist. Temporary clipping of the proximal parent artery in its clinoidal segment had to be performed on three occasions. After temporary clipping, dissection was first carried out between the aneurysm and the optic nerve and tract. The second temporary clipping allowed further dissection of the carotid ring ventrally and circumferentially. Dissection of the body of the aneurysm from the optic nerve and frontal lobe was done after direct retraction of the aneurysm with a 2 mm spatula connected to the self-retaining retractor. During the third temporary occlusion of the proximal ICA, clipping was attempted using two no. 75 ring clips with 7.5 mm curved blades. This

procedure resulted in stenosis of the parent artery and also the total length of the clips did not occlude the entire neck of the aneurysm. Further dissection was done with the clips in situ. A temporary clip was again applied and nos. 75 and 76 ring clips were applied in tandem fashion and finally a curved regular clip no. 63 was applied distally, taking care to preserve the posterior communicating and anterior choroidal arteries (Fig. 2.12b). Blood flow checked with the laser cerebral blood flow (CBF) flowmeter did not show recovery after release of the temporary clip. At the same time it was noted that the systemic pressure was also lowered by the anesthesiologist. We, however, noted that some kinking of the MCA had occurred following the use of three clips. Blood flow gradually returned to normal in the meantime. Finally the dog ear created in the distal neck was occluded by a mini-straight clip. The patency of all adjoining major arteries and their branches was checked and confirmed (Fig. 2.13). During the entire surgery direct retraction of the optic nerve was not required.

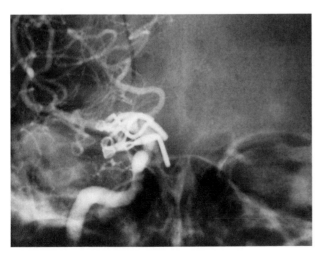

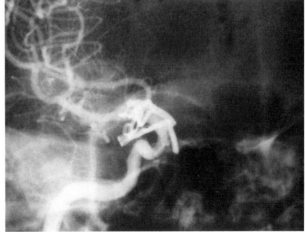

Fig. 2.13   Angiograms showing patency of all major arteries and their branches.

Comments

1. Split silastic tubes covering the optic and oculomotor nerves were helpful in preventing mechanical injury and keeping the nerves moist during the entire procedure.

2. Temporary clipping was done for less than 5 minutes each time as there was no collateral circulation from the contralateral carotid artery, although there was some supply from the vertebral system through the right posterior communicating artery. Laser CBF monitoring was done during the procedure. Whenever temporary clipping was used the flow went down and recovered when the clip was released. This was clearly observed by the laser CBF study.

3. Puncturing of the aneurysm was reserved as a last resort. This is because one frequently tends to hurry to perform the puncture even prior to complete aneurysm dissection. Once the aneurysm is punctured, temporary clipping of the parent artery cannot be released until clipping of the aneurysm is completed, and also puncture may cause clot formation in the aneurysm. Instead a repeated temporary clipping was done, permitting adequate dissection of the aneurysm from the optic nerve and the adjacent small vessels.

4. Direct retraction of the optic nerve was avoided as much as possible. Optic nerve decompression by unroofing the canal and sectioning the optic nerve sheath vertically assisted in mobility of the nerve.

5. During the dissection and clipping some small superior hypophyseal artery branches had to be sacrificed but this procedure did not result in any significant problem.

6. The patient woke up without motor weakness and noticed immediate visual recovery. There was slight oculomotor nerve paresis in the form of drooping of the eyelid and restricted upward gaze. The reason for the 3rd nerve paresis could not be clearly ascertained. However, this weakness cleared in few days' time.

CASE 2   Proximal–Lateral Variety of Large Aneurysm

A 65-year-old female was admitted with the chief complaint of rotatory nystagmus. CT and magnetic resonance imaging (MRI) showed a large aneurysm measuring 23 mm in its maximum diameter in the right ICA. The posterior communicating artery originated just distal to the aneurysm. The ophthalmic artery was opacified on the angiogram (Fig. 2.14). With the patient in the supine position, a right frontotemporal craniotomy was done (Fig. 2.15a). The dura was opened and the sylvian fissure was widely separated. The aneurysm was exposed and the distal part of the neck of the aneurysm was examined. The posterior communicating artery was seen to originate just distal to the neck from its medial aspect. The posterior communicating artery was followed up to its junction with the P1 segment of the posterior cerebral artery. The proximal end of the neck was exposed after removing the anterior clinoid process and securing the C3 portion of the ICA in Dolenc's triangle for possible temporary clipping. The dural ring was circumferentially cut and the optic nerve was unroofed. The optic nerve was seen to be compressed by the aneurysm. It was difficult to clip the aneurysm with a regular long clip without kinking the ICA. As several attempts to clip were made the whole aneurysm was dissected free and almost became a ventral type aneurysm. Clipping with multiple ring clips then became relatively easy. Because the wall of the aneurysm was so thick mere temporary occlusion did not slacken the aneurysm. Two ring clips were simultaneously placed by the surgeon and the assistant in coordination in a crossing fashion. The distal neck was additionally clipped with a curved miniclip. The ophthalmic, posterior communicating and anterior choroidal arteries were all confirmed to be spared (Figs 2.15b–d, 2.16). Because the aneurysm had rotated clockwise, the ICA at the distal side of the neck of the aneurysm was a little twisted but its lumen appeared to be of adequate size. The wound was then closed as usual. Dolenc's triangle was packed with a piece of temporalis muscle.

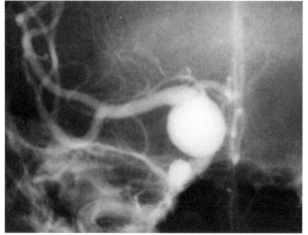

Fig. 2.14   Preoperative angiograms of aneurysm of Fig. 2.15.

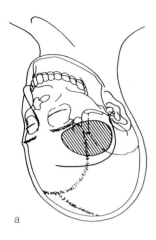

a

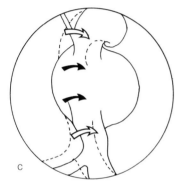

c

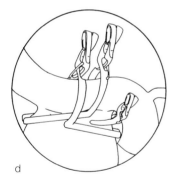

d

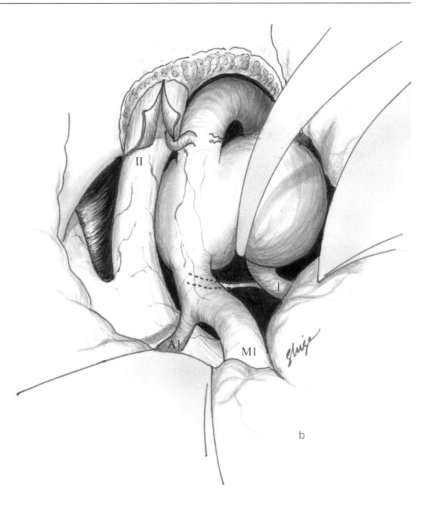

b

Fig. 2.15 **a** Right frontotemporal craniotomy. **b–d** Ophthalmic, posterior communicating and anterior choroidal arteries are all spared from clipping of the aneurysm. (1, posterior communicating artery; 2, anterior choroidal artery; black arrows, aneurysm; white arrows, 1C; II, optic nerve; A1, A1 portion of the anterior cerebral artery; M1, M1 portion of the middle cerebral artery.)

Comments

1. Laterally projecting large or giant aneurysm is usually difficult to occlude by clip. Changing of the projection of the aneurysm from lateral to ventral type was done here could be a useful alternative in such cases. However, such a procedure requires an extensive dissection of the aneurysm.

2. Postoperatively the patient lost her vision in the right eye. The exact reason for this is unclear. In some way the diameter of the ophthalmic artery may have been compromised during the manipulations.

References

Batjer H H, Frankfurt A I, Purdy P D et al 1988 Use of etomidate, temporary arterial occlusion, and intraoperative angiography in surgical treatment of large and giant cerebral aneurysms. Journal of Neurosurgery 68: 234–240

Berenstein A, Ransohoff J, Kupersmith M et al 1984 Transvascular treatment of giant aneurysms of the cavernous carotid and vertebral arteries. Surgical Neurology 21: 3–12

Drake C G 1979 Giant intracranial aneurysms: experience with surgical treatment in 174 patients. Clinical Neurosurgery 26: 12–95

Drake C G, Vanerlinden R G, Amachar A L 1968 Carotid–ophthalmic aneurysms. Journal of Neurosurgery 29: 24–31

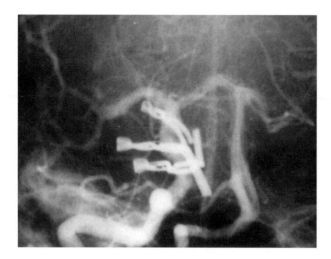
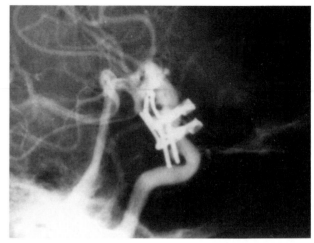

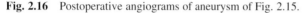

Fig. 2.16 Postoperative angiograms of aneurysm of Fig. 2.15.

Drake C G, Friedman A H, Peerless S J 1984 Failed aneurysm surgery: reoperation in 115 cases. Journal of Neurosurgery 61: 848–856

Flamm E S 1981 Suction decompression of aneurysms: technical note. Journal of Neurosurgery 54: 275–276

Fox J L 1988 Microsurgical treatment of ventral (paraclinoid) internal carotid artery aneurysms. Neurosurgery 22: 32–39

Fujita S 1986 Fenestrated clips for internal carotid artery aneurysms: technical note. Journal of Neurosurgery 65: 122–123

Heros R C, Nelson P B, Ojemann R G et al 1983 Large and giant paraclinoid aneurysms: surgical techniques, complications, and results. Neurosurgery 2: 153–163

Hongo K, Kobayashi S, Yokoh A, Sugita K 1987 Monitoring retraction pressure on the brain: an experimental and clinical study. Journal of Neurosurgery 66: 270–275

Kobayashi S, Tanaka Y 1993 Aneurysm clip design, selection, and application. In: Brain surgery. Churchill Livingstone, Edinburgh

Kobayashi S, Kyoshima K, Gibo H et al 1989 Carotid cave aneurysms of the internal carotid artery. Journal of Neurosurgery 70: 216–221

Kyoshima K, Kobayashi S, Wakui K et al 1992 A newly designed needle for suction decompression of giant aneurysm. Journal of Neurosurgery 76: 880–882

Mikabe T, Tomita S, Watanabe S et al 1991 Identification of the proximal neck of giant paraclinoid aneurysms: technical note. Journal of Neurosurgery 75: 331–332

Nutik S 1978 Carotid paraclinoid aneurysms with intradural origin and intracavernous location. Journal of Neurosurgery 48: 526–533

Nutik S L 1988a Ventral paraclinoid carotid aneurysms. Journal of Neurosurgery 69: 340–344

Nutik S L 1988b Removal of the anterior clinoid process for exposure of the proximal intracranial carotid artery. Journal of Neurosurgery 69: 529–534

Punt J 1979 Some observations of aneurysms of the proximal internal carotid artery. Journal of Neurosurgery 51: 151–154

Sekhar L N, Nelson P B 1983 A technique of clipping giant intracranial aneurysm with the preservation of the parent artery. Surgical Neurology 20: 361–368

Sengupta R P, Gryspeerdt G L, Hankinson J 1976 Carotid–ophthalmic aneurysms. Journal of Neurology, Neurosurgery and Psychiatry 3: 837–853

Shigeta H, Sone S, Kasuga T et al 1994 Digital angiotomosynthesis for preoperative evaluation of cerebral arteriovenous malformation and giant aneurysms. American Journal of Neuroradiology 15: 543–549

Sugita K 1985 Microneurosurgical atlas. Springer-Verlag, Berlin

Sugita K, Kobayashi S, Inoue T, Banno T 1981 New angled fenestrated clips for fusiform vertebral artery aneurysms. Journal of Neurosurgery 54: 346–350

Sugita K, Kobayashi S, Kyoshima K, Nakagawa F 1982 Fenestrated clips for unusual aneurysms of the carotid artery. Journal of Neurosurgery 57: 240–246

Sundt T M Jr, Piepgras D G 1979 Surgical approach to giant intracranial aneurysms: operative experience with 80 cases. Journal of Neurosurgery 51: 731–742

Tamaki N, Kim S, Ehara K et al 1991 Giant carotid–ophthalmic artery aneurysms utilizing the 'trapping–evacuation' technique. Journal of Neurosurgery 74: 567–572

Tanaka Y, Kobayashi S, Kyoshima K, Sugita K 1994 Multiple clipping technique for large and giant internal carotid artery aneurysms and complications: angiographic analysis. Journal of Neurosurgery 80: 635–642

Yasargil M G 1984 Microneurosurgery. I. Microsurgical anatomy of the basal cisterns and vessels of the brain, diagnostic studies, general operative techniques and pathological considerations of the intracranial aneurysms. George Thieme Verlag, New York

Yasargil M G, Fox J L 1975 The microsurgical approach to intracranial aneurysms. Surgical Neurology 3: 7–14

Yasargil M G, Gasser J C, Hodosh R M, Rankin T V 1977 Carotid–ophthalmic aneurysms: direct microsurgical approach. Surgical Neurology 8: 155–165

Surgical Management of Giant Intracranial Aneurysms

Michael T. Lawton   Robert F. Spetzler

Operative Approach and Exposure: The operative approach is selected to optimize exposure of the aneurysm for complete visualization of vascular anatomy and effective clip placement. Maximizing bone removal from the skull provides flat, straight routes of access while minimizing brain retraction. Maximum exposure with minimum retraction is critical for safe surgery and good surgical outcomes.

The pterional trans-sylvian approach has become the standard for most neurosurgeons who treat aneurysms of the anterior circulation. This approach provides access to the ICA, its branches, and the entire circle of Willis. The sphenoid wing is drilled extensively down to the anterior clinoid process to open the sylvian fissure route. Removal of the anterior clinoid process exposes the proximal ICA. This maneuver gains proximal control of the ICA if needed and permits ophthalmic and paraclinoid aneurysms to be dissected.

Skull Base Approaches to Aneurysms: Advances in skull base surgery have given neurosurgeons a variety of approaches to expose aneurysms at the base of the brain and to avoid retraction of vital brain structures. The orbitozygomatic–pterional approach (Al-Mefty 1992, Hakuba et al 1986) enhances the exposure obtained with the pterional approach by removing the superior and lateral orbital margins, orbital roof, and anterior zygoma. This additional bone removal increases the superior limits of the angle of exposure and thereby improves the trans-sylvian access to high upper basilar artery aneurysms (posterior cerebral artery (PCA), basilar bifurcation, and superior communicating artery (SCA)). Removing the zygoma allows the temporalis muscle to be retracted more inferiorly, improving the subtemporal access. This approach also is useful for anterior cerebral artery (ACA) aneurysms when a lower, wider exposure is required.

The subtemporal approach and its variations (i.e., the pterional–subtemporal, or 'one and a half') (Diaz 1992, Sano 1980, Sano et al 1987) were used originally for all upper basilar artery aneurysms (Drake 1979a, 1979b). Although this approach has been supplanted by the pterional approach, it is still useful with low-lying aneurysms of the basilar bifurcation that project posteriorly and with aneurysms of the distal PCA.

A variety of approaches can be used for giant infratentorial aneurysms. Transpetrosal approaches provide routes to the anterior brain stem and clivus by removing temporal bone (Hitselberger & House 1966, House 1979, House & Hitselberg 1976, Spetzler & Grahm 1990). These approaches are divided into three categories depending on the amount of bone removed: retrolabyrinthine, translabyrinthine, and transcochlear (Spetzler & Grahm 1990). These petrosal techniques can be combined with a supra- and infratentorial craniotomy to increase exposure extensively from the sphenoid ridge and cavernous sinus to the foramen magnum (Hitselberger & House 1966, Malis 1985, Spetzler et al 1992). This combined supra- and infratentorial approach divides the tentorium to connect the two compartments, allowing complete visualization of vascular structures in the posterior fossa, particularly the upper and midbasilar trunk and anterior inferior cerebellar artery (AICA).

The inferior brain stem, inferior clivus and upper cervical region can be exposed through the far-lateral approach, which is ideal for accessing vertebral artery, posterior inferior cerebellar artery (PICA) and vertebro-basilar junction (VBJ) aneurysms. The far-lateral approach removes the inferior rim of the foramen magnum, the posterior two-thirds of the occipital condyle, and the posterolateral arch of C1 to the level of the sulcus arteriosus of the vertebral artery (Hammon & Kempe 1972, Heros 1986, Sen & Sekhar 1990, Spetzler & Grahm 1990). The exposure obtained after this bony removal and dural opening requires minimal retraction of neurovascular structures.

Occasionally, a more extensive lateral exposure of the clivus is required to deal with giant aneurysms that involve the mid- and lower basilar artery. Such an exposure can be achieved by combining the far-lateral approach with either an isolated transpetrosal approach or a combined supra- and infratentorial approach. This 'combined' approach provides a wide route to the entire length of the clivus (Baldwin et al 1994).

Treatment Techniques

Direct Aneurysm Clipping: The ideal treatment for intracranial aneurysms excludes the aneurysm completely from the circulation while preserving blood flow through the parent and branch vessels. This treatment is accomplished best by direct clip placement across the aneurysm neck (Spetzler & Carter 1985). The feasibility of clipping is determined after careful intraoperative inspection of the aneurysm, its neck, and branch vessels.

Basic principles of aneurysm surgery are followed when dealing with giant aneurysms. First, proximal and distal vascular control is attained. Proximal control of ICA aneurysms may require removing the anterior clinoid process, exposing the petrous ICA in the carotid canal (Wascher et al 1993), or exposing the cervical ICA. Dissection of the aneurysm without temporary clipping of the parent vessel is best, but the decreased bulk of the aneurysm and the increased exposure gained by temporary clips are often invaluable.

Giant aneurysms typically have broad, complex necks that require either long clips with high closing pressure or multiple short clips. Booster clips may be placed across the tips of a primary clips (where the closing pressure is inherently less than at the fulcrum) to eliminate persistent flow through an unoccluded neck. Tandem clips are usually short-aperture clips placed serially across the neck until the entire base is occluded. Short clips have higher closing pressures, are less likely to slip off the neck, and can be contoured to preserve the lumen of the parent vessel. Parallel clips are applied adjacent to one another for added reinforcement. It is often safer to place a secondary parallel clip in a more optimal position on the neck rather than to reposition the primary clip and risk tearing the aneurysm. Because the aneurysmal wall is thick with layers of organized thrombus, fibrous tissue, atherosclerotic degeneration, and calcification, clips should be placed high enough on the neck to avoid compromising the parent vessel lumen. The neck is often fragile and clips must be placed delicately.

Branch vessels and perforators must be preserved. These vessels are inspected after clipping to verify patency. If patency is unclear, Doppler ultrasonography is used.

Intraoperative Cerebral Protection: Cerebral protection with barbiturates has become standard in the intraoperative management of aneurysm patients. Barbiturates reduce the metabolic demands of neural cells and extend the brain's tolerance to a decreased nutrient supply. Consequently, barbiturates help prevent cerebral injury from the focal ischemia associated with temporary occlusion of the parent vessel and dissection of giant aneurysms (Selman et al 1981, 1982, Shapiro 1985, Yatsu 1983). Patients receive intravenous barbiturate (thiopental) titrated to achieve electroencephalographic (EEG) burst suppression (Spetzler & Hadley 1989). Barbiturates are most effective when administered before the period of temporary ischemia (Selman et al 1982). Intraoperative blood pressure is maintained mildly hypertensive, especially during any temporary vessel clipping, to enhance cerebral perfusion. Patients are monitored with somatosensory evoked potentials (SSEPs) to determine tolerance to vessel occlusion.

Hypothermic Circulatory Arrest: Hypothermic circulatory arrest is a valuable surgical adjunct in the treatment of giant aneurysms (Soloman et al 1991, Spetzler et al 1988). The size of many giant aneurysms precludes adequate visualization of the anatomy. This problem is probably most dramatic when dealing with giant basilar artery aneurysms because of the limitations associated with even the most elegant surgical exposures. Additional exposure can be obtained through hypothermic circulatory arrest (Soloman et al 1991, Spetzler et al 1988). During cardiac arrest the aneurysm can be collapsed to provide more working room and easier manipulation of neurovascular structures. The anatomy is defined in a bloodless surgical field without the risk of hemorrhage.

Hypothermic circulatory arrest is complex but highly effective. The success of this tool for clipping complex aneurysms is determined by five key variables: the depth of hypothermia, the duration of circulatory arrest, the use

of barbiturates, the hemostasis, and the rate of rewarming after aneurysm clipping. In our experience, the mean brain temperature during standstill has been 14.6°C, and the mean duration of standstill 22.5 minutes (range, 2–72 minutes). The absolute maximum duration of cerebral ischemia that can be tolerated safely is unknown. Duration can be increased significantly by the use of profound hypothermia and intravenous barbiturates administered to the point of EEG burst suppression. The period of circulatory arrest should be limited to the final period of aneurysm dissection and clip application.

Meticulous attention must be given to intraoperative hemostasis, with close surveillance of the patient's clotting mechanisms. The patient must be rewarmed at a carefully controlled rate (0.2–0.5°C/min), with a mean rewarming time of 90 minutes. The potential morbidity (13%) associated with circulatory arrest stipulates that it be used only when the parent vessels and aneurysm cannot be exposed and controlled with routine surgical techniques, including such measures as the application of multiple temporary clips. However, when required, circulatory arrest provides an added measure of safety without significantly increasing the inherent morbidity or mortality associated with these lesions. The rate of direct clipping in this series (62%) exceeds the rates in other series (Drake, 39% (Drake 1979a); Sundt, 49% (Sundt 1990). This difference is attributed to the use of hypothermic circulatory arrest.

Alternative Techniques of Aneurysm Occlusion: Many giant aneurysms (38% in this series) are not amenable to direct clipping because of their size, the lack of a discrete neck, or the technical difficulty associated with the dissection. Alternative techniques for these unclippable aneurysms include proximal vessel occlusion, trapping, aneurysmorrhaphy, and excision of the aneurysm. These techniques are inferior to direct clipping because they sacrifice the parent and branch vessels. Consequently, patients are at risk for hemodynamic compromise and ischemic complications. These alternative techniques are therefore recommended only after attempts at direct clipping have failed.

Aneurysm trapping along the parent vessel completely eliminates the aneurysm from the circulation. The segment of vessel sacrificed is minimized by applying the clips as close to the aneurysm as possible. When important branch vessels are located along this segment of parent vessel and cannot be sacrificed safely (for example, along the supraclinoid ICA), it is advisable to only occlude proximally. Proximal vessel occlusion produces vascular dead space and does not prevent retrograde filling of the aneurysm, thereby making thromboembolism a potential complication. However, the reduced blood flow within the aneurysm can reduce the risk of rupture and promote thrombosis of the lumen.

Aneurysm excision is an alternative for MCA aneurysms where the vessels can be reconstructed more easily (Hadley et al 1988). Primary reanastomosis of the parent vessel is attempted but is often impossible after resection of these large lesions. When the vascular tissues around the neck are not too friable to prevent suturing, the aneurysm dome can be resected partially and the artery reconstructed with vessel wall around the neck (Bohanowski et al 1988). Aneurysmorrhaphy is technically difficult but has the advantage of reconstituting the parent vessel and maintaining CBF without a bypass procedure.

Cerebral Revascularization: Safe treatment of unclippable giant aneurysms with trapping, proximal vessel occlusion, or excision often requires revascularization to maintain CBF and to guard against ischemic complications (Spetzler & Carter 1985, Spetzler et al 1980). Most decisions regarding the need for revascularization can be made based on clinical (e.g., transient ischemic attacks and previous stroke) and angiographic information. Angiographic evidence of incompetent vessels, poor collateral circulation, and low flow distal to the aneurysm may indicate a need to revascularize. Occasionally, xenon CT–CBF studies and positron emission tomography (PET) scans are used to determine whether the region of brain in question is hypoperfused. Provocatives tests, such as balloon test occlusion with Xe CT–CBF studies, have been advocated to determine a patient's tolerance to ICA occlusion (Horton et al 1993, Linskey et al 1993, Sen & Sekhar 1992). These tests can confirm the need for revascularization. However, because these tests have a false negative rate of 7–30% (McIvor et al 1994, Sen & Sekhar 1992), they do not establish definitively the safety of vessel sacrifice, not do they address the risks of delayed ischemic deficits and de novo aneurysm formation.

Aneurysm Debulking: Compression of neural structures by the aneurysm mass caused more than a third of patient morbidity in this series. Therefore, after a giant aneurysm has been completely eliminated from the circulation – regardless of the technique – it is debulked to relieve the mass effect on surrounding structures. If the lumen is not thrombosed, simple aspiration will debulk the aneurysm. However, the lumen is filled typically with layers of thrombus that can be resected easily. Clipped or trapped aneurysms are debulked immediately. In contrast, proximally occluded aneurysms require time for thrombotic occlusion to develop and for angiographic verification of occlusion. Debulking is then performed in a separate surgical stage. The goal of aneurysm debulking is reduction of mass effect, not necessarily complete removal of the aneurysm. An aneurysm wall that is adhered densely to the brain or cranial nerves may be left behind because complete removal could injure these structures.

Postoperative Management: All patients are evaluated from postoperative angiography to confirm elimination of the aneurysm and patency of bypass grafts. Treatment cannot be considered complete until the aneurysm is eliminated. Residual aneurysm filling is treated with direct surgical or, occasionally, with endovascular techniques until the aneurysm is obliterated. Graft occlusions are treated emergently to re-establish patency. Patients with subarachnoid hemorrhage (SAH) are managed according to established protocols with hypervolemia, hypertensions, and hemodilution for 2 weeks after hemorrhage or until the symptoms resolve (Kassell et al 1982).

Summary: Patients with untreated giant intracranial aneurysms have a dismal prognosis as a result of hemorrhage, cerebral compression, and thromboembolism. Therefore, giant aneurysms should be treated. The operative approach is chosen to maximize exposure of the aneurysm. Direct clipping of the aneurysm neck, with preservation of the parent and branch vessels, is the preferred method of occlusion. Hypothermic circulatory arrest may facilitate clipping in select patients. Alternative techniques for unclippable aneurysms can be utilized, but they compromise parent arteries and require revascularization to maintain CBF. Because mass effect is an important cause of patient morbidity, giant aneurysms are usually debulked after they have been eliminated completely from the circulation. Giant aneurysms are complex lesions that demand thorough surgical planning, individualized strategies, and a multidisciplinary effort.

References

Al-Mefty O 1992 The cranio-orbital zygomatic approach for intracranial lesions. Contemporary Neurosurgery 14: 1–6

Baldwin H Z, Miller C G, Van Loveren H R et al 1994 The far lateral-combined supra- and infratentorial approach: a human cadaveric prosecution model for routes of access to the petroclival region and ventral brain stem. Journal of Neurosurgery 81: 60–68

Bohanowski W M, Spetzler R F, Carter L P 1988 Reconstruction of the MCA bifurcation after excision of a giant aneurysm: technical note. Journal of Neurosurgery 68: 974–977

Diaz F G 1992 Vertebrobasilar aneurysms: surgical management. Critical Reviews in Neurosurgery 2: 146–158

Drake C G 1979a Giant intracranial aneurysms: experience with surgical treatment in 174 patients. Clinical Neurosurgery 26: 12–96

Drake C G 1979b The treatment of aneurysms of the posterior circulation. Clinical Neurosurgery 26: 96–144

Hadley M N, Spetzler R F, Martin N A et al 1988 Middle cerebral artery aneurysm due to Nocardia asteroides: case report of aneurysm excision and extracranial–intracranial bypass. Neurosurgery 22: 923–928

Hakuba A, Liu S S, Nishimura S 1986 The orbitozygomatic infratemporal approach: a new surgical technique. Surgical Neurology 26: 271–276

Hammon W M, Kempe L G 1972 The posterior fossa approach to aneurysms of the vertebral and basilar arteries. Journal of Neurosurgery 37: 339–347

Heros R C 1986 Lateral suboccipital approach for vertebral and vertebrobasilar artery lesions. Journal of Neurosurgery 64: 559–562

Hitselberger W E, House W F 1966 A combined approach to the cerebellopontine angle: a suboccipital–petrosal approach. Archives of Otolaryngology 84: 49–67

Horton J A, Jungreis C A, Pistoia F 1993 Balloon test occlusion. In: Sekhar L N, Janecka I P (eds) Surgery of cranial base tumors. Raven, New York, pp 33–36

House W F 1979 Translabyrinthine approach. In: House W F, Luetje C M (eds) Acoustic tumors. University Park Press, Baltimore, pp 43–87

House W F, Hitselberger W E 1976 The transcochlear approach to the skull base. Archives of Otolaryngology 102: 334–342

Kassell N F, Peerless S J, Durward Q J et al 1982 Treatment of ischemic deficits from vasospasm with intravascular volume expansion and induced arterial hypertension. Neurosurgery 11: 337–343

Linskey M E, Sekhar L N, Sen C 1993 Cerebral revascularization in cranial base surgery. In: Sekhar L N, Janecka I P (eds) Surgery of cranial base tumors. Raven, New York, pp 45–68

Malis L I 1985 Surgical resection of tumors of the skull base. In: Wilkins R H, Rengachary S S (eds) Neurosurgery. McGraw-Hill, New York, pp 1011–1021

McIvor N P, Willinsky R A, TerBrugge K G et al 1994 Validity of test occlusion studies prior to internal carotid artery sacrifice. Head and Neck 16: 11–16

Sano K 1980 Temporo-polar approach to aneurysms of the basilar artery at and around the distal bifurcation: technical note. Neurological Research 2: 361–367

Sano K, Asano T, Tamura A 1987 Surgical technique. In: Sano K, Tamura A (eds) Acute aneurysm surgery: pathophysiology and management. Springer-Verlag, New York, pp 194–246

Selman W R, Spetzler R F, Roski R A et al 1981 Regional cerebral blood flow following middle cerebral artery occlusion and barbiturate therapy in baboons. Journal of Cerebral Blood Flow and Metabolism 1: S214–S215

Selman W R, Spetzler R F, Roski R A et al 1982 Barbiturate coma in focal cerebral ischemia: relationship of protection to timing of therapy. Journal of Neurosurgery 56: 685–690

Sen C N, Sekhar L N 1990 An extreme lateral approach to intradural lesions of the cervical spine and foramen magnum. Neurosurgery 27: 197–204

Sen C, Sekhar L N 1992 Direct vein graft reconstruction of the cavernous, petrous and upper cervical internal carotid artery: lessons learned from 30 cases. Neurosurgery 30: 732–743

Shapiro H M 1985 Barbiturates in brain ischaemia. British Journal of Anaesthesia 57: 82–95

Soloman R A, Smith C R, Raps E C et al 1991 Deep hypothermic circulatory arrest for the management of complex anterior and posterior circulation aneurysms. Neurosurgery 29: 732–737

Spetzler R F, Carter L P 1985 Revascularization and aneurysm surgery: current status. Neurosurgery 16: 111–116

Spetzler R F, Grahm T W 1990 The far-lateral approach to the inferior clivus and upper cervical region: technical note. Barrow Neurological Institute Quarterly 6: 35–38

Spetzler R F, Hadley M N 1989 Protection against cerebral ischemia: the role of barbiturates. Cerebrovascular and Brain Metabolism Reviews 1: 212–229

Spetzler R F, Schuster H, Roski R A 1980 Elective extracranial–intracranial arterial bypass in the treatment of inoperable giant aneurysms of the internal carotid artery. Journal of Neurosurgery 53: 22–27

Spetzler R F, Hadley M N, Rigamonti D et al 1988 Aneurysms of the basilar artery treated with circulatory arrest, hypothermia, and barbiturate cerebral protection. Journal of Neurosurgery 53: 22–27

Spetzler R F, Daspit C P, Pappas C T E 1992 The combined supra- and infratentorial approach for lesions of the petrous and clival regions: experience with 46 cases. Journal of Neurosurgery 76: 588–599

Sundt T M Jr 1990 Results of surgical management. In: Sundt T M Jr (ed) Surgical techniques for saccular and giant intracranial aneurysms. Williams & Wilkins, Baltimore, pp 19–23

Wascher T M, Spetzler R F, Zabramski J M 1993 Improved transdural exposure and temporary occlusion of the petrous internal carotid artery for cavernous sinus surgery: technical note. Journal of Neurosurgery 78: 834–837

Yatsu F M 1983 Pharmacologic protection against ischemic brain damage. Neurology Clinics 1: 37–53

INTRACRANIAL GIANT ANEURYSMS: GENERAL MANAGEMENT STRATEGIES
Issam A. Awad

Therapeutic Objectives: It is important to articulate clearly the specific and relevant objectives of any proposed treatment of an intracranial giant aneurysm (GA). The goals of aneurysm therapy may include protection from hemorrhage, limitation or prevention of thromboembolic complications, and decompression of mass effect on adjacent neural structures. These can be accomplished through palliative strategies, or by definitive exclusion of the aneurysm sac from the intracranial circulation. Such therapeutic goals also must be considered in terms of the likelihood of providing permanent protection from future clinical sequelae, i.e. durability of therapeutic benefit.

Medical management of various vascular disease risk factors, such as hypertension, theoretically may either prevent or forestall the progression of atherosclerotic changes and growth associated with GAs. There is no evidence, however, that this approach affords any reliable protection from clinical manifestations associated with atherosclerotic change (e.g., thromboembolism), and likely does not prevent lesion growth and hemorrhage. Antiplatelet and systemic anticoagulation therapies have been used in situations of acute thromboembolic brain ischemia or perforator vessel compromise associated with GAs. Additionally, superselective intra-arterial thrombolysis of acutely occluded large intracranial branches is now technically more feasible and successful in appropriately selected cases and, thus, may be complementary to potential medical management. Anticoagulation/thrombolytic management may be the only viable option in cases of acutely evolving ischemic complications in which any direct treatment of the aneurysm may be accompanied by unacceptable risk. However, such a therapeutic approach may increase hemorrhagic risk, with resulting catastrophic sequelae.

Parent artery occlusion can significantly reduce blood flow within a GA arising from that vessel, promoting intrasaccular thrombosis and involution in many cases. However, such a treatment is ineffective unless the parent vessel occlusion is performed either at or near the proximal origin of the aneurysm or in a segment of the vascular tree that has no significant branches with collaterals distal to the point of occlusion but proximal to the aneurysm (e.g., cavernous segment aneurysms). This latter point is critical, since prior experience has shown that proximal parent artery occlusion below the level of viable collaterals provides no lasting protection from the sequelae of intracranial aneurysms due to the development of collateral pathways of blood flow to the GA. This is usually the case in GAs arising at distal bifurcations of major vessels. Obviously, occlusion of the parent vessel at or near the aneurysm in these cases may result in significant risk of ischemia by compromising flow in these major branch vessels.

The most reliable and lasting treatment of GAs is the complete exclusion of the aneurysm sac from the arterial circulation. This may be accomplished by endosaccular thrombosis (with or without parent vessel occlusion) or by clip reconstruction of the parent vessel so as to trap and/or exclude the aneurysm sac. In any situation where a GA is treated with parent vessel preservation, the area of the neck remains vulnerable to aneurysm recurrence. Therefore, treatment approaches must also include a goal of durability.

Individualizing Treatment Strategies: The location of a GA, its pathoanatomical and pathophysiological features, and its previous clinical behavior must be considered in the assessment of natural history and potential treatment approaches. For certain lesions, such as GAs that are totally extradural, the natural history may be so benign as not to warrant treatment with significant morbidity. Other lesions with recent or impending hemorrhage dictate a more aggressive therapeutic tactic. The full spectrum of treatment options is considered for each lesion. At the present time, this approach requires a constant reassessment of treatment outcome with similar lesions at one's own center and in the reported experience of others. This also includes an honest appraisal of one's technical abilities and the realistic outcome of an individual technique for a given type of GA.

The experience of the past decade has demonstrated that a rigid singular modality approach is not likely to be effective, nor would it be justified in terms of risk–benefit analysis in every GA. Rather, there should be a clear articulation of treatment objectives in a particular patient in light of the specific GA and its clinical behavior and prognosis. A number of options are typically considered to achieve such an objective, and these are weighed in terms of their potential risks and benefits in the individual, clinical and pathoanatomical scenario.

Such an individualized approach to treatment requires the balanced integration of perspectives of a number of specialists, each with unique views and technical expertise. For example, neurologists may participate along with the critical care neurosurgeon in assessing the timing of treatment, medical management of acute neurological sequelae, and the assessment of natural risk. A competent neurosurgeon with specific interest and expertise in cerebrovascular surgical approaches to a variety of GAs can usually provide a realistic assessment of surgical options and risks. Similarly, the subtle diagnostic features of a particular case require the skills of an experienced vascular neuroradiologist, who is capable of gleaning important pathoanatomical information from various imaging studies that is relevant to treatment. Finally, the views of a competent and experienced interventional neuroradiologist are sought from whom an honest assessment and proposal of endovascular therapeutic options is provided.

adherent to the brain – more often to the frontal than to the temporal lobe, and more importantly these aneurysms are often fragile from neck to the dome.

The dorsal ICA aneurysm is usually small and angiographic investigation should be performed with great care. Even after careful angiographic investigation, there is still a group of patients in whom the cause of subarachnoid hemorrhage cannot be found. Four aneurysms in our series were not found on repeated angiograms preoperatively. The most probable explanation for failure in demonstrating our dorsal aneurysms appears to be their small size. An oblique view of the angiogram was frequently found to be useful to demonstrate a small wide-based dorsal aneurysm. Vasospasm may be the cause of insufficient filling of an aneurysm. Contrary to expectation, we have had two dorsal aneurysms that were not visualized on the initial angiograms when no vasospasm was present, but were seen on angiograms taken during the period of vasospasm. Forster et al (1978) also described such an aneurysm of the anterior communicating artery. This experience leads us to stress the importance of repeated examination even in the presence of vasospasm, and we should bear in mind this type of aneurysm when seeing the subarachnoid hemorrhage of unknown origin in the basal cistern.

SERIES

In the past 10 years, 20 cases of dorsal ICA aneurysms were operated upon at the Shinshu University Hospital and its affiliated hospitals (Shigeta et al 1992). During the same period there were a total of about 1600 aneurysms submitted to surgery, so that the total incidence of dorsal ICA aneurysms was about 1% of all cerebral aneurysms. There were 16 females and 4 males, with age ranging from 26 to 61 years (average 45 years). All patients presented

with subarachnoid hemorrhage, caused by rupture of the dorsal ICA aneurysm in 18 cases and of an associated aneurysm in 2 cases. The aneurysm size is generally small (average 4 mm in diameter) on the angiogram. Four dorsal ICA aneurysms were not seen on the preoperative angiograms. Six patients had multiple aneurysms.

ANGIOGRAPHIC EVALUATION

Preoperative angiograms were reviewed and the aneurysms were classified into three types with reference to the operative findings.

Type 1

Eleven aneurysms projected superiorly in the lateral view and superimposed with the ICA or projected superiorly in the anteroposterior view (Fig. 3.2). These aneurysms were found at surgery to be protruding toward the surgeon or slightly medially and to be adherent to the basal surface of

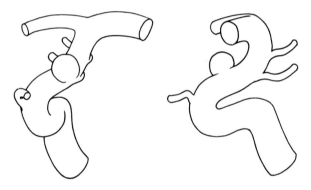

Fig. 3.2   Schematic views of a type 1 dorsal ICA aneurysm.

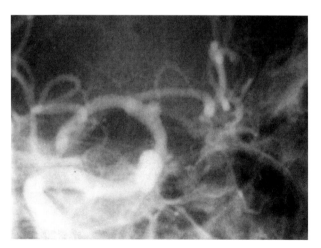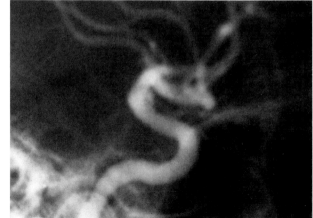

Fig. 3.3   Angiograms showing the typical type 1 aneurysm.

the frontal lobe, except, for one very small aneurysm. An illustrative case is shown in Figure 3.3.

Type 2

Five aneurysms were superimposed with the ICA in the lateral view and projected laterally in the anteroposterior view (Fig. 3.4). At surgery, these aneurysms were found to be protruding slightly laterally and adherent to the medial surface of the temporal lobe, except one very small aneurysm. An illustrative case is shown in Figure 3.5.

Type 3

Four aneurysms were not seen on the angiograms. They had no adhesion to the brain at surgery. Two of these four aneurysms were found incidentally during the approach to an associated ruptured aneurysm. The other two were operated upon because the computed tomographic (CT) scan had shown hematoma in the basal cistern, suggesting rupture of the ICA aneurysm.

In two patients the aneurysms were not seen in the initial angiograms but later were revealed by angiograms taken during the period of vasospasm.

SURGERY

The surgical tactics that we have found useful while dealing with these aneurysms include the following:

1. Care should be taken not to cause rupture during approach to the aneurysm.
2. It is important to expose the carotid artery proximal to the aneurysm at an early stage and to be prepared

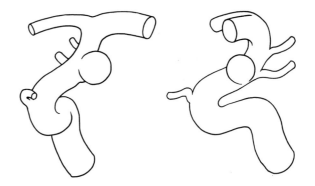

Fig. 3.4   Schematic view of type 2 dorsal ICA aneurysm.

for temporary trapping in cases with intraoperative rupture.
3. When clipping, some portion of the healthy parent artery may be included if the neck is thin.

Usually an ipsilateral pterional exposure is adequate after performing a frontotemporal craniotomy. The sylvian fissure is widely opened, care being taken such that the brain is not retracted excessively as the aneurysm may be torn in cases where it is adherent to the frontal or the temporal lobe. After exposing the aneurysm care is taken to avoid removal of blood clots plugging the site of the rupture of the aneurysm. The artery proximal to the aneurysm is exposed first and then the distal segment is exposed. Trapping of the aneurysm-bearing segment of the artery is done by application of temporary clips. Even after trapping of the artery, bleeding from the ophthalmic or posterior communicating artery can be troublesome. Adequate exposure of the posterior communicating artery should therefore always be done for possible temporary clipping. When one sees that the aneurysm is located very proximally, suggesting difficulty in exposing the parent artery

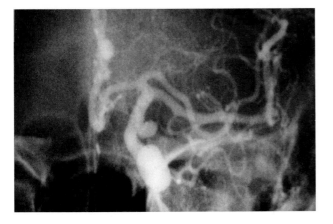 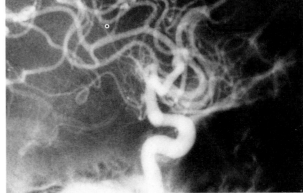

Fig. 3.5   Angiograms showing the typical type 2 aneurysm.

proximal to the aneurysm, the artery may be exposed in the neck for possible temporary occlusion. During surgery the anterior clinoid process can be drilled to obtain proximal control in such a situation. Extreme care should be taken when drilling because the aneurysm is projecting towards the drill. During removal of the anterior clinoid process for proximal exposure of the carotid artery, the ophthalmic artery may also be prepared for temporary occlusion. However, dissection and exposure of the ophthalmic artery can be difficult due to the proximity to the optic nerve and its course in the dural sheath. When the aneurysm is located distally and closer to the carotid bifurcation, distal control of the artery can be obtained by dissecting the M1 segment of the middle cerebral artery (MCA) towards the bifurcation. The actual clipping procedure can be chosen from many options (Osawa et al 1995, Shigeta et al 1992). Preferably clipping should not be repeated and should be completed at the first attempt. Repeated clipping is likely to cause rupture of the aneurysm at the neck.

1. The clip should be placed parallel to the parent artery in order to avoid unnecessary stress to the aneurysm when the clip is placed (Fig. 3.6). Perpendicular clipping carries a risk of causing neck laceration because the ICA is large and hard, often with sclerosis, and the aneurysm is not at the branching point (Fig. 3.7).
2. Whenever the aneurysm is thin walled, the clip blades may include a small portion of the normal arterial wall, thus narrowing the caliber of the artery.
3. When the aneurysm is small and fragile with a wide base, or a dissecting nature of the aneurysm is apparent, wrapping of the aneurysm is preferred. This could be done with the help of Bemsheet. The Bemsheet is used for wrapping around the portion of the artery harboring the aneurysm and a clip is applied to the sheet (Fig. 3.8).

4. When the aneurysm is dorsomedially protruded, the aneurysm can be clipped with a ring clip, with the ring portion encircling the optic nerve.
5. When the aneurysm is located dorsolaterally, the parent artery can be rotated either by direct retraction technique or by bringing the aneurysm up in the dorsal position so the clip can be placed parallel to the parent artery. Alternatively one can open the sylvian fissure more widely, retracting the temporal lobe away from the sphenoidal ridge to enable the operative field to be seen from the temporal side; the bridging anterior temporal vein may have to be sacrificed. Rotating the ICA to bring the aneurysm up into the dorsal position can be done by retracting the head of the temporary clip which is placed proximally. In cases where the aneurysm is located very proximally the dural ring may have to be cut in order to mobilize the ICA (Fig. 3.9).
6. Some cases required mutliple clipping (Fig. 3.10).

It is important to select an appropriate clip suitable for the physiological curve of the parent artery, thus avoiding mechanical stress to the thin neck and the parent artery. Temporary occlusion of the parent artery just at the time of clipping is useful in preventing intra- and postoperative rupture of the aneurysm. This technique decreases the arterial pressure and facilitates complete clipping. Care should be taken concerning the position of the clip head, because the clip may slip and cause rupture of the aneurysm when brain retraction is released on closing. The clip head should be placed on the cranial base without causing pressure on it. Embedding of the clip in the brain tissue is often advisable by tearing a small area of pia to accommodate the clip head (Fig. 3.11). Todd et al (1989) described how wrapping of an aneurysm reduced the incidence of rebleeding, particularly during the first 6 months when the risk of rebleeding is high.

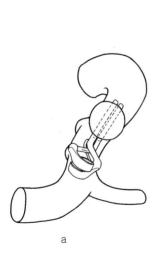

a

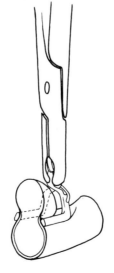

b

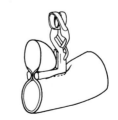

Fig. 3.6   a The clip is placed parallel to the parent artery. **b** Section of the arterial wall with the aneurysm is shown. The clip is being applied in a parallel fashion. After the application of the clip no undue stress is seen on the aneurysm or the vessel wall.

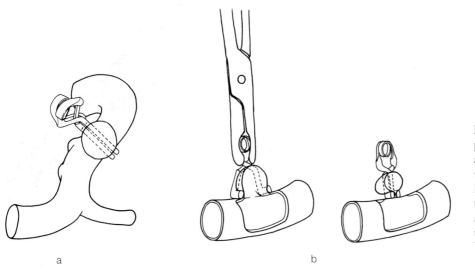

a   b

Fig. 3.7 **a** The clip is placed perpendicular to the parent artery. **b** Section of the arterial wall with the aneurysm. Perpendicular application of the clip causes stretch on the aneurysm wall, which is likely to rupture.

Intraoperative rupture

When premature rupture occurs, there are various options available to the surgeon.

First, either temporary proximal clipping or trapping of the ICA is performed. Mannitol and barbiturate may have to be additionally administered to the patient. When bleeding is under control, clip placement is attempted with a stronger clip. An L-shaped clip may be applied in a parallel fashion to the parent artery, including some portion of the normal arterial wall as well. Mild stenosis of the artery is preferable to permanent trapping of the artery. When the aneurysm ruptures, usually the dome of the aneurysm may be wiped off, leaving just a hole in the parent artery. Attempting to suture the arterial rent is difficult or impossible because the surrounding arterial wall is usually pathological. Yokoo's method (Yokoo et al 1982) and Kawase's method (Kawase et al 1994) may prove useful in such a situation. The encircling clip first described by Sundt is usually not safe as it is difficult to avoid inadvertent occlusion of branches such as posterior communicating or anterior choroidal arteries on the ventral side of the ICA.

Second, when a permanent trapping of the parent artery is necessary, additional procedures such as superficial temporal artery (STA)–MCA anastomosis or bypass with a vein graft from the neck ICA to MCA should be performed.

Regrowth of the dorsal ICA aneurysm

When the aneurysm is incompletely clipped, or when one is unable to apply the clip to the aneurysm, we have observed that the aneurysm can grow large in a few weeks' time. In our series we treated two patients who showed regrowth of the aneurysm or development of new aneurysms at the site of initial clipping. Studies on the regrowth of aneurysms after clipping are relatively few. Lin et al (1989) have presented 19 patients whose aneurysms showed regrowth at intervals ranging from 3 to 24 years after clipping of the neck. The regrowth arose proximal to the clip from a tiny portion of the aneurysm neck which remained outside the clip after the initial surgery. Ebina et al (1984) described two patients who had

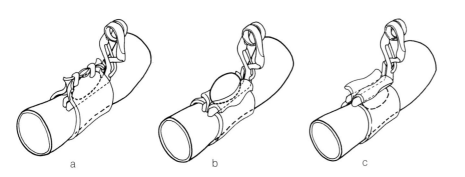

a   b   c

Fig. 3.8 Methods of application of the Bemsheet wrapping. **a** Bemsheet is wrapped around the clipped aneurysm to provide for additional safety. **b** Bemsheet and the aneurysm neck are clipped together. **c** The Bemsheet covers the aneurysm containing a segment of the vessel. The edges of the sheet are clipped.

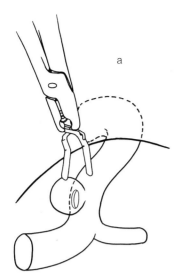

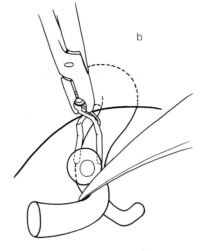

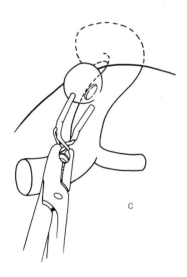

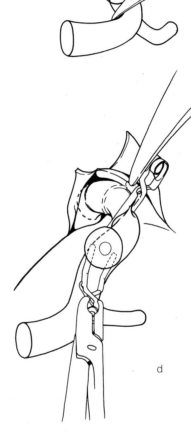

Fig. 3.9   a, b A direct retraction method of the carotid arterial wall, to rotate the aneurysm so that it can be seen better and is more suitable for clip application. **c, d** Method of temporary occlusion of the parent carotid artery and retracting the clip to expose the aneurysm into view.

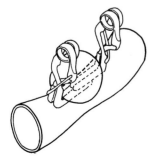

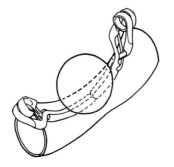

Fig. 3.10   The use of multiple clips to occlude the dorsal ICA aneurysm.

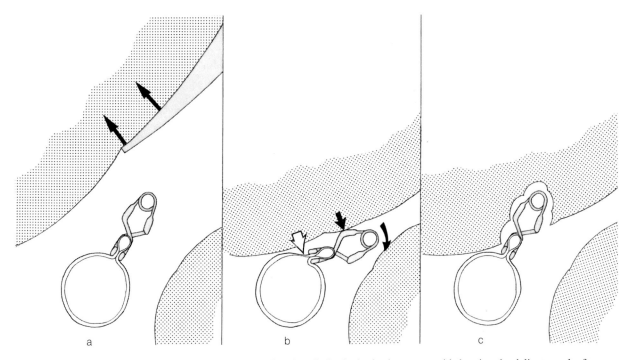

Fig. 3.11 Serial drawings showing a method of embedding the clip in the brain tissue to avoid shearing the delicate neck after restoration of normal anatomy. **a** Application of the clip. **b** The normal anatomy will distort the clip and subject the aneurysm to the danger of rupture. **c** Embedding of the clip head into the brain tissue.

a new aneurysm at the site of the initial clipping. Histological examination of the recurrent aneurysm showed that the arterial wall had been damaged by the clip edge, which resulted in thinning and disruption of both the muscle layer and internal elastic lamina. The authors suggested that local fragility of the arterial wall adjacent to the aneurysm may have been the cause of the formation of a new aneurysm and so reinforcement of the thin-walled parent artery is important. Because the parent arterial wall adjacent to the dorsal ICA aneurysm is especially thin and the aneurysm is dome shaped, the risk of its regrowth is high. Some of the aneurysms under discussion could be dissecting in nature. We emphasize the importance of complete clipping and reinforcement of the thin arterial wall as necessary.

As mentioned above, when the dorsal ICA aneurysm is located distally, it can grow larger than those located proximally, because the aneurysm wall is protected by the frontal or the temporal brain (Diraz et al 1992). The dorsal ICA aneurysm or blister aneurysm can grow in the proximal segment of the MCA as the structural relation between the aneurysm and the parent artery and hemodynamics are similar to those in the ICA. When a dissecting nature of the aneurysm is suspected, wrapping is better than the clipping of the aneurysm, as mentioned earlier.

After surgery, postoperative angiography should be performed within 1 month or relatively early in the postoper-

ative period and may be repeated in a couple of months in order to rule out regrowth of the aneurysm.

In our series all cases were operated upon by the ipsilateral pterional approach. Careful separation of the sylvian fissure was essential for prevention of premature rupture. Neck clipping of the aneurysm was performed in 17 cases, of which supplementary wrapping with Bemsheet or muscle was used in seven. Two were managed with wrapping alone because of their small size. One was managed with a bypass (superficial temporal artery to middle cerebral artery) and trapping of the parent artery due to uncontrollable intraoperative bleeding. Temporary occlusion of the parent artery was used in six cases when the aneurysm neck was markedly thin at the base.

RESULTS

Intraoperative rupture occurred in five cases. In four cases the cause of the rupture was laceration at the neck. In one case, rupture was encountered during dissection of the sylvian fissure and had to be managed by a bypass and trapping. In the remaining cases, rupture occurred at the time of completely closing the clip blades. However, clip closing was finally performed by either single or multiple clipping. In one of them the laceration was closed using two right-angled clips, and in another case using two bent clips. In the other case the cause of intraoperative rupture was slipping of the clip; reclipping was easily performed.

Postoperative rupture

Postoperative rupture occurred in two cases. In these cases the neck and the adjacent wall of the parent artery were found at surgery to be very thin. The cause of postoperative rupture is thought to be slipping off of the clip, incomplete clipping, or new growth of the aneurysm due to insufficient inclusion of the adjacent wall of the parent artery within the clip blades. One case showed a remarkable growth of the aneurysm only 21 days after the operation.

CASE 1   Large Right Dorsal ICA Aneurysm

This 25-year-old woman had suffered an episode of severe headache and nausea 4 weeks prior to her admission. Three weeks ago she suddenly became unconscious. CT scan showed subarachnoid hemorrhage and subdural hematoma. The angiogram on the same day revealed a right ICA dorsal type of aneurysm with vasospasm (Fig. 3.12). A delayed operation was performed. With the patient in the supine position the cervical ICA was exposed. A right frontotemporal craniotomy was performed (Fig. 3.13a). The dura was opened. Subdural clots in the frontal base were removed. Severe adhesions in the sylvian fissure suggested the presence of aneurysm buried in the temporal lobe. Dissection of the sylvian fissure was tedious. The distal ICA was exposed first by subpial removal of the frontal and temporal lobe base. The A1, the posterior communicating artery and the origin of the anterior choroidal were exposed. The optic nerve was unroofed and part of the anterior clinoid process was removed in order to expose the proximal ICA and the proximal part of the neck of the aneurysm. While peeling off the membranous adhesion in the

proximal neck site, a major rupture occurred at the base of the aneurysm. The cervical ICA was temporarily occluded. The bleeding, however, continued profusely. The distal ICA was then exposed by pushing the aneurysm rupture site (Fig. 3.13b) and a temporary clip was applied. The posterior communicating artery was identified in the opticocarotid space and was temporarily clipped. The ophthalmic artery was also clipped. Only after all these maneuvers did the bleeding stop. An L-shaped 1 cm long clip was applied to the neck of the aneurysm, whereby the base of the distal neck was partially left in the side of the parent artery. The proximal ICA seemed to be slightly stenotic by the tips of the clip blades. The rupture site of the aneurysm could be seen included in the clip. Replacement of the clip was considered hazardous as the field was very narrow, preventing maneuvering of the clip applicator. Temporary clips were removed (Fig. 3.13c). The total temporary occlusion time was about 20 minutes. Postoperatively the patient had mild hemiparesis which gradually cleared. The postoperative angiograms showed complete clipping (Fig. 3.14).

Comments

1. This was a large dorsal (or dorsolateral) ICA aneurysm. The dorsal ICA does not usually grow large; typically it is small, wide based, with a fragile neck. It was adherent to the temporal and frontal lobe bases.

2. Subpial dissection was useful.

References

Diraz A, Kobayashi S, Okudera H et al 1992 Suprachiasmal carotid–ophthalmic aneurysm. Neurologia Medicochirurgica (Tokyo) 32: 952–956

Ebina K, Iwabuchi T, Suzuki S 1984 A clinico-experimental study on various wrapping materials of cerebral aneurysms. Acta Neurochirurgica (Wien) 72: 61–71

Forster D M, Steiner L, Hakanson S, Bergvall U 1978 The value of repeated panangiography in cases of unexplained subarachnoid hemorrhage. Journal of Neurosurgery 48: 712–716

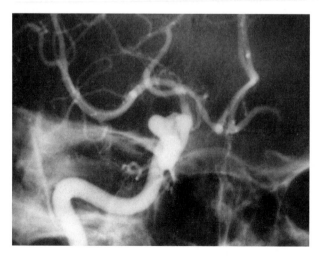 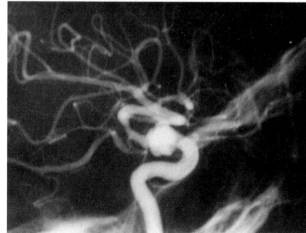

Fig. 3.12   Preoperative angiograms showing right dorsal ICA aneurysm with vasospasm.

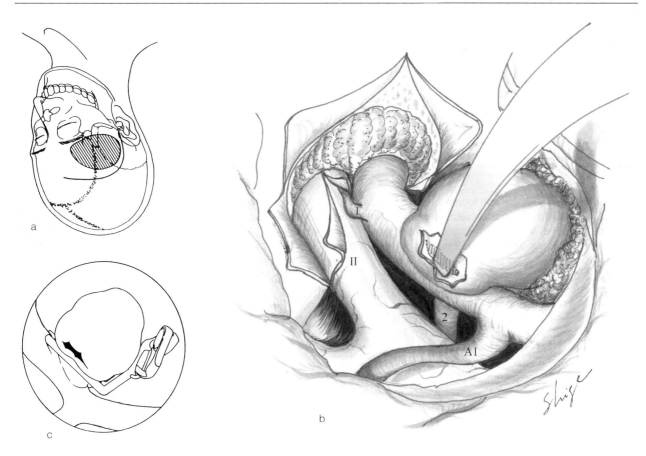

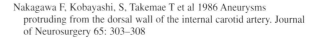

Fig. 3.13 **a** Right frontotemporal craniotomy. **b** Exposure of the distal ICA. **c** The rupture site of the aneurysm included in the clip.

Kawase T, Gotoh K, Toya S 1994 A wrapping clip combined with silastic sheet for emergent hemostasis: technical note. Neurosurgery 35: 769–770

Lin T, Fox, A J, Drake C G 1989 Regrowth of aneurysm sacs from residual neck following aneurysm clipping. Journal of Neurosurgery 70: 556–560

Nakagawa F, Kobayashi, S, Takemae T et al 1986 Aneurysms protruding from the dorsal wall of the internal carotid artery. Journal of Neurosurgery 65: 303–308

Osawa F, Obinata C, Kobayashi S et al 1995 Newly designed bayonet clips for complicated aneurysms: technical note. Neurosurgery 36: 425–427

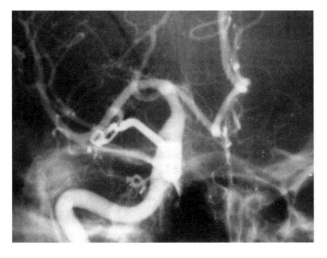

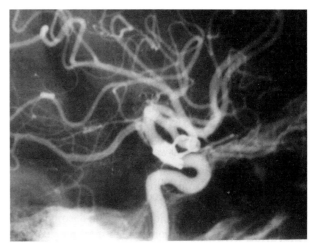

Fig. 3.14 Postoperative angiogram showing complete clipping.

CLASSIFICATION OF AComA ANEURYSM WITH SPECIAL REFERENCE TO SURGICAL APPROACH

Yasargil classified the AComA aneurysm into four types: superior, inferior, anterior and posterior (Yasargil 1984). However, in terms of selection of surgical approach, it appeared to us that three divisions, namely anterior, inferior and superior (posterior), are appropriate. If we set horizontal (x) and vertical (y) axes with the AComA as a reference (0) on the right lateral view of the angiogram, and measure the position of the AComA aneurysm clockwise from the x axis, the anterior type of aneurysm is located between 1 and 5 o'clock position, the inferior type between 5 and 9 o'clock position and the superior (posterior) type between 9 and 1 o'clock position (Fig. 4.1).

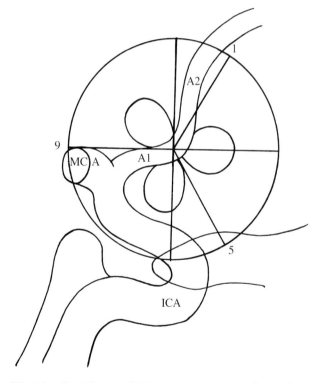

Fig. 4.1 Classification of AComA aneurysm according to the location of the aneurysm in relation to the parent arteries as seen in the right lateral view of the carotid angiogram. Aneurysms located between 1 and 5 o'clock: anterior type aneurysms between 5 and 9 o'clock: inferior type; and aneurysms between 9 and 1 o'clock: superior (posterior) type. Numbers show time on the clock. (ICA, internal carotid artery, MCA, middle cerebral artery; A1, A2: A1 and A2 segments of the anterior cerebral artery, respectively.)

Anterior type of AComA aneurysm

The majority of the AComA aneurysms correspond to this type. As the aneurysm in this situation lies away from the brain and in relationship to the arachnoid membrane, dissection and exposure of the aneurysm are relatively easy. Wide dissection of the arachnoid lessens the degree of retraction of the frontal lobe.

Inferior type of AComA aneurysm

This type of AComA aneurysm is likely to be adherent to or embedded in the chiasm and hence the retraction of the frontal lobe can be dangerous and should therefore be done very carefully. However, when the neck is exposed, clipping itself is usually easy.

Superior (posterior) AComA aneurysm

This type is difficult to clip via the pterional approach because it is hidden behind the parent arteries or the gyrus rectus. In the pterional approach, one has to confirm adequate clipping as the possibility of leaving a residual neck remains in this situation. This is because the clip and the parent arteries do not allow adequate visualization of the neck of the aneurysm. Some prefer an interhemispheric approach for this type of aneurysm.

HIGH-POSITIONED AComA ANEURYSM

If an aneurysm is located high above the clinoid process, an interhemispheric approach is preferable. This is especially so when the aneurysm is large. One can, however, expose such an aneurysm even by a pterional approach by removing a substantial amount of gyrus rectus. In the pterional approach, when it comes to the stage of clipping the aneurysm, one may have some difficulty as the field is deep, narrow and high. When the aneurysm is small, a high-positioned AComA aneurysm can be approached pterionally as well. The position of the neck in relation to the aneurysm body is important in deciding the route of approach. If the neck is positioned on top of the aneurysm, the interhemispheric approach is recommended, whereas if it is positioned lower, in inferior relationship to the aneurysm, a pterional approach can be made.

Positioning the patient

Generally speaking, the head should be kept elevated

above the level of the heart throughout the procedure. The head is fixed in the frame rotated about 45° contralaterally; the degree of rotation is changed as necessary during the procedure. For an interhemispheric approach, the head is fixed in the frame without rotation. Vertical shifting of the head position may be necessary during the procedure.

APPROACH TO THE AComA ANEURYSM

Right pterional approach

A right pterional approach is the most commonly used approach for an AComA aneurysm (Fig. 4.2). The sylvian fissure is widely opened to facilitate retraction of the frontal lobe. In order to make the brain slack, drainage of the cerebrospinal fluid (CSF) from basal cisterns is important. CSF drainage from the lateral ventricle is often helpful when the ventricle is large or the brain is tense, especially in acute-stage operation. In order to slacken the brain, intentional perforation of the lamina terminalis is sometimes helpful. This can be done easily when the aneurysm is of the anterior type. One has to be careful in doing this for an inferior type of aneurysm because the dome of the aneurysm is close to the lamina terminalis. Yasargil has advocated perforation of the lamina in the early stage of dissection for all types of aneurysms operated on via a pterional approach (Yasargil 1984). Also osmotic diuretics such as mannitol can be infused. After identification of the right optic nerve and the internal carotid artery, it is necessary to expose the origin of the right A1 for possible temporary clipping. Exposing the A1 just proximal to the aneurysmal complex may be preferred so that one can preserve the perforating arteries from the proximal portion of the A1 in case temporary clipping becomes necessary. Dissection of the prechiasmatic arachnoid is carried out, extending over to the contralateral side in most cases of the anterior type of AComA aneurysm. After dissection and exposure of the distal A1, one can partially visualize the aneurysm complex and an idea of the anatomy in the vicinity of the aneurysm can be obtained. Following this, one should expose the left (contralateral) A1. Less experienced surgeons may find difficulty in exposing the contralateral A1 because of a distorted anatomical relation encountered in the pterional approach (in the interhemispheric approach its identification is relatively easy). Usually one finds the left A1 lateral to or over the left optic nerve. In some instances the left A1 is not found crossing the left optic nerve. The left A1 is often found coursing along the ipsilateral (right) A1. In such cases one must try to expose the left A1 behind or deeper to the right A1 by retracting or resecting the right gyrus rectus.

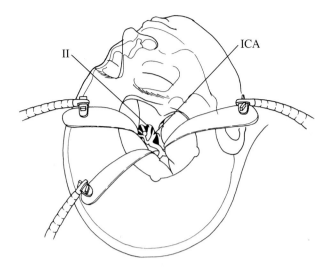

Fig. 4.2 Pterional approach (right frontotemporal craniotomy) to an AComA aneurysm, showing the patient's head position and the operative field.

Exposure of the proximal part of the two A2s is sometimes difficult because they are in close relationship to the aneurysm. In such a case, one could dissect the interhemispheric fissure distally instead of starting dissection from the aneurysmal side. After exposing the distal part of the A2 in the interhemispheric fissure it is traced proximally towards the aneurysm. One must remember that the contralateral A2 sometimes runs parallel to the ipsilateral A2. In such a case one must search the former in depth along the latter. Parallel coursing A2s may become problematic when the aneurysm is large as it is difficult to expose the origin of the contralateral A2. When the aneurysm is located high or when difficulty is encountered in finding the A2s, removal of the gyrus rectus is recommended over retraction of the frontal lobe with force.

Left pterional approach

The left pterional approach can be taken in such conditions as follows:

1. when the left A1 is dominant;
2. when the origin of the right A2 is located anterior to that of the left A2; the neck of the aneurysm is hidden by the right A2 in the right pterional approach (Fig. 4.3);
3. in the case of multiple aneurysms with other aneurysms located on the left side.

When taking a left pterional approach, the extent of craniotomy is different from that of the right pterional approach in that it needs to be extended almost to the

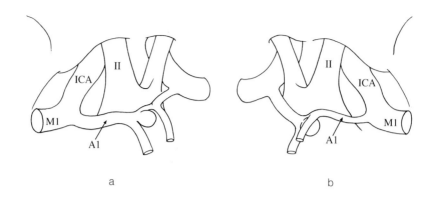

Fig. 4.3   Schematic drawings of the relation between the aneurysm and A2s in the case of the right A2 coursing anterior to the left A2. **a** Left pterional approach. **b** Right pterional approach.

frontal midline to allow the right-handed surgeon to operate easily and also to allow adequate illumination.

Interhemispheric approach

The interhemispheric approach (Fig. 4.4) is relatively infrequently used, but sometimes it can be very useful. When the aneurysm is high positioned (13 mm or more above the anterior clinoid process; Diraz et al 1993) or is of a large variety, this approach is recommended. Surgery is carried out with the patient in the supine position. A unilateral (usually right) craniotomy after a hemicoronal skin incision is sufficient. To achieve a wider exposure, the craniotomy may extend across the midline. The bridging

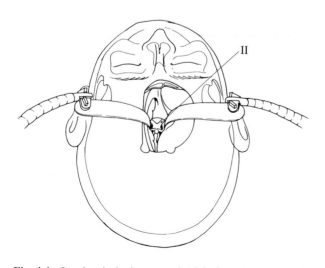

Fig. 4.4   Interhemispheric approach (right frontal craniotomy) to an AComA aneurysm, showing the patient's head position and the operative field.

veins are preserved utilizing the method described by Sugita et al (1982). Basal extension of frontal craniotomy is often helpful. By removing the orbital bar (as described elsewhere) one will be able to minimize retraction. In an interhemispheric approach, removal of CSF is difficult during the approach to a deep-seated AComA aneurysm, unlike in the case of a pterional approach where basal cisterns are relatively easily approachable.

The patient's head is initially lowered by reducing the inclination of the upper plate of the table. The genu of the corpus callosum is aproached first for the sake of orientation as well as to find and secure the two A2 segments of the aneurysm complex. This is followed by raising the patient's head by flexing the upper plate of the operating table, and the planum sphenoidale is approached. The olfactory nerves should not be unduly retracted during the procedure (Suzuki et al 1981). Once the planum sphenoidale is exposed, it is traced posteriorly to the tuberculum sellae. The optic nerves and later the internal carotid arteries and A1s can then be exposed. It is recommended that the dominant A1 be dissected first. It is not always necessary to expose both A2s. At this point, instead of dissecting around the aneurysm, one may go back to the genu of the corpus callosum and from here trace the A2s proximally, approaching the region of the aneurysm complex. It is important to completely separate both sides of the medial frontal lobe. The dissection of the fissure in proximity to the aneurysm complex should be done only after one has an idea about the anatomical situation around the aneurysm complex. One must be flexible in approaching the target (the aneurysm) as much will depend on the situation around the aneurysm. This is particularly true in cases of AComA aneurysm where the anatomical relationship tends to be variable. However, the anatomical interrelationship of the aneurysm and the parent arteries is seen to be surprisingly stereotyped after the dissection is completed.

Position of the surgeon in the interhemispheric approach

If the surgeon stands at the head end of the patient, the operating field seen under the operating microscope is a vertical opening. Also the surgeon has to work in this vertical field which is not natural. We have found it easier to operate while sitting by the ipsilateral side of the craniotomy. In this set-up, a horizontal (or near-horizontal) opening of the operating field becomes feasible and the surgeon can operate in a more natural manner. One of the disadvantages with this positioning is that it is sometimes difficult to visualize the skull base of the frontal pole unless the surgeon tilts his head excessively. Another disadvantage with the lateral positioning of the surgeon is that one can easily become disoriented in the initial stage of the approach to the aneurysm in identifying structures such as the genu of the corpus callosum, crista galli, planum sphenoidale, and other structures in the vicinity. The reason for this is that the surgeon cannot get an idea of the patient's head position, i.e. how much the head is tilted and rotated in relation to the axis of the microscope. In such a situation the surgeon can temporarily shift to the vertex end of the patient's head and continue dissection.

Number of retractors used for pterional and interhemispheric approaches

We usually use a number of 2 mm tapered spatulas held by Sugita's frame. In the right pterional approach it is important to use two spatulas on both sides of the aneurysm so that the surgeon can see the neck well. It is also advisable to place one spatula over the left gyrus rectus so as to obtain space for temporary or final clipping. In the interhemispheric approach it is important that one retractor is placed over the contralateral medial frontal lobe under the falx and two or three retractors are placed over the medial frontal lobe of the approaching side.

Combined pterional and interhemispheric approach

This approach has been rarely used. In our series we used the combined approach for giant thrombosed aneurysm and in the presence of associated aneurysms in other territories.

In the combined approach, a coronal skin incision extending from the midline to the temporal bone is used. A pterional approach either from the right or left side is performed with wide dissection of the sylvian fissure, exposing the chiasm and securing both A1s. The interhemispheric approach can be performed either ipsilateral or contralateral to the pterional approach. After the A2s are identified at the genu of the corpus callosum, the dissection is carried proximally and the interhemispheric fissure is opened anteriorly. The subsequent steps are more or less based on the same tactics previously mentioned for each individual approach.

IMPORTANT ANATOMICAL STRUCTURES AND VARIATIONS

During dissection of an aneurysm complex, it is important to keep in mind the surrounding anatomical structures and their variations. Some of the important structures beside the four parent arteries include Heubner's artery, which most often originates from the A2 and is occasionally duplicated. The hypothalamic artery is often large. It can be easily missed during dissection or clipping as it usually courses behind and under the aneurysm complex. Fenestration of the AComA is sometimes encountered and knowledge of this variation helps in terms of shortening the time necessary for dissection. The azygos A2 and median anterior cerebral artery can be detected from the preoperative angiogram. Duplication of the A1 is rare, but when it is present an aneurysm may be associated.

DISSECTION OF THE ANEURYSM COMPLEX

Some dissection techniques around the aneurysm complex which have been found useful are described. It is important to start dissecting on the lateral side of the parent arteries as the aneurysm is interposed between the parent arteries. For this reason dissection along the medial side of the parent arteries is dangerous due to the closer proximity with the aneurysm. It is also important to anticipate prior to the surgery on the basis of angiography which part of the aneurysm has bled. During surgery, inspection of the aneurysm will suggest how thick the wall of the aneurysm is. A whitish color of the wall suggests that it is thick, while a red wall generally indicates a thin wall, especially when swirling of blood is seen through the wall. However, distinction on the basis of color may not always hold. As one gains more experience, one will be able to appreciate that a 'healthy' red color of the wall usually indicates that the aneurysm has a rather thick wall which is more resistant to mechanical pressure or distortion. 'Dangerous' or 'pathological' red color is 'discolored' red (dark or grayish red). An aneurysm wall with a 'pathological' red hue often accompanies a small bleb in proximity to an uneven surface, or clots often cover the aneurysm. The location of the clot usually indicates the site of the rupture. It is wise not to peel the clots from the aneurysm unless it is absolutely necessary, and this is done after protective measures have been taken such as induced hypotension or proximal controlling. The aneurysm itself is generally dissected where the wall is thick.

It is important to try not to exert pressure on the suspected point of rupture by retracting the surrounding structures. When directly retracting the aneurysm, one must not retract the thin-walled portion of the aneurysm. During direct retraction, distortion of the portion of the aneurysm where the wall is thin should be avoided.

The general tactics are first to expose and secure both A1s and A2s. When it is difficult to isolate or identify the A2s, one may dissect in the interhemispheric fissure distally, a little away from the aneurysm complex. This procedure may appear difficult, but one can orient oneself and find the interhemispheric fissure by sufficiently changing the axis of the microscope in such a way as to look up from the orbital roof. Securing both sides of the neck at the final stage of the operation is important. This can be done in the majority of cases, but in some large or giant aneurysms, or when parent arteries are in an unusual relation to the aneurysm, complete dissection of the neck may not be possible. On such an occasion, tentative clipping to the body or dome of the aneurysm is done. With the clip in place

neck dissection can be advanced for the final clipping (Fig. 4.5).

DISSECTION OF THE ANEURYSM

Dissection of the aneurysm itself requires delicate maneuvering. We often use a silver dissector to expose the area. Dissection with the silver dissector is done parallel along the course of the parent artery. If used perpendicular to the artery, it may press upon and distort the aneurysm, which may precipitate rupture. It is also important to scrape the adventitia of the parent artery toward the aneurysm and not away from it to avoid a premature rupture. When using suction on and in the vicinity of the aneurysm, one must try always to use a small piece of cotton with it. It is recommended to use continuous suction with a shunt tube during the dissection around the aneurysm complex as it cleans the CSF as well as serving to clean the field in cases of premature rupture. Suction of part of the gyrus rectus is sometimes done. This procedure is much safer than retracting the frontal lobe with great force, a procedure which may eventually lead to contusion not only of the gyrus rectus but also of the entire frontal lobe. The gyrus rectus

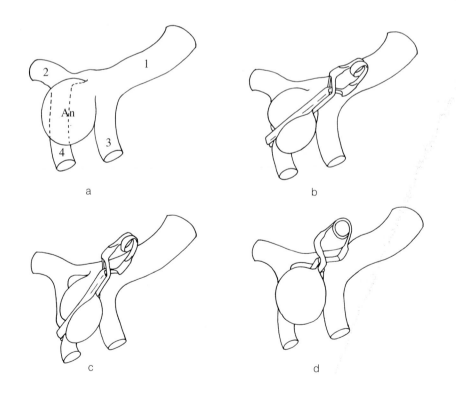

Fig. 4.5   Tentative clipping in sequence in the right pterional approach. **a** Aneurysm hiding the contralateral A2. **b** Tentative clipping of the aneurysm including contralateral A2. **c** Dissection of the aneurysm neck. **d** Final clipping. (1, right A1; 2, left A1; 3, right A2; 4, left A2; An, aneurysm.)

should be removed subpially as the pia prevents injury to the aneurysm.

CLIPPING TECHNIQUE

Whenever possible one must try to use a single clip, although in an unusual-shaped aneurysm multiple clipping may be necessary. A ring clip is sometimes useful. When using multiple clips it is better to determine the combination at the beginning of the clipping process. This helps in using a better combination of clips than if the decision was made at the time of clipping. When applying a clip, care should be taken not to injure the optic nerve or chiasm with the tip of the clip blades. It is therefore necessary to visualize the state when retraction of the frontal lobe is released after clipping. When a pterional approach is taken, some prefer a curved clip. In our practice, however, a curved clip is rarely used. Another little trick that we have found useful is 'shank clipping', whereby the shank of the bayonet clip is utilized to obliterate the part of the neck which forms the AComA itself. This shank clipping is more often used for middle cerebral artery aneurysms (Osawa et al 1995) (see Fig. 5.20.).

Temporary occlusion of the parent arteries is used when premature rupture has occurred or is likely to occur. A temporary clip (or clips) is placed to either the dominant A1, both A1s or both A1s and A2s as necessary. Tentative clipping of the aneurysm including one of the parent arteries is an alternative procedure.

Indications for double clipping

We have used double-clipping techniques whenever needed. Our indications for use of double clips are:

1. when the neck is wide;
2. when the AComA itself is forming a part of the aneurysm;
3. When the parent artery is lying over the aneurysm and is in the way of the approach;
4. for a giant aneurysm.

CASE 1   Superior type, High-positioned, Unruptured

A 69-year-old female was found to have an incidental AComA aneurysm. The angiogram showed an 8 mm aneurysm at the AComA pointing upwards and slightly posteriorly. The left A1 was dominant and the right A1 was not visualized (Fig. 4.6).

With the patient in the supine position, a left frontotemporal craniotomy was done (Fig. 4.7a). The sylvian fissure was carefully dissected and this was followed by dissection of the supraoptic arachnoid to the opposite side. After retraction of the frontal brain, the origin of the left A1 was dissected and secured. Then the right A1 was exposed, which was whitish and hypoplastic with no clear evidence of blood flowing through it (Fig. 4.7b). With further dissection around the aneurysm complex no. 8B curved clip, the aneurysmal neck was occluded between both A2s, but on inspection it was realized that a part of the aneurysm behind the left A1 had not been clipped. A no. 35 ring clip with oblique blades was used from the other side of the aneurysm with a ring over the A1 and the aneurysm was occluded completely (Fig. 4.7c). On inspection, a gap was observed in the region of the junction of the two clips. The initial clip was released and reapplied in such a way that their blades abutted on each other.

The postoperative course was uneventful. Clipping was complete (Fig. 4.8).

Comments

1. This was a superior, medium-sized aneurysm and was relatively high positioned, being about 10 mm above the anterior clinoid process.

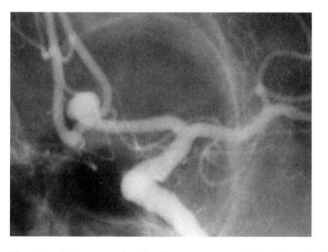
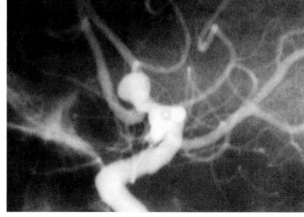

Fig. 4.6   Angiograms showing 8 mm aneurysm of the AComA, pointing upwards and slightly posteriorly.

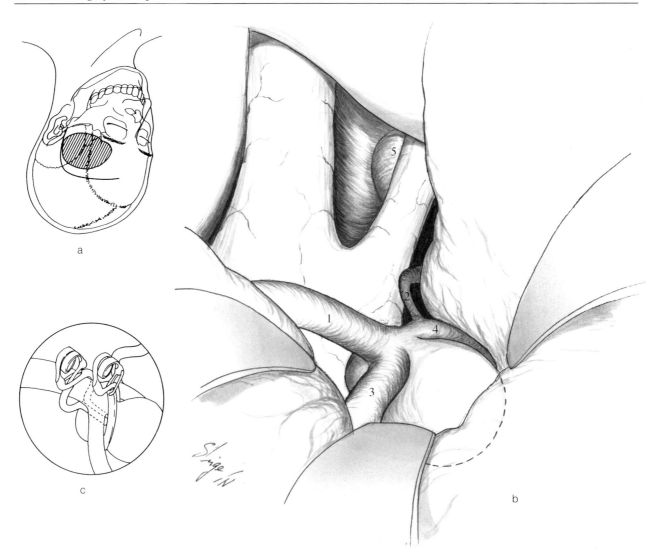

Fig. 4.7 **a** Left frontotemporal craniotomy. **b** Exposure of the right A1. **c** A no. 35 ring clip with oblique blades was applied from the other side of the aneurysm, with a ring over the A1; the aneurysm was completely occluded. (1, left A1; 2, right A1; 3, left A2; 4, right A2; 5, right ICA.)

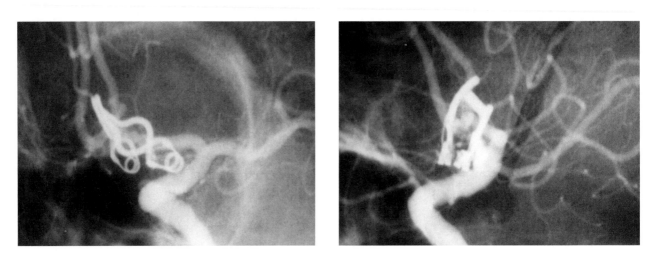

Fig. 4.8 Angiograms showing complete clipping.

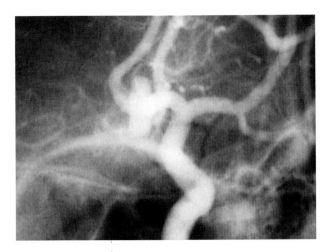

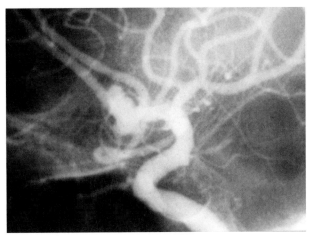

Fig. 4.9 Preoperative angiograms showing aneurysm.

2. Because there was marked brain atrophy, retraction of the brain was relatively easy.

3. The superiorly pointing aneurysm is sometimes difficult, as in this case. We used two clips, but an L-shaped clip would have sufficed.

4. During double clipping, the heads of the clips need to be aligned in a parallel fashion so as to avoid clip junctional leakage.

CASE 2

This 59-year-old male underwent the first surgery 1 month previously (Fig. 4.9). The postoperative angiogram showed that a substantial portion of the aneurysm had remained unclipped (Fig. 4.10). With the patient in the supine position the previous frontotemporal craniotomy was reopened (Fig. 4.11a) and the sphenoid ridge was drilled further. A careful, tedious dissection of the aneurysm was made. Initially both A1s, then the left A2 and later right A2 were exposed. The previously placed clip was denuded from the adhesion as much as possible. The unclipped portion was found to be at the junction between the AComA and the right A2 (Fig. 4.11b,c). Without removing the clip, a bayonet ring clip was chosen to occlude the remaining aneurysm. Under temporary clipping of both A1s, the aneurysm was further dissected to allow placing of the second clip. This was done successfully (Fig. 4.11d). As a radiolucent operating frame was being used an intraoperative angiography was performed (Fig. 4.12). The angiogram did not fill the aneurysm, but it also failed to show the filling of the right A2, even with cross compression. The aneurysm complex was exposed again and with a Doppler flowmeter the patency of the right A2 was confirmed. Anatomically the parent arteries were patent (Fig. 4.13). The postoperative condition of the patient was good.

Comments

1. A bayonet ring clip just fitted the narrow space available in the presence of a previously placed clip.

2. The intraoperative left carotid angiography did not reveal the right A2 with cross-compression. However, the Doppler flowmeter indicated the flow through the right A2.

CASE 3 Giant Thrombosed A1 Aneurysm

A 61-year-old left-handed male suffered right hemiparesis secondary to cerebral infarction 9 months before the surgery. During the investigations, an incidental partially thrombosed giant aneurysm of the A1 segment of the right anterior cerebral artery was detected on computed tomographic (CT) scan and

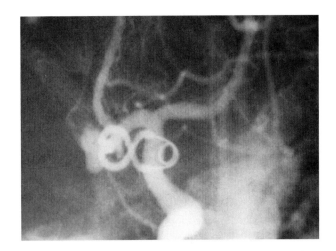

Fig. 4.10 Postoperative angiogram showing incomplete clipping of the aneurysm.

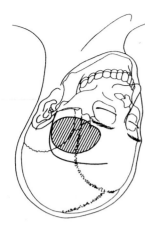

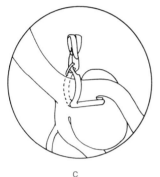

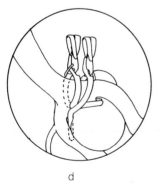

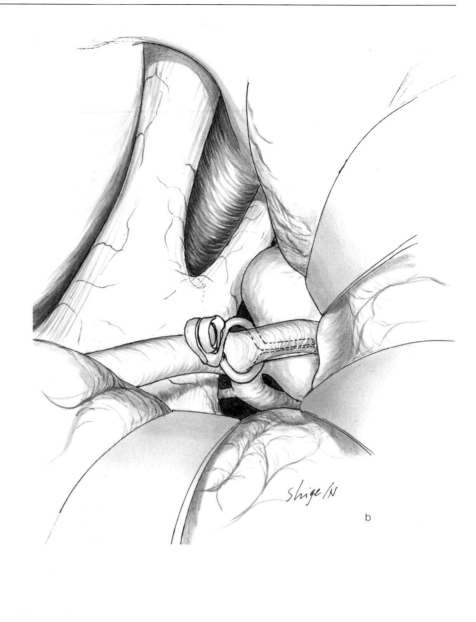

Fig. 4.11   a Frontotemporal craniotomy. **b, c** The unclipped portion was found to be at the junction between the AComA and the right A2. **d** Successful placement of the second clip.

later on magnetic resonance imaging (MRI) (Fig. 4.14) and angiography (Fig. 4.15). The aneurysm measured $34 \times 28 \times 26$ mm in size. The aneurysm arose directly from the right A1. The left A1 was hypoplastic, but the cross-flow through the AComA appeared to be satisfactory.

With the patient in the supine position, a bilateral frontal craniotomy extending to the right temporal bone was performed (Fig. 4.16a). Initially, the right sylvian fissure was widely opened to secure the origin of the anterior cerebral artery for proximal control. The aneurysm could not be seen by the pterional route. The interhemispheric approach was then adopted. The superior sagittal sinus close to the crista galli was

ligated and sectioned. The anterior interhemispheric fissure was dissected, isolating the bridging veins. The right A2 and the distal portion of A1 leading towards the aneurysm were exposed. The left A1, A2 and the AComA were also exposed. A corticotomy on the right gyrus rectus and olfactory gyrus around the distal A1 facilitated exposure of the aneurysm (Fig. 4.16b). After systemic heparinization, each side of the parent A1 was temporarily clipped (by Sugita temporary clips). The presence of blood flow in both A2 segments was confirmed by a Doppler flowmeter. The aneurysm dome was now widely opened up and the thrombosed contents were removed with a silver dissector and an ultrasonic aspirator. The aneurysm dome

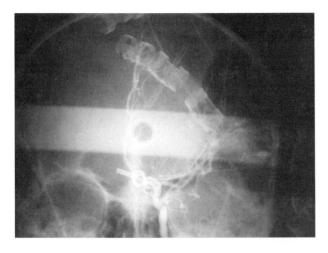

Fig. 4.12   Intraoperative angiogram.

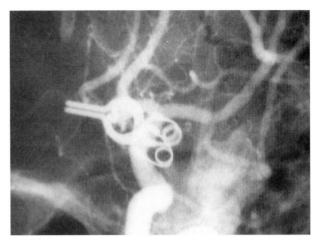

Fig. 4.13   The parent arteries were patent.

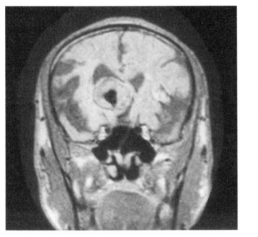

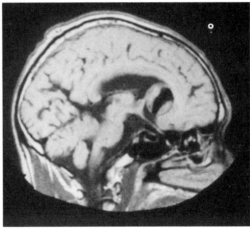

Fig. 4.14   Partial thrombosed giant aneurysm of the A1 segment of the right anterior cerebral artery was detected on CT and MRI scans (Case 3).

Fig. 4.15   Angiograms of Case 3.

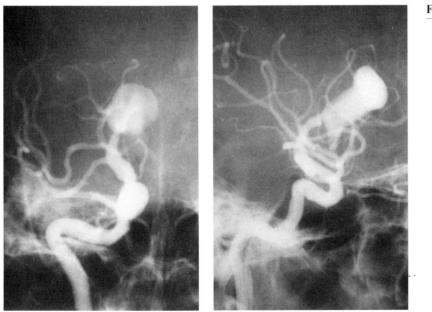

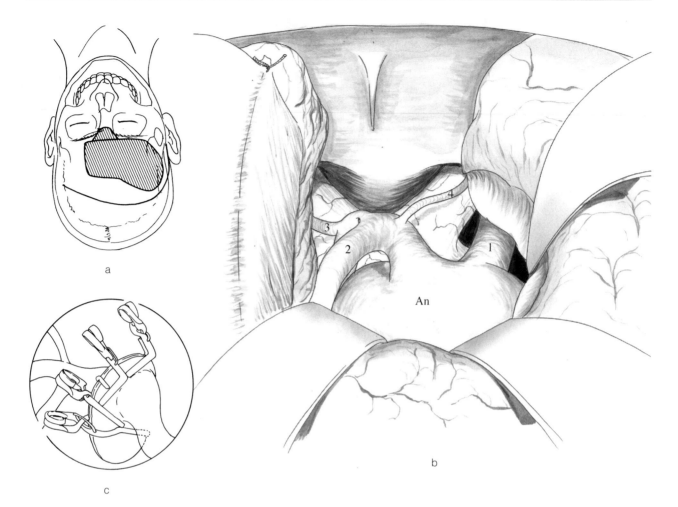

Fig. 4.16   **a** Bilateral frontal craniotomy extending to the right temporal bone. **b** Corticotomy on the right gyrus rectus and olfactory gyrus around the distal A1 facilitated exposure of the aneurysm. **c** Four clips were used: two L-shaped, one straight and one straight ring clip. (1, right A1; 2, right A2; 3, left A1; 4, Heubner's artery; An, aneurysm.)

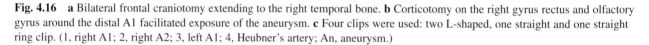

was circumferentially incised and the intraluminal surface of the aneurysm was now clearly seen. The orifices of the A1 on each side were narrow because of thickened intima. The cut edge of the aneurysm was closed by clip angioplasty with the help of three clips: an L-shaped clip, a straight ring clip and a bayonet clip. When the temporary clips were removed blood flow was not evident in the aneurysm-involved artery. The proximal A1 was trapped again and the three clips used for angioplasty were removed. The intima around both sides of the orifices was peeled off to widen the aperture. The cut edge of the aneurysm wall was reapproximated with the help of four clips: two L-shaped, one straight and one straight ring clip (Fig. 4.16c). Before the clips were finally closed, the temporary clips on each side were transiently removed to flush the thrombus and air in the parent artery and aneurysm. The patency of the A1 was confirmed with a Doppler flowmeter. A few minutes later one of the L-shaped clips slipped, resulting in profuse bleeding. After temporary trapping of the parent artery, the slipped clip was advanced a little more from the cut edge towards the aneurysm.

To avoid slippage of the clip, a hemoclip was applied at the cut edge. The aneurysm and the clips were wrapped with cottonoid patties and fibrin glue. The dome side of the aneurysm wall was not removed as it was densely adherent to the cerebral parenchyma. Total trapping time was 55 minutes. Systemic systolic blood pressure was kept around 150 mmHg during the trapping procedure.

Postoperatively the patient showed mild left hemiparesis although a CT scan and an MRI showed no evidence of fresh infarction. The postoperative angiogram showed adequate patency of the right A1 (Fig. 4.17).

References

Diraz A, Kobayashi S, Toriyama T et al 1993 Surgical approaches to the anterior communicating artery aneurysm and their results. Neurological Research 15: 273–280

Osawa M, Obinata C, Kobayashi S, Tanaka Y 1995 Newly designed bayonet clips for complicated aneurysms: technical note. Neurosurgery 36: 425–427

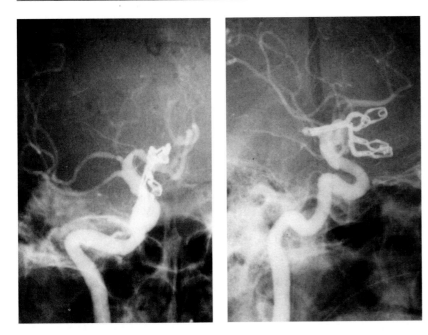

Fig. 4.17 Postoperative angiogram showed adequate patency of the right A1.

Pia H W 1978 Classification of aneurysms of the internal carotid system. Acta Neurochirurgica (Wien) 40: 5–31

Sugita K, Kobayashi S, Yokoo A 1982 Preservation of large bridging veins during brain retraction. Journal of Neurosurgery 57: 856–858

Suzuki J, Yoshimoto T, Mizoi K 1981 Preservation of the olfactory tract in bifrontal craniotomy for anterior communicating artery aneurysms, and the functional prognosis. Journal of Neurosurgery 54: 342–345

Yasargil M G 1984 Microneurosurgery II. George Thieme Verlag, Stuttgart

Technical Considerations in Anterior Communicating Artery Aneurysm Surgery
Bryce Weir

In many populations the AComA is the most common location of aneurysms. The technical conduct of the operation is based on a knowledge of the normal and abnormal anatomy of this region. The key point is a recognition of the variability in the anatomy of the AComA particularly in patients with aneurysms. While the most typical autopsy finding is a single artery about 2.6 mm in length and 1.5 mm in diameter with two small perforators emerging from the posterior aspect, this should not be counted upon with aneurysms. In 25% of cases, the AComA is larger than one of the proximal anterior cerebral (A1) segments connecting with it. Twinning or triplication of the AComA occurs in 10–15%. A network or partial duplication can occur in up to another 10% of cases. While small branches of the AComA average two in most anatomical series, the number is highly variable, as is their diameter, which is usually about ⅙ mm. Most of these small branches come directly from the AComA but they can arise at the junction with A1 or A2. The largest branch is often the subcallosal artery, which is present in more than 90% of patients and averages about ½ mm in size. It comes off the posterior dorsal surface of the AComA to run in front of the lamina terminalis, then turns rostrally and dorsally. It follows around the front of the corpus callosum, usually terminating in the genu. In about 10% of cases there is a larger branch of the

AComA which may equal the distal anterior cerebrals (A2s) in diameter, and which may travel between the right and left A2s or initially pass more posteriorly than A2, joining them at the rostrum of the corpus callosum, and going on to serve the medial hemisphere with the A2s. The technical importance of such occurrences, which should be sought on the preoperative angiograms, is that the clip may inadvertently occlude this vessel and the surgeon may feel a false sense of security by noting that two A2s are free from the clip. Also of vital importance in the surgery is the early identification of Heubner's artery. An attempt should be made to avoid occluding it in temporary clips or by the retractor blade. It may be multiple and adherent to the aneurysmal sac. Other variants of importance in AComA surgery include the possibility of a suboptic carotid–anterior cerebral artery, extreme hypoplasia of A1, fenestrations in A1, and accessory middle cerebral arteries originating from A1. The average diameter of the recurrent artery of Heubner is 1 mm. Three-quarters originate from the A2 segment and approximately one-tenth from either the exact level of the AComA or nearby A1. In almost all cases it arises within 4 cm of the AComA. In about one-sixth of cases it will be absent, and in one-tenth it will be duplicated. It is slightly more commonly situated anterior to A1 and superior to it. The recurrent artery of Heubner ends in the anterior perforated substances, the sylvian fissure, or the inferior frontal lobe, and it supplies the anterior caudate, anterior third of the putamen, anterolateral globus pallidus, and anterior limb of the internal capsule. Three-quarters of AComA aneurysms will have unequal A1 segments. About one-half of AComA aneurysms project superiorly and about one-quarter posteriorly or anteriorly, with inferior projections being relatively infrequent. AComA aneurysms are not often represented in multiple aneurysm cases. About one in 100 patients will have only a single A2 artery, the so-called azygous pericallosal artery. This single A2 is more frequently associated with aneurysms than any other anatomical anomaly. Such aneurysms are usually on the distal anterior cerebral artery.

I generally commence the operation by putting a tapered retractor down to the optic nerve and opening the arachnoid at that point. I then work laterally to open the carotid cistern and have the carotid exposed in case temporary clipping should be necessary very early in the operation. The tapered retractor is then directed more medially, following the line of the olfactory tract back to where A1 and Heubner's artery can be visualized just proximal to the aneurysm. They are cleared off so that a temporary clip can be applied on A1 for the final phases of dissection. I generally operate on the side of the largest A1 if there is a considerable degree of asymmetry. If there is not much difference, I will preferentially operate from the right side, being right-handed. It is important to be very careful during the initial phases of retraction with anterior–inferior directed aneurysms which may be adherent to the dura, since bleeding may occur as the frontal lobe is elevated.

An attempt should be made to spare the middle cerebral vein as it goes medially giving off the frontal orbital vein, the olfactory vein and the interior cerebral veins, which communicate with each other to provide a communicating vein in the approximate location of the AComA. After the olfactory vein is given off, typically the major portion of the vein goes posteriorly and medially to become the basal vein of Rosenthal. Sometimes it is necessary to coagulate these veins to gain exposure, but I try to avoid this if possible.

In acute cases with a great deal of clot, I will place a ventricular catheter early on. As much blood as possible is suctioned mechanically. In selected cases, after the aneurysm is clipped tissue plasminogen activator (t-PA) is instilled and left in situ for half an hour and then irrigated out. Further t-PA can be given postoperatively through the ventricular catheter, which is usually left in. A small incision is sometimes made in the lamina terminalis to permit further CSF removal and in the hope of reducing the chance of postoperative hydrocephalus.

One should be psychologically prepared for intraoperative aneurysmal rupture at any point in the surgery and clips should be instantly available. We have a cell saver attached to one of the suctions at the time of surgery, which is of help if there is massive rupture. Usual adjuncts to anesthesia, such as mannitol and frusemide,

are given to assist exposure. We avoid induced hypotension and, indeed, attempt to raise the blood pressure somewhat during the application of temporary clips.

Particularly in the presence of brain swelling it may be impossible to completely visualize the regional anatomy before, or indeed after, the application of a clip. Intraoperative angiography is extremely helpful in ensuring complete aneurysmal obliteration and the absence of inadvertent clipping of distal vessels. In the largest aneurysmal study reported to date about one patient in five had intraoperative rupture and one patient in 33 had inadvertent occlusion of a feeding or perforating artery demonstrated – the real incidence was doubtless higher than this since many patients can tolerate such an event without a major deficit. Premature rupture can be anticipated in at least 5% of cases, so that suitable temporary and permanent clips should be immediately available. In the event of premature rupture, it is better to use temporary clips and provisional permanent clip placement than to proceed to arterial hypotension induced by anesthesia. The latter should be a last-ditch defense in the case of torrential bleeding. If no clip or combination of clips will work, there is still some efficacy in proximal ligation of A1, but it is clearly less definitive than the clip, and it may not be as useful as intra-aneurysmal coiling. If an aneurysm ruptures at the time of clip application, the sucker tip should be brought right up to the bleeding point, the clips released and then reapplied more proximally and more deeply. If that fails to stop the bleeding additional suction may be necessary and redissection of the presumed neck performed prior to choosing a different clip.

I routinely place a ventricular drain through the frontal lobe in early aneurysm surgery. This reduces the amount of retractor pressure necessary to reach the AComA. In superiorly and posteriorly facing aneurysms it is more likely that a portion of the gyrus rectus will have to be resected. There are usually no gross psychological sequelae from this removal, but it has to be admitted that we have little data resulting from precise neuro-psychological testing.

I seldom use the interhemispheric or other transfrontal sinus approaches because of concerns regarding infection and rhinorrhea. I do recognize, however, the advantages under certain circumstances in gaining bilateral control both proximally and distally relatively easily. It is critical in these approaches, however, to avoid sacrifice of frontal veins.

The shape of these aneurysms is highly variable and they can be multilobulated, and the surgeon should be on the alert for two contiguous aneurysms masquerading as one. Important technical points in this type of surgery include checking that the correct patient and angiograms are in the theater, using rigid pin fixation of the head and proper protection of the eyes. An overhead support bar is important. I prefer to have the dura open before instituting CSF drainage via the ventricular catheter. Self-retaining retractors of just the right length and of tapered shape minimize the pressure on the brain. Generally, two or three are in place at the time of final dissection. Never move the microscope base with self-retaining retractors in place. AComA aneurysms account for about two-thirds of frontal intracerebral hematomas caused by aneurysms. Almost half of all intracerebral hematomas from aneurysms are caused by anterior cerebral artery aneurysms. The great majority of these are from the AComA location. About two-thirds of AComA aneurysms will be associated with intracerebral hematomas. If the initial CT scan demonstrates blood confined to the subarachnoid (mainly interhemispheric, chiasmatic and carotid cisterns), the outlook tends to be a bit better than if there is rupture into the frontal lobes, or worse still,

through the septum pellucidum into the ventricles. Small frontal hematomas can be left alone, whereas those larger ones associated with brain shift are probably best approached and evacuated. Anterior cerebral artery aneurysms (mainly AComA) are also the most common cause of intraventricular hemorrhage. Such intraventricular hematomas are found in about one-quarter of most clinical series of aneurysms and in about one-half of autopsy cases. Since the mortality rate from intraventricular hemorrhage associated with a ruptured AComA aneurysm approaches two-thirds without the use of any lytic agent, I use intraventricular instillation of t-PA to lead to early clot dissolution, to facilitate drainage of blood and to normalize CSF pressure.

Operative Approach for Anterior Communicating Artery Aneurysms
Nobuyuki Yasui

In this commentary, surgical strategy for AComA aneurysms and technical aspects of the interhemispheric approach performed by myself will be presented.

I routinely perform the interhemispheric approach for both ruptured and unruptured AComA aneurysms except in cases with multiple aneurysms; where there is a possibility to clip other aneurysms simultaneously a pterional approach may be preferred. But technically difficult AComA aneurysms such as large, giant or high-positioned aneurysms are operated on via the interhemispheric approach even in cases with multiple aneurysms.

The microsurgical interhemispheric approach for AComA aneurysms was first reported by Lougheed (1969), and was modified as the microsurgical anterior interhemispheric approach by Ito (1982). The difference in these two approaches is that interhemispheric dissection between bilateral cingulate gyri along the A2 portion of the anterior cerebral arteries is not necessary in the anterior interhemispheric approach. The most beneficial point of an anterior interhemispheric approach compared to Lougheed's approach is that it allows an AComA aneurysm to be visualized without exposure of cingulate gyri, with less brain retraction. However, even with this approach, the extent of brain retraction and dissection can become quite large when the aneurysm is located in a high and/or posterior position.

The other disadvantages of the anterior interhemispheric approach are a relative high incidence of olfactory dysfunction and the possibility of injury of the frontal bridging vein. For this reason the basal interhemispheric approach was developed and reported by Yasui in 1987 (Yasui et al 1986, Yasui et al 1987) to minimize operative invasion during surgery for AComA aneurysms. For the basal interhemispheric approach, subperiosteal skin flap dissection is extended to the nasion, the supraorbital foramina are exposed, and the supraorbital nerves are preserved. The craniotomy is then further extended into the anterior medial part of the

frontal base and the nasal bones using a bone saw. Laterally, the craniotomy extends just medial to the supraorbital foramen or notch and then runs down to the nasion.

The method of opening the dura differs between the two approaches. In the anterior interhemispheric approach, the dura is incised in the shape of letter W and the superior sagittal sinus is cut at its anterior end after ligation to open up the operative field while preserving the frontal bridging veins. In the basal interhemispheric approach, a small dural incision is made in the mid-basal portion of one side parallel to the superior sagittal sinus, providing an adequate operative field without sacrificing the frontal bridging veins. The extension of craniotomy to the mid-basal region allows one to approach an aneurysm 15–20 mm in length and about 20° lower than with the anterior interhemispheric approach.

The additional basal bone flap is fixed in the case of the basal interhemispheric approach, and then the defect of the opened frontal sinus is packed with bone dust mixed with antibiotic and covered with periosteum or galea stitched to the dura according to the method described by Pool (1972). In this way, no facial deformities are produced.

The beneficial points of the basal interhemispheric approach are that it requires less interhemispheric dissection and retraction, the operative field is shallower from the cortex to the AComA complex, the olfactory nerves are preserved and the subcallosal area can be more easily approached than by the anterior interhemispheric method. Also, the anterior bridging veins are avoided when a unilateral dural incision is made by the basal interhemispheric approach, because the frontal bridging veins are located more than 30 mm above the nasion in most cases and the length of the operative field required is only 16 mm. Preserving these veins is important because impairment of the frontal venous flow by cutting or damaging the anterior bridging veins will cause postoperative frontal lobe dysfunction.

Even if the aneurysm is large, it is not necessary to perform extensive brain retraction. Removal of clots from the subarachnoid space can be easily achieved in the interhemispheric, chiasmatic and pontine cisterns via the subchiasmatic route.

Although there are disadvantages such as the need for an additional craniotomy and opening of the frontal sinus, no infections or other complications due to this have been experienced so far. Moreover, no facial deformities have been produced in our patients by these additional procedures (Yasui et al 1992).

Some consider that using an interhemispheric approach can cause bilateral interhemispheric damage, resulting in Korsakoff's syndrome. With the recent development of microsurgical techniques and instrumentation, however, this approach is safe. It should be stressed that Korsakoff's syndrome should not result following an interhemispheric dissection if standard microsurgical techniques are employed.

References

Ito Z 1982 The microsurgical anterior interhemispheric approach suitably applied to ruptured aneurysms of the anterior communicating artery in the acute stage. Acta Neurochirurgica 63: 85–99

Lougheed W 1969 Selection, timing and technique of aneurysm surgery of the anterior circle of Willis. Clinical Neurosurgery 16: 95–113

Pool J L 1972 Bifrontal craniotomy for anterior communicating artery aneurysms. British Journal of Neurosurgery 36: 212–220

Yasui N, Suzuki A, Ohta H et al 1986 Microneurosurgical anterior and basal interhemispheric approaches for lesions in and around the anterior third ventricles. In: Samii M (ed): Surgery around the brain stem and the third ventricle. Springer Verlag, Berlin, pp 339–345

Yasui N, Suzuki A, Sayama I et al 1987 A new operative approach for anterior communicating aneurysm: basal interhemispheric approach. Neurologia Medicochirurgia (Tokyo) 27: 756–761

Yasui N, Nathal E, Fugiwara H et al 1992 The basal interhemispheric approach for acute anterior communicating aneurysms. Acta Neurochirurgia (Wien) 118: 91–97

Basilar bifurcation aneurysms

Shigeaki Kobayashi   Kazuhiro Hongo
Yuichiro Tanaka   Atul Goel

5

Basilar bifurcation aneurysms and basilar–superior cerebellar artery aneurysms (BA–SCA) are considered to be technically among the most difficult aneurysms to occlude. The initial attempt at directly approaching and occluding these aneurysms were made by Drake (1961) and Jamieson (1964) in the early 1960s. Their early mortality for basilar aneurysms was 55%. They both essentially used a subtemporal approach and mild hypothermia and temporary circulatory occlusion techniques. Drake employed circulatory arrest. Jamieson used temporary clipping of the basilar artery in the operative field. With the introduction of the operating microscope surgical techniques and results have improved remarkably in subsequent years. Many papers have been published, including the pioneering ones by Drake (1978, 1979), Yasargil et al (1976) and Sugita et al (1979), suggesting surgical approaches and clipping techniques for these aneurysms. Experience in dealing with the simpler variety of aneurysms, detailed anatomical information and familiarity with the instrumentation are essential before one ventures into treating this complex problem. Recent advances in skull base surgery complement the conventional procedures in various situations. The reasons for the difficulty in the surgical treatment are that the lesion is located at a depth, only a narrow operative corridor is available, and there are various critical neural and vascular structures in the area.

There are three principal surgical routes for basilar bifurcation aneurysms: the pterional approach, the subtemporal approach, and the temporopolar approach (Fig 5.1). Yasargil and Sugita primarily used the pterional approach, whereas Drake advocated and successfully used the subtemporal approach. Sano (1980) proposed the temporopolar approach. Each approach has its advantages and disadvantages. One should be familiar with the characteristics of each approach in order to select the appropriate route to individual aneurysms.

In our 112 cases of basilar bifurcation and BA–SCA aneurysms (1978–1995) pterional and subtemporal approaches were generally used (subtemporal approach in nine cases and pterional approach in 96 cases). In 11 cases the temporopolar approach was used. A combined pterional and subtemporal approach was used in three cases.

PTERIONAL APPROACH

The pterional route to the basilar bifurcation was first described by Yasargil et al in 1976. He advocated the advantages of this approach over the subtemporal approach as follows:

1. minimal retraction of the temporal lobe;
2. better appreciation of the anatomy of the interpeduncular cistern;
3. less damage to the oculomotor and trochlear nerves;
4. treatment of other aneurysms in the anterior circulation.

Yamaura et al (1982) added further points to these advantages:

1. easy exposure of the proximal basilar trunk, wider area for clot removal;
2. safer access to the laterally projecting aneurysms.

In this approach, unlike the subtemporal approach, the basilar artery apex and its major branches appear relative-

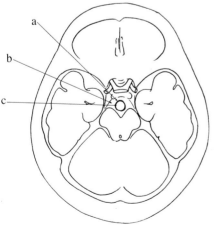

Fig. 5.1 Directions of approach to the basilar apex aneurysm. Directions of pterional (**a**), temporopolar (**b**) and subtemporal (**c**) approaches.

ly symmetrical, which makes it easier to dissect the neck away from these branches. The familiarity of this approach is an important consideration as it is used in most other aneurysms.

Dissection of the sylvian fissure

The sylvian fissure is widely opened to make space for clipping the basilar aneurysm without an excessive retraction of the frontal and temporal lobes. The sylvian fissure is usually dissected from the frontal side. A small vein occasionally found connecting the frontal and temporal lobe in the proximal sylvian fissure can be coagulated and divided. The anterior temporal artery sometimes lies in the way when it arises from the proximal M1 segment. When it is small, it can be sectioned with impunity. However, an attempt should be made to dissect a long length of the artery and to section only its distal segment.

One of the disadvantages of the pterional approach is that the route is obstructed by the internal carotid artery and the posterior communicating artery. In high-positioned aneurysms, the internal carotid or the middle cerebral artery may be retracted. Retraction of these arteries should be limited for a period of 5–10 minutes. In most cases

retraction can be done without completely occluding the artery, and with pressure which results only in mild stenosis of the artery. When retracting the internal carotid or middle cerebral artery it is recommended to use a split silastic tube to protect against mechanical injury and to keep the artery moist during the subsequent procedures (Tanaka et al 1993).

To access the basilar apex via the pterional route, the following major spaces (Fig. 5.2) should be considered (Gibo et al 1991):

1. the opticocarotid space between the optic nerve and the internal carotid artery;
2. the medial retrocarotid space between the internal carotid artery and the posterior communicating artery;
3. the lateral retrocarotid space between the posterior communicating artery and the oculomotor nerve;
4. when the intradural segment of the internal carotid artery is short, the suprabifurcation space is exceptionally used (Kobayashi et al 1983).

Opticocarotid route

The opticocarotid space is surrounded by the optic nerve,

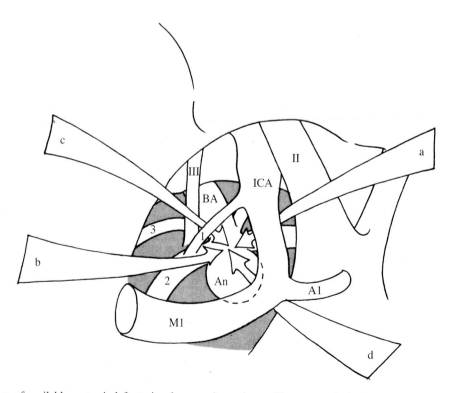

Fig. 5.2 Options of available routes in left pterional approach are shown. The arrows depict the opticocarotid (**a**), medial retrocarotid (**b**), lateral retrocarotid (**c**) and suprabifurcation (**d**) routes. (1, posterior communicating artery; 2, posterior cerebral artery; 3, superior cerebellar artery; An, aneurysm.)

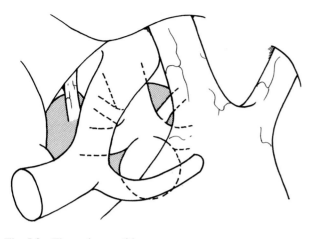

Fig. 5.3 The opticocarotid space.

the internal carotid artery, and the anterior cerebral artery (Fig. 5.3). This approach route was seen to provide a more anteriorly directed access to the aneurysms on the axial plane than the opticocarotid approach. The range of height of the aneurysm neck that can be dealt with by this approach is narrower than in the retrocarotid approach. The anterior cerebral artery forms the upper limit of the

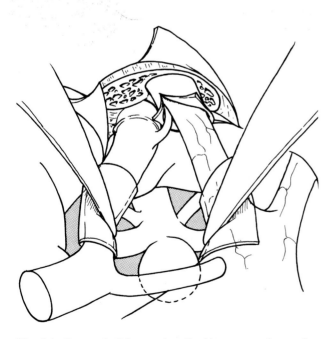

Fig. 5.4 Removal of the anterior clinoid process and retraction of the optic nerve and the carotid artery have increased the exposure of the bifurcation aneurysm.

opticocarotid space. A redundant A1 provides a wider space. It is essential to dissect the entire path of the A1 artery from the arachnoid when it is not redundant. Sectioning the artery is one of the possible options available for the surgeon when it is hypoplastic. The lower limit is the posterior clinoid process, which can be drilled to obtain an additional basal exposure. However, the space available from the opticocarotid approach is usually not wide enough to use power instruments.

The procedure to unroof the optic canal is often necessary in this approach. A simple incision of the dural fold over the optic nerve provides enough space in some cases. A silicone rubber sheet (Shibuya et al 1991) or split silicone tube (Tanaka et al 1993) is useful to protect the nerve and artery to avoid inadvertent injury or to minimize the damage when they are retracted. The tube on the carotid artery keeps its surface moist by capillary action, and is also useful to prevent an undesirable mechanical spasm. Removal of the anterior clinoid process to mobilize the internal carotid artery is another method to increase the opticocarotid space (Fig. 5.4).

Yasargil et al (1976) reported that dissection may be performed between the optic nerve and the carotid artery when a 5–10 mm space exists between them. Nagasawa et al (1987) reported that two angiographic parameters – distance of the terminal of the internal carotid artery from the midline on anteroposterior view and height of the terminal from the biclinoid line on the lateral view – are important landmarks which determine the choice of approach.

Medial retrocarotid route

Sugita et al (1979) recommended this approach (Fig. 5.5) in cases where:

1. the bifurcation is located high;
2. the P1 segment is very short;
3. the posterior communicating artery is very rigid and runs markedly concave to lateral.

Neck clipping is performed through the narrow space between the perforators from the posterior communicating artery. Therefore, a relatively longer clip blade is required because the head of the clip applicator often interferes with the surgeon's field of vision (Fig. 5.6). Although we can often create a surprising amount of room in the medial retrocarotid space between the perforators by careful dissection, attention should be paid not to cause their accidental damage and mechanical vasospasm. The posterior communicating artery was sectioned in seven cases in this series when it was hypoplastic. The artery should be sectioned finally after every effort to avoid sacrificing it, because there are no means to predict the neurological sequelae after the procedure (Regli & Tribolet 1991).

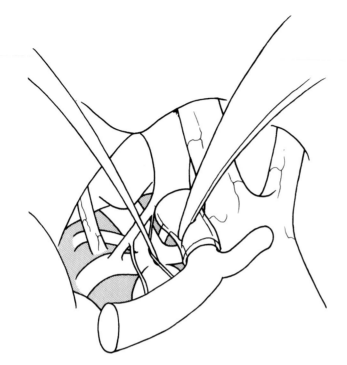

Fig. 5.5 The medial retrocarotid space. Retractors on the carotid artery and perforators are expanding the space.

Lateral retrocarotid route

This approach (Fig. 5.7) was most commonly adopted in our patients because of the wide range in the direction of the clip application and also in the height of basilar bifurcation (Figs. 5.8, 5.9). Resection of the posterior clinoid was required to expose the basilar trunk for a possible temporary clipping in the case with a low basilar bifurcation, usually less than 0 mm from the line between the anterior and posterior clinoids (Fig. 5.7b). However, this procedure was required for the aneurysm with a neck higher than 0 mm when the aneurysm was very close to the posterior clinoid. The upper limit in the height of the aneurysm in the pterional approach is considered to be 15 mm (from anterior to posterior clinoid line) in our experience, although zygomatic osteotomy and its modifications may assist surgical access to a high-positioned aneurysm (Fujitsu & Kuwabara 1985, Ikeda et al 1991, Neil-Dwyer et al 1988, Pitelli et al 1986, Shiokawa et al 1989). An alternative technique could be helpful for a high-positioned aneurysm (higher than 15 mm on the anterior–posterior clinoid line). Such alternative approaches include a trans-third ventricular approach (Kodama et al 1986) and a transcallosal approach (Abe et al 1993). Endovascular surgical treatment may also be considered in such cases.

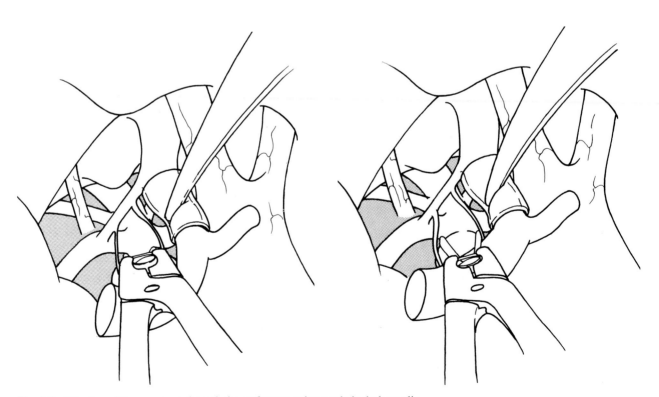

Fig. 5.6 Clipping of the aneurysm through the perforators using a relatively long clip.

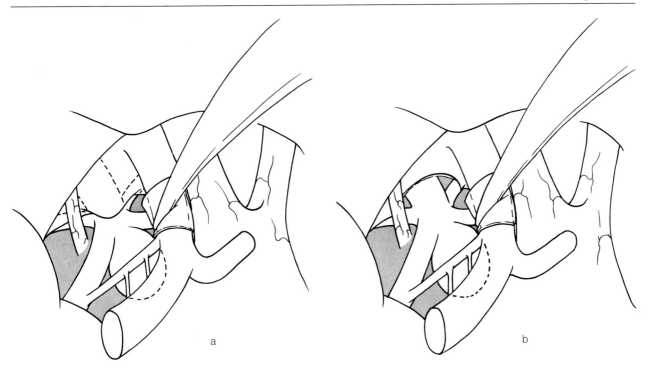

Fig. 5.7 **a** The lateral retrocarotid approach. **b** The posterior clinoid process is removed to expose the basilar trunk.

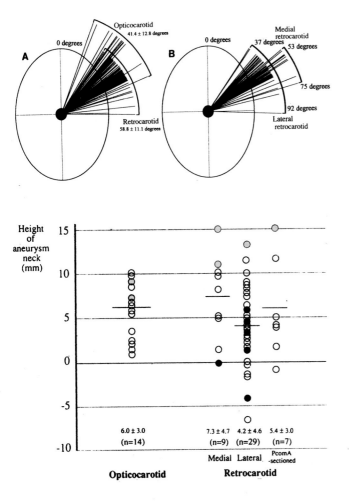

Fig. 5.8 **A** Direction of a clip application in the pterional approach (left) and in the retrocarotid approach (right), demonstrating that the distribution of the access line in the opticocarotid approach (4.14° ± 12.8°; *n*=14) is more anterior to that in the retrocarotid approach (58.8° ± 11.1°; *n*=45) with a significant difference (*p*=0.01). **B** Direction of clip application in the medial and lateral retrocarotid approach, showing that the distribution of the access line in the medial retrocarotid approach (60.4° ± 7.6°; 53–75°; *n*=9) is restricted more than that in the lateral retrocarotid approach (57.5° ± 11.9°; 37–92°; *n*=29). All of the approach routes are represented as if performed from the right side. (From Tanaka et al, with permission.)

Fig. 5.9 Relationship between the height of the aneurysm neck from the line between the anterior and posterior clinoid process on the lateral angiogram in the opticocarotid (*n*=14) and retrocarotid (*n*=45) approach routes. The dotted circle indicates a case in which zygomatic osteotomy was performed (*n*=6). The closed circle indicates a case in which the posterior clinoid was resected (*n*=7). The numbers indicate mean ± standard deviation of the height of the aneurysm neck in each group. (From Tanaka et al 1995, with permission.)

The temporopolar approach gives an additional wide space to the lateral retrocarotid approach. We section the bridging temporal polar vein especially for large aneurysms because it often disturbs the view behind the aneurysm body. On the other hand, the temporopolar approach contributes little to the high-positioned aneurysms. This procedure is not always required because an equally wide surgical area could be obtained in some cases without sacrificing the vein.

The suprabifurcation route (Fig. 5.10) (Kobayashi et al 1983) can be used when the retrocarotid and opticocarotid approaches are difficult for the following reasons:

1. the internal carotid artery is too sclerotic to mobilize;
2. the artery is unusually short; or
3. the space between the optic nerve and the internal carotid artery is narrow.

We used the suprabifurcation approach in three of the 26 BA–SCA aneurysms and one case of basilar bifurcation artery aneurysm. Care should be taken not to injure the lenticulostriate arteries and optic tract, which often obstruct the approach route in the suprabifurcation space.

SUBTEMPORAL APPROACH

The subtemporal approach is a commonly used approach and is used for low-positioned aneurysms in which the tentorium can be cut to secure the proximal basilar artery (Fig. 5.11). However, it is difficult to see the origin of the contralateral P1, especially when the aneurysm is large. The oculomotor nerve is directly in the way throughout the procedure.

The extent of temporal lobe retraction necessary for various approaches for the basilar tip is shown in Fig. 5.12. It

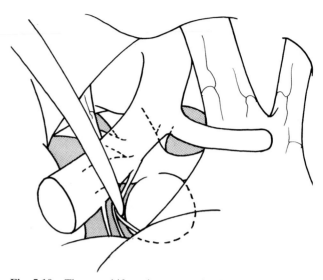

Fig. 5.10   The suprabifurcation approach. The approach is suitable in cases where the length of the supraclinoid carotid artery is short.

was observed that the maximum retraction of the temporal lobe was required for the subtemporal approach. Zygomatic osteotomy and partial removal of the middle fossa floor can be done to obtain a basal exposure. Such a basal extension of the subtemporal exposure is useful for high-positioned aneurysms. Sometimes it may be useful to resect the bone in Kawase's triangle to expose the basilar trunk for proximal control or for some low-positioned aneurysms.

Multidirectional approach

Batjer & Samson (1993) reported the use of the optico-

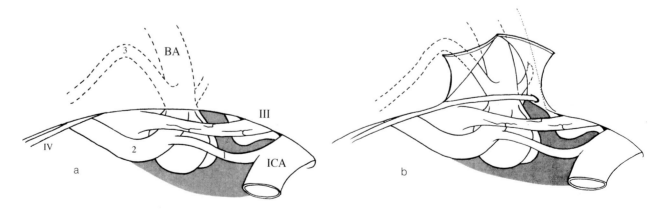

Fig. 5.11   a The subtemporal approach to the basilar top. **b** The tentorium is sectioned to widen the subtemporal exposure and to expose the basilar trunk for proximal control. (1, posterior communicating artery; 2, posterior cerebral artery; 3, superior cerebellar artery; III, oculomotor nerve; IV, trochlear nerve; ICA, internal carotid artery; BA, basilar artery.)

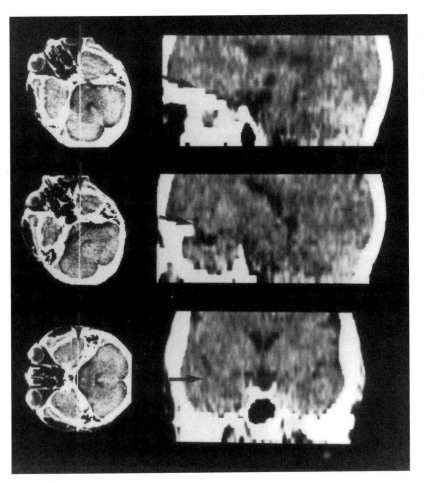

Fig. 5.12 The volume of the temporal lobe retraction required for different approaches. Upper, pterional approach; middle, temporopolar approach; lower, subtemporal approach. Note that the subtemporal approach requires the maximum retraction. (From Kobayashi & Tanaka 1994 with permission.)

carotid space for visual access, the retrocarotid space for the application of the clip, and vice versa. The optico-carotid space is useful in dissection of the opposite side of the aneurysm and is also effective in confirming the tip of the blade after clipping through the retrocarotid space (Fig. 5.13). In the pterional approach it is important to make use of all of the available spaces before and after clipping (Tanaka et al 1995).

On reviewing the directions of the clips used for basilar bifurcation aneurysms on postoperative computed tomographic (CT) scan, it was seen that the clips were applied in each approach in only a limited angle (Fig. 5.14). To make possible a wide range of clip application angles it was observed that the horizontal opening along the skull base needs to be wide. In the pterional route a rather vertical exposure is obtained, whereas in the subtemporal approach a horizontally wide opening is obtained (Fig. 5.15). With the pterional approach, the contralateral P1 is easier to expose, whereas there may be difficulty in proximal control of the parent artery. With the subtemporal approach, proximal control of the basilar trunk was easier and a better view of the posteriorly coursing perforating arteries was obtained. Currently, we prefer to perform 'a

combined exposure' or a 'multidirectional approach' to the complex basilar apex aneurysm. This procedure was previously mentioned by Drake (1978). The pterional and

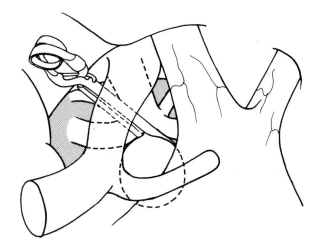

Fig. 5.13 The multidirectional approach. Clipping is performed through the retrocarotid approach and its adequacy is being observed through the opticocarotid approach.

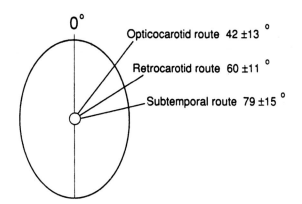

Fig. 5.14   Direction of the clips placed for basilar bifurcation aneurysms according to different approaching routes (68 case studies). The direction is expressed by degrees from the midline on the postoperative CT scan. (From Kobayashi & Tanaka 1994, with permission.)

subtemporal approaches were combined in one setting to increase accessibility to the basilar apex without sacrificing the bridging vein. The posterior edge of the regular frontotemporal craniotomy for pterional approach is extended 2–3 cm behind, and the Sugita head frame was convenient in rotating the head intraoperatively, depending on the direction of the selected approach (Sugita et al 1978). In the combined exposure it is usually effective to apply the clip from the pterional route and to confirm the preservation of perforators behind the aneurysm through the subtemporal route.

TEMPOROPOLAR APPROACH

We consider temporopolar approach a modification of pterional approach. It provides a horizontally wider space than usual pterional approach with the temporal lobe retracted posteriorly. Because the bridging veins need to be sacrificed, this approach is not applicable when the veins are prominent.

FACTORS TO BE CONSIDERED FOR SELECTING APPROACH

Height of the aneurysm neck

For a high-positioned aneurysm it was seen that the addition of zygomatic or orbitozygomatic osteotomy to the usual pterional approach provided an adequate basal approach necessary for these cases to avoid excessive frontal or temporal lobe retraction. Such an approach is recommended especially when the neck is located more than 10 mm above the level of the posterior clinoid process as seen on the lateral angiogram. In high-positioned aneurysms, a suprabifurcation approach or retrocarotid approach with the middle cerebral artery retraction after a pterional exposure may be useful; the optic tract and ipsilateral mamillary body can be retracted as necessary. In our opinion the use of a pterional approach is more appropriate for a high-location aneurysm. For low-positioned aneurysms, the subtemporal approach would be the first choice but for unusual aneurysms the pterional approach with utilization of additional skull base techniques may be useful.

Position of the aneurysm neck

The size of the neck, its deviation from the midline, and its relation to the parent artery are important variables affecting the planning of the surgery and its ultimate outcome. We prefer approaching the aneurysm from the side of its deviation, as in our experience even a few millimeters deviation provides a critical extra space necessary for clipping a deep-seated aneurysm. Handedness of the surgeon was a less significant consideration while selecting the side of the approach.

Projection of the aneurysm dome

It is important to ascertain the direction of the projection of

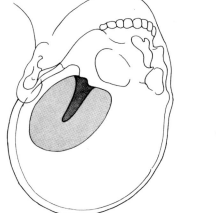

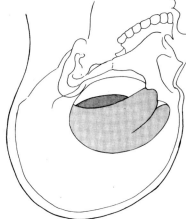

Fig. 5.15   Surgical fields obtained by pterional and subtemporal approaches. Note that the former gives a vertical opening, whereas the latter gives a horizontal opening.

the dome of the aneurysm. When the dome was projecting anteriorly, a subtemporal approach was found to be easier and it simulated to some extent the situation when an anteriorly projecting anterior communicating artery aneurysm is approached pterionally. For a posteriorly projecting aneurysm, the pterional approach is sometimes difficult, especially when the aneurysm is larger than 10 mm, as an adequate view of the perforators behind the aneurysm neck is not available by this route. In such a situation, a subtemporal approach appears to be better. The majority of regular aneurysms can be approached pterionally. However, in an unusual aneurysm, a multidirectional approach should be considered.

Size of the aneurysm

The importance of the size of the aneurysm in influencing the surgical result has been described earlier. The main problem arises as regards the relationship and distortion of the local anatomy, particularly the perforating arteries. According to our experience, aneurysms larger than 10 mm in diameter are technically more difficult to operate.

SELECTION OF THE SIDE OF APPROACH

The surgeon usually has to select one of the three approaches mentioned above. These approaches are the pterional, subtemporal, or multidirectional (combined) approach. Each of these approaches can be extended basally using a skull base technique as discussed in other chapters. The appropriate side of surgical approach also needs to be selected after a careful analysis of the angiographic study.

In choosing the side of the approach, we do not consider it important to avoid approaching from the dominant side. Although the aneurysm appears in general more or less symmetrical in the pterional approach, the local anatomy of the aneurysm in relation to the terminal branches of the basilar are subtly different in different cases, so that the easier side should be chosen with the presumed microscopic view in mind. Computer simulation can be helpful. The distance to the aneurysm in the surgical field is another important factor. By looking at the anteroposterior view of the angiogram, deviation of the aneurysm neck from the midline is determined. If it is more than a few millimeters off from the midline usually the approach is made from that side.

DISSECTION OF THE ANEURYSM

When dissecting the aneurysm, it is important to dissect on both sides of the neck, taking care not to tamper with other portions of the aneurysm complex. It may not be advisable to stick to the idea of dissecting one side completely before dissecting on the other side. It is safer to advance the dissection on both sides more or less simultaneously. The easier side may be dissected first for safety reasons. One should always be prepared for a premature rupture and in this regard exposure necessary for proximal control of the basilar artery should be made before starting the dissection of the aneurysm complex.

Identifying perforating arteries is very important (Marinkovic & Gibo 1993). This should always be done before clip application. Our cadaveric study (H. Gibo, unpublished data) indicated that the majority of the perfo-

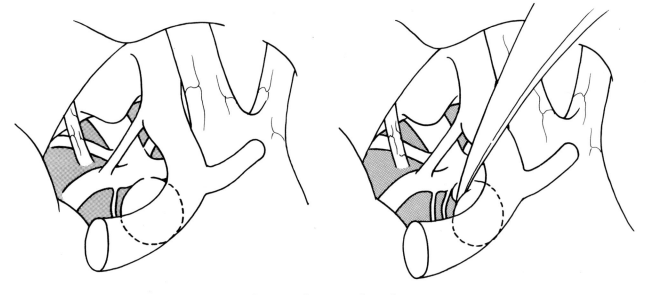

Fig. 5.16 The aneurysm or the parent artery may be retracted to expose the perforators.

rating arteries originate in the dorsal (posterior) aspect of the proximal P1. For identifying perforators, one can use direct retraction of the aneurysm or parent artery (Sugita et al 1980) (Fig. 5.16). To perform direct retraction with safety and precision, a refined retractor system such as that developed by Sugita et al (1978) is helpful. This could be done safely if a temporary clip is used for the basilar artery. Before applying direct retraction of the aneurysm, one should closely observe the face of the aneurysm to see which portion is weak and which is strong enough to permit retraction. Direct retraction of the perforators from the posterior communicating artery is often helpful in dissection of the parent artery and body of the aneurysm. These perforators are better retracted in a bundle.

CLIPPING TECHNIQUES

Temporary clipping

Temporary clipping of the parent artery can be used whenever necessary at the time of clipping as well as to facilitate dissection around the aneurysm complex. The temporary clipping time should be kept as short as possible even though we have occluded the basilar artery on two occasions for more than 15 minutes without any untoward effects. We usually perform and recommend staged clipping whenever possible, releasing the clip every 5 minutes even in situations in which rupture of the aneurysm has occurred. Whenever possible, we wait for 5 minutes for the next temporary clipping (Yokoh et al 1983). Temporary clipping should be as distal as safely possible so as to maintain blood flow through the perforating arteries. If possible temporary clipping may be done between the origins of the posterior cerebral and superior cerebellar arteries, or just proximal to the latter. One should be careful when applying a temporary clip to the parent artery which is highly sclerotic, for the fear of embolism and occasional inability to obliterate the blood flow completely.

Temporary occlusion of the basilar artery by means of intravascular technique has been shown to be useful on some of such occasions (Shucart et al 1990). Remote-controlled instruments attached to a self-retaining retractor system can be used for temporary clipping (Kyoshima et al 1993). We have found this to be safer and less troublesome. Trapping of the aneurysm by proximal and distal clipping as recommended by some was not found to be necessary in our series. This procedure could be of use when dealing with a giant aneurysm.

Tentative clipping

Tentative clipping (Fig. 5.17) is a technique of preliminary

clipping of aneurysms before completing the dissection for final clipping. Final clipping can be done either by placing another clip parallel to the tentative clip which is later removed, or one can remove the tentative clip before the dissection is completed and the final clip is placed (Fig. 5.17e). One could also place a tentative clip so as to include one of the parent branch arteries. This appears to be better than putting a temporary clip to the parent basilar artery.

Aneurysm-shifting technique

Aneurysm-shifting technique (Fig. 18) can be applied in many unruptured aneurysms, or aneurysms without adhesion to the surrounding brain tissue. By pressing with the tip of a 2 mm spatula on the parent artery, the aneurysm can be shifted to some extent for easier application of the clip. On some occasions it is even possible to retract a branching artery to suitably shift the aneurysm.

Blade dissection technique

Blade dissection (Fig. 5.19) around the neck of the aneurysm can be performed during the final stages of dissection. This method is particularly useful when further conventional dissection is considered to be risky with a possibility of premature rupture. The clip can be used for dissection by gentle opening and partial closing of the blades. During this process the clip is advanced further ahead in preparation for eventual clipping. In the event of premature rupture the blades are just closed to control bleeding.

Multiple clipping versus shank clipping

In the shank clipping method the curved portion of a bayonet clip is used to clip an irregular neck of the aneurysm (Osawa et al 1995) (Fig. 5.20). This method is most useful in cases of middle cerebral artery aneurysms. For the basilar bifurcation aneurysm, however, placing a bayonet is often difficult as the shank portion blocks the surgical view in the deep and narrow field. Multiple clipping is frequently used. Multiple clips are placed in different angles so that the clip heads do not block the view during clip placement. The use of either multiple clipping technique or shank clipping may be chosen after observing the local anatomy.

Booster clippping

In some thick-walled aneurysms, booster clipping using

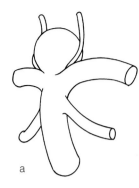

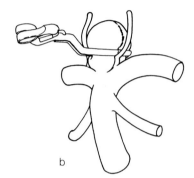

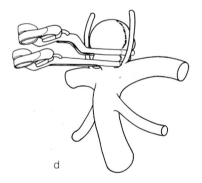

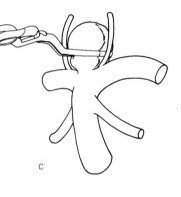

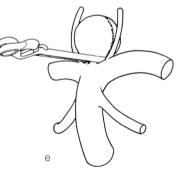

a

b

c

d

e

Fig. 5.17 Schematic drawings of the tentative clipping method in sequence. **a** The aneurysm is adherent to a perforator. **b** Tentative clipping on the dome. **c** The neck is dissected. **d** Placing the final clip. **e** The tentative clip has been removed.

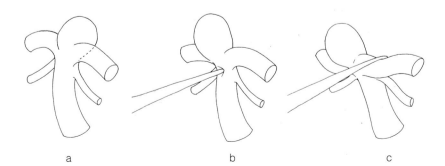

a

b

c

Fig. 5.18 Aneurysm-shifting method. **a** Inadequate visualization of the posteriorly projecting aneurysm neck. **b** Pressing the basilar trunk to shift the location of the aneurysm neck into view. **c** Retraction of the branches to get a better view of the neck.

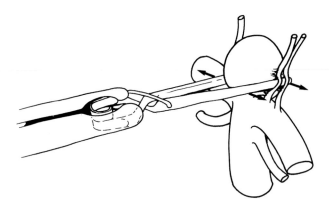

Fig. 5.19 Blade dissection technique. The clip is advanced by opening and partially closing the blades at the final stage of dissection.

more than one clip (booster clip or regular clip) was neccesary to reinforce the closing pressure (Sundt et al 1984). One should be aware of the possibility of incomplete closure of the clip blades when the clip holds additional arterial branches or perforators.

Special clips

Special clips may sometimes be necessary. A miniclip is used for small aneurysms or in the presence of multiple aneurysms in which the presence of a large clip may interfere with clipping of other aneurysms. A long clip is more frequently used in our series. The fenestration in the Drake–Sugita type of clip (Drake 1979, Sugita et al 1979) can be useful when the clip is placed during a subtemporal approach. Here the fenestration or the ring would encircle the P1, with the blades occluding the aneurysm. In our series we rarely used this variety of clip. It was felt that the alignment of P1, perforators, and the neck of the aneurysm would make the application and maneuvering of such a

clip difficult. Ring clips were successfully used by us to reinforce the closing pressure in the far side of the neck when the near side was thickened with atheroma (Fig. 5.21).

PERFORATING ARTERIES

Surgical results are intimately related to preservation of the perforators. Microneurosurgical techniques make preservation of the perforators relatively easy. Exact information of the perforators in this region is important. Preservation of the perforators is especially difficult in large or giant aneurysms. A careful observation of the preoperative angiography in various views is essential to ascertain the location, number, and course of the perforators. Before clipping, one should dissect the perforating arteries as much as possible. However, in the event of rupture, one should not stubbornly pursue this procedure. In such a situation one can check the perforators after clipping is completed or a tentative clip is placed. This may sometimes be technically difficult as the field is blocked by the head of the clip. Silastic sheet can be used to protect the perforators and avoid their inclusion in the clip (Fig. 5.22). One should observe the possible inclusion of the perforators when closing the clip as the shrinking aneurysm allows the surgeon to observe the space. When there are many perforators and one of them is originating close to the neck, one may sacrifice such a small perforator. This could be better than causing rupture of the aneurysm or damaging other perforating arteries as well. This inclusion may result in a small infarct in the thalamus. But it is usually small and unilateral, and not likely to cause a significant deficit. In our series we did not puncture or open the aneurysm after it was considered that the clipping procedure had been successfully performed. After the final clipping of the aneurysm we routinely use a micro-Doppler flowmeter to confirm the flow in the major vessels. On some occasions we have been able to observe the blood flow in larger perforators.

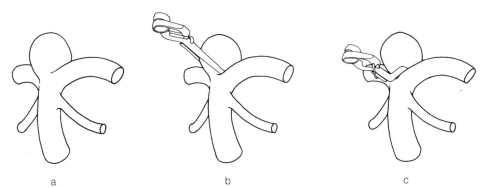

a   b   c

Fig. 5.20 Shank clipping. **a** An aneurysm before clipping. **b** Clipping using a straight clip causes incomplete occlusion of the aneurysm. **c** Shank portion of a bayonet clip is utilized to occlude a wide-based neck completely.

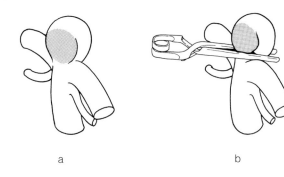

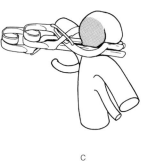

a   b   c

Fig. 5.21 Use of a ring clip to reinforce closing pressure in the far side of the neck when the near side of the neck is thickened with atheroma (shadow).

SKULL BASE TECHNIQUES

To enhance the basal exposure and to obtain additional space to manipulate instruments, we have recently used some skull basal techniques which include zygomatic osteotomy, optic unroofing, anterior clinoid removal, posterior clinoid process removal, transcavernous approach and extended pterional approach (Fig. 5.23). In order to obtain an extended view in the superior direction, zygomatic osteotomy or orbitozygomatic osteotomy may be useful. For medial extension of the field, optic nerve unroofing, for inferior extension posterior clinoid removal and a transcavernous approach, and for lateral extension we have used an extended pterional approach. With zygomatic osteotomy, a high-positioned or large aneurysm can be approached. We observed that even the mamillary bodies could be directly seen after zygomatic osteotomy was performed. With optic unroofing the optic nerve can be retracted medially and after the internal carotid artery is retracted laterally the approach through the opticocarotid space becomes wider. However, retraction of the carotid artery is safer than retraction of the optic nerve. Removal of the posterior clinoid process facilitates the approach to a low-positioned aneurysm, giving space for securing the proximal parent artery and clipping the aneurysm. The transcavernous approach, by removing the anterior and posterior clinoid processes and unroofing the optic canal, enables mobilization of the internal carotid artery, gives a wider space and facilitates an approach to a low-positioned or complex aneurysm via a pterional route.

Extended pterional approach

This requires special remarks as we have found it to be very useful not only for basilar bifurcation aneurysms but also for the juxtadural ring internal carotid artery aneurysms. This approach is essentially a pterional approach, but by adding skull base techniques one can extend the surgical view laterally as needed without sacrificing the bridging vein. After frontotemporal craniotomy,

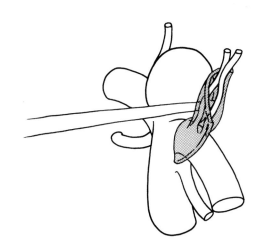

Fig. 5.22 The silastic sheaths (shadow) are protecting the artery while dissection is being carried out.

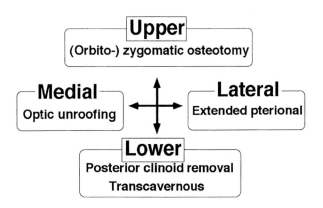

Fig. 5.23 Schematic drawing showing expansion of the pterional exposure in various directions utilizing skull base techniques.

the dura over the sphenoid ridge is cut open to remove the bone, exposing the superior orbital fissure and removing the anterior clinoid process. The dura over the superior orbital fissure is split to expose the anterior cavernous sinus. Thus the bridging vein is preserved (Fig. 5.24). Depending upon the variation in local anatomy with regard

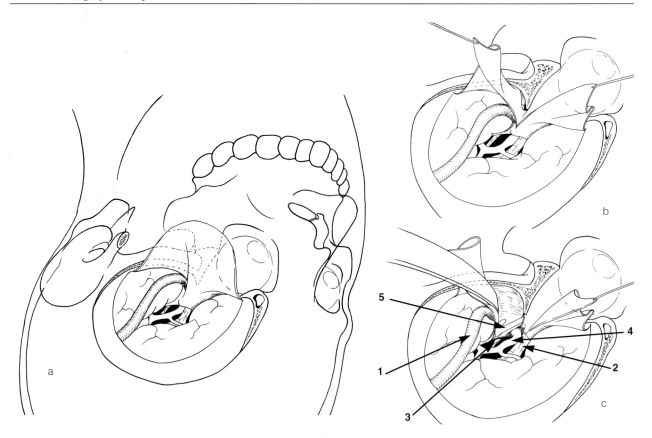

Fig. 5.24 Left extended pterional approach with dural splitting in order to preserve the bridging vein. **a** Dural opening after frontotemporal craniotomy with orbitozygomatic osteotomy. **b** The dura is cut along the sphenoidal ridge to the anterior clinoid process. **c** The dura is split and dissected from the trigeminal nerves; the temporal tip is retracted posteriorly with the bridging vein preserved. (1. sylvian vein; 2. optic nerve; 3. oculomotor nerve; 4. ICA; 5. trigeminal nerve VI)

to the bridging vein and sphenoparietal sinus, the degree of lateral extension can be altered. If one additionally utilizes zygomatic osteotomy, one can get superior extension of the field for a high-positioned or a large aneurysm.

COMPUTER-ASSISTED GEOMETRIC DESIGN OF CEREBRAL ANEURYSMS

As discussed in our other chapter computer-assisted geometric design of basilar aneurysms can be of great help in planning and executing surgery.

CASE 1   Anterior Projecting Basilar Bifurcation Aneurysm

This 70-year-old woman had been operated upon 6 months earlier for a left internal carotid–posterior communicating artery aneurysm on the third day of SAH while she was in Grade 2. An unruptured basilar bifurcation aneurysm was also detected

during investigations but was not treated at this time. Postoperative recovery was good and except for slight dementia she recovered completely. A ventriculoperitoneal shunt was done for normal-pressure hydrocephalus 4 months ago. A second-stage operation was then performed for basilar top aneurysm. The aneurysm was round in shape, pointed anteriorly and was about 2 mm to the left of the midline. The height of the aneurysm was about 8 mm from the dorsum sellae (Fig. 5.25).

With the patient in the supine position, a right frontotemporal craniotomy was performed (Fig. 5.26a). The lateral orbital rim was removed in order to obtain a wider space for approach. The sylvian fissure was opened. This procedure was difficult as there were extensive adhesions. The basilar trunk was exposed via the retrocarotid space. The dissection around the aneurysm was difficult as a sequela of the previous SAH. The SCA on both sides and the left oculomotor nerve were exposed. The left oculomotor nerve was used as a landmark to expose the aneurysm complex. The sylvian fissure was further dissected by mobilizing the anterior temporal artery in order to facilitate the retraction of the middle cerebral artery medially for exposing the P1 at depth. The right P1 was found coursing parallel to the SCA with somewhat dense adhesions between them. The right posterior communicating artery was then exposed. It was found

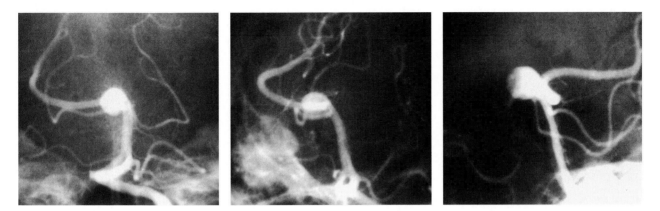

Fig. 5.25 Angiograms of basilar top aneurysm, which was round, pointed anteriorly, 2 mm to the left of the midline and 8 mm from the dorsum sellae.

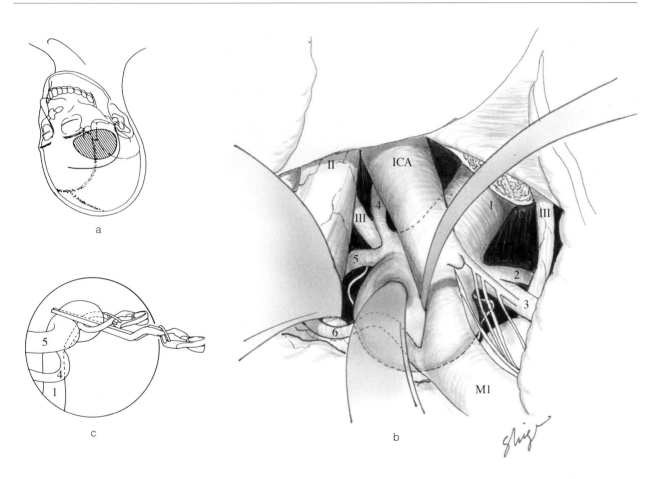

Fig. 5.26 **a** Right frontotemporal craniotomy. **b** The left P1 was exposed through the opticocarotid space. **c** No. 35 oblique angle ring clip in place. (1, basilar artery; 2, right SCA; 3, right posterior cerebral artery; 4, left SCA; 5, left posterior cerebral artery; 6, A1.)

to have been stretched due to many perforating arteries blocking the surgical view. The right P1 and the right side of the aneurysm were finally dissected and the underlying perforating arteries were exposed and protected with the help of a silastic sheet. This was done through the perforating arteries exiting from the posterior communicating artery. The left P1 was then exposed through the opticocarotid space (Fig. 5.26b). In order to make more space, the right A1 was dissected as it was of redundant type, and by freeing this A1 segment the internal carotid artery could be better retracted. The left SCA and part of

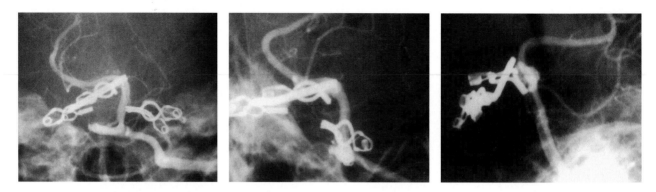

Fig. 5.27   Postoperative angiogram showing clips in place.

the left P1 were exposed with the left oculomotor nerve as the landmark. The origin of the left P1 was difficult to isolate and this was done after direct retraction of the aneurysm dome. The left P1 was found to originate a little behind the aneurysm dome and only after direct retraction of the dome did it become possible to expose the P1. Meanwhile the neck of the aneurysm and also the underlying perforating arteries were protected using a small silastic sheet. A bayonet type long clip no. 19 was used from the lateral aspect of the posterior communicating artery in the retrocarotid space whereby the M1 and the internal carotid artery were retracted medially. The blades were slowly advanced, occluding the neck of the aneurysm partially, saving the perforators from the right P1 under direct vision. Before closing the clip completely the angle of the microscope was changed so that the left side of the neck could be seen through the opticocarotid space. After confirming that all perforating arteries were spared, the clip blades were then gradually closed. On further dissection, it was seen that the tip of the clip blade was short of the far end of the aneurysm and it needed readjustment. It was noticed that the clip head was in contact with the posterior clinoid process and had resulted in kinking of the posterior communicating artery. The clip was removed and the posterior clinoid process was drilled using a diamond head, taking care not to damage the oculomotor nerve which was traversing in close proximity. The clip was reapplied to include the entire neck. As the aneurysm was round in shape and the neck partially originated from the basilar bifurcation, it became necessary to place a second clip to occlude the anterior side of the aneurysm completely. This was carried out using an oblique angle ring clip no. 35. The clipping of the aneurysm was now observed to be satisfactory (Fig. 5.26c). As the head of the second clip was somewhat compromising the stretched posterior communicating artery, a small portion of the tip of the temporal lobe was resected to accommodate the head. During the dissection a small aneurysmal dilatation of the ICA at the origin of the posterior communicating artery was detected and this was coagulated with the help of bipolar coagulation after attempts to occlude it with a mini-clip failed (Fig. 5.27).

The patient tolerated the surgery well and suffered no additional deficits.

Comments

1. Removal of the lateral orbital rim facilitated wide exposure. However, the exposure at depth was limited.

2. The short stretched posterior communicating artery hindered the surgical vision. Section of this artery was avoided.

3. The redundant A1 facilitated wider opening of the opticocarotid space.

4. Clipping from the retrocarotid space and changing the angle of the microscope were seen to be helpful.

CASE 2   Dorsally Projecting Basilar Bifurcation Aneurysm

This 55-year-old female had undergone basilar bifurcation aneurysmal clipping procedure through right frontotemporal approach (Fig. 5.28). The clipping was performed on day 27 of SAH. However, postoperative angiogram done 2 days after surgery showed that the clip had slipped from the aneurysm despite the use of a booster clip (Fig. 5.29). Reclipping was now undertaken. The aneurysm was projecting dorsally.

With the patient in the supine position, the previous frontotemporal craniotomy was reopened and it was further extended for the subtemporal approach (Fig. 5.30a). A zygomatic osteotomy was done in addition as it was observed that the aneurysm was relatively high in position. The previously used clips were observed by the transsylvian route. They had been displaced towards the internal carotid artery side (arrowhead in Fig. 5.30c) probably as a result of release of brain retraction at the previous surgery (Fig 5.30b). In order to visualize the entire aneurysm complex and the surrounding structures, the tip of the temporal lobe was retracted after coagulation and sectioning of the bridging vein that extended between it and the spenoid ridge. The aneurysm as seen from the pterional (Fig. 5.30b) and subtemporal views (Fig. 5.30d) are shown in the figures. The right oculomotor nerve was

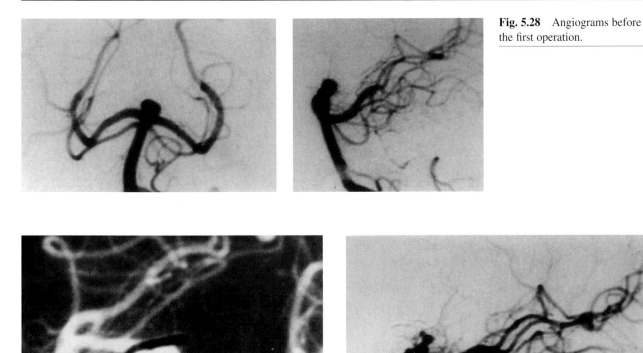

Fig. 5.28   Angiograms before the first operation.

Fig. 5.29   Angiograms 2 days postoperation of patient in Fig. 5.28 show that the clip has slipped from the aneurysm despite the use of a booster clip.

further dissected towards the uncus. A temporary clip was placed on the basilar trunk. The previously placed clips were removed. It was noticed that the clip had slipped and was now occluding the part of the dome which had probably bled. After the temporary clip was removed from the basilar trunk, bleeding started from the tip of the aneurysm. This could be easily controlled with the help of a small cottonoid placed over the rupture site. The bleeding site was bipolar coagulated with the help of a weak current. The aneurysm could now be observed between the right P1 and right SCA. The aneurysm protruded dorsally. It had many small perforating arteries around it. The perforating arteries in this region were dissected while those from the left P1 were detached from the left side of the neck. Under temporary clipping which lasted for 13 minutes, an attempt was made to clip the aneurysm with the help of a miniclip no. 84 in such a way as to clip the neck of the aneurysm at the bifurcation as well as the dome on the dorsal side of the basilar trunk. However, the length of the clip blade appeared shorter on inspection so we substituted a regular clip no. 48. The aneurysm appeared to be occluded well. But on further inspection on the lateral side of the oculomotor nerve and the tentorial edge, a considerable portion of the dome was seen to have remained unclipped. The clip was again removed and a ring clip no. 32 (ring 3.5 mm and an oblique blade) was

applied underneath and encircling the right P1. This seemed to be placed adequately but the tip of the blade was still slightly short. Hence, it was advanced further to its end (Fig. 5.30d). Because it appeared that the near side of the aneurysm neck would be short of its grip (arrowhead in Fig. 5.30d), another miniclip no. 88 was applied in parallel to the first one (Fig. 5.30). The perforating arteries on either side of the neck were found to be preserved. In order to prevent displacement of the clip after removal of the brain retraction, the tip of the uncus was sectioned to accommodate the head of the clip (Fig. 5.31).

The patient had mild oculomotor nerve paresis after the surgery.

Comments

1. The previously placed clips had displaced despite the use of booster clips, probably due to the postoperative rise in systolic blood pressure and to pulsations from the middle cerebral artery.

2. A ring clip encircling the right P1 was an appropriate choice during the present operation. This was because the neck was wide and the aneurysm protruded posteriorly.

3. Temporary clipping of the basilar trunk had to be carried out twice for 15 minutes duration.

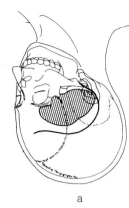

a

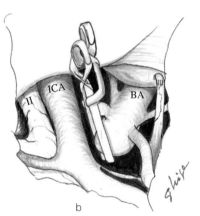

b

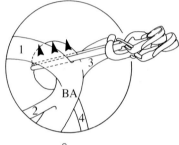

c

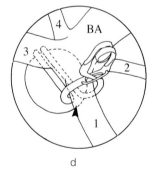

d

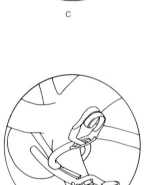

e

Fig. 5.30   a Frontotemporal craniotomy extended for the subtemporal approach. **b** Clips from first operation (patient in Figs. 5.28, 5.29) (pterional view). **c** Displacement of clips (arrowheads) from the first operation. **d** No. 32 ring clip applied encircling the right P1 (subtemporal view) (arrowhead indicates position of second clip; see Fig. 5.30e). **e** No. 88 miniclip applied in parallel to the first clip. (1, right posterior cerebral artery; 2, right SCA; 3, left posterior cerebral artery; 4, left SCA.)

CASE 3   Dorsally (posteriorly) Projecting Aneurysm

This 74-year-old female was operated on day 21 of her SAH. She was in Hunt and Hess Grade 3. The angiogram showed a high-positioned (13 mm above the posterior clinoid process) small aneurysm (Fig. 5.32). The patient was placed in the supine lateral position with the vertex turned inferiorly (Fig. 5.33a). The sylvian fissure was widely opened (Fig. 5.33b). The temporal bridging vein was dissected and preserved. The temporal lobe tip was retracted posteriorly to obtain a wider exposure than usual. The aneurysm was exposed in the retrocarotid space. It was behind the basilar terminum and the main mass was behind the right P1. An attempt to apply a ring clip was unsuccessful. After careful dissection of the dome of the aneurysm from the right P1, a no. 4 clip was applied with the P1 retracted with a silver dissector (Figs. 5.33c, 34a,b). Preservation of the perforators was confirmed via the opticocarotid space. The postoperative course was uneventful.

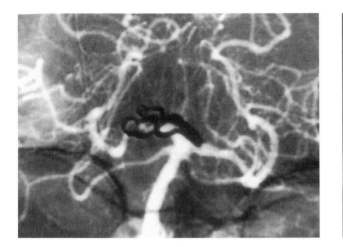

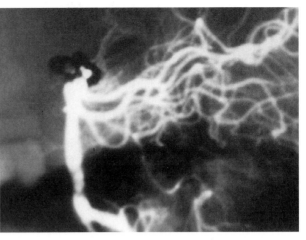

Fig. 5.31 Angiograms after the second operation.

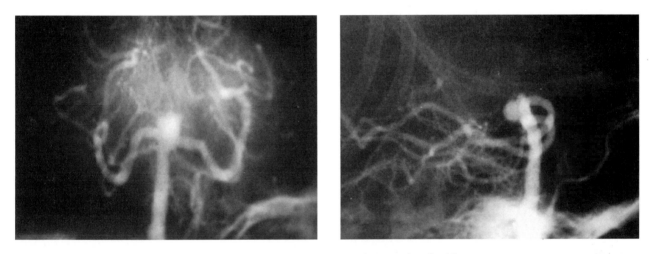

Fig. 5.32 Angiograms showing a small aneurysm located 13 mm above the posterior clinoid process.

Comments

This approach closely resembled a temporopolar approach.

CASE 4 Low-positioned Aneurysm

This 45-year-old female had experienced three episodes of SAH during the 2 months preceding the operation. The first attack 2 months previously was associated with sudden occipital headache which lasted for 2 weeks. The second and third attacks were associated with loss of consciousness lasting for a few hours. CT scan showed SAH principally in the posterior fossa. Angiogram showed an 8 mm low-positioned basilar bifurcation aneurysm (Fig. 5.35). The angiogram repeated at our university 28 days after the first SAH showed a 5 mm aneurysm located 10 mm below the biclinoid line. The aneurysm had apparently partially thrombosed.

With the patient in the supine position the cervical carotid arteries were exposed for possible temporary occlusion of the internal carotid artery during surgery. The head was then turned to the left side and fixed in a Sugita frame in the supine lateral position. A right temporal craniotomy was performed extending to the floor of the right temporal fossa (Fig. 5.36a). The external auditory canal, foramen spinosum and arcuate eminence were the landmarks for finding Kawase's triangle. Before drilling the bone of Kawase's triangle, CSF was drained by the intradural route from the basal cisterns. Kawase's triangle was drilled using a 3 mm and later a 2 mm burr (Fig. 5.36b). The superior petrosal sinus was a helpful landmark while drilling in the region of Kawase's triangle. The dura was opened in a T-fashion, first horizontally and then vertically to go through the superior petrosal sinus by coagulating and cutting and later packing the superior petrosal sinus. Meckel's cave and the ipsilateral sixth nerve and the Dorello's canal were seen. By retracting the trigeminal nerve downward we were able to get space for temporary occlusion of the basilar artery trunk just proximal to the origin of the SCA. The right SCA was single, but the left SCA was double. Both P1s were identified, which were relatively large (an unusual anatomical feature was that the oculomotor nerves were hanging down, short of the basilar

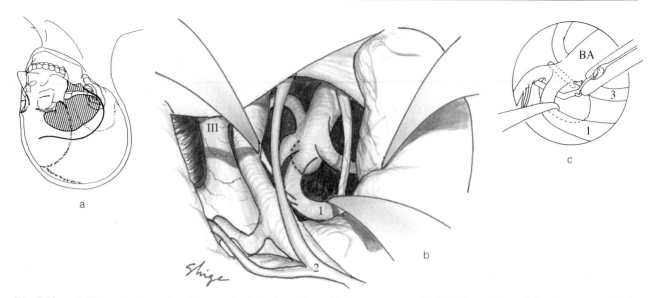

Fig. 5.33   a,b The patient was placed in a supine lateral position with the vertex turned inferiorly, and the sylvian fissure was widely opened. **c** a no. 4 clip was applied with the P1 retracted. (1, right posterior cerebral artery; 2, sylvian vein; 3, right SCA.)

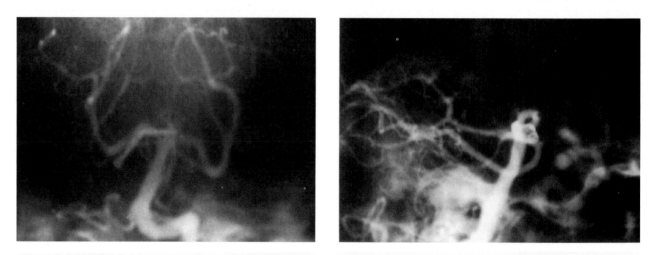

Fig. 5.34   Postoperative angiograms of the patient in Figs 5.32 and 5.33.

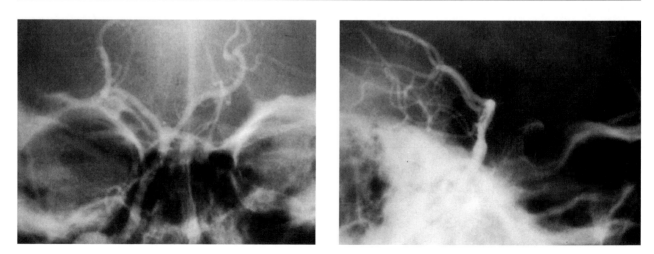

Fig. 5.35   Preoperative angiograms showing an 8 mm low-positioned basilar bifurcation aneurysm (Case 4).

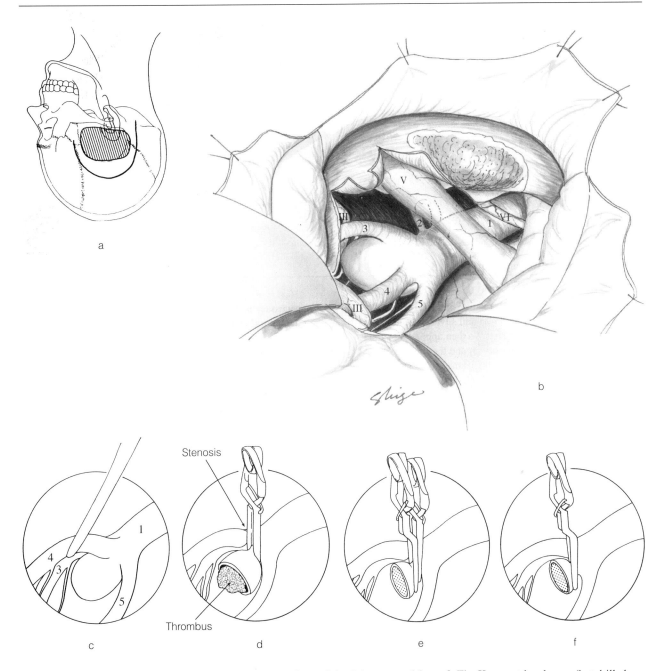

Fig. 5.36 **a** Right temporal craniotomy extending to the floor of the right temporal fossa. **b** The Kawase triangle was first drilled using a 3 mm and later a 2 mm burr. **c–f** A temporary clip was applied, the aneurysm was punctured and the thrombus was suctioned, and finally a bayonet clip was applied. (1, basilar artery; 2, left SCA; 3, left posterior cerebral artery; 4, right posterior cerebral artery; 5, right SCA.)

bifurcation). The aneurysm was red in color and the consistency implied that most of the contents of the aneurysm were soft or thrombosed. The most difficult and dangerous procedure was to dissect the perforating arteries located behind the aneurysm. Temporary occlusion of the basilar trunk was used twice during the operation for 8 and 6 minutes respectively. Most of the aneurysm could be dissected. A 15 mm straight clip was applied under temporary occlusion of the basilar artery to the neck of

the aneurysm from between the right SCA and P1. It became apparent that the dome of the aneurysm had thrombosed and it could not be collapsed. The clip was applied to the neck of the aneurysm but it resulted in kinking, with apparent partial occlusion of the right P1. It was decided to utilize step-clipping techniques after evacuating the clots from the dome of the aneurysm. The temporary clip was removed, leaving the straight clip on the neck of the aneurysm. The dome of the aneurysm

bridging veins were seen draining into the sphenoparietal sinus. As the veins were large they were not sectioned, to avoid venous congestion. The optic nerve, chiasm, left carotid artery and the left M1 and A1 segments were exposed. Figure 5.42b shows the view of the aneurysm from the subtemporal exposure and Figure 5.42c is the view from pterional exposure. The posterior clinoid process was seen and the oculomotor nerve was dissected from Liliequist's membrane. The opticocarotid space was opened in an attempt to expose the basilar trunk. However, the bulging aneurysmal sac prevented adequate exposure of the trunk. Laterally the posterior clinoid process obstructed the view of the aneurysm. From the limited exposure we decided to dissect the aneurysm as much as was possible. Through the relatively wider opticocarotid space the aneurysm was dissected. The aneurysm was whitish and relatively firm in consistency, and the dome could even be directly retracted with a 2 mm spatula. The P1 could now be seen but the perforating arteries at depth and the anatomy at the neck of the aneurysm could not be adequately visualized. The aneurysm was exposed by the retrochiasmatic route. It now appeared reddish and appeared to have a very thin wall. The right P1 and the right SCA could be seen from this angle but the basilar trunk could not be adequately exposed. The posterior clinoid process was carefully drilled with a 1 mm diamond head. There was not much bleeding from the cavernous sinus. Despite the removal of the posterior clinoid the basilar trunk could not be visualized adequately. The space between the neck of the aneurysm and the right P1 was seen, but dissection here was considered to be very dangerous as the wall of the aneurysm in this region was thin. Also numerous perforating arteries originated from this region which had to be preserved. It was now decided to shift to the subtemporal route. This was to have a better opportunity to obtain proximal control of the basilar trunk and to view the perforating arteries arising posterior and lateral to the aneurysm. Zygomatic osteotomy was helpful in minimizing temporal lobe retraction. There was some difficulty in visualizing the infratentorial space as the prominent bridging veins in the temporal polar region also had to be preserved. The tentorium was cut posterior to the entrance point of the trochlear nerve.

The third nerve was then dissected free in this space in order to expose the basilar trunk. Numerous perforating arteries were now seen in the posterior lateral space of the aneurysm neck. They were dissected carefully, but adequate space could not be obtained for clipping of the neck. A temporary clip was applied to the basilar trunk by the subtemporal route to facilitate further dissection of the aneurysm through the pterional route. After mild retraction of the internal carotid artery, the aneurysm was dissected to permit clip blades to pass through between perforating arteries and the neck, particularly on the left side. Also on the right side, the space between the neck and the right P1 was dissected. There were not too many perforating arteries seen on this side and the space was filled with old clots. Dissection at depth between the neck and the left P1 was difficult as there were many perforating arteries, some of which were lying behind the aneurysm at depth and some were adherent to the weak aneurysm wall. However, with the decrease in aneurysm tension following temporary clip application the anatomy of the perforating arteries could be seen better. Prior to further dissection of the aneurysm a tentative clip to the aneurysm was applied using a straight clip no. 18. On exploration, however, the clip was found to have included the right P1. The clip was replaced to spare the right P1 and perforating arteries. The temporary clip on the basilar trunk was released at this point and dissection was continued around the aneurysm through the pterional route. On inspection it was found that the perforating artery had been trapped by the tip of the clip blades. Under the second temporary clipping of the basilar trunk for another 15 minutes, replacement of the clip was attempted. The perforating artery which had been trapped by the clip was adherent to the aneurysm dome. This perforating artery was dissected from the body of the aneurysm for a short distance. Tentative clipping with a ring clip was done on the body of the aneurysm parallel to the previously placed clip. The temporary clip on the basilar trunk was removed. However, on further exploration this clip had also included a tiny perforating artery. A straight aneurysm clip was now used to avoid the tiny perforating artery without temporary clipping of the parent artery. This attempt was successful and the

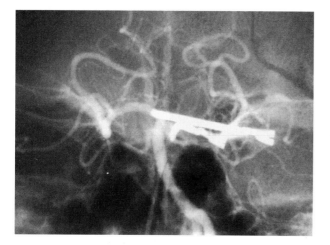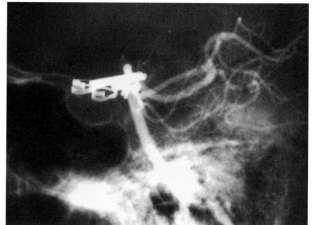

Fig. 5.43   Postoperative angiograms.

tentative ring clip which had been placed in such a way as to avoid including the posterior communicating artery was removed. The remaining portion of the aneurysm which had extended toward the posterior clinoid process was clipped with an L-shaped clip, no. 20, after shortening the blades by half using a diamond drill. This clipping was successful (Figs. 5.42d–f, 5.43).

Comments

1. This was a difficult case because the aneurysm was large and of irregular shape and the dome of the aneurysm was low positioned.

2. Because of the low position, large size and irregular shape, the pterional approach itself was not sufficient and a subtemporal approach had to be added to increase the exposure.

3. If the bridging veins were not prominent they could have been cut to obtain a wider exposure and space.

4. The posterior clinoid process restricted the exposure of the basilar trunk. Despite the removal of the process the trunk could not be satisfactorily exposed. The basilar trunk had to be exposed via the subtemporal approach.

5. Multiple clips were used.

6. Zygomatic osteotomy was helpful in minimizing temporal lobe retraction.

7. A transanterior clinoid, transcavernous approach may have been helpful. However, this approach requires significantly extra time.

8. During the subtemporal approach, the oculomotor nerve had to be manipulated to obtain exposure. This procedure probably resulted in postoperative temporary bilateral oculomotor nerve paresis. The patient also had right hemiparesis. Both these deficits rapidly cleared in a few days.

References

Abe T, Sugishita M, Yatsuzaka S et al 1993 Transcallosal interforniceal approach for posterior projecting high basilar bifurcation aneurysm: case report. Journal of Neurosurgery 78: 970–973

Batjer H H, Samson D S 1993 Basilar apex aneurysms. In: Apuzzo M L J Brain surgery: complication avoidance and management. Churchill Livingstone, Edinburgh

Drake C G 1961 Bleeding aneurysms of the basilar artery; direct surgical management in 4 cases. Journal of Neurosurgery 18: 230–238

Drake C G 1978 Treatment of aneurysm of the posterior cranial fossa. Progress in Neurological Surgery 9: 122–144

Drake C G 1979 The treatment of aneurysms of the posterior circulation. Clinical Neurosurgery 26: 96–144

Fujitsu K, Kuwabara T 1985 Zygomatic approach for lesions in the interpeduncular cistern. Journal of Neurosurgery 62: 340–343

Gibo H, Tanaka Y, Kobayashi S et al 1991 Microsurgical anatomy of approaches and perforating arteries in the surgery of basilar artery aneurysm. Surgery for Cerebral Stroke 19: 343–347

Ikeda K, Yamashita J. Hashimoto M et al 1991 Orbitozygomatic temporopolar approach for a high basilar tip aneurysm associated with a short internal carotid artery: a new surgical approach. Neurosurgery 28: 105–110

Jamieson K G 1964 Aneurysms of the vertebrobasilar system. Surgical intervention in 19 cases. Journal of Neurosurgery 21: 781–797

Kobayashi S, Tanaka Y 1994 Surgical techniques for basilar bifurcation aneurysms. Clinical Neurosurgery 41: 334–350

Kobayashi S, Sugita K, Nakagawa F 1983 An approach to a basilar aneurysm above the bifurcation of the internal carotid artery: case report. Journal of Neurosurgery 59: 1082–1084

Kodama N, Sasaki T, Yamanobe K 1986 High position basilar top aneurysm treated via third ventricle. No Shinkei Geka 14: 1277–1281

Kyoshima K, Ohigashi Y, Hokama M et al 1993 Remote-control vascular occluder: Neurosurgery 32: 322–323

Marinkovic S V, Gibo H 1993 The surgical anatomy of the perforating branches of the basilar artery. Neurosurgery 33: 80–87

Nagasawa S, Chung K J, Yonekawa Y et al 1987 Pterional approach to the basilar artery aneurysm: with special reference to the acccessibility via optic–carotid triangle. No Shinkei Geka 15: 831–835 (in Japanese)

Neil-Dwyer G, Sharr M, Haskell R et al 1988 Zygomaticotemporal approach to the basis cranii and basilar artery. Neurosurgery 23: 20–22

Osawa M, Obinata C, Kobayashi S et al 1995 Newly designed bayonet clips for complicated aneurysms: technical note. Neurosurgery 36: 425–427

Pitelli S D, Almeida G M, Nagasaki E J et al 1986 Basilar aneurysm surgery: the subtemporal approach with section of the zygomatic arch. Neurosurgery 18: 125–128

Regli L, de Tribolet N 1991 Tuberothalamic infarct after division of hypoplastic posterior communicating artery for clipping of a basilar tip aneurysm: case report. Neurosurgery 28: 456–459

Sano K 1980 Temporo-polar approach to aneurysms of the basilar artery at and around the distal bifurcation: technical note. Neurological Research 2: 361–367

Shibuya M, Sugita K, Kobayashi S 1991 Intraoperative protection of cranial nerves and perforating arteries by silicone rubber sheets. Journal of Neurosurgery 74: 677–679

Shiokawa Y, Saito I, Aoki N et al 1989 Zygomatic temporopolar approach for basilar aneurysms. Neurosurgery 25: 793–797

Shucart W A, Kwan E S, Heilman C B 1990 Temporary balloon occlusion of a proximal vessel as an aid to clipping aneurysms of the basilar and paraclinoid internal carotid arteries: technical note. Neurosurgery 27: 116–117

Sugita K, Hirota T, Mizutani T et al 1978 A newly designed multipurpose microneurosurgical head frame. Journal of Neurosurgery 48: 656–657

Sugita K, Kobayashi S, Shintani A, Mutsuga N 1979 Microneurosurgery for aneurysms of the basilar artery. Journal of Neurosurgery 51: 615–620

Sugita K, Kobayashi S, Takemae T et al 1980 Direct retraction method in aneurysm surgery. Journal of Neurosurgery 53: 417–419

Sundt T M Jr, Piepgras D G, Marsch W R 1984 Booster clips for giant and thick-based aneurysms. Journal of Neurosurgery 60: 751–762

Tanaka Y, Kobayashi S, Hongo K, Oikawa S 1993 Intraoperative protection of cranial nerves and arteries by split silicone tube. Neurosurgery 33: 523–525

Tanaka Y, Kobayashi S, Sugita K et al 1995 Characteristics of pterional routes to basilar bifurcation aneurysm. Neurosurgery 36: 533–540

Yamaura A, Ise H, Makino H 1982 Treatment of aneurysms arising from the terminal portion of the basilar artery: with special reference to the radiometric study and accessibility of trans-Sylvian approach. Neurologia Medicochirurgica (Tokyo) 22: 521–532

Yasargil M G, Antic J, Laciga R et al 1976 Microsurgical pterional approach to aneurysms of the basilar bifurcation. Surgical Neurology 6: 83–91

Yokoh A, Sugita K, Kobayashi S 1983 Intermittent versus continuous brain retraction. Journal of Neurosurgery 58: 918–923

Technical Issues in the Management of Basilar Bifurcation Aneurysms
S J Peerless

Early on, Dr Drake recognized that the basilar bifurcation aneurysm was perhaps the most hazardous vascular lesion for the neurosurgeon to treat. Of his first eight patients, only three had satisfactory results while three were poor and two died. Two of the early patients were treated with silk ligation of the neck of the aneurysm. Neither patient awakened from the anesthetic and both remained in deep coma with quadriparesis and fixed dilated pupils. Postoperative angiograms demonstrated the aneurysms were perfectly occluded and this prompted review of the anatomy of the region. The numerous, small thalamoperforating arteries arising primarily from the first part of the posterior cerebral artery and from the back of the basilar artery were noted, and seen to enter the posterior perforating substance to irrigate the midbrain, the mamillary bodies and thalamus. It was immediately apparent that injury or occlusion of these branches had been responsible for the persisting coma and paralysis.

Every effort has been made since to identify and protect these branches at all costs in the treatment of the basilar bifurcation aneurysm. Basilar bifurcation aneurysms have three typical projections. Most commonly, they project upward and align with the curve of the basilar artery; less often (14%), they project posteriorly into the interpenduncular space; least often (11%), the sac projects anteriorly, with the dome often adherent to the dorsum sellae or the back of the clivus. Very rarely, the aneurysm may be bilobed anteriorly and posteriorly as much as 90° to the projection of the basilar artery. As these aneurysms form, they typically cause an ectatic widening of the terminal basilar artery so that when viewed from the side, the P1 segment or even the SCA may seem to emerge from the sac itself. There is also a tendency for the neck to bulge anteriorly and posteriorly even when the fundus of the aneurysm is projecting directly upwards.

It is distinctly uncommon, even very rare in non-giant aneurysms, for the perforating vessels to arise from the aneurysmal sac itself. These perforators do not respect the midline so that perforators arising from the right P1 have been frequently seen to cross the midline to enter the posterior perforator substance on the left side. Most often, these perforators arise from the posterior and lateral surfaces of the P1 branch and average four per side and divide shortly after their origin. The few perforators that arise from the terminal centimeter of the basilar artery also typically arise from the posterior and lateral surfaces of this vessel. Most of the perforators arising from the basilar artery will end in the pons, but some will join with their fellows from the posterior cerebral artery to end in the mesencephalon peduncle, thalamus and mamillary bodies.

The height of the basilar artery varies a good deal in its relationship to the dorsum sellae and we feel this is very important in planning the approach to the aneurysm. Most often (40%), the artery bifurcates just at the level of the dorsum sellae or very slightly above it. In one-third of the cases, however, the bifurcation is 1 cm or more above the level of the dorsum sellae, and in 28% it is 1 cm below the dorsum sellae.

From our experience with more than 450 patients with small (12 mm) aneurysms and 280 patients with large (12–24 mm) basilar bifurcation aneurysms, we have found that the majority were operated upon in the subtemporal approach. We feel that nearly all (99%) non-giant basilar bifurcation aneurysms can be visualized subtemporally regardless of their size, height, direction or multilocularity. The tentorium can be divided easily for very low necks and for the placement of a temporary basilar clip. There is no necessity to remove the posterior clinoid or inner petrous apex from the subtemporal approach. Moreover, control of inadvertent rupture with vigorous hemorrhage from an aneurysm is much easier through the subtemporal than the transsylvian exposure. In our series, it is certain that the transsylvian exposure would have been possible in about 58% of the cases of basilar bifurcation aneurysms. It would seem to us to be most suitable for single aneurysms with small necks lying in the ideal position near the level of the dorsum sellae. It is the preferred route for those rare, very highly located, single aneurysms, with the neck lying more than 1 cm above the dorsum sellae. However, in our experience, the transsylvian approach was used most frequently in those patients where the basilar bifurcation aneurysm was one of multiple aneurysms, permitting us to clip the basilar aneurysm in the same operation as aneurysms of the anterior circulation. Aneurysms with low-lying necks and those with the fundus directed posteriorly are difficult, and often impossible, to be treated by the transsylvian route.

Because most of the troubles associated with operative repair of a basilar bifurcation aneurysms lie primarily behind the aneurysm in the form of the perforators arising off P1, the subtemporal approach has always seemed to us to be the most logical way to see these hidden dangers and protect them. With the placement of a temporary clip on the basilar artery, the surgeon can manipulate the sac, tipping it away from the interpeduncular fossa to allow the perforators to be seen and, more importantly, safely separated from the sac.

Several technical considerations need emphasizing with the subtemporal approach. First, we feel it very important that the temporal lobe should not be retracted, but rather supported by retractors after adequate CSF drainage to allow the temporal lobe to fall back. It is also essential not to injure any of the major veins draining the temporal lobe into the dura, such as the vein of Labbe or the temporal tip veins, in that many of the complications we hear about with this approach are undoubtedly due to venous infarction. The tip of the retractor should be placed over a well-padded uncus and the arachnoid of the lateral pontine cistern divided inferior to the oculomotor nerve, allowing this nerve to be gently displaced upwards with the uncus to which it is attached by its arachnoidal sheath and thereby lessening its manipulation and eventual potential damage.

Placing a suture on the edge of the tentorium and tacking it back into the middle fossa opens the visual space for the final approach by as much as 1 cm. I find it convenient to follow the SCA, easily identified on the side of the brain stem, down to the basilar artery, so as to first remove clot and expose the basilar artery well free of the filling portion of the sac. Once the SCA is identified on both sides and the basilar artery is prepared for temporary clipping, then the P1 on the right side can be exposed along with its perforators, working primarily on the posterior aspect of the aneurysm to clear the space between the aneurysm, the basilar artery and the peduncles. Occasionally, the peduncle can be gently retracted with a fine, tapered Sugita retractor to further open up this space.

The aneurysm rarely ruptures into this posterior space as it is tamponaded by the surrounding brain. The rupture sites are more likely anteriorly or superiorly – areas that need to be avoided. Particular caution must be taken when the aneurysm is projecting forward and then often fused to the dura of the clivus. Seeing across the back of the neck of the aneurysm is usually accomplished with gentle retraction of the neck of the sac with a fine sucker in the left hand, and working between the perforators and the neck and the waist of the sac with a small dissector. Occasionally, this process must be done with sharp dissection and all of this is made safer by temporary basilar occlusion. Perforators need not be completely separated from the sac, just sufficiently to allow a clip blade to slip between them and the neck of the sac and close without kinking or tearing their origins.

Only in small aneurysms does the origin and the first portion of the P1 stand free from the neck of the aneurysm. This anatomical pathological fact led Dr Drake to developing the aperture clip in1969. With this clip, the P1 can be left adherent to the sac and it, and even its perforators, protected and enclosed in the aperture. The tip of the clip must just perfectly close the sac distally, leaving the P1 and its perforators free, and the proximal portion of the blade must equally be precisely fitted to the near side. This often requires that the clip be cut (usually with a high-speed drill) and polished to a fine degree of smoothness. Often, it is not possible to seal the neck off completely with a single clip, and so always at this stage the sac is needled and, if bleeding continues, one determines the site of continued filling and then places a second tandem clip across the neck which will completely obliterate the sac.

It is always critical to immediately inspect the region to ensure that no perforators have been caught in the clip blades or deformed as the blades have closed. It is also important to precisely visualize the position of the tips on the far side to ensure that the SCA has not been misidentified as the posterior cerebral. It is surprising how often perforators are seen for the first time when trapped underneath the blade of the clip, requiring the malpositioned clip to be removed immediately. One must be as certain as possible that both the aneurysm is completely clipped and that the perforators and main branches are all free, for there is no greater calamity than to have the aneurysm rupture during the closure or in the first few hours postoperatively or to have the patient wake with a spreading infarction of the brain stem and thalamus.

Basilar Bifurcation Aneurysms: A Personal View
R P Sengupta

Aneurysms of the basilar artery are fortunately rare because surgical obliteration of these are most difficult even for the skilled aneurysm surgeon. When Drake started to challenge these aneurysms in the early 1960s three of his four patients with basilar bifurcation aneurysm died. But with perseverance and accumulative skill he proved that these aneurysms can be obliterated with outcome as good as in any other intracranial aneurysms. Yasargil and Sugita had similar success. Yet in spite of operating personally on over 1200 patients with intracranial aneurysms I could not achieve such results. Since the mortality of anterior circulation and posterior circulation aneurysms is respectively 5.1% and 15% in my own series, I do not believe that surgical skill is the only cause for such a disparity in outcome. The problem I have encountered in surgery for basilar bifurcation aneurysms include:

1. lack of experience in these aneurysms;
2. difficulty of exposure;
3. lack of proximal control;
4. difficulty in protecting the perforators;
5. disturbance of brain stem from manipulation of the vertebrobasilar artery;
6. variations in the height of the basilar artery;
7. unsuitable instruments and clips.

Lack of experience is the main cause of poor outcome. We in Newcastle at the Regional Neurosciences Centre look after 2.5 million people. Expected incidence of ruptured intracranial aneurysm in this population is 250 per year. We annually receive 160 such patients. The total number of posterior circulation aneurysm is eight and is shared by five neurosurgeons. Since the incidents of basilar bifurcation is 40% of all posterior circulation aneurysms, a surgeon deals with one basilar bifurcation aneurysm every 15 months. Since the availability of endovascular therapy the number of such aneurysms for surgery is even less.

However, endovascular therapy for basilar bifurcation aneurysms has not been able to replace surgery. It is not feasible in aneurysms with a wide neck or in a very small aneurysm. On the other hand, in spite of a successful obliteration with coils, the continuously pounding force on the basilar apex causes the coils to be pushed towards the fundus, refilling the aneurysm. Therefore the task for surgical obliteration of these aneurysms has not been overcome by endovascular therapy. For those of us who have to treat such rare aneurysms, the problems of surgery must be appreciated.

In selecting a surgical approach the following considerations are useful:

1. shortest route to avoid undue manipulation of brain or vessels;
2. access to parent artery for temporary proximal occlusion;
3. projection of aneurysm to avoid neighborhood vessels or fundus;
4. height of the basilar artery;
5. size of the aneurysm.

When the basilar bifurcation aneurysms project posteriorly, they are hidden within the cerebral peduncle, invested by the perforators and overlapped by the posterior cerebral artery and the third nerve. On the other hand, aneurysms projecting upward or anteriorly are free from these hazards.

The significance of the level of basilar bifurcation in relation to the posterior clinoid must also be appreciated before selecting a surgical approach. Since the basilar trunk varies in length the bifurcation point can be at or below the level of the dorsum sellae. In such a situation the neck of the aneurysm cannot be visualized through a pterional approach and the basilar artery cannot be exposed for temporary occlusion. It is essential to have one lateral view with bone landmark during standard digital subtraction angiography to show the aneurysmal neck in relation to the clivus.

When the aneurysm is large in size, maximal exposure is necessary to reach the parent vessel or to evacuate the sac before repairing the neck. Brain retraction for a prolonged period is very hazardous and it is much safer to carry out anterior temporal lobectomy if a lateral approach is decided upon.

Taking into account the morphological nature of the aneurysm and the basilar artery the bifurcation aneurysms can be approached through the pterional route as advocated by Yasargil, or lateral subtemporal route pioneered by Drake, with some modifications in either of these approaches. Superiorly and anteriorly projected aneurysms should be approached through the pterion, provided the aneurysm is not too large and the basilar bifurcation is not below the dorsum sellae. To overcome the problem of low bifurcation the posterior clinoid can be removed and with the experience of anterior skull base surgery removal of the fronto-orbital bar can provided additional improvement in access. For the rest of the aneurysms such as giant aneurysms, those projecting posteriorly and low bifurcation aneurysms the subtemporal route is necessary. In this approach, I prefer anterior temporal lobectomy and division of the posterior communicating artery to gain a comfortable access.

It is reassuring to know that if the aneurysms can be obliterated safely at operation, the postoperative course in those aneurysms is much less complicated since vasospasm seems to occur much less than in those in the anterior circulation.

Although the management of basilar bifurcation aneurysms remains a surgical proposition, some of these aneurysms such as those projecting posteriorly should have the first choice for endovascular therapy becauses of the relative lack of morbidity. For successful surgical outcome increased experience by pulling cases together

in a regional center is helpful. Improvement in instrumentation needed for work in a deep confined space is long overdue.

Basilar Bifurcation Aneurysm Surgery
Nobuo Hashimoto

Ruptured basilar bifurcation aneurysms used to be the only exception to indications for acute surgery. This was based on a misconception that preservation of perforating arteries might be very difficult in acute surgery of aneurysms at this particular location. My personal experience showed that this was not true and these aneurysms were prone to re-rupture when compared to aneurysms of other locations.

For patients with basilar bifurcation aneurysms, I choose a conventional pterional approach in most cases. Thus I would like to concentrate my discussion on the technical aspects of the pterional approach, including how to expose the aneurysm and how to preserve the perforating arteries in the jungle of vascular trees, branches and twigs, especially when the jungle is filled with clots.

In the pterional approach, the major obstacles are the temporal muscle and the wing of the sphenoid bone. Removal of the zygomatic arch, if necessary, and a slightly greater resection of the lesser wing than that required in cases with anterior circulation aneurysms are sufficient in most cases. When an aneurysm is located in a high position, resection of the anteroinferior portion of the temporal squama down to the level of the base of the anterior temporal fossa may be useful. It is not necessary to make a larger or more extensive craniotomy. It is necessary to make a craniotomy with a width 3 cm anterior and 2 cm posterior to the sylvian fissure at the base. And when the base of the craniotomy is extended further downwards, we can reach more rostrally without retraction of the brain or vessels. With this craniotomy, we can approach the aneurysm via the subfrontal, transsylvian or temporopolar route depending on its anatomical situation. I think one of the key points in this surgery is that the surgeon should not insist on his or her initially predecided route to reach the aneurysm. When exposure of a certain structure is difficult, this is not due to the anatomical relations in the patient but to incomplete dissection of the surrounding structures or inappropriate selection of the route by the surgeon.

After opening the sylvian fissure and basal cisterns, the structure that should be exposed initially is the proximal portion of the basilar artery. This is possible through the opticocarotid space or carotico-oculomotor space. Selection of the route depends on the length of the carotid artery. Through either space, dissection should be directed caudally to find the posterior clinoid process. Further dissection of the arachnoid structure between the posterior clinoid process and the posterior

communicating artery or oculomotor nerve creates space to place a temporary clip on the proximal basilar artery. One of the tricks in creating a wide space is cutting the arachnoid tissue on one side of the artery or nerve. Cutting of the arachnoid tissue on one side of the posterior communicating artery helps retraction of the artery to the other side.

When the prepontine cistern is filled with clots, the basilar artery is traced from the caudal to rostral direction by peeling the clots off from the surface of the basilar artery. It is not wise to aspirate clots in the prepontine cistern generously without knowing the course of fine vessels and the location of the aneurysm at this stage. Through the opticocarotid space, the proximal portion of the contralateral P1 segment and perforators from the segment are usually exposed earlier than those of the ipsilateral side. Through the carotico-oculomotor space, the P1 segment of the ipsilateral side and its perforators are identified from spaces rostral or caudal to the posterior communicating artery. Selection of the route at this stage also depends on the length of the communicating artery. Location of the aneurysmal neck is realized by observing the course of the basilar artery, oculomotor nerve, superior cerebellar arteries and P1 segments at this stage.

When both spaces medial and lateral to the carotid artery are small, this indicates that the artery is short, and the A1 and M1 segments should be freed from the surface of frontal and temporal lobes. This makes the carotid artery more mobile and usually medial retraction of the carotid artery makes the space larger to expose the neck of the aneurysm. When the anterior temporal artery or sylvian vein limits retraction, these are freed from the surface of the brain. Or we can create another space at the distal corner of the carotid bifurcation. Through this space, structures hidden by the bifurcation when seen from the carotico-oculomotor space are well seen. It is fortunate that in such a case with a short carotid artery, perforators located in the space are long and redundant, offering a nice working space.

Thus, although each space may be small, one of the advantages of this approach is that there are many spaces that can be used. When we feel that the operating space is too small, we should examine the whole operating field again under lower magnification to find other possibilities for creating a wider space. It is not uncommon that, when viewed from one route, it seems impossible to clip the aneurysm, but when approached from another direction or route the whole view of the upper basilar complex is obtained. It takes only a few seconds to change the direction of the microscope, replace the spatula and change your preconception.

For treatment of basilar bifurcation aneurysms, preservation of perforating arteries is absolutely necessary. When no perforating arteries have been identified after the efforts described above, I think that surgery should be stopped and the patient should be treated by other methods such as intravascular surgery. When perforating arteries are exposed on at least one P1 segment, the aneurysm can be clipped. Usually only the neck portion is visualized before clipping, so a tentative clip is applied near the neck and the dome is punctured to be collapsed. Coagulation or incision of the dome after clipping enables full exposure of the basilar bifurcation complex. Without collapsing the dome, it is difficult to check the perforators beneath the dome, so coagulation or cutting of the dome is mandatory. To release and reapply the initial clip correctly, complete coagulation of the dome or leaving space to apply another tentative clip is necessary. Care should be taken not to cut or coagulate perforating arteries on the surface of the other side of the dome.

I usually use microscissors with small and slightly curved blades. They are especially useful for surgery in a narrow and deep operating field. Sharp dissection is possible in a narrow space only under direct vision of the tips of the blades. Perforating arteries adherent to the dome of the basilar bifurcation aneurysm are one of the major causes of failure in this type of surgery. When we are familiar with sharp dissection techniques using instruments like such microscissors, preparation of tiny vessels from the dome of an aneurysm is possible and at least in my hand, sharp dissection under direct vision is safer than blunt dissection.

Lastly, I would like to mention a small but very useful technique for clipping the aneurysm. After exposure of the neck, we usually introduce a straight clip into the operating field. This is the best angle to see the neck of the aneurysm but this is the worst angle to see the tips of the clip because the axis of the surgeon's view and the axis of the clip are the same. Thus after confirmation of the neck, it is better to move the microscope to see the neck from a slightly different angle or from a different space. Although this is not the best angle to see the neck, we can introduce the clip from the initial route under direct vision. The neck or dome is gradually squeezed by the clip, and completeness of clipping is better confirmed from this new angle.

Basilar Bifurcation Aneurysm Surgery
Akira Yamaura

For the last 20 years, 150 patients with a basilar bifurcation aneurysm were treated in our hospital and its affiliated hospitals in Chiba prefecture. The transsylvian approach has been my favorite technique for the aneurysm at this location. Exceptions are for those aneurysms that are very large or very small in size and project posteriorly. Posteriorly projecting aneurysms were treated by the subtemporal approach. This classical approach was taken only in 10% or less of our whole basilar bifurcation aneurysm series.

Preoperative Preparation: Probably the most important preoperative management of a patient with a ruptured aneurysm would be adequate sedation, control of blood pressure within normal limits, and hydration. Restriction of fluids with an intention to prevent brain edema was an old policy, and is not currently practiced in usual cases.

Precise observation of preoperative angiography is important. In our experience, the aneurysms located 10–15 mm above the clinoid or interclinoid line (defined as a line connecting the tips of anterior and posterior clinoids) were associated with least postoperative complications. If the aneurysm neck is located below the clinoid line or higher than 15 mm from this line, access to the aneurysm becomes significantly difficult. The shape of the proximal posterior cerebral artery (PCA) is also important. If the right proximal PCA is more posterior than the left counterpart, access would be easier via the right transsylvian approach. If the right proximal PCA is present anterior to the left PCA, such cases will require more skill because the aneurysm and thalamoperforating arteries are hidden by the right PCA. A Y-shaped basilar bifurcation will be accompanied by a low-position aneurysm and a T-shaped basilar bifurcation will be often seen in a high-position aneurysm. Both of such subtypes result in additional difficulties.

Surgical Technique: The patient's head was slightly rotated to the left. I prefer to keep head rotation within 30°. The fashioning of skin incision and frontolateral craniotomy is quite similar to that used to access the anterior circulation aneurysms. The pterional bone should be sufficiently ronguered. Removal of the zygomatic arch is rarely performed. After opening of the dura mater, the first and most important step is the opening of the sylvian fissure as widely as possible. Usually the superficial arachnoid membrane is cut over 4–5 cm distance, commencing dissection posteriorly and advancing anteriorly. This direction of arachnoid incision will enable much quicker opening. The fissure is then dissected deeper to expose the middle cerebral, internal carotid (ICA) and anterior cerebral artery, and dissection proceeds to the right and left optic nerves. By this method, the frontal lobe will become well mobilized. In my technique temporal lobe dissection is minimal. Often the bridging vein at the temporal lobe tip is preserved.

Temporal lobe retraction is also minimal. The ICA is then retracted medially and the peduncular cistern is entered through opening the Kelly–Retzius arachnoid membrane. Retraction on the ICA should be regularly released. A space medial to the ICA is rarely large enough to allow placing a clip without obstructing the surgeon's view under reasonable retraction. This space is only useful for observation of the opposite PCA and its perforators. The basilar artery (BA) is dissected at its trunk just below the origin of the SCA and prepared for possible temporary clipping. The BA is then followed distally to reach the terminal portion where the aneurysm is located. Only the aneurysm neck should be dissected and the surgeon would not see its body or fundus. All possible attention should be paid to preserve the thalamoperforating arteries, not only along the right PCA, but also along the left side. If a temporary clip is placed on the BA, this should be released every 3 minutes to recirculate blood for more than 3 minutes.

A clip of the most adequate type and size should be selected for successful treatment. Often a fenestrated clip is useful to allow the right PCA and its branches to stay in the window, particularly in the cases of a large aneurysm. If there is no sizable thalamoperforating artery on the right side, there would be a well-developed one on the left side. Such single perforators occur in 10–15% of cases and perfuse both thalami and other regions.

Often the thalamoperforating arteries are adherent to the aneurysm. In such cases, dissection should be made at least at the origin of the perforators. Dissection from the aneurysm body is often quite risky. This small space could be entered using a specially designed narrow-bladed clip.

Postoperative management does not differ from any other lesions. By this transsylvian approach, third nerve paresis, including minimal or transient paresis over a few hours postoperatively, occurred only in 30% of cases.

In conclusion, there are variations in approaches to the basilar bifurcation aneurysm. My technique would be characterized by entirely mobilizing the lateral and inferior frontal lobe. Wide opening of the sylvian fissure at superficial and deeper levels and dissection of the optic nerve offer reasonably sufficient working space. If you had a very low or very high aneurysm, opening of the sylvian fissure should be much wider posteriorly. Opening the sylvian fissure more posteriorly would be the only way to obtain an adequate space to manage the lower or higher aneurysms. Successful surgery will follow from this simple procedure. Removal of the zygomatic arch will give a lower-angle access to the aneurysm. However, a superiorly or posteriorly projecting aneurysm will be hidden by the BA itself in this approach.

Basilar–superior cerebellar artery aneurysms

6

Shigeaki Kobayashi Kazuhiro Hongo Atul Goel
Yuichiro Tanaka

TECHNICAL CONSIDERATIONS

Technically speaking, basilar–superior cerebellar artery (BA–SCA) aneurysms are in general less difficult than basilar bifurcation aneurysms. This is due to the following reasons:

1. BA–SCA aneurysms are usually located lower than basilar bifurcation aneurysms.
2. They usually deviate from the midline.
3. Perforators between the SCA and P1 are fewer in number and therefore it is easier to avoid their occlusion and injury (Marinkovic & Gibo 1993).

The off-midline location makes it easier to clip the neck of the aneurysm because it is shallower in the operative field. While dissecting and clipping these aneurysms, especially the larger variety, care should be taken not to injure the oculomotor nerve, as this nerve courses between the two arteries. Usually, we prefer a pterional approach. After opening of the dura, the sylvian fissure is opened widely to facilitate retraction of the frontal and temporal lobes. Because the aneurysm can be located low, it may become necessary to drill the posterior clinoid process to secure the proximal parent artery. As it also lies laterally, it may occasionally be necessary to employ an extended pterional approach (see Ch. 5). In some cases of BA–SCA aneurysm, the neck is located in the midline as in the case of basilar bifurcation aneurysm, whereby the ipsilateral P1 and contralateral P1 and SCA are rotated and shifted so the aneurysm itself takes a position in the midline. In such a case, the approach and clipping technique are essentially the same as for the basilar bifurcation aneurysm.

CASE 1A Ruptured Left BA–SCA aneurysm, Low-positioned, Irregular-shaped (Unruptured Bilateral Middle Cerebral Artery (MCA) and Distal Left Anterior Cerebral Artery Aneurysms)

This 50-year-old male suffered subarachnoid hemorrhage (SAH). Initially the neurological grading was Grade 1. But on day 4 vasospasm developed which resulted in mild disorientation and right hemiparesis. With large doses of hydrocortisone and low-molecular-weight dextran, the

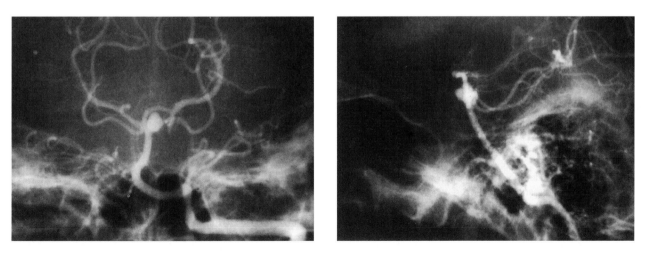

Fig. 6.1 Preoperative angiograms showing low-positioned BA–left SCA aneurysm with a bifid shape. There is an associated irregularly shaped left MCA aneurysm.

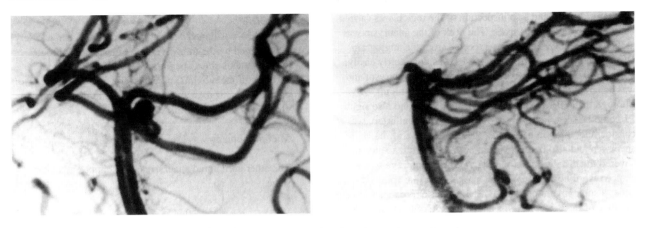

Fig. 6.4   Angiograms showing irregular domed aneurysm measuring 1 cm in maximum diameter.

was controlled with Oxycel. The dura over the temporal lobe was dissected from the structures going through the superior orbital fissure in such a way as to preserve the bridging veins (extended pterional approach, see Ch. 5). The clinoidal segment of the ICA was exposed; the carotid axilla was opened. The medial triangle of Hakuba was opened. It now became possible

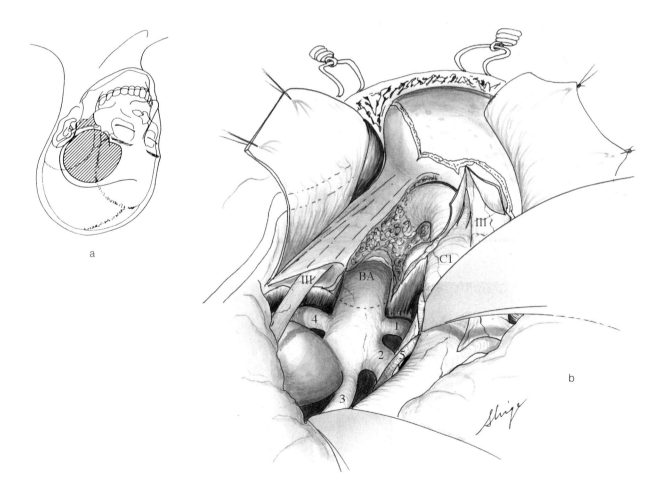

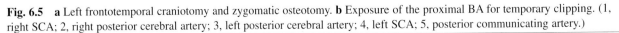

Fig. 6.5   a Left frontotemporal craniotomy and zygomatic osteotomy. **b** Exposure of the proximal BA for temporary clipping. (1, right SCA; 2, right posterior cerebral artery; 3, left posterior cerebral artery; 4, left SCA; 5, posterior communicating artery.)

to secure the proximal BA for temporary clipping (Fig. 6.5b). Under temporary clipping of the proximal BA for less than 3 minutes both proximal and distal portions of the neck of the aneurysm were dissected carefully from SCA and P1, respectively. Clipping of the aneurysm was performed with an 18 mm straight clip, but it was observed to be placed a little too deep. With a step-clipping technique (Kobayashi & Tanaka 1993), the first clip was adjusted to the right depth. Clipping was now complete on inspection. Except for mild left oculomotor paresis (which cleared in a few days) there was no postoperative problem.

Comments

We found the transcavernous extended pterional approach with preservation of the bridging temporal vein a good method to approach the proximal portion of the BA for temporary clipping. An alternative to this procedure would be a combined pterional and subtemporal approach. The subtemporal approach would have enabled a direct approach to the aneurysm and section of the tentorium could have allowed exposure of the proximal BA. However, the disadvantage would have been that as the aneurysm dome would have projected in the operating path, a premature rupture was possible during the dissection.

CASE 2 SCA Aneurysm, Buried in Clots

This 50-year-old male was seen at a local hospital immediately after suffering an SAH 6 weeks previously and was transferred to our hospital. The neurological condition was Hunt and Hess Grade 3. While he was undergoing the angiogram he bled again and worsened to Grade 4. The angiogram showed a left BA–SCA aneurysm which had become larger than that seen on angiography done on day 16 of SAH (Fig. 6.6a,b). The patient's condition somewhat improved after draining the cerebrospinal fluid via the lumbar route. Low-density areas were noticed on computed tomographic scan in both temporal lobes, probably as a result of vasospasm.

With the patient in the supine position, a left frontotemporal craniotomy was performed (Fig. 6.7a). Orbital rim osteotomy was done. The dura was opened and the sylvian fissure was separated. While dissecting the internal carotid terminal bifurcation it became necessary to further remove the lateral part of the orbital roof almost to the anterior clinoid process. As the patient had suffered repeated SAH, the interpeduncular cistern was found to be packed with hard organizing clots which made dissection here extremely difficult. Our plan was to first expose the basilar trunk and then to trace the right SCA and P1. This was successfully carried out. Exposure of the neck was difficult. The left posterior communicating artery was traced posteriorly to expose the origin of the left P1. Then, over the basilar bifurcation, the lateral side of the left SCA was finally exposed. The neck of the aneurysm was seen to be extremely thin. Doppler flowmeter indicated the location of the dome of the aneurysm. This procedure was performed entirely through the opticocarotid space (Fig. 6.7b). However, by this route the weak side of the aneurysm neck was exposed. Further dissection was made also from the left P1 side, where the neck seemed thicker. Dissection of the neck in the left SCA side was done finally. A small bleeding from the aneurysm occurred here. Under temporary clipping for about 3 minutes the neck of the aneurysm was clipped with a straight 1 cm clip. The bleeding first appeared from the neck of the aneurysm, but fortunately it stopped after clipping, indicating that the rupture had occurred from the body of the aneurysm. After confirming the top of the clip blade in a satisfactory position, the wound was closed. The orbital bone piece was replaced. The region of the anterior clinoid process was sealed with muscle and fascia. The postoperative angiogram shows complete obliteration of the aneurysm (Fig. 6.8b).

Comment

Orbitocranial craniotomy was effective as we did not need to retract the brain at all to see the mammillary body region. The hard organizing clots were difficult to deal with.

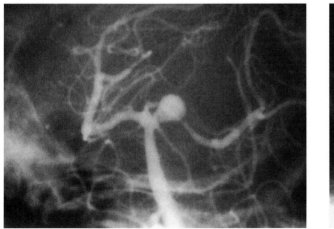
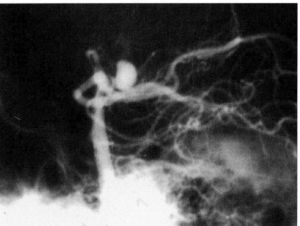

Fig. 6.6 Initial preoperative angiograms showing left BA–SCA aneurysm (day 16 post-SAH).

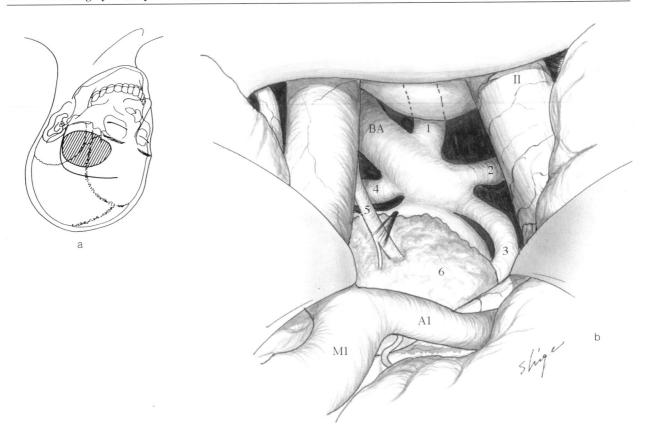

Fig. 6.7 **a** Left frontotemporal craniotomy. **b** Exposure of the aneurysm through the opticocarotid space. (1, right SCA; 2, right posterior cerebral artery; 3, left posterior cerebral artery; 4, left SCA; 5, left posterior communicating artery; 6, clots.)

References

Kobayashi S, Tanaka Y 1993 Aneurysm clip design, selection and application. In: Apuzzo MLJ (ed) Brain Surgery. Churchill Livingstone, Edinburgh

Marinkovic S, Gibo H 1993 The surgical anatomy of the perforating branches of the basilar artery. Neurosurgery 33: 80–87

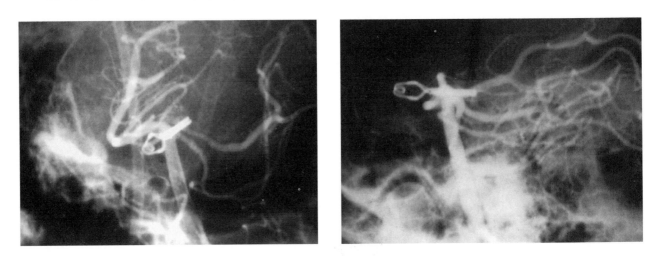

Fig. 6.8 Postoperative angiograms.

BA–SCA Aneurysm
Mamoru Taneda

A BA–SCA aneurysm is easily clippable in most cases, as compared with other aneurysms arising from the BA. Access to the aneurysm is easily possible without forceful brain retraction using either the pterional or subtemporal approach. There are usually a few small perforating arteries around the aneurysm. However, there are several problems in the operative technique that need to be emphasized. These aneurysms arise distal to the origin of the SCA. They very rarely arise from the inferior aspect of the SCA. They usually project laterally. Thus, these aneurysms lie between the SCA and posterior cerebral artery in most cases. Therefore, they have an intimate anatomical relationship with the oculomotor nerve, which is occasionally elevated and flattened by the aneurysm dome. The surgeon has to pay great attention to avoid oculomotor palsy during dissection and clipping of the aneurysm. Sometimes, the BA significantly deviates to the side of the aneurysm. In this instance, even a small aneurysm may be adherent to the oculomotor nerve. In three cases, the aneurysms were successfully operated on from the side opposite the aneurysms via a pterional approach. Those aneurysms were not covered by the oculomotor nerve in this approach, and the neck was exposed first and clipped without manipulating the oculomotor nerve.

However, in the usual case of a BA–SCA aneurysm, it is preferable to approach through a pterional craniotomy on the side of the fundus of the aneurysm. Although, with this approach, the dome of the aneurysm is not infrequently initially exposed, it is advantageous to safely dissect the aneurysm to free the SCA and posterior cerebral artery. If the aneurysmal sac is large, the BA is often hidden behind it. Using a narrow and fine spatula, the fundus has to be gently retracted and mobilized to expose the BA trunk and to prepare for possible placement of temporary clips. In some large aneurysms, application of a temporary clip to the BA may make clip application easier and safer.

The clip is, in most cases, introduced between the SCA and posterior cerebral artery, and it is closed slowly. There are two important things which should be avoided with greatest care. One is twisting or kinking of the BA, SCA, posterior cerebral and/or perforating arteries after clip application. The other is inclusion of perforating arteries between the clip blades. There are perforating branches arising from the posterior aspect of the basilar trunk. They are situated just behind the aneurysm neck and tend to be included by the tips of the clip blades. In addition, one or two perforating arteries frequently arise near the origin of the SCA. Thus, it is necessary to identify those perforators behind the aneurysm and the adjacent arteries before application of the clip.

In an aneurysm of lower position, the surgeon may use the subtemporal approach. It is important to pay attention not to injure the fourth cranial nerve.

Basilar trunk aneurysms

Shigeaki Kobayashi   Kazuhiro Hongo   Atul Goel

7

Basilar trunk aneurysms are relatively rare. The approach to the basilar trunk aneurysm has to be considered from two points:

1. the approach to the aneurysm neck and its clipping;
2. securing the proximal parent artery.

One can approach the basilar trunk aneurysm either by a subtemporal or a suboccipital route or by combining the two routes. No matter which route is adopted the cranial nerves are always located in the way. The fifth nerve is in the way during the subtemporal approach while the seventh and eighth nerves are in the way in the suboccipital approach. Some retraction of these nerves is necessary to expose the aneurysm, dissect around it and maneuver the clip into position. We have observed that the trigeminal nerve is much stronger (and safer) as regards sustaining retraction than the other cranial nerves in the region. The cochlear nerve is much weaker and does not tolerate retraction well. The facial nerve is relatively strong but its close relationship to the vestibular and cochlear nerves restricts the possibility of excessive retraction. The following approaches were considered important during surgical management.

SUBTEMPORAL (TRANSTENTORIAL), ANTERIOR TRANSPETROSAL APPROACH

The patient is placed in the lateral position. The vertex of the patient should be tilted down in order to lessen temporal lobe retraction. Usually an anterior subtemporal approach is taken, and the tentorium is cut posterior to the entry of the trochlear nerve in the tentorial dural fold. Addition of basal temporal exposure will depend on the location of the aneurysm, projection of its dome and the size of the aneurysm. Extension of the temporal craniotomy basally and transpetrosal approaches are discussed in Chapter 12 dealing with surgical approaches to the clivus. In general we do not find extensive transpetrosal approaches necessary. It is important to drill off Kawase's triangle (partial petrous apecectomy). This provides a wider space

horizontally as well as vertically to facilitate the subsequent procedure (anterior transpetrosal approach). As discussed previously (Sugita 1985), the pons can be retracted with our retractor system but, as is understandable, it is best to minimize retraction of the pons by utilizing basal exposures. Obtaining proximal control of the artery is more difficult with the subtemporal approach. One should check on the preoperative angiogram the perforating arteries in relationship to the aneurysm because by the subtemporal route the perforating arteries on the contralateral side of the aneurysm cannot be very well seen. It is especially so when the aneurysm is large. Lumbar drainage of cerebrospinal fluid (CSF) is important to reduce temporal lobe retraction. This can be performed by instituting spinal drainage and starting to remove the CSF after the dura is opened. Removing the CSF before opening the dura may cause a premature rupture of the aneurysm.

How far caudally one can reach by the subtemporal approach is a matter of debate. In our earlier publication (Sugita et al 1987) we reported that one can reach as low as 2.5 cm from the posterior clinoid process but in our present experience with skull basal exposure we have been able to reach more inferiorly.

SUBOCCIPITAL AND POSTERIOR TRANSPETROSAL APPROACH

Low-positioned basilar trunk aneurysms can be approached by the suboccipital route, avoiding the risk of damaging the temporal lobe by excessive retraction. However, this route has the disadvantage that the seventh and the eighth cranial nerves are in the way and also the basilar trunk is usually very deep in the field and retraction of the brain stem is necessary. Transpetrosal approaches are helpful in this regard. The presigmoid petrosal approach can be used for approaching the aneurysm, exposing the distal parent artery and dissecting and clipping of the aneurysm. In selected cases the presigmoid avenue can be used to approach the aneurysm while the actual clipping can be done from the retrosigmoid opening.

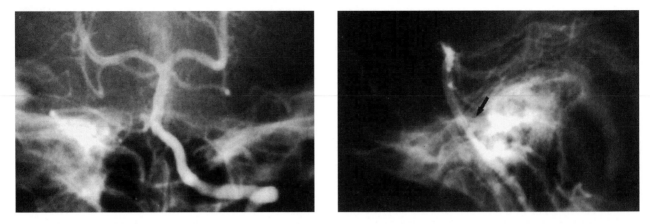

Fig. 7.1   Preoperative angiograms showing a small aneurysm at the origin of the AICA, 2.5 cm lower than the posterior clinoid process.

COMBINED SUPRA-AND INFRATENTORIAL TRANSPETROSAL APPROACH

For giant or large aneurysms with complex form, or some of the low-positioned basilar trunk aneurysms, a combined supra-and infratentorial transpetrosal approach can be adopted (see Chapter 8 on vertebral artery aneurysms).

CASE 1   Basilar Trunk Aneurysm

This 55-year-old female who suffered a subarachnoid hemorrhage (SAH) 2 weeks ago was admitted in Hunt and Hess Grade 1. The angiograms showed a small aneurysm 2.5 cm lower than the posterior clinoid process along the clivus, at the origin of the anterior inferior cerebellar artery (AICA) (Fig. 7.1).

With the patient in the lateral position, a left temporal

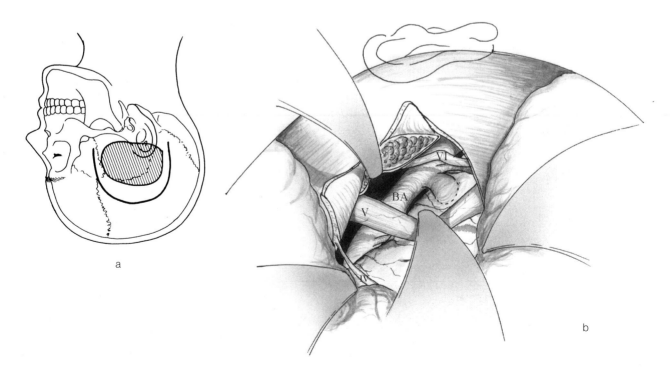

Fig. 7.2   a Left temporal craniotomy. **b** The aneurysm was projecting laterally and dorsally, with the dome buried in the pons.

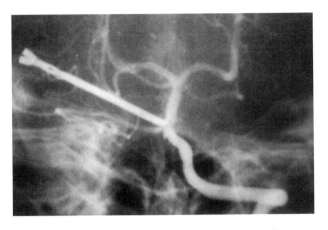

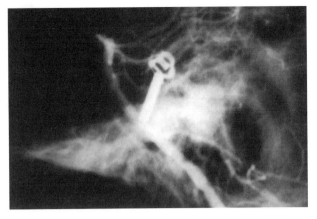

Fig. 7.3 Postoperative angiograms.

craniotomy was performed (Fig. 7.2a). After the dura was opened about 35 ml of CSF was drained from the lumbar route. The tentorial edge and the fourth nerve were identified and the tentorium was cut just posterior to the tentorial entry point of the fourth nerve. The trigeminal nerve and Meckel's cave were identified. With Meckel's cave as a landmark, an extradural approach was made to drill off the petrous apex in Kawase's triangle. The superior petrosal sinus was coagulated and cut. When seen intradurally, the trigeminal nerve was coursing obliquely in the center of the field. First, an approach was made in the space anterior to the trigeminal nerve (anterotrigeminal route). The basilar artery and the right P1 and superior cerebellar artery were exposed and identified, with the third nerve as a landmark. The aneurysm could not be seen by this approach. Then, an approach posterior to the trigeminal nerve (retrotrigeminal route) was made. The basilar trunk and the AICA and the aneurysm were found with the trigeminal nerve and pons directly retracted with a 2 mm spatula, whereby the structures were protected with thin Bemsheets. The aneurysm was projecting laterally and dorsally with the dome buried in the pons. The proximal and distal neck were dissected. Small perforators were originating nearby (Fig. 7.2b). They were protected when placing a clip. After several trials with different clips, the final clip chosen was a straight 25 mm long clip (no.

72), which was placed through the retrotrigeminal space. On exploration after clipping, the AICA and perforators appeared preserved. Postoperatively the patient had status epilepticus, but she has made a complete recovery. The postoperative angiogram showed a satisfactory clipping (Fig. 7.3).

Comments

1. The subtemporal approach with drilling of Kawase's triangle provided exposure of the aneurysm at 25 mm from the dorsum sellae; we could go down further to 3 cm. Direct retraction of the pons was still necessary.

2. A similar case of basilar trunk aneurysm located slightly lower than the present case (Fig. 7.4) could be clipped by the same approach. In this case, the aneurysm was clipped in the caudal side of the abducens nerve (Fig. 7.5).

References

Sugita K 1985 Microneurosurgical Atlas. Springer, Berlin pp 108–115

Sugita K, Kobayashi S, Takemae T et al 1987 Aneurysm of the basilar artery trunk. Journal of Neurosurgery 66: 500–505

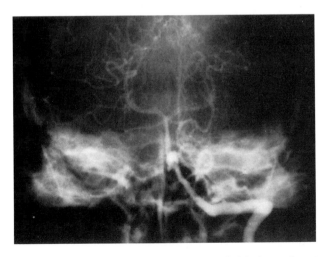

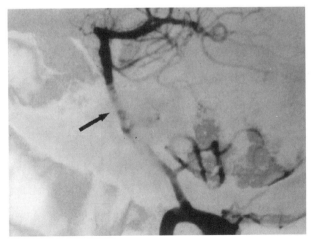

Fig. 7.4 a Basilar trunk aneurysm located slightly lower than that shown in Figures 7.1–7.3.

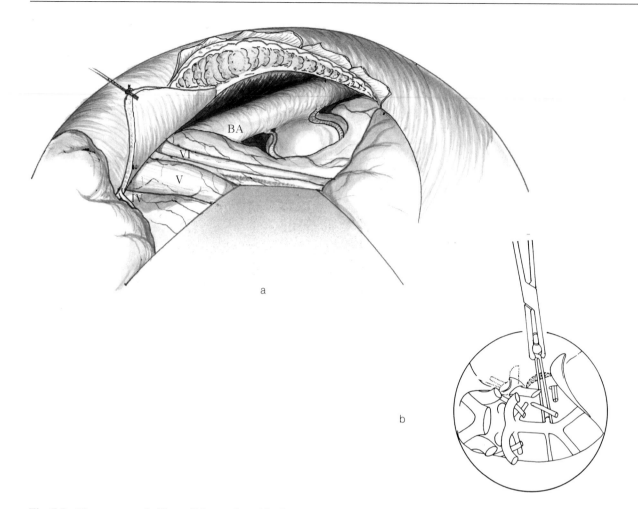

Fig. 7.5   The aneurysm in Figure 7.4 was clipped in the caudal side of the abducens nerve.

Basilar Trunk Aneurysm Surgery
Dae Hee Han, Chang-Wan Oh

Even in this era of microneurosurgery, the approach to aneurysms of the lower basilar trunk remains a formidable challenge. Historically, Dandy (1944) described a suboccipital approach to this area, but the postoperative results were often unacceptable, with a high incidence of damage to the lower cranial nerves and brain stem (Jamieson 1964). In 1965, a subtemporal transtentorial approach was described by Drake (1965, 1968), with better operative results. In some cases, however, severe temporal lobe hemorrhage and swelling occurred due to injury to the vein of Labbé or excessive retraction of the temporal lobe. In addition, with this approach, the surgical field is restricted and does not extend low enough because the petrous ridge is in the way. To overcome this problem, Sugita recommended a direct retraction of the trigeminal nerve, the pons and the aneurysm with drilling of the pyramidal edge (Sugita et al

1987). This modification facilitates visualization of the basilar artery trunk aneurysm located no more than 25 mm below the top of the posterior clinoid process. Kawase et al (1985) proposed an extradural subtemporal approach with anterior pyramidal drilling to improve the surgeon's line of sight to the lower basilar artery. These procedures, however, still provide a restricted avenue to this area, and have not been accepted widely.

The far lateral inferior suboccipital approach is a modification of the conventional unilateral suboccipital approach for aneurysms of the vertebral artery, the vertebrobasilar junction and the proximal basilar trunk (Heros 1986). This approach is good for aneurysms of the vertebral artery, with excellent exposure of its entire intracranial course to the vertebrobasilar junction, entailing minimal or no retraction of the medulla. However, it provides too long an operative distance and a restricted corridor to reach aneurysms of the lower basilar trunk, including the vertebrobasilar junction. To approach these aneurysms, retraction on the medulla oblongata is sometimes necessary and due to the bilateral vertebral arterial supply a proximal control is not possible. Possible injury to the lower cranial nerves is another concern. We have tried this approach in two patients with lower basilar trunk aneurysms, one at the vertebrobasilar junction and the other at the basilar–AICA junction, but failed to clip the aneurysmal neck in both cases. In our experience, the long distance to the aneurysm and the narrow operative field hampered appropriate small neck clipping.

Another approach to this location without retraction of the brain or cranial nerves is the transoral transclival route. Sano et al (1966) utilized this approach for vertebrobasilar artery aneurysms. The transoral approach was not adopted widely due to several serious disadvantages, including long distance to the lesion, restricted avenue, and high risk of postoperative CSF leakage and meningitis. We sometimes use this approach, but only for lesions of the clivus or the upper cervical spine.

To overcome the challenge of lesions at the anterior lower posterior fossa, several modifications of the petrosal approach have been described, including transcochlear, translabyrinthine and retrolabyrinthine approaches (Spetzler et al 1992). Of these, the presigmoid retrolabyrinthine approach described by Al-Mefty et al (1988, Al-Mefty 1993) has the following advantages over the other approaches:

1. There is minimal cerebellar and temporal lobe retraction.
2. The operative distance to the clivus is short.
3. The surgeon has a direct line of sight to the lesion and the anterior and lateral aspects of the brain stem.
4. The neural and otological structures, including cochlea, vestibule and facial nerve, are preserved.
5. The transverse and sigmoid sinuses, as well as the vein of Labbé and the basal occipital veins, are preserved.
6. Multiple axes for dissection are available.
7. In petroclival tumors, the vascular supply can be interrupted early in the procedures.

Reported complications of this approach include hemiparesis, quadriparesis, trigeminal nerve injury (facial pain and corneal anesthesia), facial palsy, hearing disturbances, CSF leakage, pseudomeningocele and pulmonary embolism. Other transpetrosal procedures, such as translabyrinthine, transchochlear, transsigmoid and various infratemporal approaches, provide a wider operative field than the presigmoid retrolabyrinthine approach (Giannotta & Maceri 1988, Sen & Sekhar 1990, Spetzler et al 1992). However, these approaches entail more destructive procedures requiring sacrifice of some neural functions, such as hearing, and carry higher risk of complications such as facial palsy, venous infarction and CSF leakage.

We have utilized the retrolabyrinthine approach in two cases of lower basilar trunk aneurysms, one at the vertebrobasilar junction and the other one at the basilar–AICA junction. This procedure provided excellent exposure of the entire basilar artery allowing proximal temporary clipping, short operative distance and ample space for dissection and clipping of the aneurysmal neck in these two patients. On the other hand, in another case with vertebrobasilar junction aneurysm, we failed to obtain enough space with the retrolabyrinthine approach. The retrolabyrinthine petrosal bone of the patient was unusually narrow and the aneurysm could not be well exposed. In this case, we should have drilled off the labyrinth down to the jugular fossa to fully expose the aneurysm.

According to our experience, we conclude that the presigmoid transpetrosal approach is excellent for aneurysms of the lower basilar trunk. The operative distance is short, there is enough space for dissection and clipping of the aneurysmal neck, safe proximal control of the parent artery is possible and there is less risk of complications. The retrolabyrinthine approach should be tried first to preserve hearing, but in cases with a narrow retrolabyrinthine space, the labyrinth should be included in petrosectomy to gain adequate space for aneurysmal neck clipping. This technique is very useful particularly in surgery carried out in acute stage.

References

Al-Mefty O, Fox J L, Smith R R 1988 Petrosal approach for petroclival meningiomas. Neurosurgery 22: 510–517

Al-Mefty O 1993 Petrosal approach to clival tumors. In: Sekhar L N, Janecka I P (eds) Surgery of cranial base tumours. Raven Press, New York, pp 307–315

Dandy W E 1944 Intracranial arterial aneurysms. Comstock, Ithaca, N Y

Drake C G 1965 Surgical treatment of ruptured aneurysms of the basilar artery: experience with 14 cases. Journal of Neurosurgery 23: 457–473

Drake C G 1968 The surgical treatment of aneurysms of the basilar artery. Journal of Neurosurgery 29: 436–446

Giannotta S L, Maceri D R 1988 Retrolabyrinthine transsigmoid approach to basilar trunk and vertebrobasilar artery junction aneurysms. Journal of Neurosurgery 69: 461–466

Heros R C 1986 Lateral suboccipital approach for vertebral and vertebrobasilar artery lesions. Journal of Neurosurgery 64: 559–562

Jamieson K G 1964 Aneurysms of the vertebrobasilar system: surgical intervention in 19 cases. Journal of Neurosurgery 21: 781–797

Kawase T, Toya S, Shiobara R et al 1985 Transpetrosal approach for aneurysms of the lower basilar artery. Journal of Neurosurgery 63: 857–861

Sano K, Jinbo M, Saito I 1966 Vertebrobasilar aneurysms with special reference to the transpharyngeal approach to the basilar aneurysm. No To Shinkei 18: 1197-1203 (in Japanese)

Sen C N, Sekhar L N 1990 The subtemporal and preauricular infratemporal approach to intradural structures ventral to the brain stem. Journal of Neurosurgery 73: 345–354

Spetzler R F, Daspit P, Pappas C T E 1992 The combined supra- and infratentorial approach for lesions of the petrous and clival regions: experiences with 46 cases. Journal of Neurosurgery 76: 588–599

Sugita K, Kobayashi S, Takemae T et al 1987 Aneurysms of the basilar artery trunk. Journal of Neurosurgery 66: 500–505

Operation on Mid-basilar Aneurysm
Hirotoshi Sano

Management of basilar trunk aneurysms is difficult because of their deep location, narrow operating space and their proximity to important perforating arteries.

There are eight approaches for a lower basilar aneurysm, namely:

1. transclinoid transcavernous approach (Dolenc et al 1987);
2. anterior temporal approach (Sano et al 1966);
3. subtemporal approach (Drake 1979);
4. subtemporal transtentorial approach (Tanabe et al 1994);
5. anterior transpetrosal approach (Kawase et al 1985);
6. presigmoid approach (Giannotta & Marceri 1988);
7. transoral approach (Hayakawa et al 1981);
8. lateral suboccipital approach or transcondylar approach (Bertalanffy et al 1995).

The former three approaches are suitable for low-situated basilar bifurcation aneurysms, especially those located more than 10 mm below the posterior clinoid process. The transclinoid transcavernous approach (Dolenc et al 1987) is good for basilar top aneurysms. The anterior clinoid process is removed extradurally following the usual frontotemporal craniotomy. The dura is opened parallel to the sylvian fissure. The anterior medial trigone of the cavernous sinus is opened and one can obtain a wider operative view than with the pterional approach. The key point to removing the anterior clinoid process is to cut the tip of the dura of the superior orbital fissure.

The subtemporal approach (Drake 1979) is good for aneurysms projecting posteriorly. The anterior temporal approach is an intermediate approach between the pterional and the subtemporal approaches. It was originally described in 1966 as the temporopolar approach (Sano et al 1966). In the original approach the temporal pole was sectioned to obtain a wider operative view. Using microsurgical techniques the sylvian fissure is opened and the temporal lobe is retracted without sectioning the bridging vein by dissecting the sphenoparietal sinus with the dura from the bone. The combination of the transclinoid transcavernous approach and anterior temporal approach is convenient.

The subtemporal transtentorial approach (Tanabe et al 1994) enables exposure up to 20 mm below the posterior clinoid process. The fourth nerve runs just below the tentorium, and the third nerve is widely visible in the operative field. Therefore there is the possibility of injury to the third and fourth nerves in this approach.

I prefer the anterior transpetrosal approach (Kawase et al 1985). For this approach, temporal craniotomy is performed following a reversed U-shaped skin incision from the zygoma to the retroauricular region. The posterior medial triangle (Kawase's triangle) of the petrosal bone is then drilled extradurally. One can see the petrosal sinus and the dura of the posterior fossa. The dura of the temporal lobe is incised to cross the petrosal sinus after coagulation. The petrosal sinus is cut posteriorly because it is easier to coagulate it in this location. The trigeminal nerve, which traverses in proximity to the sinus, is exposed. The posterior fossa dura is then cut and one can see the pons, abducens nerve, basilar artery with pontine branches, AICA, vertebral union, bilateral vertebral arteries and ipsilateral posterior inferior cerebellar artery (PICA). One can see from the jugular tuberculum to the basilar top after the tentorium is sectioned. The width of drilling of the petrosal bone is approximately 12 mm. This approach provides an anterolateral view of the basilar artery. Fenestrated clips should be applied to reconstruct the basilar artery if the aneurysm projects posteriorly. Reconstruction of the parent artery is not difficult in this case; however, preservation of pontine perforators is important. The usual type of clip (non-fenestrated type) can be applied if the aneurysm projects anteriorly. Selection of the side of approach is important. In the case of a large or giant aneurysm, one should select the neck side (contralateral side to the dome) to approach the aneurysm. In the case of a small aneurysm, one can select the dome side to approach the aneurysm. Arterial reconstruction is easier from this side of approach. One may see the whole basilar artery by the presigmoid approach. However, this approach is a posterior one; the basilar artery can be seen through many cranial nerves (V, VI, VII, VIII) and it is rather difficult to reconstruct the basilar artery without any cranial nerve damage.

The transoral approach (Hayakawa et al 1981) may be

a limited approach and applicable in only selected cases.

The lateral suboccipital or transcondylar approach (Bertalanffy et al 1995) is good for vertebral artery (VA)-PICA aneurysms and some of VA union aneurysms; however, it is difficult by this approach to see and manage the mid-basilar artery or AICA region.

These eight approaches have their own advantages and disadvantages. One must select the best approach for each case. Helical three-dimensional computed tomography is useful for preoperative simulation. One can visualize the operative view and easily decide the approach.

References

Bertalanffy H, Gilsbach J M, Mayfrank L et al 1995 Planning and surgical strategies for early management of vertebral artery and vertebrobasilar junction aneurysms. Acta Neurochirurgica (Wien) 134: 60–65

Drake C G 1979 The treatment of aneurysms of the posterior circulation. Clinical Neurosurgery 26: 96–144

Dolenc V V, Skrap M, Sustersic J et al 1987 A transcavernous transsellar approach to the basilar tip aneurysms. British Journal of Neurosurgery 1: 251–259

Giannotta S L, Marceri D R 1988 Retrolabyrinthine transsigmoid approach to basilar trunk and vertebrobasilar artery junction aneurysms: technical note. Journal of Neurosurgery 69: 461–466

Hayakawa T, Kamikawa K, Ohnishi T et al 1981 Prevention of postoperative complication after a transoral transclival approach to basilar aneurysm. Journal of Neurosurgery 54: 699–703

Kawase T, Toya S, Shiobara R et al 1985 Transpetrosal approach for aneurysms of the lower basilar artery. Journal of Neurosurgery 63: 857–861

Sano K, Jinbo M, Saito I 1966 Vertebro-basilar aneurysms, with special reference to the transpharyngeal approach to the basilar artery aneurysm. No To Shinkei 18: 1197–1203

Tanabe M, Yamasaki T, Hori T 1994 Subtemporal transtentorial approach for high position vertebral artery–posterior inferior cerebellar artery aneurysm: a case report. Surgery for Cerebral Stroke 22: 5–8 (in Japanese)

Basilar Trunk Aneurysm Surgery
H Hunt Batjer

Basilar trunk aneurysms represent a surprisingly heterogeneous collection of arterial abnormalities which share unique problems regarding their neurological implications and the techniques required for surgical exposure. These lesions collectively may produce neurological complications including the spectrum ranging from isolated cranial neuropathy, brain stem deficits, obstructive hydrocephalus and subarachnoid hemorrhage. I will attempt to group these lesions according to their pathophysiology and their anatomical location as these particular features have extreme relevance to the types of direct and indirect therapy which may be considered.

Aneurysm Configuration: The first category of basilar trunk aneurysms and the most common in my experience is the saccular aneurysm. These lesions may occur at any site from the vertebral confluens up to the basilar apex and are typically associated with either arterial anomalies such as fenestrations, major branching points, or perforating vessel origins. In addition, a number of upper basilar trunk lesions projecting anteriorly with no apparent relationship to a vessel origin may represent the vestigial termination of a trigeminal artery. These lesions commonly produce subarachnoid hemorrhage or are discovered as incidental findings in patients with SAH from another anterior or posterior circulation aneurysm. Treatment is usually definitive clip ligation of the aneurysm with preservation of associated branches and

the operative approaches will be discussed below as regards actual anatomical location.

Dolichoectasia is a condition most commonly found in the distal vertebral arteries and proximal basilar trunk. Dolichoectasia may also be found in the anterior circulation although in my experience the posterior circulation is most commonly involved. These 'aneurysms' typically produce symptoms due to mass effect. The vessel involved may become quite large and displace cranial nerves, leading to isolated cranial neuropathy, and as the disease progresses may distort the brain stem to either a minor or major extent. Not uncommonly, symptoms may result from thrombotic events within the lumen of these ectatic segments. Thrombotic material may occlude perforating arteries or may embolize and produce top of the basilar syndromes. I have also seen numerous examples of patients who had dolichoectasia of their lower basilar trunk and whose brain stem symptoms were very likely ischemic as the thickening of the arterial wall and atheromatous changes occluded the origins of vital pontine perforating vessels. Unfortunately, these ectatic segments can also become extremely attenuated at specific sites and SAH is an unusual but highly dangerous complication. Mass effect symptoms can occasionally be improved by innovative operative procedures. Patients with trigeminal neuralgia or other compressive cranial neuropathy can occasionally be benefited by placing Merocell or other padding material between the arterial tissue and the involved cranial nerve. Additionally it is occasionally possible to place a fenestrated clip with the actual blade removed around the artery and suture the clip itself to the clival dura, thus displacing the involved arterial segment from the cranial nerve and the brain stem itself. Over the years we have also tried proximal ligation or resection of a distal vertebral that was involved in an attempt to accomplish this same goal. The outcome of patients treated with dolichoectasia with mass effect symptoms (as well as ischemic complications) has been relatively poor. While it is attractive to consider intraluminal thrombolytic therapy or anticoagulation for patients with thrombotic complications, one must keep in mind the very definite possibility that attenuated portions may be present which are quite capable of producing SAH in the setting of thrombolysis or anticoagulation. All things considered, dolichoectasia of the lower basilar trunk remains an extremely morbid and difficult disease to manage.

Aneurysms reaching giant size may have a predominantly saccular form or may be fusiform. A number of lesions, particularly of the lower basilar trunk, may also have a saccular component together with a fusiform origin or termination leading into the parent trunk. These hybrid forms may produce SAH, thrombotic disease or mass effect. The therapeutic strategies that have proven to be of benefit include definitive clipping of the saccular and ruptured component, with wrapping or reinforcement of the fusiform lesion. Hunterian ligation for giant aneurysms in this region remains a viable alternative if adequate collaterals are either congenitally present or can be established by surgical revascularization.

Temporary Arterial Occlusion: Temporary arterial occlusion should be considered in most, if not all, aneurysms of the basilar trunk being attacked surgically. In treating small saccular aneurysms, while temporary arterial occlusion may not be truly necessary to allow definitive clipping, the morbidity associated with intraoperative rupture during dissection or closure of a clip is so severe that the use of temporary clips seems to be a very helpful adjunct. Temporary clipping is needed for the purposes of aneurysm decompression and vessel reconstruction in large and giant aneurysms with great regularity. Patients with adequate posterior communicating arteries may tolerate quite protracted temporary arterial occlusion of the basilar trunk but our experience has been that the safe interval of iatrogenic ischemia for lesions in this area using brain protective strategies is between 15 and 20 minutes. Bench research in canine brain stem ischemia in our laboratories has demonstrated that thiopental and the other barbiturates are probably the most effective pharmacological agents that we have available and also that hypothermia may be an extremely helpful adjunct. For the most complex lesions circulatory arrest procedures should be considered due to the decompression achieved by the procedure and the additional time, up to 1 hour, afforded

by the use of profound hypothermia at 16°C.

Trial Arterial Occlusion: Recent progress in interventional radiology has allowed the use of non-detachable balloons in the performance of trial arterial occlusion analogous to the commonly performed procedures for the cervical internal carotid. Anticoagulation is typically used during these procedures. A trial occlusion, with an awake patient, of approximately 30 minutes should be adequate to assess collateral flow. While tolerance of balloon occlusion gives very helpful evidence that adequate collaterals exist should basilar occlusion be entertained as definitive therapy, failure to tolerate such trial occlusion may not accurately reflect distal hemodynamics. The size of the balloon itself during inflation can occlude the orifice of numerous perforating vessels, leading to focal brain stem ischemic dysfunction that can be quite difficult to distinguish from upper basilar ischemia. Therefore, a tolerated trial occlusion yields very helpful information but a failed occlusion test must be evaluated very carefully and, if at all possible, a detailed neurological assessment must be performed very quickly prior to balloon deflation.

Proximal and Distal Control: While the early acquisition of proximal and distal arterial control is a fundamental component of all aneurysm surgery, the importance of early assurance of definitive vascular control is heightened in lesions of the basilar trunk. Premature rupture can be extremely difficult to deal with due to the deep exposure and the eloquence of surrounding neurovascular anatomy that can be obscured in a bloody field. Therefore, regardless of the anatomical site being attacked the surgeon is obliged to plan the operative procedure such that wide exposure is obtained and early acquisition of proximal and subsequently distal control achieved.

Location and Specific Operative Exposure: For the purposes of this discussion three general locations will be considered: the vertebral confluens or basilar origin, mid-basilar trunk, and upper basilar trunk. Each anatomical site is unique regarding the surgical exposures which have been found adequate to manage the various types of aneurysms.

Aneurysms of the vertebral confluens should be studied carefully angiographically to determine if there is an associated anomaly of the proximal basilar artery such as a fenestration and to determine on the lateral, subtracted angiogram the height of the lesion as regards the bony clivus. Typically vertebral confluens aneurysms are located either at the level of the lower third of the clivus or at the junction of the lower and middle thirds. They are also typically eccentrically located due to the asymmetry of the vertebral arteries, which seems to be contributory toward the formation of aneurysms at this site. Typically a standard suboccipital craniectomy with wide lateral exposure with the head in the lateral position is most successful for these lesions. If an aneurysm is displaced unilaterally, my preference is to approach from the side of the aneurysm itself. After wide dural opening, proximal control unilaterally can be achieved at the level of the spinal fibers of the eleventh cranial nerve. Once that landmark has been noted, dissection should be performed to minimally dissect the important tenth nerve fibers entering the jugular foramen. With minimal manipulation of these fibers the dissection can be deepened just superior to the jugular foramen and the ninth nerve fibers and deepened along the ipsilateral vertebral to identify the contralateral vertebral artery. Dissection in this fashion minimizes the risk of postoperative aspiration. Once the contralateral vertebral is seen and isolated for potential clipping, the direction proceeds distally in the space between the ninth nerve inferiorly and the seventh and eighth nerve superiorly. The definitive portion of the procedure is dictated by the regional anatomy and the type of aneurysm under attack.

Mid-basilar trunk aneurysms are historically the most difficult to expose. These lesions may originate from the origin of the AICA or in their giant forms from perforating origins. Not infrequently fusiform variants may be encountered. Recent experience would suggest that a critical portion of the preoperative evaluation concerns the level of the clivus involved on the lateral unsubtracted view and the pattern of venous sinus drainage noted during the anterior circulation injections. Typical surgical approaches which optimize laterally and bony exposure are achieved above and below the level of the transverse and sigmoid sinuses. A formal mastoidectomy is performed and the sigmoid sinus is widely exposed, with care to avoid inner ear structures and the facial nerve. Not infrequently aggressive bony exposure anterior to the sigmoid sinus can allow an infratentorial and supratentorial dural opening which is extended to divide the superior petrosal sinus. The microscope is then used to divide the tentorium in parallel to the petrous pyramid to the level of the tentorial incisura just posterior to the insertion of the fourth cranial nerve. In unruptured aneurysms this presigmoid approach is usually more than adequate to expose the full basilar trunk in the middle third of the clivus and the lower portion of the upper third of the clivus. For ruptured lesions it has been my preference to divide the sigmoid sinus sparing the vein of Labbé if the superior sagittal sinus and torcular drain adequately contralaterally. This true lateral approach to the mid-basilar trunk results in definitive arterial exposure without brain stem retraction.

Aneurysms of the upper basilar trunk may typically project either posteriorly or anteriorly and only rarely do they project laterally. One could also include in this designation very low-lying superior cerebellar aneurysms associated with a very low basilar bifurcation. Particular scrutiny should be given to the lateral unsubtracted arteriogram to determine the relationship of the aneurysm neck to the sellar floor. Aneurysms located below the mid-sellar depth are quite difficult to expose through a pterional approach. My preference has been to expose these lesions from a non-dominant, subtemporal

procedure through a temporal craniotomy with medial to lateral division of the tentorium posterior to the insertion of the fourth cranial nerve. The resultant exposure is limited somewhat by the contents of Meckel's cave but the relevant anatomy can virtually always be dissected from this viewpoint. In very unusual cases associated with a very high basilar bifurcation, an upper basilar trunk lesion can occasionally be exposed through a pterional route. A helpful landmark to determine whether this will be feasible or not is the mid-sellar depth. The pterional view gives a beautiful demonstration of anatomy at and above the mid-sellar depth. This exposure can be extended somewhat by conversion to a 'half-and-half' view with displacement of the uncus.

GDC Coils: Due to the inherent surgical difficulty in accessing and definitively occluding numerous lesions of the basilar trunk, GDC coils have been felt to offer a striking therapeutic benefit. North American experience with GDC coils to date would suggest that coil placement in lesions of the basilar trunk is quite feasible but that complete occlusion of the aneurysm is obtainable in a striking minority of cases and is virtually never accomplished in the large broad-based and giant aneurysms. Small aneurysms with small necks can be definitively occluded in the early phase in approximately two-thirds of cases and the likelihood of complete obliteration decreases markedly as the complexity of the aneurysm increases. Recurrence of aneurysm following GDC coil placement is a major concern and also increases markedly in likelihood as the size and complexity of the aneurysm increase. It should also be noted that follow-up on patients so treated to date is quite brief. It is my opinion that the incidence of recurrence of basilar trunk and other aneurysms will be extremely high as these patients are followed up for 5–10 years.

Therefore, it is my feeling that endovascular therapy should be entertained in three specific clinical situations: (1) saccular aneurysms in poor-grade SAH patients; (2) saccular aneurysms in patients with prohibitive medical complications such as acute myocardial infarction; (3) aneurysms found to be untreatable by experienced cerebrovascular surgeons. The use of GDC coil placement in poor-grade patients following SAH appears to be a very valuable strategy as a palliative maneuver. The interventional radiologist can treat the ruptured lesion with the luxury of not having to achieve definitive occlusion. Occlusion of the majority of the fundus should protect against subsequent hemorrhage and allow medical or interventional treatment of vasospasm should it develop. If the patient recovers from acute illness, delayed angiography can be performed 3 or 4 weeks later and a surgical procedure entertained at that time.

Summary: Basilar trunk aneurysms are diverse in their anatomical characteristics as well as their location within the cranial vault. Technical misadventure is extremely unforgiving due to the vital nature of surrounding neurovascular anatomy. In general the three above-mentioned operative exposures provide excellent access to the overwhelming majority of lesions and, in the peculiar high-lying lesions, a variant of the pterional view may also be employed. It is my opinion that these difficult and morbid aneurysms should be treated by surgeons experienced in cerebrovascular surgery and in centers with access to skilled and experienced endovascular therapists.

Vertebral artery aneurysms

Shigeaki Kobayashi Kazuhiro Hongo Atul Goel

8

The surgical strategy for vertebral artery aneurysms depends on the location of the aneurysm on the vertebral artery, its size and its nature (saccular, dissecting, fusiform, giant thrombosed), dominance of the involved vertebral artery and other factors. The symptoms are usually those related either to subarachnoid hemorrhage, mass lesion or ischemia, or rarely patients present with hemifacial spasms and trigeminal neuralgia. For a saccular aneurysm clip occlusion of the neck is advocated. For dissecting aneurysms, proximal ligation by clip or by a balloon or trapping of the aneurysm can be performed (Zhang et al 1994). For a fusiform aneurysm clipping can be performed (Sugita et al 1988). For the giant aneurysm or giant thrombosed aneurysm, special techniques and approaches should be considered especially from the point of view of reducing the mass effect (Hopkins et al 1983, Wakui et al 1992). Preoperative angiographic study is important in determining whether the aneurysm can be clip occluded. The exact location and size of the neck in relation to branching arteries need to be adequately assessed, more particularly to the posterior inferior cerebellar artery (PICA). Balloon occlusion test may be performed during the angiographic study. The exact nature of a given vertebral aneurysm is often difficult to determine on the basis of angiography or even at surgery.

APPROACH TO THE ANEURYSM

Usually a lateral suboccipital approach is chosen. On the basis of the preoperative study of the angiograms, the deviation of the neck from the midline and the height of the aneurysm from the foramen magnum level are important factors in deciding whether a regular lateral suboccipital craniotomy or a modified lateral approach such as a far lateral approach or transpetrosal approach would be necessary. The displacements of the brain stem and lower cranial nerves should be adequately analyzed so as to avoid damage to these important structures. A far lateral approach is useful in avoiding or minimizing handling of cranial nerves and retraction of the brain stem.

Unilateral lateral suboccipital approach

For a small-sized and laterally located aneurysm, the usual lateral suboccipital craniotomy with partial removal of the foramen magnum is sufficient. The patient is positioned in a lateral 'park bench' position. During this position the head should be elevated so that the surgical field is higher than the patient's heart level. The neck should not be excessively flexed or laterally rotated so as to avoid obstruction of the jugular venous flow. Skin incision could be either S-shaped, reverse U-shaped or a linear incision depending on the location and size of the aneurysm. After opening the dura the proximal vertebral artery is secured and the aneurysm is exposed. Care should be taken not to injure the filaments of the lower cranial nerves. The origin of the PICA is dissected in order to establish its relation to the aneurysm. The hypoglossal nerve is also exposed and its location ascertained. The segment of the vertebral artery distal to the aneurysm is then exposed. In small-sized saccular aneurysms regular or ring clips are usually sufficient.

Far lateral approach

For most large or medially located vertebral artery aneurysms a far lateral approach is necessary. The laterality of the bone exposure depends on the nature of the aneurysm. Medially and superiorly located aneurysms require additional lateral exposure. The patient's position is basically the same as in the unilateral suboccipital approach. The skin incision is made either in a large J-shaped, S-shaped or paramedian straight fashion. The occipital muscles are incised and reflected laterally as much as possible to obtain an operative view from a lateral perspective. Condyle removal is rarely necessary and only a posterior third of it may be removed. In such a case, when dealing with the aneurysm intradurally, the aneurysm dome and the neck are often hidden by the bulge of the jugular tubercle, making it difficult to dissect and clip. The jugular tubercle is removed as much as needed.

Transpetrosal approach

For giant aneurysms of the vertebral artery, the transpetrosal approach is used. This can be combined with the far lateral approach. The far lateral approach enables proximal control of the parent artery (and the contralateral vertebral artery) and also exposing the caudal side of the aneurysm. The posterior petrosal approach, by drilling the mastoid process and whenever necessary partial or complete labyrinthectomy, may be done to obtain a presigmoid avenue for access to the distal parent artery. With some large and distal type aneurysms, working space for dissecting and clipping of the aneurysm could be obtained by the help of a combined supra- and infratentorial approach.

CASE 1 Giant Vertebral Artery Aneurysm

This 53-year-old male noticed numbness of the right hand and fingers a year ago. Six months ago he felt numbness in the sole of the right foot and left hand. Recently he noted numbness of the right hand and hypesthesia of the parieto-occipital region associated with severe nuchal pain. Computed tomographic (CT) scan showed a large enhancing mass in the posterior fossa (Fig. 8.1a). Angiography revealed a 26 mm aneurysm arising from the left vertebral artery and pressing the medulla posteriorly (Fig. 8.1b,c). Both vertebral arteries opacified equally. At the time of balloon occlusion test of the vertebral artery, the patient developed a small infarct in the region of the left thalamus from which he developed transient right hemiparesis which lasted for several days.

With the patient in the prone position, a reverse J-shaped skin incision was made. A left suboccipital craniectomy extending to the foramen magnum with removal of the C1 lamina was performed (Fig. 8.2a). The left lateral edge of the foramen magnum was substantially removed to view the anterior surface of the medulla. On opening the dura special care was taken to avoid untoward prolapse of the medulla which had been thinned and pushed posteriorly. The aneurysm was immediately seen on the left side of the thinned medulla. The proximal and distal vertebral arteries were exposed. The proximal intracranial vertebral artery was rather short. The distal vertebral artery was in the depth and the PICA was originating about 6 mm away from the distal neck, as we had anticipated from the preoperative angiogram. Securing the vertebral artery extradurally between the C1 lamina and the foramen magnum was attempted but it was difficult and unsuccessful because it had been buried in the fibrous soft tissue. We decided to go ahead with an intradural procedure. A bolus of 5000 units of heparin was given intravenously. The vertebral artery was temporarily clipped both proximally and distally to the aneurysm with Sugita no. 1 clips. Cessation of the intraluminal flow was confirmed with a Doppler flowmeter. The aneurysm was punctured with the aneurysm puncture system (Kyoshima et al 1992) (Fig. 8.2b). After 5 ml of blood was suctioned the aneurysm became soft and flaccid. It was easily dissected from the medulla and the surrounding tissue.

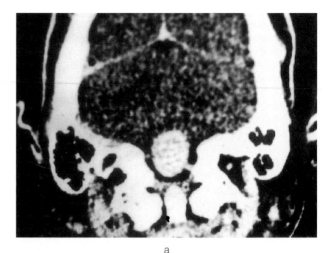

a

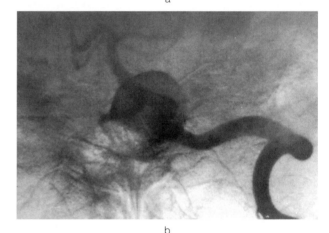

b

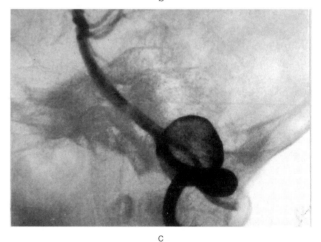

c

Fig. 8.1 **a** CT scan showing a large enhancing mass in the posterior fossa. **b,c** Angiograms showing a 26 mm left vertebral artery.

The aneurysm neck appeared to be about 1 cm in length. First a 19 mm straight clip was applied which did not occlude the neck completely. Before applying a longer clip, the aneurysm was flushed by releasing the distal and then the proximal clip. A 25 mm straight clip was then applied. On releasing the temporary clips, it was found that the clipping was incomplete, apparently

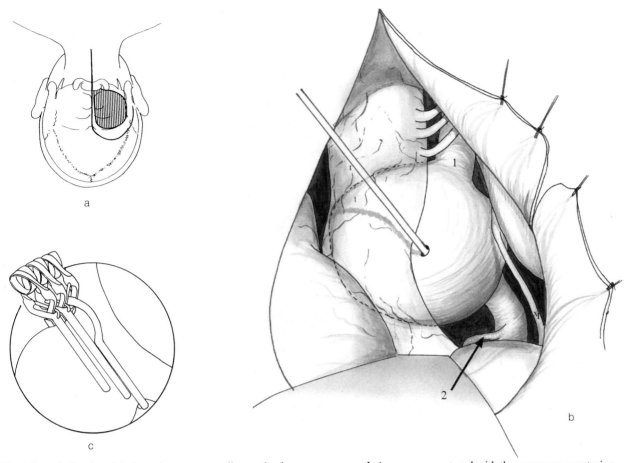

Fig. 8.2 **a** Left suboccipital craniectomy extending to the foramen magnum. **b** Aneurysm punctured with the aneurysm puncturing system. **c** Nos. 15, 18 and 37 clips in parallel. (1, vertebral artery; 2, PICA.)

leaving the distal part of the neck incompletely occluded. A couple of application trials with straight clips were unsuccessful. After further dissection of the deepest (distal) portion of the aneurysm, a longest (no. 37) ring clip was applied in the deeper portion and then a straight (no. 18) clip was applied in parallel fashion to the dome side to occlude the shallower portion of the aneurysm. Prior to closure of the second clip, the aneurysm was flushed by releasing the proximal temporary clip. In order to prevent slippage of the second clip to the dome side, another 15 mm straight clip (no.15) was applied to the dome, parallel to the second clip (Fig. 8.2c). The temporary clip was now released. Clipping was now complete. The patency of the parent artery was confirmed by the Doppler flowmeter. The postoperative course was uneventful.

Comments

1. Use of the puncture system was successful in this case to obtain decompression of the aneurysm. Heparin was used to prevent distal embolization from the punctured aneurysm.

2. Complete occlusion of a giant aneurysm with clips was often difficult because of the giant size of the aneurysm and sclerotic thick (uneven wall of the neck).

3. The period of temporary clipping was 55 minutes without causing deficits.

CASE 2   Large Vertebral Artery (Dissecting) Aneurysm

This 61-year-old female presented with a progressive quadriparesis starting with left hemiparesis over the past 5 years. Recently she could only move her right upper limb well and was almost bedridden. Magnetic resonance imaging (MRI) showed a mass in the right ventral side of the medulla (Fig. 8.3a,b). An angiogram showed a large right vertebral artery aneurysm, while the left vertebral artery was patent (Fig. 8.3c,d).

With the patient in the lateral position, a lateral suboccipital craniectomy was performed (Fig. 8.4a). The dura was opened. The vertebral artery was first exposed on the proximal side of the aneurysm and then with the aid of direct retraction of the aneurysm the distal part of the vertebral artery was exposed (Fig. 8.4b). The wall of the aneurysm was whitish. The PICA appeared to originate directly from the body of the aneurysm. As the contralateral vertebral artery was large we went ahead with trapping of the aneurysm with three clips, applied to the

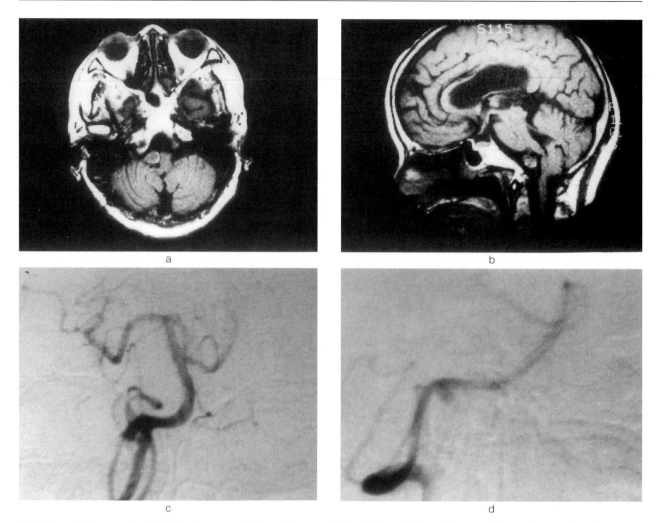

Fig. 8.3 **a,b** Preoperative MRI showing a mass in the right ventral side of the medulla. **c,d** Preoperative angiograms showing a large right vertebral artery aneurysm.

vertebral artery proximal and distal to the aneurysm and PICA. The aneurysm was cut at its dome; observation of the content of the aneurysm indicated that it was a dissecting type of aneurysm. The ostium to the aneurysm was well visualized (Fig. 8.4c). By flushing the proximal vertebral artery and PICA, it was found that they were opened to the same lumen of the distal VA. A bolus of 5000 units of heparin was injected intravenously and organized clots inside the aneurysmal lumen were removed as much as possible. Under temporary trapping, three clips were used to completely occlude the aneurysm as the wall of the aneurysm was uneven and partly calcified and thick (Fig. 8.4d). A small perforator from the aneurysm was torn; its bleeding was controlled by cutting and coagulating it. The postoperative course has been uneventful.

Comments

1. The aneurysm appeared dissecting in type at surgery.

2. The best way of treating this particular case is yet to be determined (Yamaura 1988). Suturing or patch-grafting the

hole, reinforced with clipping, would be the treatment of choice. Although clipping of a dissecting aneurysm is generally not used, fortunately the patient has done well since the operation performed 5 years previously.

CASE 3 Giant Thrombosed Vertebral Artery Aneurysm

A 46-year-old man first complained of headache and visited the hospital where CT scan revealed a large enhancing mass of 50 mm in maximum diameter with a calcified wall and a dilated vessel in the posterior fossa. The symptoms included truncal ataxia and dysphasia but no motor or sensory deficits. MRI revealed the mass clearly displacing the medulla posteriorly, with a small flow-void area in the ventral side (Fig. 8.5a,b). Vertebral angiograms showed a serpentine aneurysm of the left vertebral artery (Fig. 8.5c,d). The right vertebral artery terminated solely in the PICA. The posterior cerebral arteries

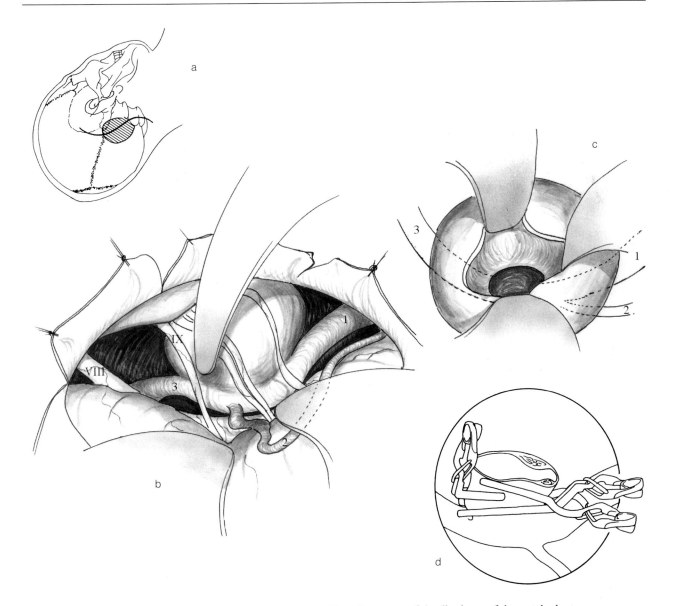

Fig. 8.4 **a** Large suboccipital craniectomy. **b** Direct retraction allowed exposure of the distal part of the vertebral artery. **c** Visualization of the ostium to the aneurysm. **d** Three clips were used to completely occlude the aneurysm.

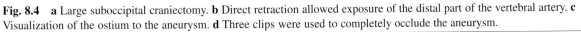

were filled only by the affected vertebral artery. Two operations were performed prior to the final procedure.

In the first operation, a bypass surgical procedure with saphenous vein graft was performed between the left external carotid artery to the left superior cerebellar artery. The graft was found occluded on the angiogram taken on the following day, with worsening symptoms necessitating tracheostomy.

The second operation was designed to accomplish decompression of the mass because of the progression of the symptoms. With the patient in the lateral position, a right temporosuboccipital craniotomy extending to the foramen magnum was performed. A partial mastoidectomy was carried out. The sigmoid sinus was unroofed to the jugular foramen. An extreme lateral approach (Sen & Sekhar 1990) was made with C1 hemilaminectomy and by drilling the posterior half of the

occipital condyle. The right vertebral artery was mobilized by cutting the dura on both sides of its dural penetration; the left vertebral artery was visualized. The distal left vertebral artery and the basilar artery were visualized via the presigmoid route. Both the proximal and distal parent arteries were thus secured. The ipsilateral cranial nerves seen had all been stretched by the underlying giant aneurysm. The thinned medulla was partly seen overriding the aneurysm, and the pons displaced cranial to the fifth nerve. The aneurysmotomy was done between the seventh and twelfth nerves. The content of the thrombosed aneurysm was removed carefully using an ultrasonic aspirator under the guidance of a Doppler flowmeter for determining the course of the vertebral artery inside the aneurysm. As oozing of blood started inside the aneurysm, debulking was stopped here. The aneurysm was decompressed to a depth of 2.5 cm. The

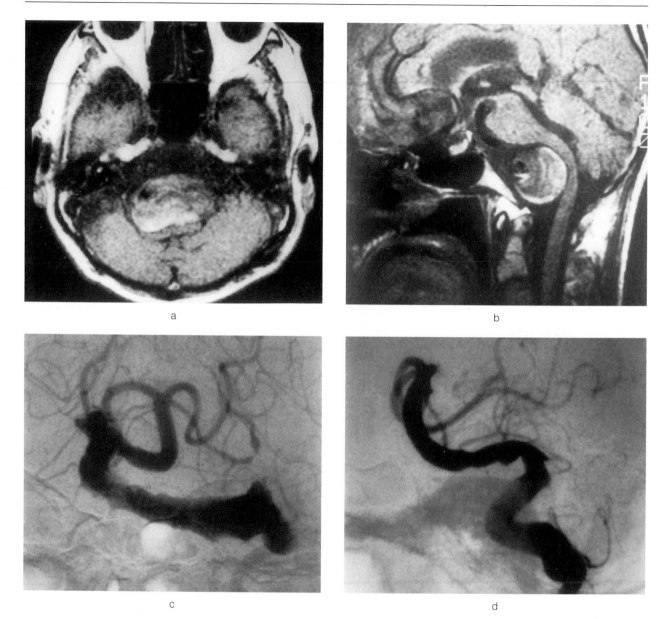

a   b

c   d

Fig. 8.5 Preoperative radiographic studies. Upper: axial (**a**) and sagittal (**b**) MRI. The aneurysm is markedly displacing the medulla posteriorly. A flow-void area is recognized in the ventral side of the aneurysm. Lower: left vertebral angiograms, anteroposterior projection (**c**) and lateral projection (**d**). The serpentine aneurysm is recognized. The vertebral artery is running from the left to the right upper side. (From Wakui et al 1992, with permission.)

lower medulla was considered to be well decompressed. The aneurysmotomy wound was closed by suture.

The patient's consciousness disturbance was slightly better postoperatively but the symptoms did not improve much. A radical aneurysmectomy for complete decompression was designed as a final procedure because additional progressive neurological deficits appeared in the course.

In a third operation, with the patient in the supine lateral position, the wound from the second operation was reopened and a radial artery bypass was performed from the right neck external carotid artery to the right posterior cerebral artery (P2

segment); graft patency was confirmed intraoperatively with the Doppler flowmeter. The previous operative wound was densely adherent and it was extremely difficult to find and confirm the important structures. First, the right vertebral artery and PICA were found; they had thrombosed and were black. Then, the contralateral (left) vertebral artery was found. The basilar artery was separated from the aneurysm and the right anterior inferior cerebellar artery (AICA) was found and dissected free. The aneurysm was trapped with temporary clips placed on the left vertebral artery and basilar artery. The aneurysm was entered and the content of the aneurysm was removed, mostly by

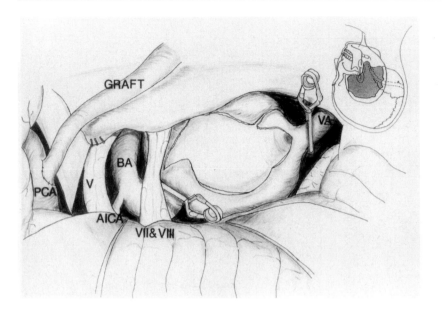

Fig. 8.6 Schematic drawing of the third operative view, the aneurysm was trapped with clips and the content of the aneurysm removed. The wall of the aneurysm was resected. (Va, left vertebral artery; GRAFT, radial artery graft; PCA, posterior cerebral artery; BA, basilar artery; V, VII and VIII, trigeminal, facial and acoustic nerves; AICA, anterior inferior cerebellar artery.) (From Wakui et al 1992, with permission.)

ultrasonic aspirator. As we decompressed the aneurysm it became possible to further visualize the inlet and outlet ostia. The trapping clips were replaced closer to the aneurysm. During this process, both AICAs were found and spared from clipping, together with a couple of perforating arteries. These procedures were facilitated by cutting the aneurysm wall. Except for the dorsomedial wall of the aneurysm, which had been attached to the medulla and was mostly calcified, the remaining aneurysm wall was thinned from the inside as much as possible, thus achieving complete decompression (Fig. 8.6). Patency of the radial arterial graft and the retrograde blood flow of the basilar artery were confirmed with the Doppler flowmeter.

POSTOPERATIVE COURSE

The patient showed a gradual improvement of his preoperative deficits, but severe dysphagia persisted. A CT scan, MRI and right carotid angiograms showed the posterior fossa well decompressed and good patency of the radial artery graft through which the basilar arterial system was well opacified (Fig. 8.7).

Comments

1. We feel that in the treatment for giant thrombosed vertebral artery aneurysm it is extremely important to reduce the mass substantially or completely to relieve symptoms, although simple ligation of the proximal vertebral artery may yield a good result without complications (Ishii et al 1983, Sugita 1985). Mere external decompression may aggravate the symptoms because the brain stem gets displaced more.

2. Surgical exposure of the aneurysm and all parent arteries was excellent in this case with a combined right

transmastoid, petrosal, suboccipital, extreme lateral approach utilizing pre- and postsigmoid routes.

3. Almost all the intraluminal clots were evacuated by the ultrasonic aspirator. The Doppler flowmeter is also useful for identifying the course of the blood compartment inside a thrombosed aneurysm or detecting the ostia to the parent artery.

4. As to the bypass surgery between the external carotid artery and the superior cerebellar artery, the radial artery graft may have remained patent in part because it may be a better graft than a saphenous vein (Yasui et al 1985), and in part because the vertebral artery occluded simultaneously.

REFERENCES

Hopkins L N, Budney J L, Castellani D 1983 Extracranial–intracranial arterial bypass and basilar artery ligation in the treatment of giant basilar artery aneurysms. Neurosurgery 13: 189–194

Ishii R, Tanaka R, Koike T et al 1983 Computed tomographic demonstration of the effect of proximal parent artery ligation for giant intracranial aneurysms. Surgical Neurology 19: 532–540

Kyoshima K, Kobayashi S, Wakui K et al 1992 A newly designed needle for suction decompression of giant aneurysm. Journal of Neurosurgery 76: 880–882

Sen C N, Sekhar L N 1990 An extreme lateral approach to intradural lesions of the cervical spine and foramen magnum. Neurosurgery 27: 197–204

Sugita K 1985 Microneurosurgical atlas. Springer-Verlag, Berlin, pp 116–135

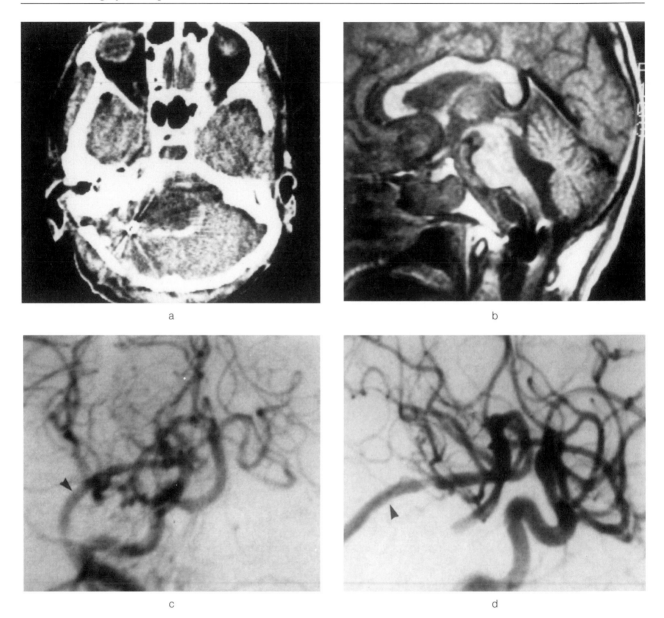

Fig. 8.7 Radiographic studies after the third operation. **a** CT scan. Space created by the aneurysmectomy showing a large low-density area. The remaining wall of the aneurysm is seen as a linear high-density area. **b** MRI showing the medulla markedly decompressed. Lower: right carotid angiograms, anteroposterior view(**c**) and lateral view (**d**). There is good patency of the radial arterial graft (arrows) and the basilar arterial system is well opacified. (From Wakui et al 1992, with permission.)

Suguta K, Kobayashi S, Toshiki et al 1988 Giant aneurysms of the vertebral artery: report of five cases. Journal of Neurosurgery 68: 960–966

Wakui K, Kobayashi S, Takemae T et al 1992 Giant thrombosed vertebral artery aneurysm managed with extracranial–intracranial bypass surgery and aneurysmectomy. Journal of Neurosurgery 77: 624–627

Yamaura A 1988 Diagnosis and treatment of vertebral aneurysms. Journal of Neurosurgery 69: 345–349

Yasui N, Ohta H, Suzuki A et al 1985 Cervical carotid artery to middle cerebral artery anastomosis with interposed radial artery graft. In: Spetzler R F, Carter L P, Selman W R et al (eds) Cerebral revascularization for stroke. Thieme-Stratton, New York, pp 379–385

Zhang Q J, Kobayashi S, Gibo H et al 1994 Vertebrobasilar junction fenestration associated with dissecting aneurysm of intracranial vertebral artery. Stroke 25: 1273–1275

Vertebral and vertebral basilar junction aneurysm
Steven L. Giannotta

Aneurysms of the distal vertebral artery and vertebral basilar junction present some of the more interesting challenges for the vascular neurosurgeon. Due to their relative infrequency, true expertise in their surgical management is difficult to attain in a timely manner. Because of the constricted space in which they reside, surgical access is complicated. Surgical complications which result in ischemia to this area may result in devastating neurological deficits. Lower cranial nerve dysfunction, a frequent concomitant of complex surgical procedures in this area, may also result in potentially life-threatening conditions.

The discipline of cranial base surgery has probably contributed the most clinically significant advances in the treatment of vertebral and vertebral basilar junction aneurysms over the past few years.

Principles employed include:

1. shortest trajectory to the lesion;
2. bone removal in lieu of brain retraction;
3. maximization of extradural exposure;
4. cranial nerve preservation;
5. skeletonization/decompression of cranial nerves and arteries;
6. reconstitution of all dural openings.

Utilizing these tenets, three cranial base approaches are available for consideration in the treatment of complex vertebral and vertebral basilar junction aneurysms. It should be noted that the traditional lateral suboccipital craniectomy may be satisfactory for the exposure and treatment of vertebral PICA aneurysms and small proximal vertebral lesions. For giant or complex vertebral aneurysms a more extended portal is necessary. The extreme lateral inferior transcondylar approach (ELITE) is an expansion of the far lateral approach initially proposed by Heros. The trajectory of this approach is virtually anterior to the medulla and upper cervical spinal cord, sacrificing bone in lieu of lower brain stem and upper cervical cord retraction. By the extradural removal of the mastoid tip, jugular tubercle, rim of the foramen magnum and lateral third of the occipital condyle, in association with a retrosigmoid dural incision, the sigmoid sinus and jugular bulb are reflected laterally. The visualization and sight line of the operating microscope are parallel to the course of the intradural vertebral artery. The extradural portion of the vertebral artery is available for either temporary occlusion or transposition. One then has an expanded view superiorly to the vertebral basilar junction and lower basilar trunk.

A purely lateral approach to the upper vertebral artery and vertebral basilar junction can be obtained using the retrolabyrinthine transsigmoid approach (RLTS). A mastoidectomy is performed undercutting but preserving the labyrinth. The sigmoid sinus is exposed from the junction with the lateral sinus to its junction with the jugular bulb. A small retrosigmoid craniectomy completes the bony exposure. The sigmoid sinus is ligated with ligature clips at the superior and inferior limits of exposure and the dura is opened across the sigmoid sinus. The benefits of such an approach are the lack of brain stem retraction, a line of sight in working plane parallel to the lower cranial nerves, and the ability to gain proximal and distal control for temporary occlusion. Non-giant aneurysms of the distal vertebral artery, vertebral basilar junction or lower basilar trunk, including AICA lesions, are most appropriate for this approach. For lesions that point dorsally or ventrally, the site of the approach is predicted on the relative size of the dome. In the event that the dominant sigmoid sinus occurs on the side of the approach, temporary occlusion with measurement of proximal sinus pressure can be used as a guide as to whether or not the sinus can be sacrificed. If the pressure rises by more than 5 mmHg, an alternative approach such as the ELITE approach or the transpetrosal approach might better be selected.

Completing the various trajectories to the vertebral artery and vertebral basilar junction is the so-called transpetrosal approach. This strategy allows a more superomedial trajectory and is best selected for giant lesions of the lower basilar trunk or in the case of a high-riding vertebral basilar junction. The features of this approach include the following: retrolabyrinthine presigmoid bone removal, modest temporal craniotomy with extradural retraction of the mid-portion of the temporal lobe, ligation of the superior petrosal sinus with division of the tentorium to the tentorial hiatus, posterior retraction of the sigmoid sinus and gentle superior traction of the temporal lobe along with the severed leaves of the tentorium. The benefits of such an approach include reduced brain retraction due to a more lateral to medial and superior to inferior trajectory. Further, the sigmoid sinus is preserved and using a retrolabyrinthine technique hearing may also be preserved.

With each of the aforementioned approaches, mastoid air cells are opened. This raises the specter of spinal fluid otorhinorrhea. As an adjunct to each of these approaches, autologous fat is harvested and placed in the mastoid defect. This reduces the CSF leakage rate to less than 5%.

Lower cranial nerve injury is probably the most life-threatening of the potential complications of these approaches. The surgeon must develop a strategy of working above and below each of the nerves with bayoneted slim-lined instruments. Slim-line aneurysm clip applicators are an important adjunct to surgical success. In lieu of a slim-line applicator, extra-long clips can be utilized so as to reduce the chances of a wide clip applicator injuring the cranial nerve as it is passed along the line of sight toward the aneurysm.

The utilization of these cranial base approaches may

require some additional skills and review of certain regional anatomical features. All of these approaches involve a trajectory through the mastoid. Practice in the cranial base laboratory, enrollment in one of several temporal bone courses, or enlisting the aid of an otological colleague can facilitate skills acquisition.

Vertebral Artery Aneurysms
Bernard George

Vertebral artery (VA) aneurysms include different types of lesions, each one having a particular prognosis and requiring a specific treatment.

The VA aneurysms are of extracranial or intracranial variety. The clinical presentation varies in these two varieties. Extracranial aneurysms are caused by many pathologies, as in the following list, of which dissecting hematoma is the most frequent:

Dissecting hematoma
Fibromuscular dysplasia
Collagen disease (Ehlers–Danlos)
Neurofibromatosis
Atherosclerosis
Trauma
Radionecrosis

Dissecting hematoma generally induces tubular stenosis of the vertebral artery but can also be associated with aneurysm. The two usual locations for vertebral artery aneurysms are at the site of its entry into the foramen transversarium at the level of C6 vertebral level and in its suboccipital segment (C2–C0).

Stenosis generally heals spontaneously in a few weeks or months. On the contrary, aneurysms have a very low tendency to decrease their size. Therefore like aneurysms of any other cause, the risk of embolism persists and must be prevented by surgical exclusion. Treatment is better achieved by bypassing the common carotid artery to the VA, distal to the aneurysm, using a saphenous vein graft. Direct repair is not recommended since the arterial wall is dysplasic and therefore difficult to suture.

In general intracranial aneurysms are of two main types: saccular and dissecting aneurysms. Intracranial dissecting aneurysms are recognized by the usual angiographic features of dissecting hematoma and by their generally more or less fusiform shape. Their most common mode of presentation is not ischemia from embolism as in extracranial aneurysms but subarachnoid hemorrhage. Their evolution is often associated with a high risk of bleeding. They should therefore be treated as soon as possible, with the goal of excluding the arterial segment involved. This can be achieved surgically or by interventional radiological means. The VA may be occluded proximal to the aneurysm or the arterial segment can be trapped. As for the extracranial aneurysm, the complete wall of the VA is involved and thus reconstruction by clips or direct arterial repair is not a lasting or safe method of treatment. Occlusion or trapping must be discussed according to the size of the

VA and to the site of origin of the PICA and of branches for the medulla. Proximal occlusion with coil or balloon is in the vast majority of our cases the chosen treatment since the placement of a distal coil is often hazardous. The balloon is placed distal to the PICA whenever possible. Obviously, definitive occlusion is only decided after a tolerance test with clinical and angiographic control in normal and hypotensive conditions. In case of poor tolerance, the balloon is moved backwards and placed more proximally. In our experience, it is always possible to find a place (even extracranial) where the occlusion will be well tolerated. The patient must receive anticoagulant therapy for the following 8 days and a steady normal (or slightly increased) arterial pressure should be maintained. The problem is puzzling when the dissection is bilateral or involves the PICA. When dissecting hematoma extends to the PICA the best solution, if well tolerated, is to occlude the VA both proximal and distal to the origin of the PICA. When the dissecting aneurysm is bilateral, there is no good way since simultaneous bilateral VA occlusion cannot be safely performed.

Saccular aneurysms of the VA have the same presentation as in any other localization. However, VA aneurysms, like internal carotid artery aneurysms, are more commonly observed in women and associated with fibromuscular dysplasia. Multiplicity is also a very common feature. Our policy for treatment of VA aneurysms is similar to any other location. Endovascular technique is the first choice if the case is suitable for this technique after angiographic studies are evaluated. More than 70% of the intracranial saccular aneurysms appear good candidates for endovascular treatment. In other cases which are often difficult for both surgical and endovascular treatment, the technique with the least risk is chosen. Therefore, according to the aneurysm and also the patient characteristics, it may be decided to occlude the VA at the level of the aneurysm or proximally with balloons or coils.

Surgery has been chosen in our experience when the risks were similar or smaller and when without increasing the risks a major artery (VA or PICA) could be preserved by surgery but not by endovascular treatment. This is particularly the case for VA–PICA junction aneurysms where the endovascular material often cannot completely treat the aneurysm without stenosing or occluding the parent vessels.

For surgery, the more or less distal localization on the VA is the main point to consider. Proximal aneurysms up to the lateral side of the medulla oblongata are easy to reach. On the contrary, distal aneurysms anterior to the medulla oblongata are difficult to treat surgically. In fact, the two most frequent locations of vertebral artery aneurysms are the VA–PICA junction and the VA–basilar trunk junction. Aneurysms located on intermediate segments are rather dissecting aneurysms than saccular forms. The exposure is always done by the posterolateral approach we designed to expose lateral and anterior tumors of the foramen magnum. The patient is in the sitting position. The incision is median vertical up to the occipital protuberance, then curved laterally more or less towards the mastoid process. The lower part of the occipital bone and posterior arch of the atlas are exposed, including the VA in its groove. The more distal the aneurysm, the more lateral the opening is extended. For proximal ones, the posterior arch is resected up to the lateral mass of the atlas, which is almost not drilled. For distal ones, the VA is exposed up to the transverse foramen of the atlas and the bone opening is extended as far as the sigmoid sinus, with more drilling of the occipital condyle and lateral mass of the atlas. Then, the dissection progresses along the VA; with the posterolateral approach, the axis of work is quite lateral and there is no need to retract the neural axis. Therefore, the main problem is the lower cranial nerves. VA–PICA aneurysms are most commonly located at the level of the crossing of the VA by the nerves and thus nerve rootlets must be displaced superiorly or inferiorly to properly place the clip. To reach distal VA aneurysms, one must find the most appropriate space between the lower cranial nerves. The space is sometimes very easily opened. However, in some cases, one is faced with multiple rootlets and arterial branches; they must be dissected free all along from the brain stem to the jugular foramen so as to be able to displace them upwards or downwards without stretching. Exposure of the aneurysmal neck and separation from the PICA origin may be difficult in the VA–PICA variety of aneurysm, and in VA–basilar trunk junction aneurysms if they point inferolaterally over the distal VA and thus hide the neck. It is often very useful to have selective digital angiography to anticipate the anatomical disposition and clip placement. Fenestrated clips are often used to deal with the cranial nerves or the PICA.

In conclusion, with the development of endovascular techniques surgical treatment is less often applied. The posterolateral approach, which can be enlarged laterally, generally provides a wide exposure of the distal VA. The major problem is the control and clipping of the neck while preserving the lower cranial nerves, PICA and small brain stem vascular branches.

Arteriovenous malformation

9

Kazuhiro Hongo   Shigeaki Kobayashi
Toshiki Takemae

GENERAL CONSIDERATIONS

The operation for an arteriovenous malformation (AVM), other than for a small and superficial one, is still considered to be one of the more difficult neurosurgical procedures. The technical difficulty in surgery of an AVM depends on its size, location, and also on the relation between the feeding arteries and draining veins. The larger the AVM, the more difficult is the operation. Even when it is small, it is difficult to operate these lesions when they are located in the depth, especially in proximity to eloquent and critical neural areas.

In recent years, by introduction and refinement of endovascular techniques and gamma knife surgery, surgical indications of AVM have changed significantly. Yet, direct surgical treatment of AVM is still an important choice of treatment. Treatment of AVM is generally divided into two broad categories: conservative and non-conservative. Non-conservative treatment includes direct operation, endovascular embolization followed by surgery and gamma knife therapy. The gamma knife treatment can be performed after an operative treatment. It is generally agreed that the AVM smaller than 3 cm can be treated by gamma knife. Whether gamma knife treatment can eradicate a small AVM is still a matter of debate and the results of long-term follow-up of these patients is awaited. Presently, it appears that gamma knife treatment is indicated especially for AVMs in an eloquent area. Embolization followed by direct surgical removal is now a commonly practiced procedure.

SURGICAL CONSIDERATIONS

The purpose of AVM surgery is to remove the nidus to prevent future hemorrhage and also to improve the neurological status caused by the presence and effects of AVM. It is known that if a small part of the nidus is left unremoved following surgery, it is likely that the AVM will develop into a bigger one in the future. After proper embolization of the feeding arteries by intravascular technique, final removal is made by surgical intervention. It is very important that the surgical exposure provides access to important feeding arteries and also draining veins. Therefore preoperative embolization is primarily performed to target the feeding arteries which are difficult to approach at the time of surgery and/or the major feeding arteries to minimize intraoperative bleeding. It is also performed to reduce postoperative vascular overload to the surrounding brain, as described later.

Recently, we have utilized preoperative embolization in most cases. Embolization should not be performed just because it is possible. The procedure has potential complications such as cerebral infarction and bleeding. After the surgical strategy is planned, preoperative embolization is carried out especially where the surgical procedure is difficult. A feeding artery located behind the nidus in the operating view of the surgeon is a good indication for preoperative embolization wherever it is possible. For the AVM in an eloquent area, its exact location in relation to the surrounding gyri or other structures should be analyzed on magnetic resonance imaging (MRI).

INDICATIONS FOR SURGERY

There are no strict guidelines suggesting definite indications for surgery on AVMs. The advisability and feasibility of surgery greatly depend on the skill and experience of the surgeon as well as on the patient's condition and on the size and location of the AVM. Whenever surgical therapy is chosen, total resection or occlusion of the nidus should be performed. Either direct surgery only or a combination of direct surgery in association with preoperative embolization may be carried out. Gamma knife is another rapidly emerging option, especially for AVMs which are small in size (nidus size of less than 3 cm) or are located at depth or in eloquent areas.

For AVMs in association with hemorrhage, direct surgical resection of the AVM is usually performed along with removal of the hematoma. In non-hemorrhage cases, however, indications for surgical treatment might be variable.

PREOPERATIVE EVALUATION

Careful and detailed evaluation of the preoperative angiogram is essential for successful treatment of AVM. The neural structures around the AVM, exact location of the nidus, especially when it is located near the eloquent area, feeding arteries and draining veins should be well studied.

Digital angiotomosynthesis was observed to be an extremely useful method for recognizing the three-dimensional and detailed vascular topography of the AVM. Using this technique, fine feeders, which are difficult to trace on the conventional angiogram, were relatively easily recognized (Shigeta et al 1994) (Fig. 9.1).

SURGICAL TECHNIQUES

Maintaining an ideal position during the entire surgical procedure is very important. To lessen intraoperative bleeding, the head plate of the operating table should be raised around 30°. In our studies on this subject we recognized that in this position the jugular venous pressure was almost 0 mmHg. The patient's head is rotated depending on the location of the operative field; however, too much rotation can result in interference of the venous return with the possibility of resultant intracerebral hemorrhage from the fragile nidus or even cerebral swelling. Another important point concerning the patient's position is that the operating field should be maintained in such a way that the axis of the operating microscope is directed more or less perpendicularly to the floor. Using the microscope at this angle, the surgeon can perform the surgical procedure comfortably. During surgery, not only is the patient's head rotated, but also the operating microscope should be frequently shifted as needed and/or the surgeon should change position to obtain a good operative view so that safe and comfortable surgery can be performed.

As in any neurosurgical procedure, selection of an appropriate approach is a matter of great importance. This

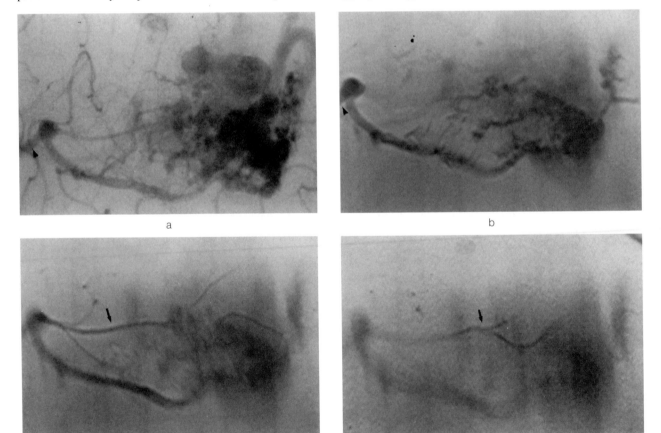

a

b

c

d

Fig. 9.1 Angiotomosynthesis clearly showing the feeding arteries which are not seen in usual angiograms. Case with an AVM in the right parietal lobe. **a** Lateral view of the conventional left internal carotid angiogram. The arrowhead indicates the anterior pericallosal artery. **b–d** Reconstructed angiotomograms in the mid-sagittal plane (**b**), 5 mm to the left (**c**), and 10 mm to the left (**d**), clearly showing many feeders originating from the left anterior pericallosal artery and a passing artery (arrows) in close proximity to the nidus. The arrowhead indicates the interior pericallosal artery. (From Shigeta et al 1994, with permission.)

is especially so with a deep-seated AVM or an AVM close to eloquent areas. Regardless of the approaches adopted, a large craniotomy should be performed. After inspecting the cortical surface, feeding arteries and/or cortical draining veins, it is important to get adequately oriented prior to beginning the dissection.

It is a well-known principle of the AVM operation that all feeders are obliterated before the main drainer is sacrificed. Generally, the approach should be such that the feeding artery is exposed early in the operation. Malis (1982), on the other hand, recommended an approach to the AVM by exposing and following the draining vein towards the nidus. The venous anatomy should be carefully evaluated on the preoperative angiography and functional studies during endovascular study. When there is more than one draining vein, the draining vein can be obliterated in the event of inadvertent rupture without provoking a disaster. Following the vein is an option; however, considering the possible presence of so-called C-type nidus (described later), we prefer approaching feeding arteries first.

During dissection of the nidus, the cortical sulcus in which the feeding arteries enter is carefully followed and opened by sharp dissection of the arachnoid membrane. Once the surface of the nidus is reached, dissection of the nidus is started along its surface. In hemorrhagic cases, dissection of the nidus is relatively easy. Even when there is no apparent hematoma on the preoperative computed tomographic (CT) scan and/or MRI, a thin zone with evidence of prior bleeding is often present. Identification of this plane of cleavage is frequently the key to further dis-

section. When small feeding arteries and/or small draining veins are encountered, those can adequately be coagulated and cut. It is important to coagulate the vessels long enough before cutting them (Fig. 9.2). It is also important not to pull the vessels on coagulation to avoid their avulsion. Once the cut end of the vessel retracts into the parenchyma, it is difficult to isolate it and coagulate. When we are in doubt as to whether a particular vessel is normal or a feeder, it is exposed along its course for an adequate distance or is left untouched until the nidus is widely exposed. When the length of a feeder between the parent artery and the nidus is short or when a nidus is attached to the parent artery, dissection of the nidus from the parent artery is very difficult; the feeder should not be coagulated, but should instead be ligated with a suture or obliterated with a small titanium hemoclip. The surface of the nidus is dissected free from the surrounding cerebral tissue. It is important that one should dissect the nidus just over the surface and not inside the nidus. Dissecting in the correct plane is important as, if one enters the inside of the nidus, bleeding occurs which can sometimes be difficult to control. The nidus should not be dissected at a single spot, but should be dissected all around. The parenchymal side of the dissected plane is covered with cottonoid patties to protect the brain. The dissected nidus can be retracted using a spoon retractor (Fig. 9.3). The spoon retractor is occasionally a useful instrument for AVM surgery. The curvature of the retractor, which can be of variable shapes and sizes, is selected to suit the size of the nidus. Using this type of retractor, the nidus can be dissected without slip-

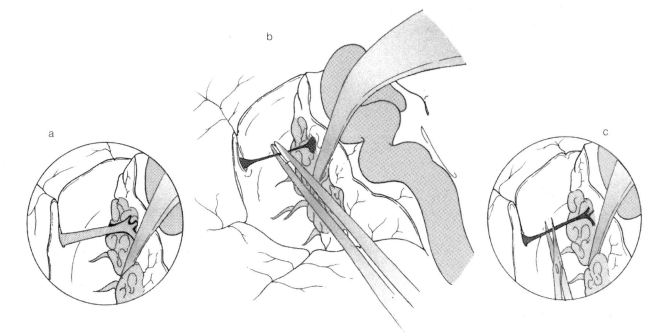

Fig. 9.2 Schematic drawings showing how to coagulate and cut a feeding artery. **a** Dissecting the feeding artery for a long distance. **b** Coagulating the feeding artery sufficiently. **c** Cutting the artery.

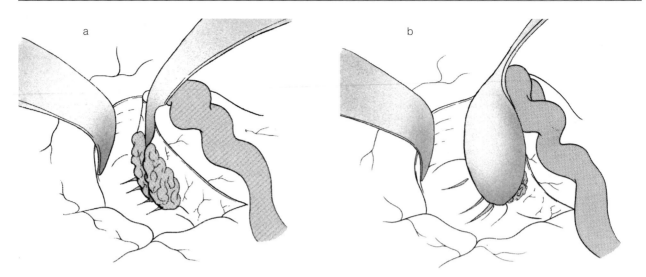

Fig. 9.3 Schematic drawings of a spoon retractor holding the nidus. **a** Retracting a nidus by a tapered spatula. **b** Retracting a nidus using a spoon retractor. Note that the spoon holds the nidus better, without obstructing the draining venous circulation.

ping and also without causing obliteration of the draining veins inside the nidus. A spoon retractor can be connected to a self-retaining retractor. Both hands of the surgeons are now available for further dissection. Although the main drainer should be preserved until the final stages of the dissection, small draining veins can be conveniently coagulated and cut during dissection of the nidus.

During dissection in the vicinity of the nidus, it is often difficult to distinguish between feeding arteries and draining veins. The color of the feeding artery is usually whiter than that of the draining veins. However, distinguishing by color is sometimes difficult as the vessels are small. Test

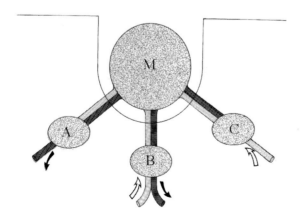

Fig. 9.4 Schematic drawing showing various types of daughter nidus. (A, B, C, types A, B and C nidus, respectively; M, main nidus; open arrow, feeding artery; black arrow, draining vein. For details see the text.)

bipolar coagulation is sometimes helpful; the artery shrinks readily with bipolar coagulation, while the draining vein does not coagulate and may easily rupture.

It is important to determine which draining veins can be sacrificed early in the course of dissection on the basis of the preoperative study and also on intraoperative judgment. On the basis of the preoperative angiogram one should determine whether the AVM has single or multiple compartments as regards the feeding and draining system. A large AVM or an AVM in the sylvian fissure or deep temporal lobe is likely to be multicompartment in type, being fed from different arterial trunks, such as anterior, middle and posterior cerebral arteries (Sugita et al 1987). From intraoperative judgment during the course of dissection of the nidus and occlusion of feeding arteries, one can tell which compartment of, or what part of, the AVM is obtaining arterial supply: one can judge by the change in color of the nidus or by detecting the flow with the aid of a Doppler flowmeter.

CLASSIFICATION OF THE RESIDUAL DAUGHTER NIDUS

As proposed by Sugita (Sugita 1985), there are three types of residual daughter nidus connected to the main nidus by a band containing both feeders and draining vessels (Fig. 9.4). The residual portion of type A has only a drainer; it disappears postoperatively. Type B has both feeder and drainer; it is found as a residual AVM on the postoperative angiogram. Type C has only feeders and it is the most dangerous. If such a daughter nidus is left unresected severe bleeding is bound to occur either intra- or postoperatively. Although it is possible to remove a type B nidus by a second operation, one must never leave a type C nidus. Such a nidus is most likely to be missed when a large AVM is dissected close to its coils in a critical area. In these cases, intraoperative angiography is helpful. The nature of a nidus should be determined cautiously. Careful temporary clipping for a short duration may be helpful. When one encounters bleeding after removal of the main nidus, one should suspect the presence of a type B or type C nidus in the vicinity. This daughter nidus needs to be dissected and removed.

When sectioning a large draining vein, temporary clipping should be attempted first. The drainer can then be cut after confirming that no swelling of the nidus occurs. Small-sized feeders and drainers can be coagulated and cut without using hemoclips, but larger feeders need to be ligated or clipped to prevent postoperative bleeding. When bipolar coagulation is not effective, bleeding from the nidus is controlled by covering the area with Oxycel and cotton, which are pressed against the nidus with a tapered spatula.

AKA-MUSHI ('BLOOD-WARM') VESSELS

Utmost care should be taken while dealing with small red fragile veins, which we call 'blood-warm' (aka-mushi) vessels. This is especially so when they are behind the nidus deep in the operating field, where control of bleeding is relatively difficult. Difficulty in the control of bleeding is usually observed during the final stages of the removal of a large AVM when the remaining vessels, both arteries and veins, are often under high pressure. In this situation the following points may be helpful:

1. Bipolar forceps with tips composed of a metal that has high heat conductance should be used. Forceps made of titanium are avoided. The forceps should be insulated except for the tips. A weaker current should be used than when coagulating an aneurysm wall. Coagulation with wider-tipped forceps should be done with a different current from that employed while using narrower forceps because the former has lower impedance. The output current should be changed frequently. We use a small sterilized output controller near the operating field which is controlled by an assistant surgeon as needed.
2. Transient hypotension, induced at about 70 mmHg systolic, is often useful to control bleeding and to coagulate the thin-walled vessels.
3. Although bleeding from the nidus can usually be controlled with Oxycel covering, bleeding from the normal cerebral side should not be controlled only with

Oxycel except for an occasional very small bleeding. Instead, the bleeding point should be coagulated completely.

When bleeding occurs from a small artery and it is difficult to coagulate, the area may be covered with Oxycel and cotton and the area pressed with a brain spatula connected to a self-retaining retractor. The surgeon can then work in another field until the bleeding stops.

Another way for controlling bleeding from a fragile vein is to use an ultra-miniclip. This is a miniature Sugita aneurysm clip with a blade length of 2 mm. When one encounters difficulty in controlling bleeding from fragile vessels, one may have to consider staging of the operation.

SINGLE OR STAGED SURGERY

One can plan a staged surgery according to the size of the AVM and the problems expected in accessing the feeding arteries and draining veins. Or one can perform a staged operation using intraoperative judgment as stated above when one encounters difficulty in controlling bleeding with the aka-mushi ('blood-warm') vessels. A staged operation can include preoperative embolization, occluding feeding arteries or some of the nidus by liquid material. However, during the waiting period the possibilities of bleeding from the AVM are probably higher as there is a change in hemodynamic status. Staging of the surgery also reduces the possibility of the postoperative overload to the surrounding brain.

In our practice the indications for staged surgery are as follows:

1. An AVM where the nidus is bigger than 5 cm and a volume index is greater than 60. The index is expressed as follows: volume index (V.I.)$=X \times Y \times Z$, where X is the maximum diameter (cm) of a nidus on the lateral angiogram, Y is the diameter (cm) perpendicular to X, and Z is the maximum diameter (cm) on the anteroposterior angiogram (Fig. 9.5). The actual volume of a nidus would be about $0.4 \times$ V.I. cm^3.
2. Very high-flow AVM.
3. Intraoperative judgment of rapid increase in feeder pressure.
4. Rapid increase in cortical blood flow as determined by cortical thermoplate or laser plate measurement.

INTRAOPERATIVE MONITORING

There are several modalities of monitoring during AVM surgery, some of which were originally described from our institute. Intraoperative monitoring is important for the safe and smooth conduct of AVM surgery.

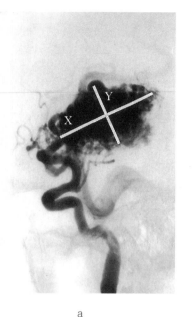
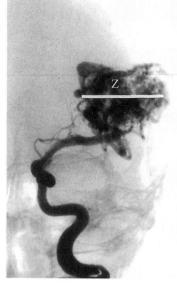

a   b

Fig. 9.5 Schematic drawings indicating volume index. **a** X and Y indicate the maximum diameter of the nidus and a diameter perpendicular to X in the lateral view, respectively. **b** Z indicates the maximum diameter of the nidus in the anteroposterior view.

Intraoperative angiography

To confirm complete resection of the nidus, intraoperative angiography is extremely useful. Currently we are using a radiolucent head frame made from super engineering plastic (Okudera et al 1994a). The method for the intraoperative angiography is reported previously (Okudera et al 1994b). A catheter is placed in the intracranial internal carotid artery during surgery and cerebral angiography is performed. Even during surgery, when the patient's head is fixed in the frame, a good-quality angiogram can be obtained.

The purpose of the intraoperative angiography may be summarized as follows:

1. to identify the feeding artery by placing a small clip on it during surgery. Angiography helps in delineating the relationship of the clip to the nidus. This is especially useful for AVMs located deep in the brain.
2. to confirm the extent or completion of resection of the nidus.
3. residual nidus can be detected. Once residual nidus is found, further dissection can be performed until total excision of the nidus is achieved.

Intraoperative measurement of cortical cerebral blood flow

Intraoperative cortical cerebral blood flow (CBF) is recorded with a thermoplate and, recently, with a laser plate placed near the nidus of the AVM.

Simultaneous pressure recording is made from each of the feeding arteries and draining veins. Generally, the feeding arterial pressure gradually rises and the draining venous pressure decreases as the dissection of the nidus is advanced.

Intraoperative use of Doppler flowmeter

The Doppler flowmeter now appears to be indispensable while surgically treating AVMs. Feeding arteries can be identified using the flowmeter. A possible feeding artery is temporarily clipped and the flow is checked on the nidus. Decrease in intranidal flow suggests that the clipped vessel could be the feeding artery. As the Doppler flowmeter can suggest the direction of flow in a vessel, one can decide the direction in which the dissection should proceed. This is especially useful when the feeding arteries are tortuous just before entering the nidus. The feeding artery should be coagulated and incised as close to the nidus as possible. When it is obliterated too proximally, or away from the nidus, branches to the normal cerebral tissue might be compromised. An artery passing through or sometimes running inside the nidus should be preserved. The Doppler flowmeter is also helpful in identifying the passing through artery.

Intraoperative monitoring using thermography

Intraoperative use of thermography is another way of monitoring the feeding arteries and the draining veins. This helps in the resection of the nidus (Okudera et al 1994c). Changes in the surface temperature of the cortical draining vein and the surrounding cortical surface have been observed intraoperatively before and after occlusion of the main feeder. Intraoperative functional thermography with cold physiological saline solution demonstrated a change in the heat clearance of the draining vein after complete obliteration of the feeder.

POSTOPERATIVE MANAGEMENT

An important issue in postoperative management is to keep the systolic blood pressure relatively low, to around 100 mmHg. This is especially important after resection of a large AVM. Systolic blood pressure can be reduced by the use of antihypertensive drugs or barbiturates during the first few days after surgery. Postoperative angiograms should be taken 1 week after surgery even in cases where complete resection of the nidus was confirmed by intraoperative angiography. The overload phenomenon (mentioned later) might be observed. Induced hypotension should be maintained until the overload phenomenon disappears. After resection of a giant or large AVM, the overload phenomenon may occur (Sugita & Takemae 1988, Takemae et al 1993).

LARGE AVM

A large AVM is characterized as one with a maximum diameter greater than 5 cm. Our clinical data indicates that an AVM with a volume index greater than 60 carries a high risk of causing the overload phenomenon. The technical points regarding the dissection of the nidus are not much different from in the smaller AVM. In these AVMs there are many feeding arteries coming from various directions and the veins drain into the superficial and deep venous systems. Careful analysis of the preoperative angiogram is therefore essential. Intraoperative angiography is also more helpful in such cases than for the smaller AVM.

OVERLOAD PHENOMENON

A hypervascular network appears in the vicinity of the resected nidus when seen on the capillary and venous phases on the immediate postoperative angiogram. There are associated contrast-filled stagnant large arteries, which roughly correspond to the arteries described by Hassler (1986). We have named these vessels as the network of

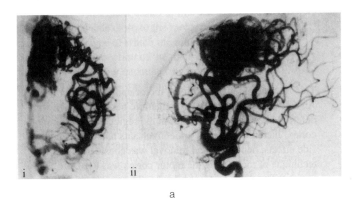

a

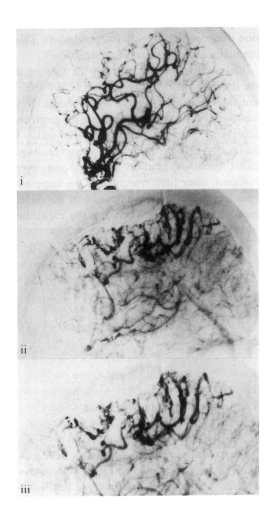

b

Fig. 9.6 Angiograms showing stagnating artery ('modja-modja' vessels). **a** Preoperative left carotid angiograms: **i** anteroposterior view, **ii** lateral view. **b** Immediate postoperative angiograms: **i** arterial phase, **ii** venous phase, showing contrast material remaining in the arteries around the removed nidus (stagnating arteries) and a hypervascular network composed of shaggy staining. **iii** Higher magnification of **ii**; note that the caliber of the vessels in the hypervascular network is irregular and varied in size. (From Takemae et al 1993, with permission.)

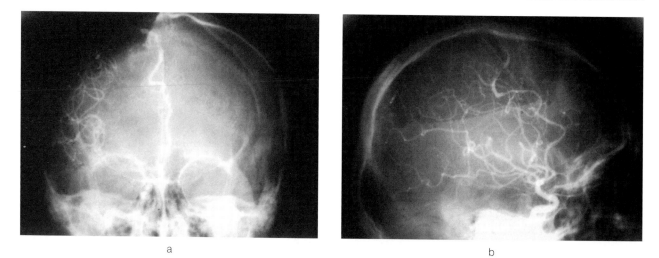

a

b

Fig. 9.9   Postoperative angiograms. **a** Anteroposterior view. **b** Lateral view.

3. C-type nidus was encountered in this case which had a separate feeder. The draining vein had been entangled with the main nidus. This was probably the reason we encountered difficulty in controlling bleeding from the C-type nidus after removal of the main nidus.

4. Barbiturate and induced hypotension were used during the procedure of controlling bleeding.

CASE 2

This 56-year-old male had a focal motor seizure followed by weakness of the left leg. CT, MRI and angiogram showed a large right parietal AVM fed mainly by the posterior parietal and pericallosal arteries. The AVM drained into the superior sagittal sinus (SSS). The size of the nidus was about 4 cm (Figs 9.10, 9.11). Three days before surgery on the AVM, preoperative embolization with Aviten and polyvinyl alcohol was carried out. An approximately 50% reduction in the size of the AVM was achieved (Fig. 9.12). With the patient in the supine position a large U-shaped skin incision was made in the

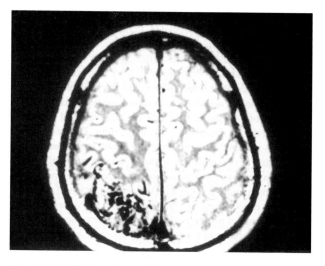

Fig. 9.10   MRI showing a nidus at the right parietal lobe.

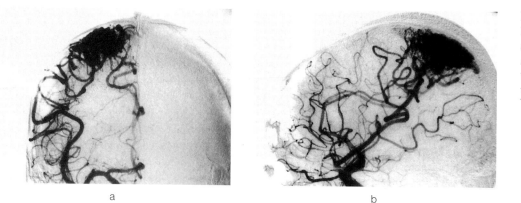

a

b

Fig. 9.11
Preoperative angiograms. **a** Anteroposterior view. **b** Lateral view.

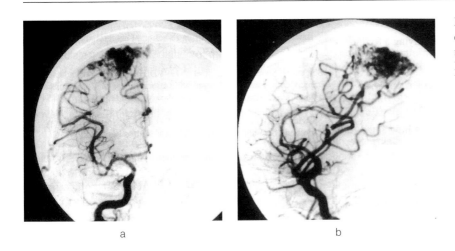

a

b

Fig. 9.12 Angiograms after embolization showing reduction in nidus size. **a** Anteroposterior view. **b** Lateral view.

right parietal region which extended to the contralateral side. A large parietal craniotomy was made which also extended to the left side, crossing the SSS. The dura mater was partly adherent to the surface of the arachnoid membrane. The arachnoid membrane was thick at and around the nidus. Arachnoid dissection was started from the anterior border of the nidus to the lateral side. On inspection, the nidus was seen to be partly embolized, with only mild pulsations. Feeding arteries from the middle cerebral artery were confirmed to be partly embolized. First, only the embolized arteries were cut. Dissection was performed on the anterior and lateral sides and the nidus, which was retracted medially. With the aid of a Doppler flowmeter, feeding arteries and draining veins were evaluated and cut. A titanium hemoclip was used to occlude the large feeding arteries.

Probably because of the preoperative embolization, bleeding from the nidus was minimal and was easily controlled with electrocoagulation. Several small feeders from the anterior cerebral artery (ACA) were coagulated and cut. Main feeders from the ACA were later found through the interhemispheric fissure. Dissection was done gradually, and the dissected nidus was retracted and held by a tapered spatula or a spoon retractor. Several large vessels were seen while dissecting through an interhemispheric approach. Two of these large vessels were feeders and one was a large draining vein, as was observed on the Doppler flowmeter. Even after the temporary clips were applied to the feeding arteries, flow to the nidus did not reduce significantly. After further dissection another set of feeders from the ACA were identified. After occluding these feeding vessels, tension of the nidus dramatically decreased and the nidus was dissected and removed. Intraoperative DSA was performed at this stage. A catheter was introduced into the right common carotid artery through the right brachial artery. The angiogram revealed that the nidus was removed completely. The flow in the SSS anterior to the nidus draining vein was patent, but was relatively slow. After confirming hemostasis the dura mater and wound were closed. Estimated blood loss was about 600 ml. Immediate postoperative CT scan showed no postoperative hemorrhage or infarction. Systemic blood pressure was maintained at around 90–100 mmHg throughout the procedure. Postoperative angiography showed no residual nidus (Fig. 9.13), and the patient did well, without neurological deficits.

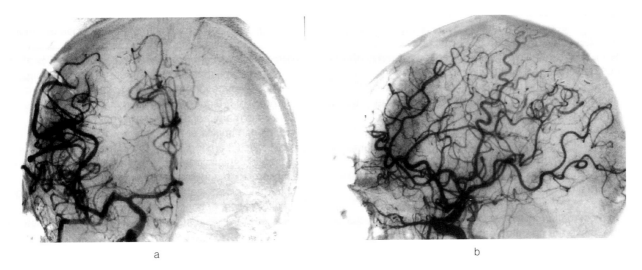

a

b

Fig. 9.13 Postoperative angiograms. **a** Anteroposterior view. **b** Lateral view.

In patients with Grade 5 lesion, the result of treatment was unsatisfactory. In our series neurological worsening was observed in 50% of cases of which two patients died. There were three sylvian and four temporal AVMs. Hemorrhage caused the trouble in almost all cases. In one case it occurred from the dilated pial vessels on the surrounding brain after the nidus was removed. They spontaneously ruptured due to the increase of intravascular pressure after the large arteriovenous shunt was closed. In large AVMs intravascular pressure in these dilated small vessels is considerably lowered because of the presence of a large arteriovenous shunt. These may easily rupture, therefore, by the increase in intravascular pressure after the removal of AVMs.

Bleeding from the surrounding brain due to the change of hemodynamics after removal of the AVM may be avoided by adopting the strategy of staged operation. However, the resection of the AVM even after many staged procedures may cause hemorrhage in Grade 5 AVMs for the hemodynamic reason inherently associated with occluding a large AV shunt.

In conclusion, microsurgery should be the treatment of choice in Grade 1 and 2 patients. Cases of Grade 3 can be treated with microsurgery alone with an acceptable risk, but improvement of the treatment result can be expected by embolizing deep-feeding perforators preoperatively. Radiosurgery can be indicated for several deep-seated lesions. For Grade 4 patients, preoperative embolization would be of help by obliterating lesions in critical locations and where the feeders are difficult to access. Treatment of Grade 5 patients still has many problems to be solved.

The Role of Preoperative Embolization in the Treatment of Arteriovenous Malformations
Takashi Yoshimoto

It is challenging to treat brain AVMs because of their vast anatomical complexity and varied clinical presentations. Even though modern therapeutic modalities including microneurosurgery, intravascular surgery, and stereotactic radiosurgery are available, each modality itself raises some controversy that must be resolved. However, combining each of these three modalities with the participation of its respective specialist would provide maximum clinical benefits. A special effort should be made to utilize these three available methodologies of treatment because any one of these modalities used alone may not be able to solve the complex clinical problems associated with treatment of AVMs. During the past several decades surgery has been the principal thrust of treatment. Intravascular neurosurgical technology was introduced in 1986 and gamma knife stereotactic radiosurgery in 1991 for the treatment of AVMs. Combining these treatment modalities, we have tried to improve the ultimate clinical outcome in our patient results over the past 10 years.

In this report, we will discuss our experiences of the successful excision of extensive basal ganglia AVMs, with special emphasis on the role of intravascular neurosurgical techniques, in the context of a multidisciplinary approach.

Preoperative Embolization: The recent development of small, highly flexible catheters has greatly increased the role of preoperative embolization in the treatment of AVMs. Preoperative embolization of AVMs is now routine at many institutions. Extensive embolization of the AVMs would diminish the complexity of their vascular supply, allowing them to become more accessible to surgical resection which can then often be performed in a single-stage operation. Staged preoperative embolization can reduce the number of deep-feeding vessels and prevent major bleeding during the dissection of the nidus. An additional subtemporal approach for obliteration of feeding vessels from the posterior cerebral artery was not required, because these vessels had been almost completely interrupted preoperatively. We are convinced that the AVMs in our series could not have been operated upon as safely without the preoperative embolization.

The selection of material for embolization is crucial, particularly when resection of the AVM is planned. Many groups have recommended the use of polyvinyl alcohol particles (Ivalon) for preoperative embolization. However, it is well known that recanalization frequently occurs within a relatively short period after embolization with Ivalon. Conversely a liquid embolization material has the merit of less possibility for recanalization compared to Ivalon. However, a conventional liquid material such as a cyanoacrylate glue makes the lesions hard and could make surgical resection more difficult. We have developed a new liquid embolization material, estrogen alcohol (EA) and polyvinyl acetate (PVac) solution (Mizoi et al 1992, Takahashi & Suzuki 1988, Takahashi et al 1991). This is a soft gel and the occluded vessels and the nidus maintain their flexibility, so that dissection and retraction of the lesions are quite easy. We believe PVac is the material of choice for staged preoperative embolization.

Surgical Approach and Intraoperative DSA: The safest route should be selected to approach a deep-seated AVM. The malformations located in the anterior thalamus or the head of the caudate nucleus are best approached through an interhemispheric transcallosal approach. However, there has not yet been any description in the literature concerning the best approach for removal of the malformations located in the corpus striatum.

A transsylvian approach has been described previously, used by several authors for removing malformations in the region of the insular cortex, lentiform nucleus or medial temporal lobe. We believe that striocapsular malformations are best exposed through an extended transsylvian approach. This approach has the merit of adding less intraoperative injury to eloquent cortical areas, such as the sensorimotor strip and speech areas. However, in the resection of deep AVM, the most serious postoperative morbidity would be caused by damage not to the cortical areas but to the pyramidal tract. Accordingly, during dissection on the medial side of the lesions, it would be critically important to preserve the paraventricular white matter, which frequently includes the internal capsule.

Preoperative study of the magnetic resonance image is useful to define the topographical anatomy of the malformation. However, in the case of large or giant deep-seated AVMs, it is difficult to predict preoperatively whether the malformation directly involves the internal capsule, or the nidus immediately adjacent to it. One must try to minimize damage to the paraventricular area by making the dissection plane as close as possible to the nidus. This is crucial in preservation of motor function in such AVMs.

Use of intraoperative DSA is helpful. Information about the status of AVM during surgery sometimes cannot be obtained by intraoperative visual inspection alone. DSA during surgery helps in avoiding unnecessary dissection, facilitates safe resection and avoids permanent postoperative neurological deficit. We believe that it is not necessary to remove the compartment of the nidus obliterated with our liquid embolic material (EA and PVac), as we are convinced that this region would never recanalize.

The disadvantage of an extended transsylvian approach is the possibility of damage to the superficial sylvian veins. The sacrifice of the veins may cause venous infarction of the frontal lobe. This will not occur if the veins are widely dissected free from the surrounding arachnoid. The veins should be dissected as long as possible using a microdissection technique. For such a sharp dissection, we prefer to use the tip of a no. 27 gauge needle as the arachnoid knife.

In conclusion, our experience supports the use of combined intravascular and surgical treatment for complex AVMs, which a few years ago were considered as inoperable lesions. In our case, however, clot cavities formed by previous hemorrhage were apparently helpful for surgery. It is difficult to arrive at a uniform philosophy of management for giant ganglia AVMs unless the lesion had previously bled. It is our opinion that asymptomatic patients with giant basal ganglia AVMs do not require aggressive operative treatment.

References

Mizoi K, Takahashi A, Yoshimoto T et al 1992 Surgical excision of giant cerebellar hemispheric arteriovenous malformations following preoperative embolization. Journal of Neurosurgery 76: 1008–1011

Takahashi A, Suzuki J 1988 Nonsurgical treatment of AVM: development of new liquid embolization method. In: Suzuki J (ed) Advances in surgery for cerebral stroke. Springer-Verlag, Tokyo, pp 215–224

Takahashi A, Yoshimoto T, Sugawara T 1991 New liquid embolization method for brain arteriovenous malformations: combined infusion of estrogen-alcohol and polyvinyl acetate. Neuroradiology 33 (Suppl): 190–192

Bilateral Parafalcine Approach for Arteriovenous Malformations Located in the Interhemispheric Fissure
Atul Goel

AVMs located in the interhemispheric fissure are supplied by the pericallosal arteries and their branches arising from either the anterior or posterior cerebral arteries. These AVMs frequently drain into the superior sagittal sinus and some drain into the deep venous system. In larger AVMs the veins draining into the superior sagittal sinus can be large and multiple. Retraction of the hemisphere to expose the nidus widely can be severely limited by the presence of the veins draining into the superior sagittal sinus. Attempted hemispheric retraction can lead to tearing of the large vein, a procedure which can result in profuse bleeding, necessitating its coagulation. Venous coagulation may have an adverse effect on the nidus of the AVM, which can also bleed and complicate the surgery. We propose a bilateral exposure on both sides of the superior sagittal sinus and the falx (Fig. 9.14). The craniotomy is preferably a single large one which extends widely on both sides of the midline. The contralateral hemisphere is retracted first. The retraction of this side is relatively safe as there is no obstruction from the veins draining into the superior sagittal sinus. A large window is made into the falx and after adequate dissection the principal feeding artery to the AVM is isolated and coagulated. Other large feeding vessels are more easily exposed from this side and dissection of the nidus in the line of vision is carried out. On some occasions entire nidus resection can be carried out from the contralateral side transfalcine approach. The ipsilateral side is exposed if necessary. After section of the principal feeding arterial channels dissection around the veins draining into the superior sagittal sinus becomes safe and relatively easily possible. The entire nidus can thus be dissected and resected by working from both sides of the falx.

advances in microneurosurgical technology and techniques, more and more of these lesions, which were hitherto considered inoperable, are being treated surgically. The anatomical issues concerning the cavernous sinus have been a subject of controversy (Inoue et al 1990,

Dolenc 1989, Goel 1996b, Sekhar et al 1987, 1992, 1993, Parkinson 1965, Umansky & Nathan 1982). Its nature and function, exact topographical location, relationship to the dural envelope and to the carotid artery and cranial nerves remain controversial. Despite these issues, it is important

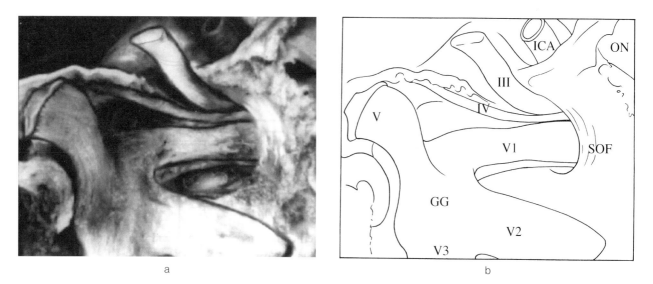

a   b

Fig. 10.5   a Anatomy of the lateral wall of the cavernous sinus after removal of the dural layers. The third, fourth and first divisions of the Vth nerve enter into the superior orbital fissure. The VIth nerve is not seen. The anterior clinoid process is not removed. **b** Key. ICA, internal carotid artery; ON, optic nerve; GG, Gasserian ganglion; V1, first division of trigeminal nerve; V2, second division of trigeminal nerve; V3, third division of trigeminal nerve; III–VI, cranial nerves.

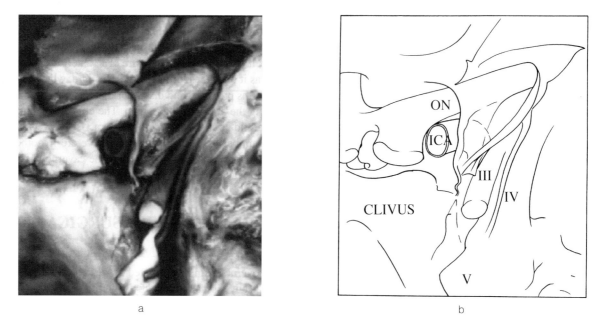

a   b

Fig. 10.6   a Anatomy of the lateral wall of the cavernous sinus after resection of the anterior clinoid process. Note the relationship of cranial nerves II, III and IV, and the carotid artery and dural rings. **b** Key. ICA, internal carotid artery; ON, optic nerve; III–V, cranial nerves.

for a neurosurgeon to know the gross features of anatomy in a three-dimensional perspective.

Anatomical considerations

The cavernous sinuses are paired structures situated on each side of the sella turcica, approximating the sphenoid bone. The cavernous sinus extends from the superior orbital fissure anteriorly to the petrous apex posteriorly (Figs 10.5–10.8).

Walls

The cavernous sinus has posterior, medial, superior, inferior and lateral dural walls. The latter four walls merge at the anterior clinoid process. Its dimensions are approximately 2 (length) × 1 (width) × 1 (height) cm. Cranial nerves III and IV enter the dural covering of the cavernous sinus in its superior wall and course in the superior aspect of its lateral wall. The Gasserian ganglion, its V1 and V2 divisions, are located in the dural sheath of the lateral wall. The cranial nerve VI traverses 'within' the cavernous sinus.

The dural envelope of the cavernous sinus is complex to understand. In the present study, it was seen that the lateral wall of the cavernous sinus had three well-defined and manually separable layers of dura. The internal two layers of dura were formed by the incurving of layers of the dura along the cranial nerves III–V as they entered the cavernous sinus, in the IIIrd nerve cave (discussed later), IVth nerve dural sheath and in Meckel's cave respectively. The dural cover of each of these nerves (thick around the Vth nerve and thin around other nerves) is continuous with each other by a reticular membrane which varies in thickness. The arachnoid layer was also identified to accompany the cranial nerves, being more well defined around the Gasserian ganglion and cranial nerve III. The outer dural layer of the lateral wall of the cavernous sinus is thick and often can be separated by sharp dissection into two or more

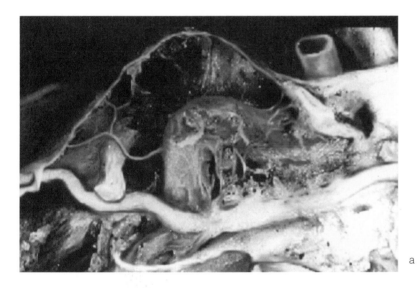

a

Fig. 10.7 **a** Anatomy as seen after removal of the cranial nerves of the lateral wall of the cavernous sinus. The IIIrd, IVth and all the three divisions of the Vth nerve have been removed. The intracavernous course of the carotid artery is seen. The clival dural entry point of the VIth nerve, its course in Dorello's canal and lateral to the carotid artery is seen. The VIth cranial nerve traverses under the sectioned petroclinoid ligament. **b** Key. ICA, internal carotid artery; ON, optic nerve; Clival a, clival artery; VI, VIth cranial nerve; PC lig, petroclinoid ligament.

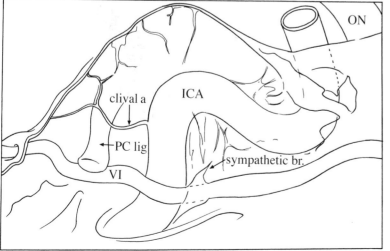

b

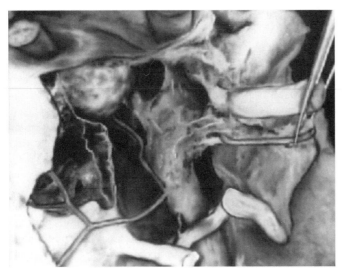

Fig. 10.8   a Anatomy as viewed from a posterior perspective. Cranial nerves III–V are retracted laterally, exposing the posterior bend of the intracavernous carotid artery. The meningohypophyseal trunk and its inferior hypophyseal and clival dural branches are seen. **b** Key. ICA, internal carotid artery; III–VI, cranial nerves; PC lig, petroclinoid ligament; MGH, meningohypophyseal trunk; IHA, inferior hypophyseal artery; Pit, pituitary gland.

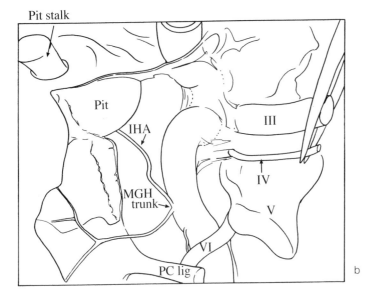

layers. The embryological and anatomical significance of the multiple layers of the thick lateral wall dura is not clearly understood. This thick dural layer can be dissected from the inner dural layers covering cranial nerves III–V and the reticular layer between them by gentle sharp dissection in a relatively bloodless plane. Brisk venous bleeding can, however, occur in the region of Parkinson's triangle as the reticular membrane is often deficient at this site. The two-layered middle fossa dura divides to encase the cavernous sinus, the inner (cerebral) layer forming the outer layer of the lateral wall and the outer (periosteal) layer forming the inferior wall of the cavernous sinus and later continuing as its medial wall. This description of the dural layers suggests that the cavernous sinus is like other venous sinuses (e.g. the superior sagittal sinus), with the exception that cranial nerves and carotid artery traverse in

close proximity during their course in the base of the skull. The dura of the medial wall of the cavernous sinus is very thin and closely adherent to the body of the sphenoid bone. The wall of the sphenoid bone separating the pituitary gland from the cavernous sinus is also thin. This explains the frequent spread of the pituitary tumors into the cavernous sinus. The lateral wall of the cavernous sinus, being thick and resilient, restricts further lateral spread of pituitary tumors. The thinner outer (endosteal) layer of the middle fossa dura separates from the thicker inner (cerebral) layer at the lateral aspect of the Gasserian ganglion and its division. At the various foramina, this layer folds out with the nerves and carotid artery. It thickens in the form of a firm ring at the entry of the carotid artery into the cavernous sinus. It also curves along the carotid artery into its petrous segment and forms the 'periosteal sheath'. It forms the medial wall of the cavernous sinus, where it is thin and relatively firmly stuck to the bone.

The outer, thicker layer of the dura of the lateral wall of the cavernous sinus continues laterally as the inner layer of the middle fossa dura, and medially as the superior wall of the cavernous sinus. The superior wall dura continues medially as the dura over the planum sphenoidale, wraps around the anterior clinoid process, covers the tuberculum sellae and forms the diaphragma sellae. It also forms the roof of the proximal part of the optic canal in the form of a thick dural fold called the falciform ligament. The dural layer is markedly thickened at the anterior and posterior petroclinoid folds and moderately thickened at the interclinoid dural folds. It is firmly adherent at the tip of the clinoid processes but is separable by blunt and occasionally sharp dissection. The same layer of dura is also continuous with the dura of the tentorium and clivus.

The superior wall of the cavernous sinus is triangular in shape, the sides of the triangle being formed by thickened dural folds, which are anterior extensions of the dura of the tentorium and the dura of the lateral wall of the cavernous sinus. The apex of the triangle is formed by the anterior clinoid process. The smaller posterior side is formed by the posterior petroclinoid fold extending from the petrous apex to the posterior clinoid process. The lateral side is formed by the anterior petroclinoid dural fold, extending from the petrous apex to the anterior clinoid process, while the medial side is formed by the interclinoid dural fold. The space enclosed by these three dural folds is called the oculomotor trigone.

Cranial nerve III

In the center of the oculomotor trigone cranial nerve III enters the dural wall of the cavernous sinus. This nerve forms a smooth crater for itself along the superior wall of the cavernous sinus and posterior petroclinoid dural fold. The dura of the superior wall curves with and traverses along the IIIrd nerve. A relatively large subarachnoid space covers the IIIrd nerve for about 6 mm after its entry into the superior wall. The appearance of the nerve at its entry into the cavernous sinus from a superior view is that of entering into a cave of dura. Paracavernous tumors can enter into this cave along with the IIIrd nerve. The dura, being separate from the nerve in this region, also provides the surgeon a plane to make an incision in the lateral wall of the cavernous sinus. The IIIrd nerve (and similar other cranial nerves of the cavernous sinus being surrounded by the dural layers) itself is not in direct contact with the venous blood in the cavernous sinus. The directions of the IIIrd nerve and the anterior clinoid process are important surgical landmarks. The inferolateral surface of the anterior clinoid process is in direct contact with and frequently grooved by the IIIrd nerve. The nerve can therefore be injured during procedures involving drilling of the anterior clinoid process.

Cranial nerve IV

This nerve enters the oculomotor trigone at its lateral angle. The IVth cranial nerve, after its course in the ambient cistern just underneath the tentorial edge, enters the leaves of dura of the tentorium at a distance of 10–18 mm from the posterior clinoid process. To save the IVth cranial nerve during sectioning of the tentorium, one should incise the tentorium at least 15 mm posterior to the posterior clinoid process, keeping the IVth nerve in view during this process. The IVth cranial nerve than traverses in the walls of the edge of the tentorium for 8–10 mm before turning to course parallel to the IIIrd nerve. Just before its entry into the superior orbital fissure the nerve turns superiorly to cross the IIIrd nerve.

Cranial nerve V

The two dural layers which enclose the Gasserian ganglion and its three divisions (after the Vth nerve enters Meckel's cave) are free and can be easily dissected from it until the semilunar ganglion divides into three, the space between the dura and ganglion being occupied by cerebrospinal fluid (CSF) during life. After the semilunar ganglion, the accompanying arachnoid layer becomes thinned out, and the dura is relatively firmly fixed to the divisions of the nerves and becomes continuous with the epineurium. The dura is more densely stuck to the V1 division of the nerve, from which it is relatively difficult to dissect free. The upper two-thirds of the Gasserian ganglion and its V1 division, and often the upper part of the V2 division, are located in the lateral wall of the cavernous sinus. The V3 separates from the ganglion and after a short intracranial course exits from the foramen ovale. The V2 exits from the foramen rotundum and its initial segment forms the lateral wall of the cavernous sinus and is the longest segment of the Vth cranial nerve in direct relation with the cavernous sinus. The superior ophthalmic vein drains into the cavernous sinus through the angle between the V1 and V2 nerves.

Cranial nerve VI

This nerve enters the cavernous sinus via Dorello's canal. This canal is situated in the two layers of the dura of the petroclival region. It is located between the petroclinoid ligament and the superior surface of the medial part of the clivus, which is covered by the dural layer forming the medial wall of the cavernous sinus. The entry point of the nerve into the clival dura is situated 15 mm below the tip of the posterior clinoid process. The two nerves enter the dura parallel to each other and at a distance of 12–15 mm from each other. The nerve enters the clival dura carrying with it a very thin dural and arachnoid sheath. It courses superiorly in the basilar venous sinus of the clivus, then takes a smooth bend over the petrous apex. At the petrous apex it traverses under the medial part of the petroclival ligament (Gruber's ligament), which is a bow-tie shaped ligament extending from the petrous apex to the clival dura. It is wider at its attachment and relatively thin at the center. This ligament is situated in the venous pool and demarcates the cavernous sinus from the large basilar venous plexus. There are multiple rootlets of the VIth nerve which join to form a single bundle at its entry into the clival dura. These rootlets may divide in Dorello's canal into two to five. Some of these rootlets may even course above the petroclival or petrosphenoid ligament (Gruber's ligament), which can always be identified by its large size, its tough and elastic character (unlike the relatively weak dural folds in the surroundings), and its shiny silvery appearance. Dorello's canal is an osteofibrous conduit located over the clivus, measuring about 3–4 mm in length (the floor being bony, formed by the lateral edge of the clival bone and roof by Gruber's ligament), and is about 3.5 mm anteromedial to the petrous apex. The VIth nerve traverses Dorello's canal to reach the cavity of the cavernous sinus. After the VIth nerve exits from under the petroclival ligament it turns superolaterally to traverse lateral to the carotid artery at its posterior ascending segment. It is sometimes important to identify and dissect the VIth nerve during surgery. It can be traced during its course medial to Meckel's cave and the inferior aspect of the V1 division of the Vth nerve. It is usually situated between the axilla of the horizontal segment of the intracavernous carotid artery and the artery of the inferior cavernous sinus. The nerve traverses lateral to the carotid artery at its posterior ascending segment, and is then inferolateral to it.

The average distance between the points of entry of the cranial nerves in the cavernous sinus was found to be as follows: between III and IV, 6.16 mm; between III and V, 12.34 mm; between IV and V, 10.52 mm; and between V and VI, 6.50 mm. The mean length of intracavernous cranial nerves was as follows: III, 12.26 mm; IV, 14.40 mm; V, 16.38 mm; and VI, 20.44 mm.

Venous sinuses

There has been considerable controversy as to whether the cavernous sinus is made up of large sinusoidal venous spaces or of a plexus of veins. The recent opinion based on histo-architectural studies confirms the plexus pattern. However, in cadaveric studies large venous sinusoidal spaces are seen. The description of the plexus venous pattern does not appear to be relevant from the surgical point of view. The plexus pattern is more distinct in fetal cavernous sinuses and in the cavernous sinuses of lower animals. The main venous drainage of the cavernous sinus comes through the superior ophthalmic veins via the superior orbital fissure draining in the cavernous sinus between V1 and V2. The cavernous sinuses also communicate anteriorly with the sphenoparietal sinus and the superficial sylvian vein; laterally with the venous sinuses

accompanying the middle meningeal artery; and posteriorly with the basilar sinus. The pterygoid venous plexus communicates with the cavernous sinus via the emissary sphenoidal foramen situated medial to the foramen ovale. The anterior and posterior intercavernous sinuses, named from the relationship to the pituitary gland, connect the two cavernous sinuses. The posterior intercavernous sinus is larger than the anterior. These interconnections are situated between two layers of dura. There is a large venous connection between the two cavernous sinus via the basilar clival venous plexus. The basilar venous plexus contains a large pool of venous blood. This blood pool can significantly affect transclival surgical approaches. The basilar venous plexus communicates with the cavernous sinus via a large venous communication at the petrous apex. There is a larger superior petrosal sinus and smaller inferior petrosal sinus draining the cavernous sinus. The superior petrosal sinus is situated over the petrous ridge. It traverses over the root of the Vth nerve within two layers of dura. The inferior petrosal sinus travels inferior to the root of the Vth nerve. The venous spaces in the cavernous sinus have been named by Rhoton et al from their relationship to the carotid artery. The main venous spaces are medial, lateral, anteroinferior and posterosuperior venous spaces. All the specimens studied were medial space dominant, the largest venous pool of blood being situated in the posteromedial aspect of the cavernous sinus.

Carotid artery

The carotid artery traverses the petrous apex region underneath the Gasserian ganglion. A dural ring under the Gasserian ganglion marks the entry point of the artery into the cavernous sinus. The artery under this dural ring is relatively fixed and the segment in the cavernous sinus beyond this ring is relatively mobile. The carotid artery is also fixed to the skull base at the anterior clinoid process by the dural rings. In about 70% of specimens the bone separating the carotid artery from the lateral half of the Gasserian ganglion is absent. It was seen during our dissections that there are membranous adhesions of the carotid artery, VIth nerve and IIIrd–IVth nerves to each other and to the dural wall of the cavernous sinus. The artery encounters many twists and turns and spins around its longitudinal axis during its course in the cavernous sinus, which may in some way be responsible for the temperature regulation of cerebral blood flow (Dolenc 1989). The intracavernous carotid artery has been divided into posterior ascending segment, posterior genu, horizontal segment, anterior genu and anterior ascending segment. The dome of the posterior genu can sometimes, particularly in the elderly with atherosclerotic vessels, be very close to the posterior clinoid process. This relationship has to be properly understood while doing surgery for basilar tip aneurysms as sometimes there is a need to drill the posterior clinoid process. The distal part of the anterior ascending segment of the carotid artery is situated medial to the anterior clinoid process. Removal of the anterior clinoid process permits an additional exposure of approximately 6 mm of the internal carotid artery (ICA) without entering the cavernous sinus. The juxtaclinoid carotid artery is surrounded by bone almost in its entire circumference. Laterally it is related to the medial surface of the anterior clinoid process, anteriorly it is in close proximity to the posterior surface of the optic strut, while medially it lies on the body of the sphenoid bone. The posterior border of this segment of the carotid artery is in relation to the cavity of the cavernous sinus. However, sometimes the middle clinoid process may form a bony division between the artery and the cavernous sinus. The anterior clinoid process is separated from the carotid artery by a dural sheath. There are two prominent dural folds lateral to the carotid artery after the anterior clinoid process is drilled off. These are called the proximal and distal dural rings of the carotid artery. The dural sheath covering the artery is continuous with the dura covering the nerves of the superior orbital fissure and the dura over the planum sphenoidale and tuberculum sellae and with the lateral wall of the cavernous sinus. The supraclinoid carotid artery courses over the superior wall of the cavernous sinus. Lateral or medial retraction of this segment of the carotid artery can lead to the exposure of the superior wall. The exposure of the intracavernous lesions via the superior wall is an important surgical avenue.

There are two main branches of the intracavernous carotid artery. The meningohypophyseal trunk emerges from the posterior aspect of the ascending segment of the cavernous carotid artery about 4–6 mm below the dome of the posterior genu of the artery. The artery was seen to divide into multiple branches immediately after its origin. The tentorial artery (of Bernasconi and Cassineri) after its short course in the cavernous sinus enters into the tentorial dural fold. The dorsal meningeal artery and inferior hypophyseal artery have a relatively long course in the venous pool. The dorsal meningeal artery traverses in a posteromedial direction near the clival end of the petroclival ligament (coursing over the clival dural surface) and then divides into superior and inferior clival branches. Branches of this artery are seen to anastomose with the branches of the contralateral artery. The inferior hypophyseal artery travels medially, in a relatively straight course, to the posterior lobe of the pituitary gland. Branches of the meningohypophyseal trunk are seen going to cranial nerves III–VI. The artery of the inferior cavernous sinus (inferolateral trunk) is the other branch of the intracavernous carotid artery. This artery arises from the horizontal segment of the carotid artery and traverses over the VIth cranial nerve. It corresponds to the proximal remnant of the embryonic dorsal ophthalmic artery. In one speci-

men, however, the artery coursed under the VIth nerve. It supplied the dura of the inferior wall of the cavernous sinus and also small branches supplied cranial nerves III–VI. McConnel's capsular artery has been seen to arise in 18% of specimens from the medial surface of the distal half of the horizontal segment of the artery, supplying the dural sheath around the pituitary gland. The ophthalmic artery has sometimes been seen to arise from intracavernous carotid.

A sympathetic plexus of nerves accompanies the carotid artery in the petrous bone. After the artery enters the cavernous sinus by passing under the dural ring the sympathetic nerves separate from the carotid. Some branches initially join the VIth nerve and then the V1 division of the Vth nerve, and ultimately exit the cavernous sinus, with each division of the trigeminal nerve providing sympathetic innervation to the skin in the respective territory. A ganglion of the sympathetic nerve has been seen between the VIth cranial nerve and the carotid artery.

Occasionally some fat globules may be seen in the cavernous sinus. The fat was commonly situated in the anterolateral end adjoining the orbital adipose tissue and in the posterior end near the petrous margin of the cavernous sinus. In the middle part scattered fat deposits around the pituitary fossa are often seen. It is frequently difficult to differentiate fat globules from sympathetic fibers and ganglion on routine microscopic examination.

Triangles

Various triangles have been described by Dolenc and others to clarify and simplify an understanding of the anatomy of the cavernous sinus. These triangles often become distorted by the presence of intracavernous pathology. However, the entry and exit points of the nerves and artery into the cavernous sinus are via a relatively fixed site and even if the triangles may become distorted a general idea and orientation during surgery can be had from the fixed entry and exit points of these nerves and the carotid artery.

Dwight Parkinson described an important triangle for approaching the cavernous sinus through its lateral wall. The boundaries of this triangle are the IIIrd/IVth nerve complex superiorly, the V1 division of the Vth nerve inferiorly and the clival dura posteriorly. The maximum distance between the V1 division of the Vth nerve and the IVth cranial nerve was 4 mm. The VIth nerve is not seen in this triangle. The V1 division of the Vth nerve has to be retracted inferiorly to expose the VIth nerve. Occasionally the medial surface of the V1 division of the Vth nerve may be indented by the VIth nerve. The posterior ascending segment of the carotid artery and its meningohypophyseal trunk can be exposed in this triangle. Parkinson described this triangle for exposure of the carotid artery and the meningohypophyseal trunk, for this is an important site of development of intracavernous carotid artery aneurysms and caroticocavernous fistulae. The triangle is an important landmark for exposure of intracavernous lesions.

Prior to actually incising the walls of the cavernous sinus it is important to get oriented to the local anatomy. Important bony landmarks are the anterior clinoid process, posterior clinoid process, foramen ovale, foramen rotundum, superior orbital fissure and the petrous apex. Soft tissue landmarks are the exit point of carotid artery from the roof of the cavernous sinus, optic nerve, divisions of the Vth nerve, greater superficial petrosal nerve and the entry point and direction of the various cranial nerves.

CONCLUSIONS

The complex anatomy of the cavernous sinus can be made relatively clear by systematic and repeated cadaveric anatomical study. The present study can be useful for surgeons operating in and around the region of the cavernous sinus.

REFERENCES

Inoue T, Rhoton A L Jr, Theele D, Barry M E 1990 Surgical approaches to the cavernous sinus: a microsurgical study. Neurosurgery 26: 903–932

Dolenc V V 1989 Anatomy of the cavernous sinus. In Dolenc V V (ed) Anatomy and surgery of the cavernous sinus. Springer-Verlag, New York, 1989

Goel A 1996a Cavernous sinus: a speculative note. Journal of Clinical Neuroscience 3: 281

Goel A 1996b Surgical anatomy of the cavernous sinus. In Torrens M J, Al-Mefty O, Kobayashi S (eds) Operative skull base surgery, Churchill Livingstone, Edinburgh (in press)

Parkinson D 1965 A surgical approach to the cavernous portion of the carotid artery: anatomical studies and case report. Journal of Neurosurgery 23: 474–483

Sekhar L N, Burgess J, Atkin O 1987 Anatomical study of the cavernous sinus emphasizing operative approaches and related vascular and neural reconstruction. Neurosurgery 21: 806–816

Sekhar L N, Goel A, Sen C N 1992 General neurosurgical operative techniques and instrumentation in cranial base surgery. In Sekhar L N, Janecka I P (eds) Atlas of skull base surgery. Raven Press, New York

Sekhar L N, Goel A, Sen C N 1993 Cavernous sinus surgery. In Appuzo M (ed) Brain surgery: complication avoidance and management. Churchill Livingstone, Edinburgh pp 2197–2219

Umansky F, Nathan H 1982 The lateral wall of the cavernous sinus, with special reference to the nerves related to it. Journal of Neurosurgery 56: 228–234

The Surgical Anatomy of the Cavernous Sinus and Dural Folds of the Parasellar Region

Felix Umansky   Alberto Valarezo   Elen Piontek   Sergey Spektor

The continuous development of microsurgical techniques to treat lesions in and around the cavernous sinus emphasizes the need for an accurate understanding of the microanatomy of this complex region (Dolenc 1989, Harris & Rhoton 1976, Inoue et al 1990, Sekhar et al 1987, Umansky and Nathan 1982, Umansky et al 1994).

The surgical anatomy of the cavernous sinus walls including the dural folds and ligaments of the parasellar region will be described in a concise manner.

1. Lateral Wall (Fig. 10.9): The lateral wall of the cavernous sinus was consistently found to be formed of two layers: a smooth superficial layer formed by the dura mater, and a deep layer containing nerves III, IV, and V1. The two layers of the wall were only loosely attached to each other and could therefore be easily separated.

The deep layer was less defined than the superficial layer and was more irregular and variable in its texture and morphological characteristics. It was found to be formed by the sleeves or sheaths of dura mater accompanying the corresponding nerves from their points of penetration into the sinus walls.

The sheaths around nerves III and V1,2 were rather thick and constantly distinct, while that of nerve IV was thin and often inconspicuous. A membrane of a reticular texture extended between the sheaths of the nerves, thus completing the deep layer. This membrane seemed to be composed of the connective tissue forming the trabeculae of the sinus cavity. It was found as a thin but definitely complete membrane in 60% of the specimens. In 40% it was incomplete, and often missing in the space between nerves III and V1. In these cases, a kind of window between these two nerves appeared when the superficial layer was dissected and reflected; through this window, the cavity of the sinus was revealed with its trabeculae and blood remnants. When these were cleared away, the ICA and nerve VI could be seen in the cavity. The window was generally triangular in shape, with its base situated posteriorly, corresponding to the posterior border of the wall. The superior border of the triangle corresponded to nerve III with its meningeal sheath, and the inferior border to nerve V1 with its sheath. The apex of the triangle corresponded to the point where the two nerves met and decussated in the

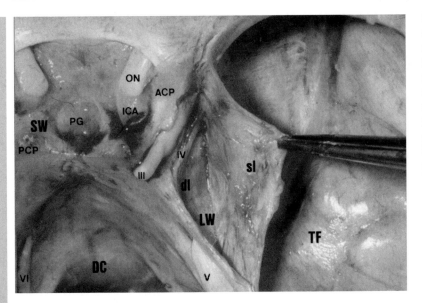

anterior part of the sinus wall. Nerve IV generally ran parallel with and close and inferior to nerve III at the superior limit of the window.

In the area of the window, the lateral wall of the sinus was much thinner than at the level of nerves III and V, since it was formed here only by the superficial layer. Due to its transparency, it could generally be recognized even by direct observation before the wall was opened because of the darker color of its area.

This space between nerves III and IV above and V1 and VI below corresponds to Parkinson's triangle (Parkinson 1965) (Fig. 10.13).

2. Superior Wall (Fig. 10.10): The superior wall of the cavernous sinus, trapezoidal in shape, is limited laterally by the anterior petroclinoid ligament, medially by the dura of the diaphragma sellae, anteriorly by the endosteal dura of the carotid canal and posteriorly by the posterior petroclinoid ligament. A line parallel to the interclinoid ligament divides this wall into two triangles: the carotid trigone anteromedially and the oculomotor trigone posterolaterally. Similar to the lateral wall of the sinus, its superior wall is formed by two layers: a smooth superficial dural layer and a thin, less-defined deep layer. For didactic purposes, the superior wall of the cavernous sinus has been divided into three areas: the oculomotor trigone, the carotid trigone, and the clinoid space.

Oculomotor Trigone: Cranial nerves III and IV entered the cavernous sinus in this area of the superior wall. The dural foramen of the oculomotor nerve, elliptical in shape (maximum diameter 4.9 ± 1.1 mm), was larger than the nerve crossing it in most cases. The dural opening for the trochlear nerve was located in the angle between the anterior and posterior petroclinoid ligaments and in a large number of cases (63%) the diameter of the opening was equal to the diameter of the nerve.

In the oculomotor trigone the dural layers (superficial

and deep) could be easily separated. The superficial layer continued laterally with the superficial layer of the lateral wall, medially with the superficial layer of the carotid trigone, and posteriorly with the superficial layer of the petroclival dura in the posterior wall of the cavernous sinus. The deep layer, thinner than the superficial layer, continued laterally, medially, and posteriorly with the deep dural layer of the lateral wall, carotid trigone, and posterior wall of the cavernous sinus, respectively.

Carotid Trigone: This area of the superior wall was limited laterally by a line overlying the interclinoid ligament, medially by the dura of the diaphragma sellae, and anteriorly by the endosteal dura of the carotid canal. The anterior portion of this trigone presented the opening for the ICA at the beginning of its supraclinoid segment. The ICA foramen had a diameter of 6.86 ± 0.9 mm, and on its medial side the dura mater could be easily separated from the artery, revealing a semilunar space known as the 'carotid cave' (Kobayashi et al 1989).

In the area of the carotid trigone, dissection between the superficial and deep dural layers was more difficult than in the oculomotor trigone. The superficial dural layer continued laterally with the similar layer of the oculomotor trigone and with the dura that covered the superior aspect of the anterior clinoid process, medially with the dura of the diaphragma sellae, and anteriorly with the endosteal dura of the carotid canal. This superficial layer contributed to the formation of the distal ring of the ICA. The deep dural layer was very thin and friable and was usually incomplete in the posterior half of this area. This layer ended medially at the level of the diaphragma sellae. The deep layer of the carotid trigone dura mater contributed to the formation of the medial ring of the ICA. This ring is described in more detail in the area of the clinoid space. The deep layer continued posteriorly with the deep layer of the oculomotor trigone.

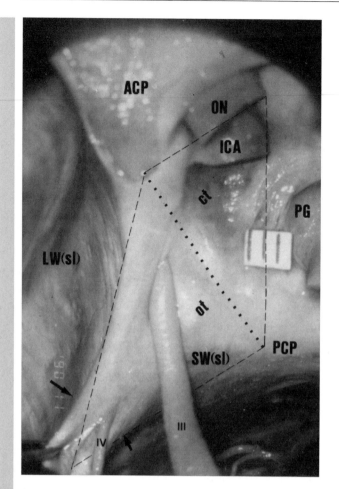

Fig. 10.10 Superior view of the left cavernous sinus. The superior wall of the sinus (broken line) is divided into two triangles by a dotted line overlying the interclinoid ligament: the oculomotor trigone (ot) posterolaterally and carotid trigone (ct) anteromedially. The third (III) and fourth (IV) cranial nerves enter the sinus through the oculomotor trigone while the internal carotid artery (ICA) exits the sinus in the area of the carotid trigone. The dura mater over the anterior clinoid process (ACP) has been removed. The superficial layer of the superior wall of the sinus SW(sl) continues laterally with the superficial layer of the lateral wall of the sinus LW(sl). The long arrow points to the anterior petroclinoid ligament and the short arrow to the posterior petroclinoid ligament. (ON, optic nerve; PCP, posterior clinoid process; PG, pituitary gland, scale in millimeters.)

Clinoid Area or Space (Fig. 10.11): The removal of the anterior clinoid process revealed an interdural space between both dural layers, which separated at this level to wrap the bone process. Beyond this interdural space, the paraclinoid or clinoid segment of the ICA could be clearly seen. There was a small area anterior to the artery frequently occupied by an extension of the ethmoid or sphenoid air cells. Inadvertent opening of these cells

during surgery may cause rhinorrhea. There was another small triangular area posterior to the ICA covered by the deep layer of the dura mater. Opening this thin membrane would lead to the interior of the cavernous sinus. In some of our specimens, this membrane was incomplete. At the level of the ICA, the deep layer of the dura mater became thicker to form the medial ring of the artery.

This deep layer continued laterally with the deep layer of the lateral wall of the cavernous sinus and with the dura mater of the superior orbital fissure.

3. Posterior Wall (Fig. 10.12): This wall, which belongs to the petroclival dura mater, is limited superolaterally by the posterior petroclinoid ligament, medially by the dorsum sellae and inferiorly by the petrous apex and Dorello's canal. Similar to the lateral and superior walls of the sinus, its posterior wall was found to be formed by two layers: a smooth superficial dural layer and a thin and less-defined deep layer. This wall covers not only the posterior aspect of the cavernous sinus but a venous confluence joined also by the basilar sinus and the inferior petrosal sinus. The anatomy of this wall becomes important when dealing with lesions in the petroclival area.

Dural Folds of the Parasellar Region: The parasellar dural folds have been classified into three groups: tentorial, carotid and interdural.

1. Tentorial Group (Fig. 10.10): *Anterior petroclinoid ligament:* this ligament, which is the extension of the free edge of the tentorium, runs from posterior to anterior and from lateral to medial toward the anterior clinoid process. Fibers of this ligament contribute to the formation of the superficial layer of the lateral and superior cavernous sinus walls.

Posterior petroclinoid ligament: this ligament is related to the attached border of the tentorium and runs anteromedially toward the posterior clinoid process. Its fibers contribute to the formation of the superficial layer of the superior and posterior walls of the cavernous sinus.

In the angle between the origin of both petroclinoid ligaments cranial nerve IV pierces the dura mater of the superior wall of the cavernous sinus.

2. Carotid Group (Fig. 10.13): The three dural folds partially encircling the ICA in the parasellar region are called the proximal, medial, and distal carotid rings.

Proximal carotid ring: this is located at the level of the endocranial opening of the foramen lacerum where the ICA enters the cavernous sinus.

This ring is 'V' shaped and surrounds the ICA except for its anterior aspect. The lateral fiber of this ring constitutes the petrolingual ligament. This ligament is the anatomical landmark between the intrapetrous and cavernous ICA.

Medial carotid ring: this ring is related to the deep layer

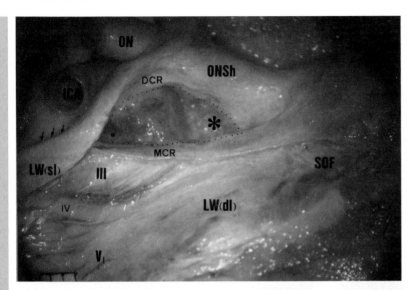

Fig. 10.11   Lateral view of the right cavernous sinus after removal of the anterior clinoid process. The superior oribital fissure (SOF) has been exposed and the optic nerve (ON) unroofed. The clinoid space is circumscribed by a dotted line. An extension of the sinus air cells is visible (asterisk). The triangular space posterior to the internal carotid artery (ICA) is marked by an open dot. The superficial layer of the lateral wall of the sinus LW(sl) contributing to the anterior petroclinoid ligament (arrows) has been peeled upward, exposing the oculomotor (III), trochlear (IV) and ophthalmic (VI) nerves embedded in the deep dural layer of the lateral wall LW(dl). (DCR, distal carotid ring; MCR, medial carotid ring; ON, optic nerve; ONSh, optic nerve sheath; scale in millimeters.)

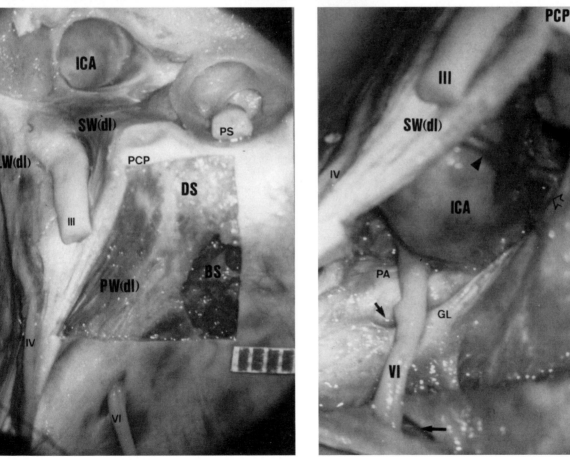

a

b

Fig. 10.12   Posterosuperior (**a**) and posterior **b** view of the left cavernous sinus after superficial **a** and deep **b** dissection. **a** The superficial dural layer of the petroclival region, lateral and superior walls of the cavernous sinus have been removed. The basilar sinus (BS) has been exposed by partial removal of the deep dural layer of the superior wall SW(dl) and that of the lateral wall LW(dl) of the cavernous sinus. (DS, dorsum sellae; ICA, internal carotid artery; PS, pituitary stalk; III, oculomotor nerve; IV, trochlear nerve; VI, abducens nerve; scale in millimeters.) **b** Further dissection of this region has been performed, bringing into view the posterior aspect of the cavernous sinus. In this particular specimen the abducens nerve (VI) is coursing over Gruber's ligament (GL) on its way to the cavernous sinus. (C, clivus, DS, dorsum sellae; ICA, oculomotor nerve; IV, trochlear nerve. The long black arrow points to the dural foramen of the abducens nerve; short black arrow indicates Dorello's canal; arrowhead points to the meningohypophyseal trunk; open arrow points to the dorsomeningeal artery; scale in millimeters.)

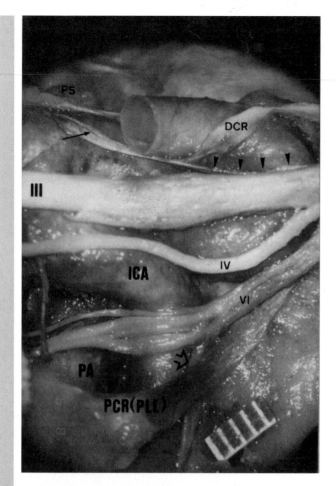

Fig. 10.13 Lateral view of the right cavernous sinus. The lateral wall of the sinus has been completely removed, disclosing the contents of the sinus. (DCR, distal carotid ring; ICA, internal carotid artery; PA, petrous apex; PCR (PLL), lateral fibers of the proximal carotid ring formed by the petrolingual ligament; PS, pituitary stalk; III, oculomotor nerve; IV, trochlear nerve; VI, abducens nerve; arrow points to the interclinoid ligament; arrowheads indicate the medial carotid ring; the open arrow shows the sympathetic nerve; scale in millimeters.) The space between the trochlear and abducens nerve corresponds to the area of Parkinson's triangle.

of dura mater of the superior wall of the cavernous sinus and becomes visible after drilling the anterior clinoid process. The ring surrounds the posterolateral aspect of the carotid artery and posteriorly gives origin to the interclinoid ligament. Anteriorly and medially the ring fuses with the endosteum of the carotid canal.

Distal carotid ring: the fibers of this ring belong to the superficial layer of the superior wall of the cavernous sinus. The ring courses over the superior aspect of the ICA just anterior to the region of its ophthalmic branch. Medial to the carotid artery the ring is loose, leaving a

small space described by Kobayashi et al as 'carotid cave' (Kobayashi et al 1989).

3. Interdural Group: Gruber's ligament (Fig. 10.11b): also called the petrosphenoidal ligament, this extends from the spina sphenoidalis located on the superior border of the petrous apex to the lateral border of the dorsum sellae and clivus. This ligament appears as a fibrous trabecula within a large venous lake formed by the confluence of the cavernous, basilar and inferior petrosal sinuses.

Interclinoid ligament (Fig. 10.10): this ligament becomes apparent after removing both the superficial and deep layers of dura mater of the superior wall of the cavernous sinus. Its fibers run from the posterior to the anterior clinoid processes but its anterior insertion is at the level of the medial ring of the ICA. The length of the ligament was 9.75 ± 0.5 mm. It was found partially ossified in 10% and totally ossified in another 10% of the specimens.

In Conclusion: From our anatomical studies we found a common dural architecture consistent with two dural layers (superficial and deep) in the lateral, superior and posterior walls of the cavernous sinus. These membranes are also involved in the formation of ligaments and rings and the anatomy of these structures should be known by the surgeon working in this area. These dural membranes participate in the formation of the sheaths of some of the cranial nerves (mainly III and IV) coursing through the lateral wall.

The study of the complex dural anatomy of the cavernous sinus and parasellar region is not only of academic interest. Benign tumors like meningiomas may spread over long distances through the virtual space existing between both dural layers and through the dural foramina of the cranial nerves.

From a surgical point of view, most of the approaches to the cavernous sinus are through its lateral or superior wall or a combination of both. Cavernous sinus tumors and aneurysms of the ICA in its intracavernous course and at the level of its ophthalmic branch have been treated through these approaches. The relatively easy dissection of both layers of dura mater in the lateral wall of the sinus allows peeling of the outer layer with the extracavernous portion of the tumor and, in cases of pure intracavernous lesions, evaluation of the adhesion of the cranial nerves to the tumor. Schwannomas which grow in the 'interdural space' between both layers will be also removed in this way. The approach through the superior wall has the advantage of having the ICA and the oculomotor nerve as the only structures exiting and entering this wall and combined with the lateral wall approach allows a very good exploration of the sinuses. The posterior wall is infrequently used as an entry gate to the sinus but is usually involved in lesions of the petroclival area.

References

Dolenc V V 1989 Anatomy of the cavernous sinus. In: Dolenc V V (ed) Anatomy and surgery of the cavernous sinus. Springer-Verlag, New York, pp 3–7

Harris F S, Rhoton A L Jr 1976 Anatomy of the cavernous sinus: a microsurgical study. Journal of Neurosurgery 45: 169–180

Inoue T, Rhoton A L Jr, Theele D et al 1990 Surgical approaches to the cavernous sinus: a microsurgical study. Neurosurgery 26: 903–932

Kobayashi S, Kyoshima K, Gibo H et al 1989 Carotid cave aneurysm of the internal carotid artery. Journal of Neurosurgery 70: 216–221

Parkinson D 1965 A surgical approach to the cavernous portion of the carotid artery: anatomical studies and case report. Journal of Neurosurgery 23: 474–483

Sekhar L N, Burgess J, Akin O 1987 Anatomical study of the cavernous sinus emphasizing operative approaches and related vascular and neural reconstruction. Neurosurgery 21: 806–816

Umansky F, Nathan H 1982 The lateral wall of the cavernous sinus: with special reference to the nerves related to it. Journal of Neurosurgery 56: 228–234

Umansky F, Valarezo A, Elidan J 1994 The superior wall of the cavernous sinus: a microanatomical study. Journal of Neurosurgery 81: 914–920

Surgical strategy in tumors involving the cavernous sinus

11

Atul Goel   Trimurti Nadkarni   Shigeaki Kobayashi

Surgery of the cavernous sinus is amongst the most complex neurosurgical challenges. Despite the advances in skull base surgery, few series outlining the operative strategy on tumors involving the cavernous sinus are seen in the literature. Magnetic resonance imaging (MRI) has been a major factor in the advancement of cavernous sinus tumor surgery. It has not only increased the sensitivity in detecting these lesions, but by clarification of the tumor–carotid artery relationship it guides the surgeon in adequately planning the operative strategy (Goel 1995a, 1995b, 1996a, 1996b, 1996c).

HISTOLOGICAL NATURE OF THE LESION

Most of the tumors involve the cavernous sinus secondarily. Intracavernous origin of a tumor is rare. Spread of a primarily extracavernous tumor into the cavernous sinus is usually along the dural folds at the site of the entry of the cranial nerves. Direct spread of a tumor through the dural walls is rare. On most occasions it is possible for the surgeon to make a reasonable guess about the histological nature of the lesion on the basis of the clinical and radiological studies. The age and sex of the patient, acuity of the presentation, principal presenting signs, size of the tumor, extent of cranial nerve involvement, nature of carotid artery displacement and/or encasement, imaging characters on computed tomographic (CT) scanning and MRI and other such features are helpful in estimating the consistency and vascularity of the lesion, site of origin and direction of its spread, and the extent and nature of cavernous sinus involvement. Such information is critically important in guiding the direction of the approach to the lesion and the cavernous sinus, need for carotid artery control, extent of the surgical resection that would be necessary and possible, and prognosticating the ultimate outcome.

CAVERNOUS SINUS INVOLVEMENT: FEATURES OF SOME MORE COMMON LESIONS

Nasopharyngeal angiofibromas

The age, sex, and presentation with epistaxis are characteristic. These lesions are primarily extracranial and extradural (Goel et al 1994). In larger lesions the basal bones are eroded, thinned out and elevated superiorly. In our large series of massive tumors cavernous sinus invasion was not seen. Dural invasion has been recorded in rare cases and is in the form of small tail-like invaginations. Cavernous sinus involvement is in the form of superior displacement and seldom as invasion (Figs 11.1, 11.2). The entire cavernous sinus with its contained vascular and neural structures is pushed superiorly by the tumor. This character of the tumor assists in developing a plane between the tumor and the basal dura even with a blunt dissection. On CT scan it may appear that the entire cavernous sinus is involved by the tumor, but MRI and angiography usually clarify the picture. Due to their location most tumors present when they are large in size despite their expansive growth characters. In rare cases proximal exposure of the carotid artery for the purpose of control may be necessary.

Trigeminal neurinomas

These lesions are located within the confines of dura in the lateral wall of the cavernous sinus. The location has sometimes been termed 'interdural' (Dolenc 1994, Goel 1995). Despite the massive growth of the lesion in some cases, the confines of the dura are not eroded (Figs 11.3, 11.4). The dura is relatively free from the Gasserian ganglion in the region of Meckel's cave. Normally, there is a large subarachnoid space in this region. Beyond the Gasserian ganglion the dura is adherent to the divisions of the nerve and

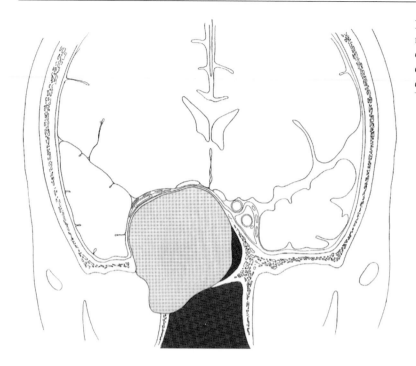

Fig.11.1 Line drawing showing the massive nasopharyngeal angiofibroma. The ipsilateral cavernous sinus and its contained structures are elevated on the dome of the tumor. Note the eroded basal bone.

later it is continuous with their epineurium. Adhesion of the dura to the divisions is more firm in its first division than in the second and third. The tumor usually arises in the region of the Gasserian ganglion. The growing tumor can be accommodated within the confines of Meckel's cave, which becomes bloated. Anterior extension along the root, into the infratemporal fossa, or into the dural sheath

of the lateral wall of the cavernous sinus, is rare, probably due to the natural adhesions of the dura and nerve. The intracavernous carotid artery is displaced medially and the precavernous carotid at the petrous apex inferiorly by the lesion. Due to the characteristic location and protection provided to the carotid artery by the dura medially in relation to the cavernous sinus and inferiorly in relation to the

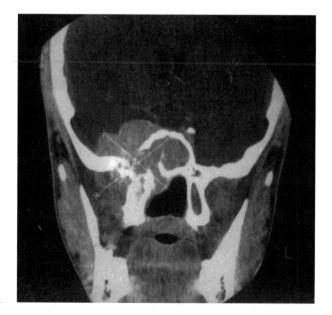

Fig. 11.2 CT scan showing the massive nasopharyngeal angiofibroma. The displaced contents of the cavernous sinus can be seen. The tumor is essentially extradural and extracranial.

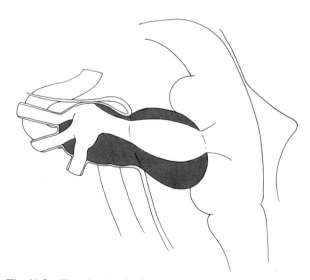

Fig. 11.3 The trigeminal neurinoma filling up and dilating Meckel's cave. The tumor extends into the posterior cranial fossa, displacing the brain stem. The ICA is displaced by the tumor. The Vth nerve itself is splayed. The part of the tumor in Meckel's cave is shown to be interdural while the part in the posterior cranial fossa is intradural.

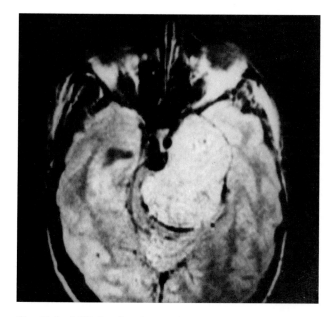

Fig. 11.4 MRI showing the massive trigeminal neurinoma. Despite the large size the tumor only dilated Meckel's cave.

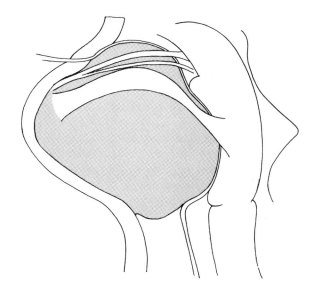

Fig. 11.5 The more typical variety of petroclival chordoma. The lesion displaces the carotid artery anteriorly while the cavernous sinus is displaced superiorly.

petrous apex, working within the dural boundary is relatively safe and effective. Opening up of the outer dural sheath of the Gasserian ganglion without exposing the temporal brain, for excision of the tumor, may be carried out. There is seldom any need to have a proximal arterial control for tumor excision in these cases.

Chordomas

Although various authors have noted cavernous sinus invasion by chordomas and chondrosarcomas, it was observed that even in massive tumors the cavernous sinus involvement by these lesions was in the form of displacement rather than invasion (Goel 1995a, 1995c). The tumor arises from the spheno-occipital synchondrosis and grows eccentrically into the subcavernous sinus' region and elevates it on its dome (Figs 11.5, 11.6). The tumor destroys the bone and displaces the soft tissues. The functional involvement of the nerves of the cavernous sinus is apparently due to the stretch. The precavernous and cavernous segments of the carotid artery are displaced anteriorly by the tumor. The tumor is primarily extradural and actual transgression of the dura is a rare feature. Even in large lesions a layer of dura separates the tumor from neural and vascular structures, providing a plane of cleavage for surgical resection. The displacement of the carotid artery and Gasserian ganglion and destruction of the petrous apex and clivus make an intradural subtemporal sub-Gasserian ganglion approach a suitable alternative for resection of these lesions.

Pituitary tumors

The anatomic relationship of the pituitary gland to the cavernous sinus is quite intimate. The medial wall of the cavernous sinus almost touches the pituitary gland. The dural wall that separates the pituitary gland from the cavernous sinus is thin. The ease with which the medial dural layer of the cavernous sinus gives way to the growing tumor raises

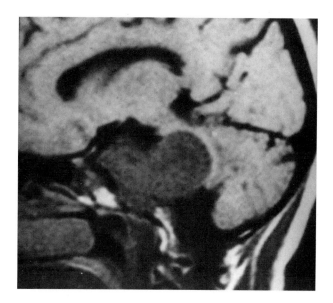

Fig. 11.6 MRI shows the massive chordoma. The arrow shows the carotid artery displaced along the anterior surface of the tumor. The brain stem is displaced posteriorly.

suspicion as to the 'dural' nature of the layer. The soft pituitary tumor invades into the cavernous sinus through its medial wall (Figs 11.7–11.9). The tumor mushrooms into the available venous spaces in the cavernous sinus, surrounds the carotid artery and bloats up the cavernous sinus. But the lesion, being soft, does not possess the strength required to invade and extend through the thick lateral wall. The tumor encases the carotid artery but usually cannot squeeze its lumen. The tumor frequently has an eccentric spread. The tumor bloats the cavernous sinus and stretches on its nerves. Any lateral approach therefore has the danger of injuring these nerves. A midline approach appears to be a better alternative. A contralateral subfrontal approach was noted to be the most suitable direction of approach to the tumor (Goel & Nadkarni 1995a, 1995b, 1996).

Meningiomas

Meningiomas are amongst the more common lesions encountered in relation to the cavernous sinus. The relatively firm consistency and vascularity of the lesion pose a surgical challenge. These tumors seldom arise within the cavernous sinus, which is more frequently only secondarily involved. Intracavernous sinus origin and presence in this location in isolation is rare. Involvement of the cav-

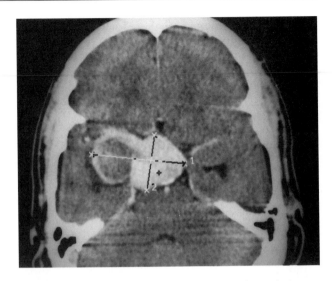

Fig. 11.8   Contrast-enhanced CT scan shows a large pituitary tumor which has invaded into the cavernous sinus. The medial temporal extension is entirely intracavernous. A contralateral subfrontal approach was suitable to radically resect this tumor.

ernous sinus in meningiomas is frequently in the form of thickening of the dural cover and its displacement. Sometimes the tumor grows on both sides of the dura of the lateral wall of the cavernous sinus. The tumor usually invades into the cavernous sinus through the dural folds of the cranial nerves. Displacement of dural wall of the cavernous sinus by the tumor rather than direct transgression through the dural wall is a more frequent event. Involvement of the carotid artery varies with the nature of the tumor. It is usually displaced along with the dura in a direction which depends on the site of origin of the lesion.

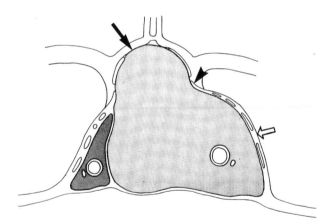

Fig. 11.7   The more typical extensions of a giant pituitary tumor. The tumor invades through the medial wall of the cavernous sinus and engulfs the carotid artery and the VIth nerve and displaces the lateral wall with its contained nerves. The white arrow shows that in a lateral approach to the cavernous sinus the markedly stretched cranial nerves are encountered early and possibility of damage is greater. The arrowhead shows an ipsilateral subfrontal approach. The tumor involving the cavernous sinus is difficult to approach due to the angulation necessary. Black arrow shows a contralateral subfrontal approach. The angle of approach provides a better opportunity to deal with intracavernous extension of the tumor.

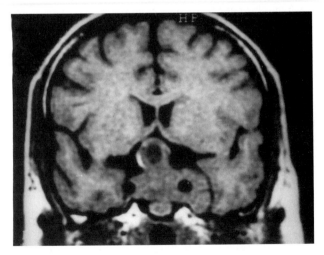

Fig. 11.9   MRI showing the encasement of the intracavernous sinus ICA by the tumor. The lumen of the artery is not narrowed in size.

In cases where the intracavernous carotid artery is completely surrounded or even squeezed by the tumor, a plane of cleavage can usually be developed between the tumor and the artery.

Cavernous hemangiomas

Cavernous hemangiomas are the only true intracavernous sinus lesions. The spread of the tumor 'opens' up the cavernous sinus and clarifies the anatomical characters of the cavernous sinus. The tumor occupies the venous spaces and dilates the dural walls. They progressively increase in size, bloat the cavernous sinus, displace the carotid artery and spread into the sellar region from the region of intercavernous sinus connections and displacement of the medial dural wall. This pattern of growth has been uniformly observed in the reported cases (Goel & Nadkarni 1995a). The similarity on MRI of the lesions reported in the literature is remarkable. The dumbbell-shaped tumor involved the cavernous sinus completely and had a tail-like extension towards the sella in all cases (Figs 11.10, 11.15). In the two cases encountered by us no definite tumor blush was identified on angiography. The vascular supply of the tumor has been reported to be from the meningohypophyseal trunk, middle meningeal artery or both. In both our cases it appeared that the inferolateral trunk of the carotid artery supplied the tumor. On CT the isodense tumor enhanced markedly. On T1-weighted images the lesion is iso- to hypointense but turns almost white on T2-weighted images. As the lesion arises from the region of the VIth cranial nerve the cavernous carotid is displaced medially.

SURGICAL STRATEGIES IN CAVERNOUS SINUS LESIONS

Indications for surgery

The problem of identifying the need for surgery seldom arises for lesions located around the cavernous sinus, such as trigeminal neurinoma, chordoma or pituitary tumor. These lesions should be resected radically. The question arises regarding the indication for resection of small intracavernous lesions or of the part invaginating into the cavernous sinus. Progressive functional disability, large and increasing size of lesion, and feasibility of radical operation in the available conditions are the indications for operation. Considering the intensity of surgery, lesions with subtle symptoms and signs can be conserved. It is a universal experience that radiation treatment results in adhesions of the tumor to the adjoining nerves and vessels

(which also become friable and more prone to trauma) and consequently results in difficult and hazardous surgery. Hence, irradiation of a benign lesion which is likely to grow and would then need an operation should be avoided. The lesion may be observed with serial scanning and if a definite growth is seen on radiology and the clinical symptoms are compelling, surgery could be performed.

Investigations

All cases should be thoroughly investigated with CT scanning, MRI and arterial DSA studies. Angiography should include bilateral studies to determine the side of dominance of the circulation and sizes of the posterior and anterior communicating arteries. In our study we concluded that these investigations, although suggestive, are not absolutely reliable as regards the patency and dominance of the carotid artery. In one of the author's cases, angiography showed a complete occlusion of the intracavernous carotid artery, an impression which proved to be wrong during surgery, resulting in torrential blood loss and adversely affecting the functional outcome. The balloon occlusion test to indicate the dominance of the carotid artery and feasibility of its occlusion during surgery is a helpful but not foolproof investigation. Although this investigation was done in the early phase of our experience, due to its unreliability it has currently been abandoned.

Consistency and vascularity of the tumor

The consistency of the tumor to a considerable extent, and vascularity of the tumor to a significant extent, determine the extent of tumor resectibility and outcome. It is important therefore to determine the consistency of the lesion on the basis of available clinical parameters and investigations. Subtle signs, despite the large size and short duration of symptoms, are usually seen with soft tumors. Presentation and detection of a tumor when it is only of small size are suggestive of a firm nature of the tumor. Displacement of the major arteries without encasement is frequently encountered in firm tumors. Smooth borders of the tumor are suggestive of a firm tumor while irregular borders indicate a soft tumor. Encasement of the carotid without compromise of the caliber is usually seen with softer tumors. Hypointensity on T1 and marked hyperintensity on T2 is usually seen in soft tumors. Multiple punctate hypointense areas of flow void suggest an intensely vascular tumor. Firmer tumors are frequently less vascular. Angiography is necessary to know the vascularity of the lesion.

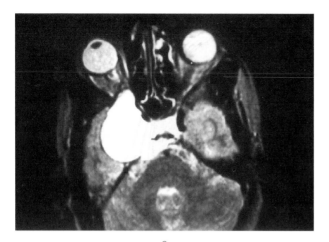

a

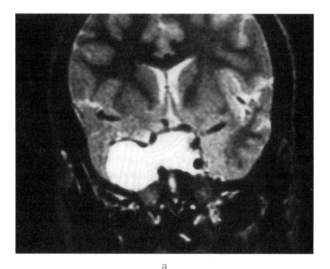

a

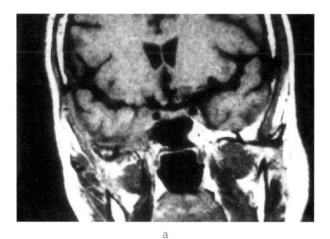

a

Fig. 11.15   a (Case 3) T-2-weighted image of a large intracavernous sinus cavernous hemangioma extending across the midline. **b** (Case 3) Coronal section shows the large intracavernous sinus tumor extending across the midline to reach the contralateral cavernous sinus. **c** Postoperative scan showing complete resection of the tumor. The tumor was removed essentially en masse.

ganglion and its divisions could not be adequately identified in continuity and saved.

The sixth case was an intracavernous sinus tuberculoma (case 6, Fig. 11.19). This lesion also involved Meckel's dural cave and had a relatively smaller intracavernous sinus extension. The entire tumor was resected by opening up the dural sheath of Meckel's cave and following the tumor into the cavernous sinus. The lesion was relatively avascular but merged markedly with the fibers of the Gasserian ganglion.

In none of the cases was there an injury to the carotid artery during dissection. Venous bleeding from the cavernous sinus did not impose any significant problem during surgery.

The temporalis muscle was rotated to the middle fossa base in its entirety in two cases for reconstruction. In all other cases the region of the cavernous sinus was stuffed lightly with Surgicel prior to closure of the wound. No fibrin glue or any free fascia or soft tissue was used.

Results

All six tumors were completely excised. Removal of the tumor was confirmed on postoperative MRI study in all cases. In the case with meningioma a dural incision was made to confirm the continuity of the intradural course of the IIIrd nerve. In other cases dural opening was unnecessary. There was no surgical complication. The cranial nerve outcome is shown in Table 11.1. In the relatively short duration of follow-up (ranging from 1 to 28 months) four patients improved in their cranial nerve function. In one case recovery was complete while in the other three only minimal to moderate but definite recovery of extraocular muscle function was observed. In one case (case 2) tumor recurrence was noted 24 months after surgery. The patient with fungal granuloma died following acute basilar artery thrombosis due to infiltration by *Aspergillus* fungus 1 month after the surgery, despite being on antifungal drugs.

Discussion

Various authors have stressed the need to understand the three-dimensional anatomical topography of the cavernous sinus for surgery in this region. There are some recent reports suggesting an extradural and 'interdural' approaches to lesions involving the Vth nerve located within the dural leaves of the lateral wall of the cavernous sinus (Dolenc 1994, Goel 1995b). The surgical approach towards cavernous sinus surgery as recommended by Dolenc provides an additional opportunity to work in the extradural compartment. In the wide extradural corridor,

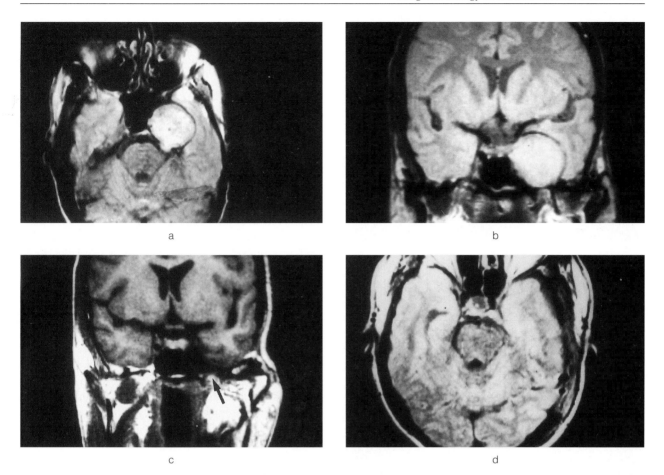

Fig. 11.16   **a** (Case 1) MRI image showing a large intracavernous meningioma (angioblastic variety). **b** Coronal section showing the large intracavernous tumor. **c** Arrow showing the region of the cavernous sinus from where complete excision of a vascular meningioma was achieved. **d** Postoperative scan showing tumor resection.

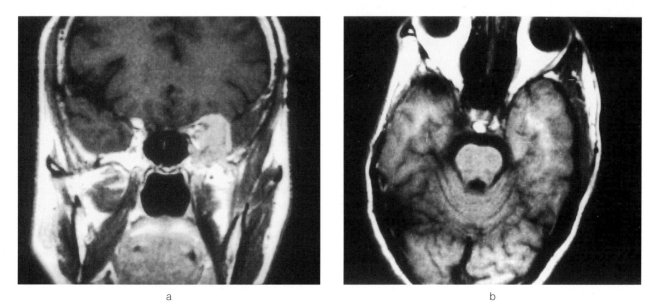

Fig. 11.17   **a** (Case 2) Contrast-enhanced picture showing intracavernous meningioma. **b** Scan showing complete resection of the tumor.

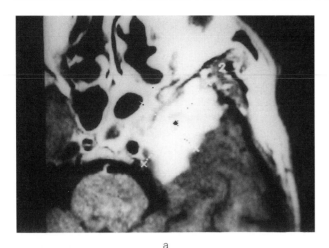

a

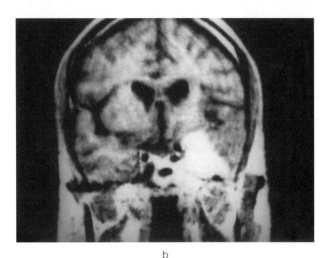

b

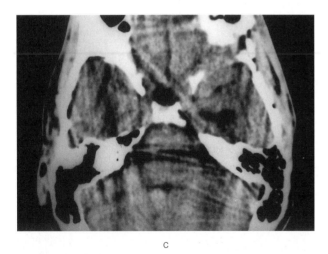

c

Fig. 11.18 **a** (Case 5) CT scan showing the large fungal granuloma (aspergilloma) in relationship to the cavernous sinus. **b** Coronal view of contrast-enhanced MRI shows the large cavernous sinus tumor displacing the ICA medially. **c** Postoperative scan showing complete resection of the lesion.

after adequate mobilization of the lateral dural wall of the cavernous sinus the medial triangles, namely the antero-medial, paramedian and Parkinson's triangle, as well as the anterolateral, lateral, Glasscock's and Kawase's triangles, can be exposed. Working in the extradural space, after an adequate bony exposure, avoids the need to work in a deep and narrow field. The surgical distance from the surface is reduced, providing an opportunity to work nearer to the tumor. During the approach to the tumor there is no compromise of or need to displace any arterial, major venous channel, neural structures or joints. One of the major concerns during cavernous sinus surgery is to avoid retraction of the brain as surgery could be relatively prolonged. Basal bone resection that would facilitate a low exposure has been recommended. In the technique described, the operation is performed in an extradural compartment, avoiding the need for use of a brain retractor during the procedure. The preserved dura, through an extradural dissection, provides additional protection for the brain during the procedure. The approach is anatomically relevant as the dural sheaths may be peeled off. The bulge of the cavernous sinus as a result of the presence of tumor helps in the dissection. The carotid artery is under control in the petrous apex and is exposed, although with a thin dural cover, in the paraclinoid segment. In all cases the intracavernous carotid was displaced medially, suggesting a lateral origin of the tumor. The arterial relationship to the tumor was an important indicator in deciding the direction of surgical approach and also in assessing the consistency and histological nature of the lesion (Goel 1995). The displacements of the IIIrd cranial nerve superolaterally by the tumor and splaying apart of the fibers of the Vth cranial nerve assisted in dissection between the fibers. The fibers of the first division of the Vth nerve are relatively firmly adherent to the dura and need to be protected during the dural dissection. The dura was opened in only one case to confirm the course of the distorted IIIrd nerve. In the six cases presented three tumors (two cavernous hemangiomas and one meningioma) were extensively vascular. However, after the control of major feeding vessels, the removal of these tumors became relatively easy as they were essentially of a soft nature. In case additional exposure from the superior wall of the cavernous sinus was felt necessary the dura could be opened as a frontotemporal craniotomy had already been done. An exposure from the superior or the medial wall of the cavernous sinus may be preferred in cases where the intracavernous carotid is shifted laterally. In none of the presented cases was additional exposure of the cavernous sinus necessary. It appears that with further experience with the extradural avenue, the exposure necessary to approach tumors involving the cavernous sinus could be minimized. In the appropriate case, frontotemporal craniotomy exposing the convexity dura could be avoided.

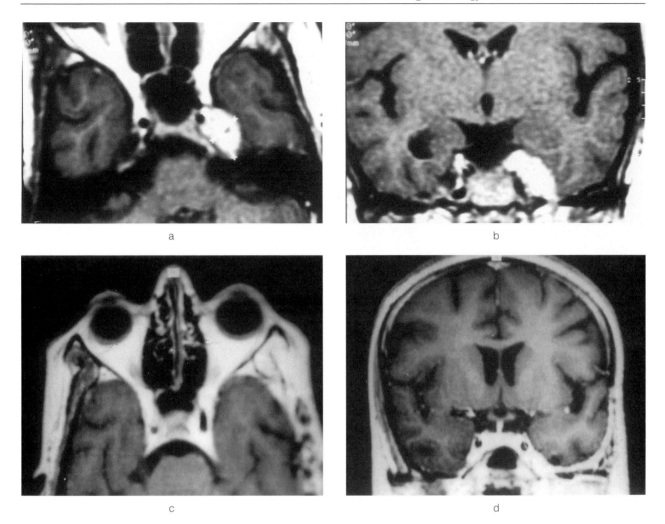

Fig. 11.19 **a** Contrast-enhanced MRI shows the posterior intracavernous sinus lesion, displacing the ICA medially. **b** Coronal section showing the tumor and its relationship to the carotid artery. **c** Postoperative contrast-enhanced MRI shows complete resection of the tumor. **d** Coronal image shows the tumor resection. There is no evidence of temporal lobe insult.

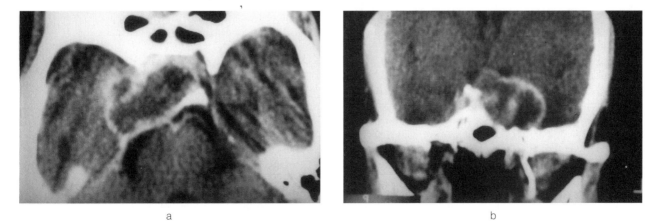

Fig. 11.20 **a** CT scan showing a large intracavernous sinus tumor extending towards the sellar region. **b** Coronal section shows the extensions of the tumor. A pituitary tumor was suspected. However, a tuberculoma was a surprise histological finding.

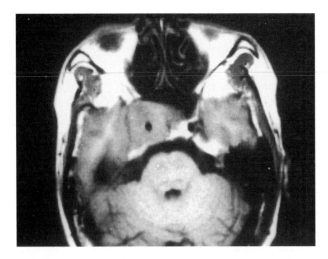

Fig. 11.21   T1-weighted MRI shows the large intracavernous sinus lesions squeezing the carotid artery. Histology was a tuberculoma.

Case   Cavernous Hemangioma in the Cavernous Sinus (Goel & Nadkarni 1995a)

This surgery was carried out in 1992–93. Presently the author would adopt an extradural approach to treat such lesions.

A 38-year-old woman presented with left hemifacial pain for 1 year. She developed rapidly progressive complete ptosis in 4–5 days 6 months prior to her admission to hospital. On examination she had complete ophthalmoplegia of the left eye. There was Vth nerve involvement in the form of numbness over the left half of the face and absence of corneal reflex and wasted temporalis and masseter muscles. There was no other neurological deficit. CT scan showed a well-defined isodense, brilliantly enhancing cavernous sinus tumor extending into the sella. MRI delineated the extension of this dumbbell-shaped mass clearly and defined the relationship of the completely encased carotid artery. The lesion was hypointense to isointense on T1-weighted image (Fig. 11.10a) and was very hyperintense on proton density and T2-weighted images (Fig. 11.10b). The left ICA angiogram revealed no tumor circulation or blush (Fig. 11.10d). The patient tolerated the balloon occlusion test of the carotid artery for 15 minutes without ill effect.

The preoperative diagnosis was of a meningioma or a trigeminal neurinoma. A frontotemporal craniotomy and orbitozygomatic osteotomy was done. This was followed by resection of the middle fossa floor to provide for basal exposure and isolation of the ICA at the petrous apex for proximal control. The dura of the lateral wall of the cavernous sinus was expanded and pushed laterally by the intracavernous lesion. A cruciate incision was made in its lateral wall. A bright red tumor was seen just underneath the dura. It was extremely vascular and would not tolerate even the slightest touch without bleeding. Small pieces were taken for histology and bleeding was controlled with great difficulty. In view of the extensive vascularity of the tumor and because a malignant lesion was considered possible, it was not considered safe to proceed

further and the surgery was terminated. However, the histology was of a benign lesion – a cavernous hemangioma.

Reoperation was then carried out. The basal exposure was further widened and ICA was exposed at the petrous apex. Distal control of the carotid was obtained at the supraclinoid segment. Adequate arrangements were made to bypass the cavernous segment of the ICA with a saphenous vein graft. The incision over the dura was extended further. The tumor was identified, and dissected from the markedly displaced cranial nerves and the carotid artery. The tumor was excised en masse. The ease of handling this vascular tumor, and its dissectibility from the displaced nerves and carotid artery, made surgical resection easily possible with preservation of the cranial nerves and the carotid artery. The VIth nerve could not be identified during surgery. As the tumor was dissected from the nerves and vessels it shrank progressively. During surgery it appeared that the tumor was supplied by the inferolateral trunk of the cavernous segment of the carotid artery. The postoperative recovery was uneventful. The patient showed marginal but definite recovery of IIIrd and Vth nerve function when she was seen 3 months after the operation. She was free of facial pain. A postoperative scan confirmed complete resection (Fig. 11.10e).

Comments

1. Cavernous hemangiomas involving the cavernous sinus are rare. The lesion has been most frequently reported in the fourth decade and female predominance has been noted. In the reported cases the presentation has been in the form of ocular symptoms related to the nerves traversing the cavernous sinus. Although extension of the lesion into the sella has been seen, symptoms related to pituitary dysfunction have not been seen.

2. The similarity of the MRI appearances in this case to those reported earlier was remarkable. The dumbbell-shaped tumor involved the cavernous sinus completely and had a tail-like extension into the sella in these cases. Tumor blush has been reported on angiography. However, in our case no definite tumor circulation was identified. The vascular supply of the tumor has been reported to be from the meningohypophyseal trunk, middle meningeal artery or both. In our case it appeared that the artery of the inferolateral trunk of the carotid artery supplied the tumor. On CT the isodense tumor enhanced markedly.

3. Histologically, cavernous hemangiomas are collections of vascular channels lined by endothelial cells and connective tissue. The histological picture in our case was similar to those reported earlier.

4. In most of the reported cases tumor resection was carried out in a piecemeal fashion. In one case the advantage of using a Cavitron ultrasonic aspirator (CUSA) was shown (Kudo et al 1989). The tumor in the presented case was excised en masse. The tumor could be handled 'easily' and a well-defined plane of resection could be developed within the cavernous sinus. From this experience, we observed that piecemeal resection of this tumor is excessively bloody, and carries a danger of injuring the cranial nerves

of the cavernous sinus and the carotid artery. Dissection of the tumor by gentle separation from the adjoining structures was found to be easy and safe.

5. Preoperative embolization has not been found to be useful. Hypothermia, vascular occlusion and intraoperative hypotension have been recommended. These special anesthetic measures were not found to be necessary in the present case.

Granulomas of cavernous sinus

Granulomas involving the cavernous sinus are rare. However, the close proximity of the cavernous sinus to the sphenoid sinus, extensive venous drainage from the orbit and face and venous connections to the infratemporal fossa and to Batson's venous plexus of the extradural spinal veins predisposes it to development of infectious lesions. Apart from fungal granulomas (Fig. 11.18) some tuberculomas of the cavernous sinus were encountered by us which completely encased in the intracavernous carotid artery. These lesions are shown in Figures 11.19–11.21.

References

Day J D, Fukushisma T, Gianotta S L 1994 Microanatomical study of the extradural middle fossa approach to the petroclival and posterior cavernous sinus region: description of the rhomboid construct. Neurosurgery 34: 1009–1016

Dolenc V V (1994) Frontotemporal epidural approach to trigeminal neurinomas. Acta Neurochirurgica (Wien) 130: 55–65

Goel A 1994 Extradural approach to lesions involving cavernous sinus. Paper presented at the Fifth Advanced Course in Head and Neck Cancer Surgery, 21–23 November 1994, Singapore

Goel A 1995a Chordoma and chondrosarcoma: relationship to the internal carotid artery. Acta Neurochirurgica (Wien) 133: 30–35

Goel A 1995b Infratemporal fossa interdural approach for trigeminal neurinomas. Acta Neurochirurgica (Wien) 136: 99–102

Goel A 1995c Middle fossa sub-Gasserian ganglion approach to clivus chordomas. Acta Neurochirurgica (Wien) 136: 212–216

Goel A 1995d Extended middle fossa approach to petroclival tumors. Acta Neurochirurgica (Wien) 135: 78–83

Goel A 1996a Cavernous sinus: a speculative note. Journal of Clinical Neuroscience 3: 281

Goel A 1996b Extradural approach to lesions including cavernous sinus. British Journal of Neurosurgery (in press)

Goel A 1996b Surgical anatomy of the cavernous sinus. In: Torrens M J, Al-Mefty O, Kobayashi S (eds) Operative skull base surgery. Churchill Livingstone, Edinburgh (in press-b)

Goel A, Nadkarni T D 1995a Cavernous hemangioma in the cavernous sinus. British Journal of Neurosurgery 9: 77–80

Goel A, Nadkarni 1995b Medial compartment of the cavernous sinus. Journal of Neurosurgery 83: 763–764

Goel A, Nadkarni T 1996 Surgical management of giant pituitary tumors – a review of 30 cases. Acta Neurochirurgica (Wein) (in press)

Goel A, Sheode J, Bhayani J 1994 Extended transcranial approach to nasopharyngeal angiofibroma. British Journal of Neurosurgery 8: 593–597

Kudo T, Ueki S, Kobayashi et al 1989 Experience with the ultrasonic aspirator in a cavernous hemangioma of the cavernous sinus. Neurosurgery 24: 628–631

Parkinson D (1965) A surgical approach to the cavernous portion of the carotid artery: anatomical studies and case report. Journal of Neurosurgery 23: 474–483

Sekhar L N, Goel A, Sen C N 1992 Middle fossa approaches for invasive tumors involving the skull base. In: Rengachary S, Wilkins R (eds) American Association of Neurological Surgeons Fascicle, Vol 2. Williams & Wilkins, Baltimore, pp 221–232

Sekhar L N, Goel A, Sen C N 1993a Cavernous sinus surgery. In: Appuzo M (ed) Brain surgery: complication avoidance and management, Vol II. Churchill Livingstone, Edinburgh, pp 2197–2219

Sekhar L N, Goel A, Sen C N 1993b General neurosurgical operative techniques and instrumentation in cranial base surgery. In: Sekhar L N, Janecka I P (eds) Atlas of skull base surgery. Raven Press, New York, pp 1–10

Taptas J N 1982 The so-called cavernous sinus: a review of the controversy and its implications for neurosurgeons. Neurosurgery 11: 712–717

Direct Cavernous Sinus Surgery Has a Future
Vinko V. Dolenc

During the last 15 years cavernous sinus surgery has been regularly exposed to criticism, and is still not properly accepted as the first choice of treatment of tumorous and vascular lesions in the cavernous sinus. The reasons for this are manifold, important ones being the complexity of the normal anatomy and – even more so – the pathological anatomy. Another very important reason for unfavorable attitudes toward direct surgical approaches to the cavernous sinus is lack of experience in dealing with lesions in this region. The many arguments against direct surgical approaches to cavernous sinus pathologies, generated also by some world neurosurgical authorities, speak for themselves; i.e. the new generation of neurosurgeons will not be able to survive without also knowing the normal and pathological anatomy of the parasellar region in every detail. A better understanding of the surgical anatomy automatically helps us to adopt reasonable and less complex approaches to the region. Less traumatization of the brain is achieved with no retraction of the temporal lobe, and a higher percentage in radicality of tumor removal is only possible with appropriate compilation of knowledge of the anatomy and hence understanding of the relevant approach to the lesion. It is difficult to understand why, in spite of the available knowledge, it took so long before it became clear that some of the cavernous sinus lesions could be removed completely using an exclusively extradural approach, e.g. in dealing with Vth nerve tumors (Dolenc 1994). It is probable that the complexity of the architecture of the cavernous sinus, as well as its position on the inferior aspect of the brain, have caused us to overlook the only logical (extradural) approach. While it may be difficult for a neurosurgeon to agree to undertake a complex neurosurgical intervention in the extradural space, it is also frustrating for other specialists if they have to enter the cavernous sinus from its outer side when the tumor does not remain within the boundaries and invades the parasellar space. These two latter facts indicate the need for cooperation between experts of different specialities, which is essential in cases of malignant diseases of the skull base, as well as in some cases of benign lesions when these do not conform to the anatomical boundaries. There is no doubt that the team approach to the pathologies of the skull base will ultimately lead to a complete resolution of all problems which still exist in this area. Furthermore, dispersal of the myths surrounding the cavernous sinus will help neurosurgeons to become radical in many more intradural pathologies, provided they do not hesitate to enter the cavernous sinus when treating the tumors. For the new generation of neurosurgeons, there will be no reason for not removing a tumor which also partially invades the cavernous sinus, by using the excuse that this would be 'too dangerous'. The level of risk at surgery is proportionally reduced by improved practical knowledge of surgical anatomy. A thorough study of the anatomy of the parasellar region, and anatomical dissections of the specimens of the central skull base, are nowadays a vital requirement for all neurosurgical residents as well as practitioners in neurosurgery, and in particular for those who declare themselves to be 'skull base surgeons'.

With appropriate study and practice in the laboratory, the new generation of neurosurgeons will be able to include direct surgical procedures within the cavernous sinus in the list of regular neurosurgical interventions in the near future.

Reference

Dolenc V V 1994 Frontotemporal epidural approach to trigeminal neurinomas. Acta Neurochirurgica 130: 55–65

Surgical approaches to clival lesions 12

Atul Goel   Junpei Nitta   Shigeaki Kobayashi

Advances in skull base surgery have resulted in development and refinements in approaches to petroclival and clival lesions (Al-Mefty et al 1989, Bochenek & Kukawa 1975, Bonnal et al 1964, Fay 1930, Fisch & Kumar 1985, Goel 1995, Hakuba et al 1988, House 1961, Kawase et al 1991, Malis 1985, Morrison & King 1973, Rosomoff 1971, Samii et al 1989, Sekhar et al 1987, Shiobara et al 1988, Spetzler et al 1992, Stieglitz et al 1986, Symon 1982, Tarlov 1977). With the availability of modern radiological technology, in most cases the histopathological nature of the lesion can frequently be known. The surgery is therefore undertaken with the aim of radical excision and decompression of the region, helping in relieving the symptoms and aiming for a cure. To achieve this goal, the planning and execution of the surgery should be meticulous and should take advantage of advancing technology in radiology, neurophysiology, operative instrumentation, and neurointensive care. Wherever necessary, the combined effort of a neurosurgeon and otolaryngologist could prove to be helpful.

Petroclival meningiomas are described as those which arise from the dura in the region medial to the entry of the trigeminal root in Meckel's cave (Figs 12.1–12.6). Frequently these and other lesions situated in this region involve the cavernous sinus and extend down to the mid or low clivus, encasing and/or displacing critical arteries and perforators. For satisfactory and safe excision of these tumors an adequate exposure is necessary. Meningiomas in proximity to the clivus are amongst the most difficult surgical problems. The difficulty in resection of these lesions stems from the following facts:

1. These benign lesions are frequently of large size at the time of presentation.
2. Patients present with relatively subtle neurological symptoms and signs.
3. Tumors may encase vital major arteries and perforators, sacrifice of which could result in permanent neurological deficit or even death. Such an eventuality could have taken years in the natural course of tumor growth.
4. Alternative methods of treatment like radiosurgery, chemotherapy, photodynamic therapy etc. are of no proven value in the management of these cases.

5. If left alone, in all probability the tumor will grow and lead to a slow and crippling death.

Once the decision regarding surgery is made, one has to understand that in most cases the operation is not being carried out to obtain a histological confirmation regarding the nature of the lesion, as such information is usually available with reasonable certainty on clinical evaluation and radiological studies. The approach for the lesion involves retraction of vital brain and the operation needs prolonged microsurgical dissection to isolate the lesion from vital structures. A low or basal approach to avoid or limit retraction is necessary as prolonged and excessive retraction may not be well tolerated by the brain. The approach to such deep-seated tumors is difficult and fraught with possibilities of various complications by itself. A small or limited excision may be of very little help to the patient. It only means that clival lesions should be approached when the operating team is reasonably confident that a total or a large excision may be made on the basis of their experience and level of confidence.

Clival region surgery has emerged from a state where it was considered to be an unapproachable zone or a 'no man's land'. There are various approaches described to deal with the lesions present in this location. However, for a particular tumor there is only one approach which is ideal and can be performed. It is for the surgeon to decide which is the ideal route of approach for a particular lesion. Familiarity with all the available approaches is therefore essential so that the best possible route can be selected. Expertise in one particular route and an attempt towards performing surgery on all lesions with the same approach may sometimes lead to problems. Some modifications of the described approaches may be appropriate for a particular case. The issues in the decision regarding the approach should include consideration for the approach which could be performed in the shortest time, is least difficult and safest for the patient. The exposure must be wide and it must also provide with avenues for dealing with disasters like major arterial tears, and for reconstruction of nerves and arteries whenever necessary.

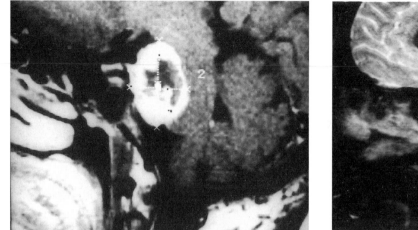

a

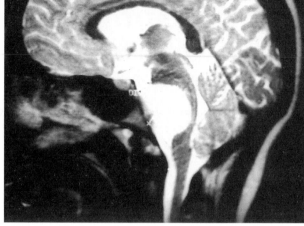

a

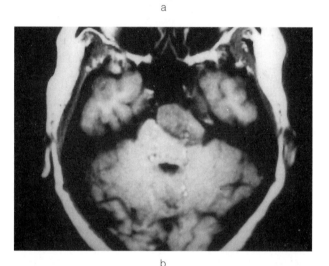

b

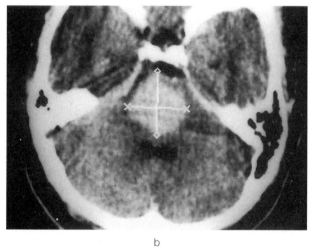

b

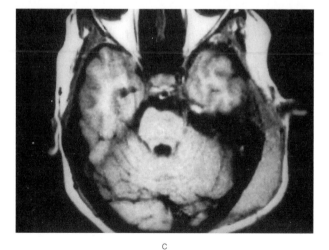

c

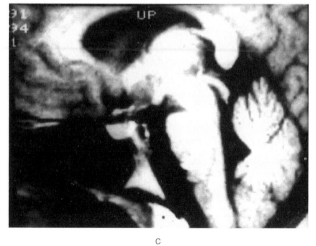

c

Fig. 12.1 **a** Contrast-enhanced MRI shows a large clival meningioma. **b** Transverse cut showing the tumor indenting into the pons. **c** Postoperative scan showing complete resection of the tumor. Basal extension of the subtemporal craniotomy was used to resect the tumor. Resection of the rest of the petrous bone was not necessary.

Fig. 12.2 **a** T2-weighted MRI shows a large hyperintense midclival tumor deeply indenting the pons. **b** Contrast-enhanced CT scan shows the large tumor involving the pons. **c** Postoperative MRI showing complete resection of the tumor.

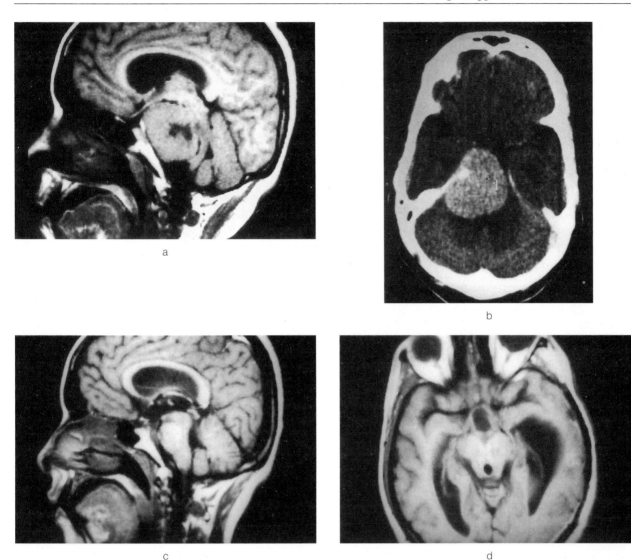

Fig. 12.3 **a** MRI scan shows the massive petroclival meningioma. The tumor was vascular being fed by the branches of the meningohypophyseal trunk and middle meningeal artery. (From Goel 1995, with permission.) **b** Contrast-enhanced CT scan showing the large petroclival meningioma. **c** Extended middle fossa approach was used to resect this tumor completely. **d** Axial scan showing the resection of the tumor.

SURGICAL APPROACH DECISION MAKING

The following important characters of the tumor determine the nature of approach.

Size of the tumor, its relationship to arteries and nerves, and to the adjacent bone: the larger the size of the tumor, the more difficult is the surgery and consequently the outcome can be affected. The vertical height of the tumor in relation to the petrous bone and tentorium is also an important consideration when deciding an approach. In cases of large tumors, the approach itself may not be extremely wide, as the tumor makes space for itself, and when the ini-

tial intratumoral debulking is started more and more working space can be obtained around the area.

Nature of the tumor: in most cases the arterial displacements as a result of growth of the tumor differentiate meningiomas from other tumors. The trigeminal neurinoma displaces the intracavernous carotid medially, while the chordoma and chondrosarcomas displace the internal carotid artery at the petrous apex anteriorly. Soft tumors like the chordomas and pituitary tumors displace the artery but only rarely narrow its lumen. On the other hand firmer tumors like meningiomas rarely encase the artery, and when they do they frequently narrow its lumen. Such and other characters help in histologically classifying the

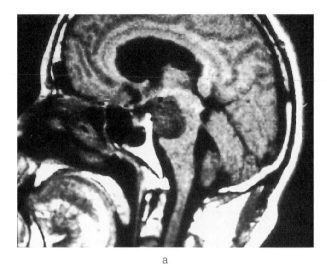

a

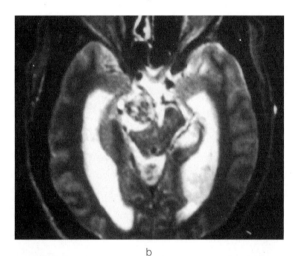

b

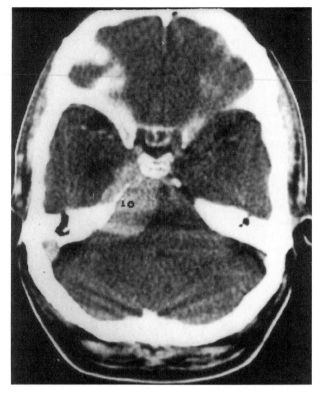

Fig. 12.5 CT scan showing the more usual extensions of a petroclival tumor. Note the involvement of the cavernous sinus and extension along the petrous apex. The histopathology of the tumor was meningeal sarcoma.

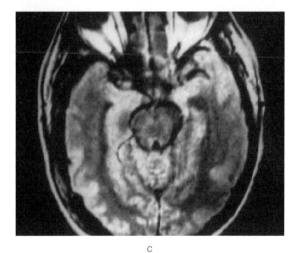

c

Fig. 12.4 **a** Sagittal view of T1-weighted MRI showing the large hypointense tumor located on the anterior surface of the pons. **b** T2-weighted image showing the hyperintense tumor indenting the pons. **c** Postoperative scan demonstrating the tumor excision. Basal extension of the subtemporal craniotomy was used to resect the tumor.

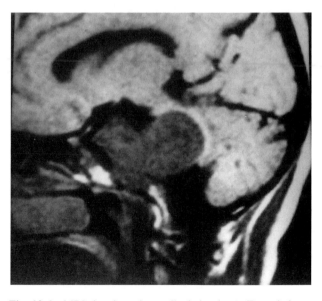

Fig. 12.6 MRI showing a large clival chordoma. Extended middle fossa approach was used to radically resect this tumor.

tumors, and thus assist in deciding about the route of approach and the extent of resectibility and for prognosticating the ultimate outcome.

Consistency of the tumor: on the basis of radiological imaging and presenting clinical features a reasonable idea regarding the consistency of the tumor can be made. Longstanding symptoms and symptomatic involvement of adjacent cranial nerves suggest presence of a firm tumor. Signal characters on T1- and T2-weighted images can guide towards the nature of the tumor. This character determines to a considerable extent the ease of surgical resection and the extent of exposure that may be necessary to resect the lesion. The consistency of the tumor and its vascularity are important variables on which the course of surgery depends. Encasement of the vessels signals difficulties in resection. Narrowing of the encased vessels suggests the firm nature of the tumor. Resection of such tumors may be a formidable surgical problem.

Vascularity of the lesion: this can be observed on angiography. Multiple punctate spots in the tumor on magnetic resonance imaging (MRI) also suggests high vascularity. The more vascular the lesion, the larger is the exposure that is necessary.

Presence of an arachnoidal plane of dissection around the tumor can be determined on MRI scanning. Such information can be critically important. Presence of arachnoidal lakes around the tumor should be carefully analyzed.

Patient-related factors like age or presence of other major illnesses can also guide towards the extent of the surgery that would necessary.

OPERATIVE TECHNIQUE

The direction of the approach should be towards the base or site of the attachment of the tumor in an attempt to devascularize it early. In larger tumors, approaching the base may sometimes be difficult, due to the presence of the tumor bulk and the stretched adjoining nerves and vessels. In the majority of cases intratumoral debulking near the base, devascularizing the lesion by coagulating at the site of attachment to the dura, followed by further debulking and later removal of the thin residual shell by carefully separating the adjacent structures under vision can lead to successful resection of the lesion. In cases where the tumor has encased a particular major vessel, the first aim is to either isolate the parent artery early in the operation, or debulk the tumor with the primary aim of isolating the parent artery and the tumor-encased vessel. Once the artery is isolated and dissected the rest of the operation becomes relatively safe. More often there is a clear plane of cleavage between the artery and the tumor and the dissection can proceed in that plane. In case the arachnoidal plane is lost, one should consider the risks of further dissection vis-à-vis problems of leaving residual tumor behind. Extensive dissection around arteries is fraught with risks of vascular occlusion by laceration or thrombosis. It is usually safer to avoid prolonged dissection of the tumor from the arteries. Tumoral coagulation should be avoided as such a procedure makes the tumor firmer and resection more difficult. A combination of sharp and blunt dissection with the help of bipolar (with irrigation) and graded suction is necessary in the proximity of major arterial channels. Traction over the tumor should be avoided during the entire operation. Kobayashi et al use pronged self-retaining retractors to handle the tumor during surgery. Leaving tumor residue remote from the site of attachment is safer than leaving tumor in the region of attachment (or origin) regarding the possibility of recurrence.

Frequently lumbar puncture and drainage of cerebrospinal fluid (CSF) is an important preoperative adjuvant to help relaxation of the brain and to permit safe and adequate retraction of the lesion. In subtemporal approaches retraction of the temporal lobe is much easier and safer when CSF drainage is performed. CSF drainage may always be considered when a bulging brain restricts manipulations. For this reason a complete lateral position is better than a supine position with head turned on the other side. Lumbar drainage of CSF can be done with ease whenever it is indicated in this position. CSF drainage for facilitating retraction of the brain may be avoided in cases of large tumors where herniation may occur.

BONE WORK

Drilling of the petrous bone to obtain basal and wider exposure is frequently necessary. However, such a procedure should be done only when it is absolutely necessary. The drilling should be minimal and only in sites where it is necessary to expand the exposure. In more difficult varieties of lesions extensive temporal bone drilling may be required.

IDEAL APPROACH

It is necessary to consider various issues while selecting an ideal approach for a particular tumor. The ideal approach has the following features:

1. The working distance between the surgeon and the tumor should be minimal. The direction of the approach selected should therefore be such that the tumor is closest to the surface. Temporal bone drilling may be done on some occasions only to reduce the operating distance.
2. The approach should be quick to perform. The time

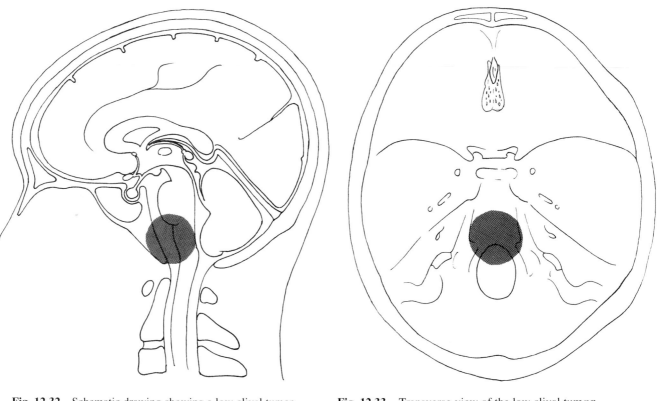

Fig. 12.32   Schematic drawing showing a low clival tumor.

Fig. 12.33   Transverse view of the low clival tumor.

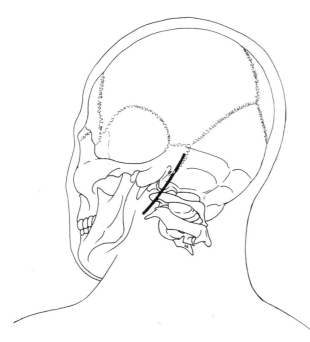

Fig. 12.34   Line drawing showing the incision for supracondylar infrajugular bulb keyhole approach to anterior medullary, low clival lesions.

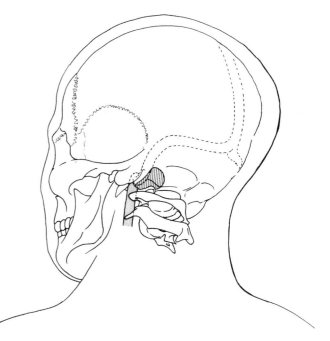

Fig. 12.35   The shaded area shows the site of keyhole exposure. The bone lying between the condyle and the jugular bulb is removed. Bone removal is extended posteriorly to include the anteroinferior part of the occipital squama.

extends inferiorly into the upper cervical region. The lateral rim of the foramen magnum and the occipital squama is exposed. The part of the occipital squama including the rim of the foramen magnum is removed carefully (Fig. 12.34). Bone removal is extended anteriorly to include the bone of the supracondylar and infrajugular bulb region. The condylar vein can sometimes result in troublesome bleeding and has to be adequately dealt with. The exposure obtained is of a key shape (Fig. 12.35). A dural incision is made as shown in Figure 12.36. The lateral edge of the cisterna magna is opened. The intradural segment of the vertebral artery is identified and its relationship to the tumor analyzed. The tumor is then inspected. If it is of a soft and suckable variety, no additional exposure may be necessary. The exposure may be widened inferiorly by drilling off the condyle as much as is necessary, preserving the hypoglossal nerve which travels in the superior half of the condyle. The bone on the inferior aspect of the jugular bulb can be widely removed. In cases where the dura of the jugular bulb is thick the jugular bulb can be compressed superiorly and the exposure widened (Fig. 12.37). In most cases no significant further increase in exposure is necessary. Whenever necessary various complex maneuvers such as exposure of the extradural vertebral artery, its mobilization, condylar resection, obliteration of the jugular bulb and other such procedures may be employed (Figs 12.38–12.40).

SURGICAL STRATEGY FOR HYPOGLOSSAL NEURINOMAS

Most of the intracranial neurinomas arise from sensory divisions of the cranial nerves. Tumors arising from motor nerves are less common. Fewer than 50 cases of hypoglossal nerve tumors have been reported in the literature. Due to their rarity, the surgical approach, operative strategy and management problems in such cases have not been discussed at length in the literature. Less than one-third of these tumors present with a dumbbell configuration, with one end intracranially anterolateral to the medulla and the other extracranially, with the two connected to each other by the part in the condyle. More commonly, entirely intracranial hypoglossal neurinomas have been seen. The site of the tumor matches the anatomical situation of the nerve. The intracranial part of the tumor is located medial to the IX–XI cranial nerves, anterolateral to the medulla and inferomedial to the intracranial part of the vertebral artery. The extracranial tumor is usually located medial to the jugular bulb and vein, exiting IX–XI cranial nerves and the distal cervical carotid artery. Such extensions make radical surgical excision an apparently formidable task. Due to the benign nature of the disease, usual presentation with unilateral progressive involvement of multiple lower

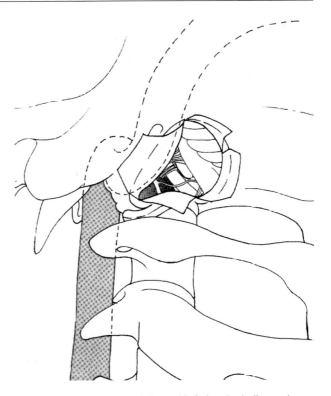

Fig. 12.36   The supracondylar and infrajugular bulb area is exposed after making a cruciate dural incision and reflecting the dural flaps. The large condylar vein can sometimes cause troublesome bleeding.

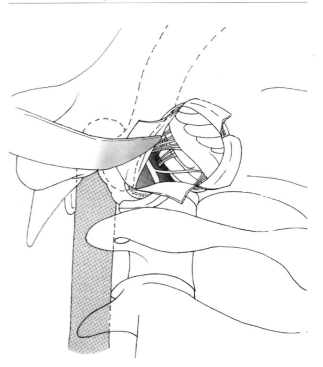

Fig. 12.37   The jugular bulb is being retracted superiorly to enhance the exposure. In cases where additional exposure is required the jugular bulb can be sacrificed and packed after adequate preparations.

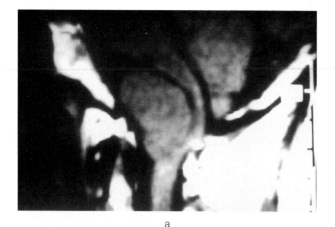

a

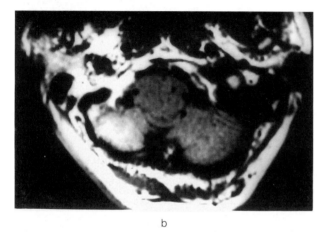

b

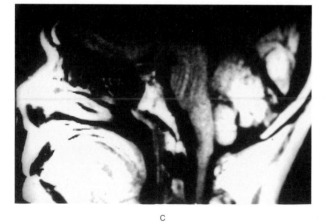

c

Fig. 12.38 a T1-weighted MRI shows a large anterior medullary meningioma. **b** Tranverse cut showing partial encasement of both vertebral arteries. **c** Postoperative scan showing complete resection of the tumor. A lateral suboccipital subsigmoid sinus approach was used to resect the tumor.

cranial nerves and low recurrence rate after surgical excision, attempted radical surgical resection is the only available option for the surgeon. Widening and erosion of the

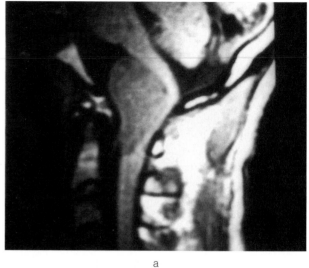

a

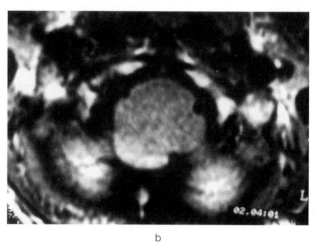

b

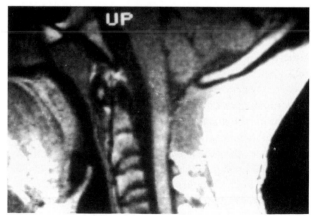

c

Fig. 12.39 a T1-weighted MRI shows the low clival meningioma. **b** Transverse section shows the midline location of the tumor, involvement of both vertebral arteries and deep indentation of the medulla. **c** Postoperative scan shows complete resection of the tumor. A supracondylar, infrajugular bulb keyhole approach was used to resect the lesion.

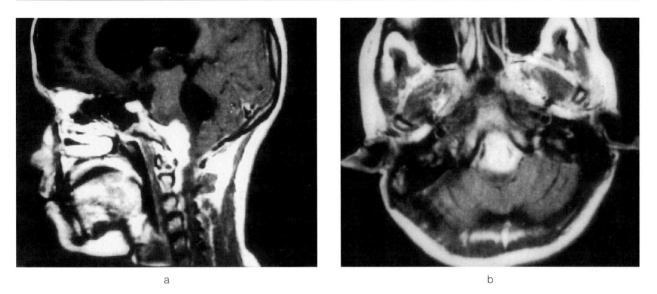

a   b

Fig. 12.40   **a** Contrast-enhanced MRI shows the large premedullary lesion. **b** Transverse section showing that both vertebral arteries are traversing within the tumor. On exploration by supracondylar, infrajugular bulb keyhole approach the lesion was detected to be a tuberculoma. A partial resection followed by antituberculous drugs were used to successfully treat the lesion.

hypoglossal canal in association with other radiological and clinical parameters help in preoperative assessment of the nature of the lesion. Widening of the condylar canal can be best seen on CT scan (Fig. 12.41a). MRI not only shows the extensions of the tumor clearly, but also delineates clearly the vascular relationship (Fig. 12.41b). In most instances atrophy of the tongue is clearly defined on radiological examination. Hyperintensity of the involved tongue on both T1- and T2-weighted images was seen in our cases (Fig. 12.41c).

Our experience with three cases of large and typical dumbbell-shaped hypoglossal neurinomas was encouraging. All three tumors were soft and eminently amenable to excision by suction, and were relatively avascular. The tumors were much softer when compared to the usual consistency of acoustic neurinomas. The capsule of the tumor was not very well defined. Intratumoral excision followed by removal of the capsule was safe and relatively easy. A large exposure was achieved in the first case in which tumor resection was performed in two stages. A low retro-jugular bulb and subsigmoid craniectomy and removal of the lateral wall of condyle exposed the intracranial and condylar part of the tumor. In the second stage a transcervical approach was needed to excise the extracranial portion. The tumor was soft and could be decompressed, and later was easily separable from the surrounding structures. With the experience of the first case, the exposure in the other two cases was limited to transcervical anterior approach only. After the excision of the extracranial part the exposure was widened and the smaller condylar and intracranial parts could also be removed. In the third case

a combined exposure for both the intracranial and extracranial components of the tumor was made. By working anterior and posterior to the jugular vein the entire tumor was resected. In all three cases a total excision of the tumor could be achieved with satisfactory outcome.

However, it is presumed that all tumors may not be soft and avascular as was seen in our cases, and a staged surgery is recommended.

The feasibility of excising the entire tumor in a single exposure has been described. However, the ramus and condyle of the mandible, styloid process, passage of the lower cranial nerves, jugular vein and the carotid artery can severely limit the exposure.

Operative steps

The approach selection should be such that there is no compromise of venous and arterial circulation, with minimal need to retract the lower cranial nerves. The lateral half of the tumor-involved condyle is drilled off to expose the tumor. However, it seems that if the opposite condyle is intact there is no need for a fixation procedure after the tumor resection. The operation can be performed in one stage when one works anterior and posterior to the jugular vein and IX–XI cranial nerves. Alternatively if either the extracranial or the intracranial portion of the tumor is small in size a single-stage approach in either direction can be adopted and the tumor exposed by suitably altering the direction of the angle of the microscope.

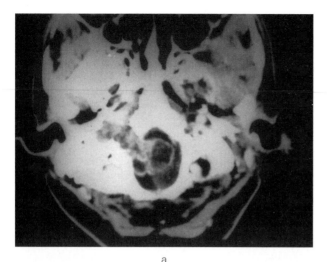

a

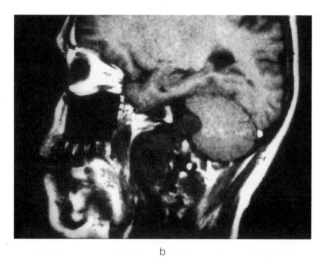

b

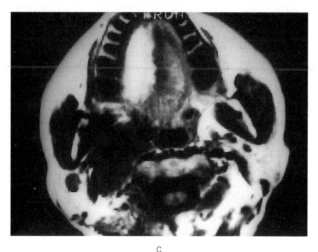

c

Fig. 12.41   a CT scan showing the intra-and extracranial tumor traveling through an enlarged condylar canal. **b** T1-weighted MRI shows a large dumbbell-shaped hypoglossal neurinoma. The intracranial part of the tumor is relatively small in size. **c** T1-weighted MRI shows hyperintensity of the right half of the tongue suggesting its fatty degeneration. Atrophy of the tongue can thus be detected with the help of MRI. The large hypointense hypoglossal neurinoma can be seen in the retropharyngeal region.

CASE 1   Unattached Petroclival Region Extra-axial Schwannoma (Goel et al 1995)

A very unusual case of an intracranial extra-axial petroclival schwannoma is presented. The lesion was not arising from any

cranial nerve, nor was it attached to brain parenchyma or dura.

A 43-year-old male patient without stigmata of von Recklinghausen's disease presented with a 6-month history of right frontotemporal headache, intermittent giddiness and occasional visual blurring. Except for bilateral papilloedema, there was no neurological deficit. Computed tomographic (CT) scan showed an isodense enhancing, right petroclival tumor indenting the pons and midbrain. There was moderate supratentorial hydrocephalus. On T1-weighted MRI the lesion was hypointense, while on T2-weighted images it was hyperintense (Fig. 12.4a,b). MRI clearly showed the mass to be extra-axial. The lesion was completely excised by a right subtemporal transtentorial approach (Fig. 12.4c). The tumor was well circumscribed, moderately vascular and soft. The IVth to VIIIth cranial nerves were displaced on the dome but were entirely free from the tumor. There was no dural attachment and the arachnoidal plane separating the tumor from the brain stem was well preserved. Histopathological examination showed the structure of a tumor consisting of spindle-shaped cells with elongated nuclei arranged in compact interlacing fascicles. There was a suggestion of nuclear palisading. However, no characteristic Verocay bodies were seen. There was no nuclear pleomorphism, hyperchromatism or mitosis. There was hyalinized connective tissue stroma and thick-walled blood vessels. No Antoni B area was seen. These features and the completely extraparenchymal nature of the lesion favored a histological diagnosis of a schwannoma. Immunostaining could not be performed due to lack of facilities. At 6-month follow-up the patient was asymptomatic. There was no cranial nerve dysfunction.

Comments

Schwannomas are benign neoplasms of the peripheral nerve sheath and are believed to have their origin in embryonic neural crest cells. They account for approximately 8% of all brain tumors and 25% of all spinal tumors. Intraparenchymatous schwannomas of the central nervous system have also been rarely reported (Deogaonkar et al 1995, Sharma & Gurusinghe 1993). In the presented case the tumor was neither attached to any cranial nerve, nor to the brain parenchyma or dura. Literature search failed to reveal any report of a similar case.

The most common site for intracranial schwannomas is the vestibular portion of the VIIIth nerve. Although uncommon these tumors have been reported to occur on every cranial nerve except the optic nerve. Intraparenchymatous schwannomas have also been reported though rarely. Goebel et al (1979) reported a case of an extra-axial schwannoma not connected to any cranial nerve but attached to the dura in the region of the tuberculum sellae and simulating a meningioma. Our patient's clinical presentation, radiographic as well as operative findings suggested an extra-axial situation in the vicinity of the anterior surface of the pons. The tumor did not have any attachment to the cranial nerves which were in the vicinity. It was also clearly free of the dura and brain that was around it. The absence of cranial nerve and brain stem dysfunction both prior to and after surgery corroborated this impression. The occurrence of a nerve sheath tumor in such a location raises the important question of its histogenesis. Various theories have been proposed for the origin of intraparenchymal schwannomas. Redekop et al 1990 supported the theory of distorted embryogenesis. Riggs & Clary (1957) postulated that these tumors could arise from proliferation of Schwann cells in perivascular plexuses. Russell & Rubenstein (1977) suggested that conversion of pial cells to Schwann cells was the possible mode of histogenesis. Prakash et al (1980) suggested misplaced myelinated nerve fibers as the site of origin. Ramamurthi et al (1958) suggested displaced neural crest cells in the developing nervous system to be the origin of these tumors. Differentiation from multipotent mesenchymal cells has also been suggested (Feigin & Ogata 1971). Some cases associated with neurofibromatosis have been reported (Russell & Rubenstein 1977). We believe that the origin of the tumor in the present case is most easily explained by the theory of disordered extracerebral ectopic neural crest cell migration with subsequent neoplastic transformation, the other possibilities of its origin being from Schwann cells in the perivascular plexus (Riggs & Clary 1957) or misplaced myelinated nerve fibers not attached to any of the cranial nerves (Prakash et al 1980). The benign nature of this tumor indicates the need for radical tumor excision. Histopathologically these tumors should be differentiated from microcystic meningiomas and pilocytic astrocytomas (Sobel & Michaud 1985).

CASE 2 An Unusual Case of Extra-axial Clival Blastomycosis Granuloma (Goel et al 1996)

A 25-year-old female patient was admitted with complaints of tingling numbness and weakness of the left side limbs for 6 months. She had occasional associated giddiness and neck pains. Her voice was noted to have changed for about a month. On examination her speech had a nasal twang and sensations over the left side of the face and the corneal reflex were depressed. In addition she had left-sided deafness, depressed palatal and gag reflexes, a wasted left trapezius, as well as a left-sided wasted tongue. She also had spastic quadriparesis, with a weaker left side. The sensations, however, were normal. There was no history of any major infection nor was there any evidence of an immunocompromised state. MRI and CT showed a large enhancing anterior foramen magnum tumor (Fig. 12.2a,b). The tumor was excised through a left suboccipital basal craniectomy (Fig. 12.2c). The tumor was firm, vascular and had a large attachment to the dura in the region of the occipital condyle. It was entirely extra-axial and had displaced the adjoining cranial nerves, vertebral artery and brain stem posteriorly. The operative impression was that of a meningioma. Histopathology revealed that the

lesion was a fungal granuloma. Hematoxylin and eosin staining revealed thick-walled budding yeast-like forms. Gracott's methenine silver(GMS) staining confirmed that the fungus was *Blastomyces dermatitidis*. The patient recovered, with return of palatal reflexes, clearance of nasal twang and return of full power. She is undergoing therapy with amphotericin B.

Comments

Blastomyces dermatitidis infection rarely involves the central nervous system. Chronic meningitis is the frequent form of presentation. Cerebral and extradural abscesses, intraparenchymal granulomas and cerebritis have also been rarely reported (Buechner & Clawson 1967). To the best of our knowledge intradural extra-axial granuloma caused by *Blastomyces dermatitidis* has not been reported (Goel 1995b).

Fungal infections of the brain are rare. They usually occur as opportunistic infections in immunosuppressed individuals. *Blastomyces dermatitidis*, a dimorphic fungus, is predominantly found in central North America (Kinkel 1984). Sporadic cases from other parts of the world have also been reported. Infection of the central nervous system is frequently a secondary manifestation of the systemic disease. Hematogenous spread of infection to the brain has been suggested. Chronic meningitis, multiple small abscesses, cerebritis, intraparenchymal granulomas and epidural abscesses have been the reported lesions attributed to *Blastomyces dermatitidis*. Intracranial lesions rarely occur in isolation and are usually associated with meningitis. The diagnosis is made by direct demonstration of the fungus in the infected tissues. Amphotericin B is the drug of choice and has been reported to be effective in 90% of cases. The mortality from central nervous system blastomycosis is high.

In the presented case there were various unusual features. The patient was young and otherwise in good health. The radiological appearance strongly suggested a meningioma. The operation findings of an extra-axial tumor, fibrovascular in nature with a wide dural attachment, supported the diagnosis of a meningioma. The histological diagnosis of a fungal granuloma came as a total surprise. Absence of meningeal infection and failure to find the primary focus of infection were other unusual features. Administration of amphotericin B is necessary to eradicate any residual infection that may be present.

The lesion was extra-axial and well circumscribed. There was no clinical or operative evidence of meningeal infection. The source of infection and the nature of its spread to the lower clivus remain obscure. The lesion was excised surgically and the patient showed rapid neurological recovery. The long-term outcome of the patient will be monitored.

CASE 3 Huge Benign Osteoblastoma of the Clivus and Atlas (Goel et al 1994)

A 50-year-old well-built male had pain in the neck and torticollis for 2 years. For 4 months he had noticed a progressively enlarging swelling in the right occipitocervical region. For 10 days prior to admission he started developing a rapidly progressive neurological deficit. First the right-sided limbs became weak and in 3 days he developed right hemiplegia. This was followed by left-sided weakness and symptoms of lower cranial nerve palsies. He was unable to speak or swallow and respiration was labored with the help of accessory muscles. Gag and palatal reflexes were absent and there was a right hypoglossal nerve palsy. There was spasticity in all four limbs, the deep tendon reflexes were exaggerated and the plantar reflexes were extensor. The patient was virtually quadriplegic with only feeble movements remaining at the left hip. The right occipitocervical external swelling measured about 17 cm × 12 cm and appeared to be arising from the underlying bone. It was free from the overlying skin.

X-rays and tomograms of the craniovertebral region (Fig. 12.42a) showed a large multiloculated radiolucent mass overlying the occipital bone and upper cervical vertebra. An eggshell-like appearance was seen along its posterior suboccipital and right-sided walls. The central part overlying atlas, axis and mastoid bones was irregularly, densely sclerotic, suggesting new bone formation and/or calcification. There was evidence of destruction of a large part of the atlas (arches, anterior and posterior tubercles and right lateral mass), adontoid process, lower clivus and right lateral margin of the foramen magnum. A large soft tissue mass was seen in the retro- and right parapharyngeal regions. An MRI scan (Fig. 12.42b,c) showed the massive tumor with extensions into the cervicomedullary junction and cerebellum, the former displaced to the left and the latter elevated. The tumor extension into the neck and parapharyngeal region was also vividly shown. The signal intensity of some of the cystic spaces suggested the presence of blood. Vertebral angiography showed the right vertebral artery to be narrowed up to the basilar artery and showed irregularity of its lumen from above the third cervical

vertebra. The tumor was vascular, deriving its blood supply from the muscular branches of the vertebral artery. Carotid angiography showed the common carotid and their bifurcations displaced anteriorly by the mass. There was no contribution of the blood supply from the carotids. The patient's precarious state warranted immediate surgery. In the left lateral position, a long incision was taken over the bulge of the tumor extending from just lateral to the occipitocervical region near the midline to the anterior border of the sternocleidomastoid region. The incision was deepened into the tumor which had displaced and stretched the muscles of the region. It was moderately vascular and largely cystic. The cysts were filled up with blood-stained yellow fluid. The walls of the cyst were made up of tumorous bony shell. As the cysts were evacuated and the bony shells removed, a large exposure was obtained enabling excision of the diseased bone around the craniocervical junction on the right side and anterior to the brain stem, including the rim of the foramen magnum, lower one-third of the clivus, arch and lateral mass of the atlas, lateral mass of the axis and the odontoid process. The vertebral artery was free and pulsatile from the point of its exit from the foramen transversarium of the third cervical vertebra to its dural entry into the posterior fossa. Thus a radical gross total excision of the extradural tumor was performed. Fusion of the grossly unstable craniovertebral region was not performed at this stage. A firm cervical collar was applied. The patient showed rapid neurological improvement following the surgery. He started talking, and the power of the left side improved to grade 4 and to grade 1 in the right side within 2 days. On the third day when the patient was being turned to one side he complained of a crackling sound in the neck and within a few minutes developed quadriplegia, followed by respiratory arrest. The collar had been inadvertently

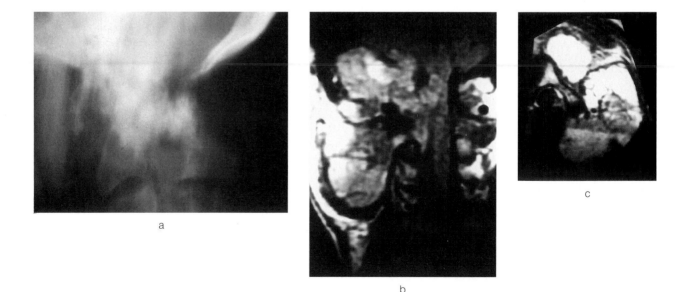

a

b

c

Fig. 12.42 **a** X-ray of the craniovertebral junction showing destruction of the atlas and lower clivus. Arrowheads show the faintly ossified border of the tumor. (From Goel et al 1994, with permission.) **b** Coronal cut of the MRI scan (T1-weighted image) of the craniovertebral region showing the massive tumor with compression of the spinomedullary junction. (From Goel et al 1994, with permission.) **c** Transverse cut showing the massive anteroposterior extensions of the tumor.

removed at this time. He was placed on assisted ventilation. However, he died 24 hours later.

Histopathology showed normal bony trabeculae destroyed by the tumor, which consisted of islands of osteoid tissue rimmed by osteoblasts with collagenous stroma. There were also large vascular spaces lined by endothelium and osteoblastic giant cells. There was no evidence of malignancy.

At autopsy there was no residual tumor, but there was a central hemorrhage within the cervical cord and the medulla. This primarily occurred during the unguarded turning of the patient.

Comments

This is a case of massive benign osteoblastoma involving the clivus and atlas. Usually these tumors involve the posterior elements of a vertebra and are detected when they are small due to the usual presenting symptom of pain. The unusual site, massive size and presentation with neurological deficits are rare for benign osteoblastomas.

The bone-forming 'benign osteoblastomas' are rare and account for less than 1% of primary bone tumors. The appendicular skeleton and the vertebrae are more commonly affected. There is a tendency for them to occur in the posterior elements of the spine. Few cases with involvement of the skull bone have been reported, the base being more frequently involved than the vault. Our literature review on this subject revealed only isolated cases with involvement of the clivus and atlas (Gelberman & Olson 1974). There was no neurological involvement or deficit in any of these cases. Predilection for males under the age of 30 years has been shown. Benign osteoblastomas are slow-growing tumors and rarely may acquire a giant size. The usual presentation is in the form of a slow-growing swelling and local pain. The pain is characteristically relieved by aspirin and other cyclooxygenase inhibitors. The radiological appearance of a well-circumscribed, essentially radiolucent, multiloculated tumor with areas of mottled calcification and ossification is common with other bone-forming tumors, more commonly giant cell tumors, osteogenic sarcoma and aneurysmal bone cysts. The usefulness of pre- and intraoperative localization of the lesion by radionuclear techniques has been reported. Radical surgical treatment has been advocated and long-term cure from the disease has been reported. The tumors are usually vascular. Considering that multiple cystic areas are encountered and the tumor is well circumscribed, excision of the tumor is not difficult. Although radiotherapy has been advocated by some for residual tumor, malignant transformation of the lesion following it has been reported.

The large size of the tumor and extensive involvement of the craniocervical region added to the problems in the patient presented. A radical excision necessarily resulted in an unstable spine. In retrospect it is quite evident that fusion with internal or external stabilization was absolutely necessary.

References

Al-Mefty O, Anand V K 1990 Zygomatic approach to skull-base lesions. Journal of Neurosurgery 73: 668–673

Al-Mefty O, Fox J L, Smith R R 1989 Petrosal approach for petroclival meningiomas. Neurosurgery 22: 510–517, 1988.

Bochenek Z, Kukawa A 1975 An extended approach through the middle cranial fossa to the internal auditory meatus and the cerebellopontine angle. Acta Otolaryngologica 80: 40–414

Bonnal J, Louis R, Combalbert A 1964 L'abord temporal transtentoriel de l'angle ponto-cerebelleux et du clivus. Neurochirurgie 10: 3–12

Buechner H A, Clawson C M 1967 Blastomycosis of the central nervous system: II. A report of nine cases from the Veterans Administrative cooperative study. American Review of Respiratory Diseases 95: 820–826

Deogaonkar M, Goel A, Nagpal R D et al 1995 Intraparenchymal schwannoma of the frontal lobe. Journal of Postgraduate Medicine (in press).

Fay T 1930 The management of tumors of the posterior fossa by a transtentorial approach. Surgical Clinics of North America 10: 1427–1459

Feigin I, Ogata J 1971 Schwann cells and peripheral myelin within human central nervous tissues: the mesenchymal character of schwann cells. Journal of Neuropathology and Experimental Neurology 30: 603–612

Fisch U, Kumar A 1985 Infratemporal surgery of the skull base. In: Rand R W (ed): Microneurosurgery, 3rd edn. Mosby, St Louis pp 421–454

Gelberman R H, Olson C O 1974 Benign osteoblastoma of the atlas: a case report. Journal of Bone and Joint Surgery 56: 808–811

Goebel H H, Shimokawa, Schaake Th et al 1979 Schwannoma of the sellar region. Acta Neurochirurgica 48: 191–197

Goel A 1995a Middle fossa sub-gasserian ganglion approach to clivus chordomas. Acta Neurochirurgica (Wien) 136: 212–216

Goel A 1995b Extended middle fossa approach for petroclival lesions. Acta Neurochirurgica (Wien) 135: 78–83

Goel A 1995c Tentorial dural flap for transtentorial surgery. British Journal of Neurosurgery 9: 785–786

Goel A 1996 Basal lateral subtemporal approach. British Journal of Neurosurgery (in press)

Goel A, Bhayani R, Nagpal R D 1994 Massive benign osteoblastoma of the clivus and atlas. British Journal of Neurosurgery 8: 483–486

Goel A, Bhayani R, Nagpal R D 1995 Unusual extra-axial schwannoma. British Journal of Neurosurgery (in press)

Goel A, Deogaonkar M, Nagpal R D 1996 Extra axial clival blasto-mycosis granuloma: a case report. British Journal of Neurosurgery 10: 97–98

Hakuba A, Nishimura S, Jang B J 1988 A combined retroauricular and preauricular transpetrosal transtentorial approach to clivus meningiomas. Surgical Neurology 30: 108–116

House W F 1961 Surgical exposure of the internal auditory canal and its contents through the middle cranial fossa. Laryngoscope 71: 1363–1385

Kawase T, Shiobara R, Toya S 1991 Anterior trans-petrosal–transtentorial approach for sphenopetroclival meningiomas: surgical method and results in 10 patients. Neurosurgery 28: 869–876

Kinkel W 1984 North American blastomycosis. Surgery Gynecology and Obstetrics 99: 1–26

Malis L I 1985 Surgical resection of tumor of the skull base, Vol 1. In Wilkins R H, Rengachary S S (eds) Neurosurgery, McGraw Hill, New York, pp 1011–1021

Morrison A W, King T T 1973 Experience with a translabyrinthine–transtentorial approach to the cerebellopontine angle: technical note. Journal of Neurosurgery 38: 382–390

Prakash B, Roy S, Tandon P N 1980 Schwannoma of the brain stem: case report. Journal of Neurosurgery 53: 121–123

Ramamurthi B, Anguli V C, Iyer C G S 1958 A case of intramedullary neurinoma. Journal of Neurology Neurosurgery and Psychiatry 21: 92–94

Redekop G, Elisevich K, Gilbert J 1990 Fourth ventricular schwannoma. Journal of Neurosurgery 73: 771–781

Riggs H E, Clary W U 1957 A case of intramedullary sheath cell tumor of the spinal cord: consideration of vascular nerves as a source of origin. Journal of Neuropathology and Experimental Neurology 16: 332–336

Rosomoff H L 1971 Subtemporal transtentorial approach for cerebellopontine angle. Laryngoscope 81: 1448–1454

Russell D S, Rubinstein L J 1977 Pathology of tumors of the nervous system, 4th ed. Edward Arnold, London, 51–52: 372–379

Samii M, Ammirati M, Mahran A et al 1989 Surgery of petroclival meningiomas: report of 24 cases. Neurosurgery 24: 12–17

Sekhar L N, Schramm V L Jr, Jones N F 1987 Subtemporal–preauricular infratemporal fossa approach to large lateral and posterior cranial base neoplasms. Journal of Neurosurgery 67: 488–499

Sekhar L N, Pomeranz S, Janecka I P et al 1992 Temporal bone neoplasms: a report on 20 surgically treated cases. Journal of Neurosurgery 76: 578–587

Sharma R R, Gurusinghe T N 1993 Intraparenchymatous schwannoma of cerebellum. British Journal of Neurosurgery 7: 83–90

Shiobara R, Ohira T, Kanzaki J et al 1988 A modified extended middle cranial fossa approach for acoustic nerve tumors. Journal of Neurosurgery 68: 358–365

Sindou M P, Fobe J 1991 Removal of the roof of the external auditory meatus in approaching the tentorial notch through a low temporal craniotomy. Journal of Neurosurgery 74: 520–522

Sobel R A, Michaud J 1985 Microcystic meningioma of the falx cerebri with numerous palisading structures: an unusual histological pattern mimicking schwannoma. Acta Neuropathologica 68: 256

Spetzler R F, Daspit P D, Pappas C T E 1992 The combined supra- and infratentorial approach for lesions of the petrous and clival regions: experience with 46 cases. Journal of Neurosurgery 76: 588–599

Stieglitz L, Gerster A G, Lilienthal H 1986 A study of three cases of tumor of the brain in which the operation was performed: one recovery, two deaths. American Journal of Medical Sciences 111: 509–531

Symon L 1982 Surgical approaches to the tentorial hiatus. Advances in Technical Standards in Neurosurgery 9: 69–112

Tarlov E 1977 Surgical management of tumors of the tentorium and clivus. In: Schmidek H H, Sweet W H (eds) Operative neurosurgical techniques, Vol 1. Grune & Stratton, New York, pp 381–388

Yasargil M G, Mortara R W, Curie M 1980 Meningiomas of basal posterior cranial fossa. Advances in Technical Standards in Neurosurgery 7: 1–15

Middle Fossa Transpetrosal Approaches for Lesions of the Clivus and Cerebellopontine Angle

Takeshi Kawase

Surgical removal of the pyramidal bone has been used mainly for cerebellopontine angle (CPA) tumors since 1970 (extended middle fossa approach, posterior transpetrosal approach, or presigmoid transpetrosal approach) (King 1970, House 1973, Bochenek and Kukawa 1975, Kanzaki et al 1977, Hakuba 1978, Shiobara et al 1989). This approach is a combination of the subtemporal and translabyrinthine approaches, and gives the surgeon the possibility of reaching the CPA and mid-frontal portion of the pons from the drilled pyramidal bone. In 1977, the transpetrosal approach was applied to the clival meningioma (Hakuba et al 1977). Advantages of the approach were wider surgical exposure and minimal brain damage because it is accessed epidurally from the space of the resected pyramidal bone to spare brain retraction and sacrifice of the bridging veins. Direct observation of the pontine surface reduced the risk of arterial injury. A higher tumor radicality was expected in meningiomas removed with attached dura below the resected bone by the transpetrosal approach, compared with that by the suboccipital approach. Disadvantages were long operation time, sacrificed hearing and risk of rhinorrhea. In 1985, limited pyramidal resection anteromedial to the auditory organs (anterior transpetrosal approach) was reported for preservation of hearing in clipping of aneurysms of the lower basilar artery (Kawase et al 1985). This approach decreased the operation time, giving further direct observation toward the clivus and prepontine space without manipulation of the VIIth and VIIIth cranial nerves. Another advantage of the anterior approach was easy access to the parasellar area from a small middle fossa craniotomy, being indicated for petroclival meningiomas with parasellar invasion (Kawase et al 1991, 1994). Thus the transpetrosal approaches, even modified by surgeons (Al-Mefty et al 1988, Samii and Ammirati 1988, Samii et al

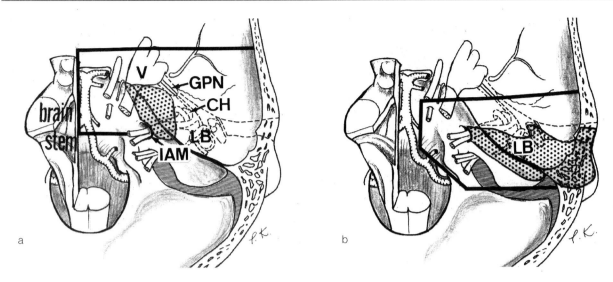

Fig. 12.43   a Line drawing with dotted areas showing the region of bone resection in the anterior transpetrosal approach. GPN = greater superficial petrosal nerve, CH = cochlea, IAM = internal auditory meatus, V = Gasserian ganglion, LB = labyrinth. **b** Line drawing with dotted areas showing the region of bone resection in the posterior transpetrosal approach. LB = labyrinth.

1989, Sen & Sekhar 1990), became relevant surgical approaches to the upper clivus and brain stem.

1. Anterior Transpetrosal Approach

Advantages
1. Direct surgical field to the clivus by minimal pyramid resection, giving access to both the middle and posterior fossae.
2. Minimal retraction damage and venous complication.
3. Low risk of facial or lower cranial nerve injury.
4. Hearing preservation.

Disadvantages
1. Limited surgical field.
2. Risk of CSF rhinorrhea.

Indication
1. Petroclival tumors located anterior to the internal auditory meatus, with or without parasellar extension (meningiomas, trigeminal neurinomas, chordomas and prepontine epidermoids).
2. Small acoustic tumors with useful hearing.
3. Basilar trunk aneurysms located between the sellar floor and the internal auditory meatus on the lateral projection of the angiogram, and especially that projected posteriorly.

Surgical Technique: Above the mandibular joint, a small craniotomy of the same size to the squamous suture is made, and the anterior petrous pyramid is accessed epidurally. The middle meningeal artery is coagulated and detached at the foramen spinosum. Periosteal adhesion on the GSPN is sharply dissected from the meningeal dura, and the apical petrous pyramid is exposed. Bone resection is limited anterior to the auditory

organs, such as cochlea and labyrinth. The area of bone resection is surrounded by the trigeminal impression anteriorly, the eminentia arcuata posteriorly, GSPN, the carotid artery (C6) and cochlea laterally, and internal auditory meatus (IAM) inferiorly (Fig. 12.43a). For small acoustic tumors, the roof of the IAM is selectively opened without sacrificing the cochlea or labyrinth. A dural incision parallel to the superior petrosal sinus, which is ligated and detached thereafter, is followed by complete incision of the tentorium. By retraction of the leaflets of the tentorium, the surgical field is opened directly toward the clivus, anterior surface of the pons and to the basilar artery between the IIIrd and VIIth cranial nerves. Meckel's cave is opened from its orifice, and the cavernous sinus can be accessed if necessary, from the enlarged Parkinson's triangle by mobilization of the trigeminal nerve. A large petroclival tumor can be removed by further resection of the pyramid including the labyrinth, resulting in the sacrifice of hearing. The drilled pyramidal bone is covered with a temporal periosteo-fascia flap with fibrin glue to avoid CSF leakage.

2. Posterior Transpetrosal Approach

Advantages
1. Low risk of arterial and brain damage by direct observation of the CPA from the side of bone resection.
2. High tumor radicality by removal of the dural attachment in meningioma.

Disadvantages
1. Long operation time.
2. Hearing sacrificed.
3. Risk of CSF rhinorrhea.

Indication: Patients with CPA tumors, whose hearing is already lost, or hearing preservation is not anticipated (meningiomas, neurinomas).

Surgical Methods: A horseshoe scalp incision and craniotomy are made above the external auditory meatus. The upper mastoid process with air cells and the posterior pyramid including the labyrinth are resected until the internal auditory meatus is opened (Fig. 12.43b). The roof of the geniculate ganglion of the facial nerve is not resected, to spare nerve injury. The dural incision including detachment of the tentorium is the same as that of the anterior approach: retraction of the tentorial leaflets offers a direct surgical field to the CPA and IAM without retraction of the cerebellum. Total resection of the pyramid including the anterior part (total petrosectomy) offers a wide surgical field from IIIrd to XIth cranial nerves, and is indicated for large petroclival tumors covering the total ridge of the pyramid. CSF leakage is prevented with a free muscle piece plunged into the orifice of the Eustachian tube, and with the periosteo-fascia flap or with a piece of abdominal fat tissue.

The transpetrosal approach is comparable to the suboccipital approach in acoustic tumors. The average morbidity is not different between the two (Shiobara et al 1989), and the advantage may depend on each case. The former may have an advantage in the tumor with anterior extension, and the latter in posterior extension. The surgeon's experience of the approach may be another factor. In trigeminal neurinomas or meningiomas, however, the transpetrosal approach has further advantages. Tumor resection away from cranial nerves VII–XI decrease the manipulation injury of these nerves. Tumor resection with dural attachment on the pyramid and the tentorium may decrease tumor regrowth. A disadvantage of the transpetrosal approach may be the complicated anatomy, and training on the cadaver may be important. By either approach, however, complete tumor resection did not always produce good surgical results. Total tumor resection was risky in patients with the tumor adhesive to the brain stem, or tumor encasing the basilar system (Kawase et al 1994). Radiosurgery will be the best tool after subtotal removal.

References

Al-Mefty O, Fox J L, Smith R R 1988 Petrosal approach for petroclival meningiomas. Neurosurgery 22: 510–517

Bochenek Z, Kukwa A 1975 An extended approach through the middle cranial fossa to the internal auditory meatus and the cerebellopontine angle. Acta Otolaryngologica 80: 410–414

Hakuba A 1978 Total removal of cerebellopontine angle tumors with a combined transpetrosal–transtentorial approach. No Shinkei Geka 6: 347–354 (in Japanese)

Hakuba A, Nishimura S, Tanaka K et al 1977 Clivus meningioma: six cases of total removal. Neurologia Medico Chirurgica 17: 63–77 (in Japanese)

House W F 1973 Surgery of acoustic tumors. Otolaryngol Clin Nose Am 6: 245–266

Kanzaki J, Kawase T, Sano H et al 1977 A modified extended middle cranial fossa approach for acoustic tumors. Archives of Otorhinolaryngology 212: 119–121

Kawase T, Toya S, Shiobara R, Mine S 1985 Transpetrosal approach for aneurysms of the lower basilar artery. Journal of Neurosurgery 63: 857–867

Kawase T, Shiobara R, Toya S 1991 Anterior transpetrosal–transtentorial approach for sphenopetro-clival meningiomas: surgical method and results in 10 patients. Neurosurgery 2: 869–876

Kawase T, Shiobara R, Toya S 1994 Middle fossa transpetrosal–transtentorial approaches for petroclival meningiomas: selective pyramid resection and radicality. Acta Neurochirurgica 129: 113–120

King T T 1970 Combined translabyrinthine–transtentorial approach to acoustic nerve tumors. Proceedings of Royal Society of Medicine 63: 780–782

Samii M, Ammirati M 1988 The combined supra-infratentorial presigmoid avenue to the petroclival region: surgical technique and clinical applications. Acta Neurochirurgica (Wien) 95: 6–12

Samii M, Ammirati M, Mahran A et al 1989 Surgery of petroclival meningiomas: report of 24 cases. Neurosurgery 24: 12–17

Sen C N, Sekhar L N 1990 The subtemporal and preauricular infratemporal approach to intradural structures ventral to the brain stem. Journal of Neurosurgery 73: 345–354

Shiobara R, Ohira T, Kanzaki J et al 1989 A modified extended middle cranial fossa approach for acoustic nerve tumors. Journal of Neurosurgery 68: 358–365

Surgery on Clivus Meningiomas
Hideyuki Ohnishi

Clivus meningiomas have been terra incognita for neurosurgeons. There have been a few pioneers who have attempted to improve the approaches to these tumors. Prior to the era of microsurgery, the mortality rate was about 50% (Mayberg & Symon 1986). In the recent past, there has been a considerable increase in the interest in these previously considered untreatable tumors. The development of new skull base approaches has helped to decrease the overall surgical morbidity. However, the reported incidence of neurological morbidity and mortality associated with clivus meningioma surgery is still higher than most benign tumors at other locations. The postoperative motor deficits ranged from 7% to 45% and cranial nerve deficit ranged from 12% to 91% in some of the recently published series (Al-Mefty et al 1988, Bricolo et al 1992, Spetzler et al 1992). Postoperative mortality ranged from nil to 10% (Al-Mefty et al 1988, Bricolo et al 1992, Cantore et al 1994, Kawase et al 1994, Mayberg & Symon 1986, Nishimura et al 1989, Saleh et al 1994, Sami & Tatagiba 1992, Sekhar et al 1990, 1994, Spetzler et al 1992). It is important for neurosurgeons to know some common risk factors associated with surgery in these cases. Information regarding the available operative techniques to deal with these tumors is essential.

General Considerations: The important considerations during surgery on clivus meningiomas are proper selection of an operative candidate, selection of the appropriate operative approach and judgment on the degree of tumor removal possible. Operative candidates are decided on the basis of age of the patient and general preoperative condition. Total excision without causing additional neurological deficit is the goal of surgery. Among the clivus meningiomas, the risk of morbidity is higher with large or giant-sized tumors than that accompanying small or medium-sized tumors. The decision making as to whether to remove tumors totally or subtotally and/or to consider gamma knife surgery is important, especially in cases where the tumor invades into the cavernous sinus.

While dealing with skull base meningiomas, its devascularization, dissection from adjacent structures and tumor debulking are key issues. Preoperative embolization of the feeding arteries is beneficial for devascularization of tumors. It is easy to embolize feeding arteries from the external carotid artery but it is difficult to embolize branches from the meningohypophyseal artery. Epidural approaches such as the transpetrous presigmoid approach may decrease blood loss as feeding arteries can be cauterized close to the origin of tumor. Dissection of the tumor from the brain stem, cerebellum, cranial nerves and blood vessels is difficult and time-consuming and requires a high level of technical skill. With continuous saline irrigation and bipolar cautery, shrinking of the tumor while dissecting it off the brain stem or cerebellum is a useful maneuver. The arachnoid plane is an important and useful guide during the dissection. It is important not to lose this plane. Various shaped dissectors may be useful while dissecting the tumor from cranial nerves or blood vessels. The ring-shaped bipolar cautery and ultrasound surgical aspirator are useful, especially in cases of fibrous tumors. It is important to have an orientation of critical arteries and cranial nerves which have been compressed and deviated from their normal position and/or encased before starting debulking the tumor.

A subtemporal or a conventional lateral suboccipital approach are not recommended for large-sized clivus meningiomas because of the need of strong brain retraction, high risk of cerebral contusion and narrow and poor operative exposure obtained. The selection of an appropriate skull base approach is important according to the location of tumors. Adequate precautions for prevention of postoperative CSF rhinootorrhea are necessary. In some cases, a two-staged operation is useful. In such cases, after the bony decompression and devascularization of the tumor the operation may be terminated after reposition of normal structures. Actual tumor resection may be carried out during a second-stage operation.

Operative Techniques

1. Petroclival Meningiomas: Petroclival meningiomas which arise from the posterior clinoid and the petrous apex are difficult surgical challenges. They distort the brain stem and involve the basilar artery and its branches. They frequently involve cranial nerves III–XII. They may extend anteriorly and invade the cavernous sinus.

Small-sized tumors are removed by a retrosigmoid approach or by an anterior transpetrous approach via the middle fossa. Large or giant-sized petroclival lesions are usually resected by a transpetrous presigmoid approach, performed with or without partial labyrinthectomy according to the preoperative hearing status. In this approach, preservation of the anteriorly placed vein of Labbé, the inferior temporal veins and the sphenopetrosal vein is important to prevent postoperative intratemporal hemorrhages. The traditional subtemporal approach is not recommended due to the dangers involved to these veins. The first step is to identify all of the cranial nerves if possible. It is not unusual for these tumors to involve cranial nerves II–XII. Intraoperative monitoring, such as somatosensory evoked potential (SEP), ABR and direct cranial nerve monitoring are useful. The portions of the tumor adherent to brain stem and basilar arteries should be removed last to minimize the need for brain stem retraction. The abducens nerve is most likely to be injured during surgery because of the fact that these tumors often arise from the area of Dorello's canal. A thin rim of tumor on the brain stem may be left behind if the arachnoidal cleavage plane cannot be adequately defined during surgery. When the vertebrobasilar arteries and their branches are encased by a tough and fibrous tumor, tumor resection can result in vascular injury as tumor may invade into the wall of the vessels. It is especially difficult to dissect the tumor at the second operation or after radiation therapy.

2. Lower Clival and Foramen Magnum Meningiomas: These lesions are resected by an extreme lateral transcondylar approach. One-third to one-half of the lateral mass of the atlas and the occipital condyle are removed, exposing at least 1 cm of dura anterior to the entrance of the vertebral artery. Great caution must be exercised with the anterior spinal arteries, which may be encased. When bilateral lower cranial nerves are involved, postoperative severe dysfunction, such as dysphonia, dysarthria and dysphagia can occur. Postoperative respiratory care and prevention of aspiration pneumonia are important.

3. Panclival Meningiomas: Panclival lesions are removed by a combination of the posterior transpetrous and transcondylar approaches. In these patients, tumors are usually enormous and postoperative clinical deterioration should be anticipated. The key point in such cases is to estimate how much tumor can be removed safely.

Factors Influencing Surgical Outcome: Preoperative patient condition (Karnofsky scale score) is directly related to early postoperative functional deterioration. Male gender seems to have a significant correlation with the outcome. In our experience the age factor does not significantly affect the outcome (Sekhar et al 1994). As a tumor grows in size, it compresses and distorts the brain stem. In the initial stage of brain stem compression by tumors, the arachnoid plane is preserved. In this stage, the dissection of the tumor is relatively easy. In the second stage, the arachnoid plane is lost, particularly at the site of maximum compression. Tumor dissection becomes difficult in the region of the damaged arachnoid plane. In the terminal stages, tumors become large or giant and the pia mater is invaded. The vertebrobasilar arteries can be encased by such a tumor. Brain stem edema, appearing as a high-intensity area on T2-weighted images of MRI, occurs because of a breakdown of the tumor–brain barrier. The tumor is fed by branches of the vertebrobasilar artery. In such cases, total excision of the tumor is extremely difficult. In some instances, the tumor at the site of the brain stem invasion and the vertebrobasilar artery encasement should not be removed completely, in order to preserve these neurovascular tissues. Reoperation and preoperative radiation therapy are also important risk factors because the arachnoid plane is frequently lost in these cases. Tumor nature also affects the radicality of removal. In the case of soft and suckable tumors, it is easy to remove tumors from the brain stem, cranial nerves and blood vessels. But in the firm fibrous tumor, the dissection is difficult.

Conclusion: In addition to knowing some common risk factors and mastering skull base techniques, decision making about selection of operative candidates, appropriate skull base approach, and estimation of the degree of safe tumor removal is important in clival meningioma surgery. Symptomatic patients with small-sized tumors should be encouraged to undergo surgery. Patients with large or giant-sized tumors have a greater likelihood of postoperative dysfunction and have a need for postoperative rehabilitation. Especially in these patients, an integrated therapy is beneficial if patients are to lead a useful life.

References

Al-Mefty O, Fox J L, Smith R R 1988 Petrosal approach for petroclival meningiomas. Neurosurgery 22: 510–517

Bricolo A P, Turazzi S, Talacchi A et al 1992 Microsurgical removal of petroclival meningiomas: a report of 33 patients. Neurosurgery 31: 813–828

Cantore G, Delfini R, Ciappetta P 1994 Surgical treatment of petroclival meningiomas: experience with 16 cases. Surgical Neurology 42: 105–111

Kawase T, Shiobara, R, Toya Sh 1994 Middle fossa transpetrosal–transtentorial approaches for petroclival meningiomas: selective pyramid resection and radicality. Acta Neurochirurgica (Wien) 129: 113–120

Mayberg M R, Symon L 1986 Meningiomas of the clivus and apical petrous bone: report of 35 cases. Journal of Neurosurgery 65: 160–167

Nishimura S, Hakuba A, Jank B et al 1989 Clivus and apicopetroclivus meningiomas: report of 24 cases. Neurologia Medicochirurgia 29: 1004–1011

Saleh E A, Taibah A K, Achilli V et al 1994 Posterior fossa meningioma: surgical strategy. Skull Base Surgery 4: 202–212

Samii M, Tatagiba M 1992 Experience with 36 surgical cases of petroclival meningiomas. Acta Neurochirugica (Wien) 118: 27–32

Sekhar L N, Jannetta P F, Burkhart L E et al 1990 Meningiomas involving the clivus: a six-year experience with 41 patients. Neurosurgery 27: 764–781

Sekhar L N, Swamy N K S, Jaiswal V et al 1994 Surgical excision of meningiomas involving the clivus: preoperative and intraoperative features as predictors of postoperative functional deterioration. Journal of Neurosurgery 81: 860–868

Spetzler R F, Daspit C P, Pappas C T E 1992 The combined supra- and infratentorial approach for lesions of the petrous and clival regions: experience with 46 cases. Journal of Neurosurgery 76: 588–599

Anterior skull base tumors

Atul Goel   Shigeaki Kobayashi   Kazuhiro Hongo

13

GENERAL CONSIDERATIONS IN TUMOR SURGERY

Patient and head position and the site and size of the scalp incision should be planned meticulously as these factors will be important to decide the course of the surgery.

In general the head of the patient should be placed in a manner that the entire operation can be carried out without the need for alterations in the head or table position. However, during the operation, whenever it is necessary the head and table position should be changed without hesitation. The principal operating surgeon should himself observe and approve the patient and head position and mark the incision before painting and draping is allowed. The patient needs to be placed in a natural position, as if 'sleeping' comfortably, so that no undue stretch to any body part is caused. The placement of the operating area should preferably be in the superior – most part of the field so that the surgeon operates in a comfortable sitting position without the need of twisting his own body or neck. While pin fixation of the head is helpful in firmly holding the head into position, whenever feasible it should be avoided. Considerations of adequate venous drainage, and whenever possible and necessary provision for an avenue for lumbar cerebrospinal fluid (CSF) drainage, should be made.

Scalp incision

The incision over the scalp should not only be cosmetically acceptable, but should also provide an adequate exposure for the entire lesion in one field. It should be possible to excise the tumor in one operative field. It may be necessary to achieve this by expanding the exposure. It is seldom necessary to plan an operation such that only a part of the tumor will be excised on the first occasion and part will be excised on the second utilizing a separate exposure.

There are various papers written on the subject of preservation of the facial nerve branches supplying the region of the forehead in the basal pterional approach.

Preservation of the trunk and branches of the superficial temporal artery should also be emphasized.

Anatomical considerations

The frontal and temporal branches of the facial nerve, after their course through the lobes of the parotid gland, traverse superiorly over the anterior aspect of the zygomatic arch. The nerve traverses superficial to the superficial layer of temporalis and masseteric fascia; by remaining deep to these layers a subperiosteal dissection over the zygomatic arch provides the best chance of preservation of these tiny nerve branches. Subperiosteal exposure of the zygomatic arch should be in a posterior to anterior direction. It is also advisable to avoid using cautery while exposing the zygomatic arch as the heat can result in compromise of neural function. Retraction of the everted scalp with hooks or stitches needs to be gentle and avoid the region of the course of the nerve. While elevating a bifrontal scalp flap, it is preferable to elevate the flap in the subpericranial plane. Branches of the supraorbital nerves can be inadvertently damaged if the dissection is in the subgaleal plane. The thicker the elevated scalp flap, the better is its vascular nourishment and also better are the chances of preservation of thin nerves which travel within the scalp layers.

The incisions for pterional exposure posterior to the superficial temporal artery have been recommended so the scalp can receive vascular supply from the artery (Fig. 13.1). Such an incision can result in compromise of the major anterior branch of the superficial temporal artery. It is recommended that in situations where there is no danger of compromise of the scalp circulation an incision taken anterior to the course of the superficial temporal artery and its anterior branch and posterior to the course of the facial nerve branches over the zygomatic arch may be suitable. Such an incision may be about 20 mm anterior to the tragus. This incision may be placed posterior to the hairline (Fig. 13.2). The preservation of the entire superficial temporal artery can be crucially important in some instances where there is a possibility of operative trauma to the

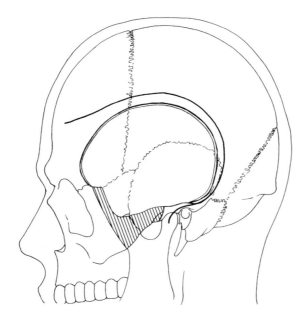

Fig. 13.1   Conventional scalp incision for a frontotemporal craniotomy. The zygomatic bone is shaded to show the area of osteotomy to enhance the basal exposure.

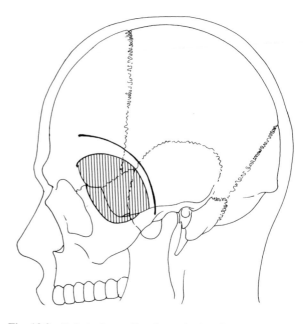

Fig. 13.2   Relatively small and anterior basal exposure for a pterional craniotomy. The posterior half of the lateral and superior walls of the orbit and the entire lesser wing of the sphenoid bone are removed.

major middle cerebral artery branch and the need for vascular anastomosis is considered.

Keyhole approaches

With the advances in microsurgical techniques the extent of the surgical incision has reduced and keyhole exposures have been successfully employed. These measures should be employed if there is no compromise over the extent of the tumor excision or the safety of the patient as regards provision for control of vessels and exposure of major nerves.

For lesions in the sellar and parasellar areas where a pterional approach is selected, there may not be the need to expose extensively the temporal or the frontal lobes. Thus the incision can be moved anteriorly towards the lesser wing. The basal extension of the approach can be obtained by removal of the entire lesser wing and part of the roof and lateral wall of the orbit (Figs 13.2, 13.3). This keyhole approach can provide a basal view to the lesion and also avoids unnecessary scalp incision or bone work.

Estimation of the histological nature of the lesion

It is on various occasions critically important to have a fair idea about the histological nature of the lesion on the basis

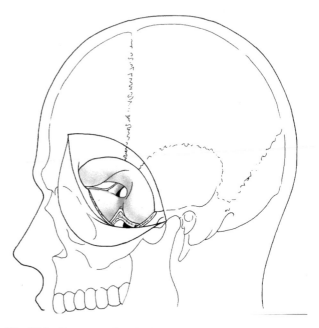

Fig. 13.3   Exposure after the bone work. The orbit, optic nerve, paraclinoid carotid artery, frontal and the temporal lobes are exposed. Surgery in the region of the clinoid process can be carried out with minimal need to retract the brain.

of symptomatology and radiology. This would not only help to plan the nature of required exposure, need for arterial dissection and control, surgical strategy and the extent of excision, but also to prognosticate the ultimate outcome. Careful analysis of history of the symptoms and signs can provide some clues regarding the nature of the lesion on various occasions. For example, in a case of a suprasellar tumor it is sometimes difficult to distinguish on the basis of radiology between an optic nerve glioma, craniopharyngioma, pituitary tumor and a meningioma. The history of presentation of each of these lesions has some peculiar features which can lead to a diagnosis. The age of the patient, duration of the symptoms, nature of neurological involvement, presence or absence of symptoms of increased intracranial pressure secondary to tumor growth and hydrocephalus, in addition to radiological pictures, can in most cases provide a fair idea about the histological nature of the lesion. The type of tumor lobulations, cystic changes, intratumoral necrosis, calcification, peritumoral edema, and nature of vascular displacement can provide clues regarding the histological nature of the lesion. The nature of the arterial and cranial nerve relationship also varies with the variety of the tumor. To have such an idea prior to the operation can help in planning the surgical strategy.

Massive optic nerve/chiasmatic glioma often simulates meningioma on radiological examination. Their consistency also matches. However, the optic nerve/chiasmatic gliomas present more frequently in children or in young adults. Involvement of the visual pathway and hormonal dysfunction are the principal presenting symptoms. Headaches or other symptoms of raised intracranial pressure are seldom predominant. The tumor is homogeneously enhancing in nature with an irregular and lobulated border. Intratumoral calcifications are not present. The lobulations of the tumor are characteristic. Association of hydrocephalus is late in optic nerve gliomas. It is crucially important to have a preoperative cognizance of an optic nerve glioma as the operative strategy varies significantly in these lesions. An attempt towards radical total excision of an optic nerve/chiasmatic glioma could be life threatening.

DIAGNOSING THE HISTOLOGY ON BASIS OF ARTERIAL DISPLACEMENTS

The site of origin and the character of the spread of the tumor can usually be gauged from the nature of arterial displacements. The arterial displacement in relationship to the tumor can be clearly seen on magnetic resonance imaging (MRI). The arterial displacements and the nature of encasement can assist in providing clues regarding the histological nature of the tumor. The direction of approach to the tumor depends on the site of displacement of the artery. The direction should not be such that the maximally dis-

placed segment of the artery is exposed early in the operation.

Estimation of consistency of the tumor

Tumor consistency dictates on most occasions the extent and ease of possible surgical excision and the ultimate outcome. Estimation of consistency of the tumor on the basis of clinical and radiological features can guide the planning and execution of the operation. Duration of symptoms and the extent of neural involvement provide useful clues. For example, in cases of meningiomas in the region of the anterior clinoid process, the longer the duration of symptoms and worse the visual impairment, the firmer is the consistency of the tumor. Intensities on T1- and T2-weighted images can provide a reasonable clue as to the consistency of the lesion. Hypointensity on T1- and hyperintensity on the T2-weighted images suggest that the tumor is soft. Softer varieties of tumors frequently encase the tumor, while firmer varieties will displace the tumor. A softer tumor will encase the artery but may not narrow its lumen. When the lumen is narrowed the tumor is likely to be firm.

Estimation of vascularity of the lesion

The vascularity of the tumor can be an important variable which may decide the course of the operation. Unless extremely vascular (as in cases of angioblastic meningiomas, or hemangioblastomas), consistency of the tumor can be as important a factor as vascularity. Although contrast enhancement on computed tomographic (CT) scanning is not a guide, some idea about the degree of vascularity can be had from the extent of enhancement. Presence of punctate or linear flow voids in and around the tumor as seen on MRI can give a fair idea about vascularity. Angiography gives exact information about the vascularity of the tumor, and the nature, size, direction and source of the feeding vessels. Usually firm tumors are less vascular. In firm tumors delayed films in angiography may be more useful, as the contrast takes time to enter into and clear from the tumor.

Estimations of tumor surrounding arachnoidal plane

Presence or absence of arachnoidal plane around the tumor can usually be seen on a good-quality MRI. The rounded or irregular borders of the tumor, tumor bossilations, encasement of surrounding vessels and peritumoral edema can provide a clue as to the presence of an arachnoidal plane which could affect the surgery. The arachnoidal plane was always preserved in the authors' practice and a plane of cleavage for dissection was available between the tumor and the neural and vascular structures. It appears that the arachnoid membrane is a firm membrane which meningiomas can never 'pierce' and enter into the subpial plane. The arachnoid around the subarachnoid vessels can sometimes fold around the vessels along with the tumor, which then encases the artery, while remaining extraarachnoid.

Anatomy of tumors

Tumors arise and spread along specified planes. Growth of the tumor proceeds by opening up the anatomical planes. The tumor never traverses through or pierces an anatomical layer. By studying the anatomical spread of the tumors, the anatomy of the area can be better appreciated. The anatomy of the cavernous sinus, and the controversy of its dural cover, is clarified if the tumors growing in and around the cavernous sinus are studied. The cavernous hemangioma growing inside the cavernous sinus opens its dural walls and provides a clear picture of the shape, extensions and communications of the cavernous sinus. Tumors arising around the cavernous sinus displace the dural walls in a very specified manner displaying clearly the anatomy of the area. Bone anatomy, on the other hand, can modulate itself on the basis of the growth of the tumor.

Proposed modification of the Simpson grading (Kobayashi et al 1994)

Grade I: Complete microscopic removal of the tumor and dural attachments with any abnormal bone.
Grade II: Complete microscopic removal of the tumor with diathermy coagulation of its dural attachment.
Grade III: Complete microscopic removal of intradural tumor without resection or coagulation of its dural attachment or any extradural extensions.
Grade IVA: Intentional subtotal removal to preserve cranial nerves and/or blood vessels with complete microscopic removal of attachment.
Grade IVB: Partial removal leaving tumor less than 10% in volume.
Grade V: Partial removal leaving tumor more than 10% or decompression with or without biopsy.

In the modified Simpson grading system the word 'macroscopic' is changed to 'microscopic'. We divide the original Grade IV into two: Grade IVA is defined as intential subtotal removal to preserve cranial nerves and/or blood vessels with complete removal of the attachment. The modified

Simpson Grade IVB is partial removal of the tumor by less than 10%.

The original Simpson (1957) grading is based on macroscopic surgery.

Original Simpson grading:

Grade I: Complete macroscopic removal of the tumor and dural attachment with any abnormal bone.
Grade II: Complete macroscopic removal of the tumor with diathermy coagulation of its dural attachment.
Grade III: Complete microscopic removal of intradural tumor without resection or coagulation of its dural attachment or of any extradural extensions.
Grade IV: Partial removal leaving intradural tumor in site.
Grade V: Simple decompression with or without biopsy.

Residual lesion

On some occasions we have noticed that resection of the tumor near the site of its origin and dural attachment is relatively easily possible, but resection of the tumor in proximity to critical neural structures like the brain stem, cranial nerves and major vessels may be difficult. Although the exact incidence of difference of recurrence rates between the residual lesions left at the site of origin and that left away from the origin has not yet been analyzed adequately, it appears that recurrence rate is much less in the latter. This may be due to the fact that these tumor cells are deprived of circulation and act essentially as a mass of dead cells. It implies that the difficult part of the tumor entangled in blood vessels or close to vital neural structures can be relatively safely left behind.

Indications for spinal drainage during operation

In general, drainage of CSF from the lumbar cul-de-sac or from ventricles should be avoided. Adoption of a basal surgical exposure, early drainage of subarachnoid cisternal spaces and intratumoral decompression can relax the brain sufficiently. However, there are some situations where a lumbar drainage may be useful in providing a lax brain which could avoid retraction-related damage to the brain. Such a drainage procedure can be useful whenever a subtemporal approach is adopted. Occasionally for other approaches and varieties of lesions such a lumbar drainage may assist in adequate exposure.

Pretumor resection arterial bypass

One can never presume on the basis of preoperative investigations that the narrowed artery will not be dissectible from the tumor. To perform a pretumor resection major arterial bypass operation is an ill-conceived surgery. It may be advisable to leave tumor remnants with the involved artery rather than take the risks of the bypass. It may, however, be advisable to be prepared for a bypass operation in cases where operative tears or compromise to the circulation has taken place.

Direction of approach to the tumor

In general, the direction of the approach should be such that the part of origin of the tumor is exposed in the initial phase of the operation rather than the dome of the tumor. This policy holds good not only for meningiomas but also for most other tumors like craniopharyngiomas, pituitary tumors, chordomas etc. The dome is the region where the normal neural and vascular tissues are stretched maximally and are liable to get injured. To detach the tumor from the site of origin and debulk it in the direction of the growth provides a better opportunity to preserve the function and integrity of the stretched vessels and nerves.

Staging of surgery

One should never plan a staged operation. The first operation should be planned with the idea to excise the entire tumor. In rare cases where for some reason complete tumor excision is not possible, the operation may be staged. In cases of meningiomas where significant excision has been achieved, the second-stage surgery may be performed about 8–10 weeks after the first operation. By this time the brain normalizes and settles from the insult from the first operative procedure.

Radiation treatment to residual meningiomas

In some cases it is not possible to resect the entire meningioma for various reasons. Some advise radiation treatment to the residual lesion. In general the author is not in favor of any form of radiation therapy for any benign or even some low-grade malignant tumors. In meningiomas and neurinomas in particular, radiotherapy is not indicated. There are only isolated reports showing successful results following focused radiation treatment. In cases with small residual meningiomas, it is advisable to observe the lesion with serial scanning. In case a definite growth is observed one may reoperate the lesion. In cases where the residual tumor has been subjected to radiation treatment reoperation can be difficult and hazardous. An attempt to completely resect irradiated meningiomas in proximity to vital

nerves and vessels may be difficult and dangerous. The arteries become adherent to the tumor and their walls become fragile. The surrounding brain becomes excessively adherent to the tumor, which could affect safe excision.

Selection of the approach

Selection of the approach for a particular case will depend on the histological nature of the tumor in question, consistency and vascularity of the lesion and major arterial and cranial nerve relationships. The selected approach should be wide enough that the entire tumor may be excised safely and in case of intraoperative arterial tears the surgeon has avenues for control and reconstruction. However, the approach should be as short as possible, should avoid bone drilling as much as possible, avoid entry into air sinuses wherever possible, and avoid arterial, venous sinus and neural manipulation. There should be no compromises whenever the approach is selected. For any tumor only one approach is ideal and is possible. Proper anatomical analysis and approach selection are therefore crucial for the success of the operation.

Reconstruction

Reconstruction should be as adequate and as complete as the exposure. In most instances the reconstruction should be planned at the time of exposure. In general terms the closure should be dura for dura and bone for bone. Whenever possible vascularized pedicle graft should be used. In potentially infected spaces free grafts may fail. All empty spaces should be filled up. Fat, meshed muscle and bone dust are good filler material, in that order. One has to take note of the potential herniation of the brain matter into the large bone defects created at the base, and the reconstruction should be carried out accordingly. Remote flaps with microvascular anastomoses are seldom necessary.

ANTERIOR CRANIAL BASE SURGICAL APPROACHES

Subfrontal approaches are used for midline lesions generally located in the sellar and parasellar areas. More frequently the conventional approaches wherein the craniotomy is placed above the frontal air sinus or including its upper half are adequate for safe and radical resection of the lesions. Retraction of the frontal lobes is usually safe and after the drainage of CSF from basal subfrontal, chiasmal and sylvian cisterns a large space can be obtained for a comfortable dissection in the sellar area. Extensive manipulation of the frontal air sinuses and the supraorbital rims may be avoided and should not be performed as a routine. For some lesions which involve a prolonged microsurgical dissection, anterior cranial 'basal' approaches can be useful. Basal extension of the conventional frontal craniotomy can be done in various ways. Resection of the superior half of the frontal air sinus can provide an effective increase in the basal exposure.

Dealing with air sinuses

Air sinuses are practically sterile but potentially infective spaces as they may contain commensal organisms. The sinuses communicate ultimately with the nasal cavity. Opening up of the sinuses during intracranial surgery is like providing a communication of the intracranial compartment to the nose. Opening of the air sinuses should be avoided as much as possible. Frontal air sinuses are frequently opened during basal frontal exposures. Whenever opened it is pertinent, therefore, that the communication of the air sinus with the exterior be adequately sealed. The frontal sinus communicates with the nose through the frontonasal duct. Some use a small bone strut or muscle piece to pack the frontonasal duct. Sealing of the duct and leaving residual mucosa in the sinus can lead to collection of secretions in the sinus which could accumulate and form a mucocele or a pyocele. Disconnection of the opened sinus from the exterior would avoid CSF leakage and ascending infections. Placement of subgaleal drains after the operation to assist evacuation of collected blood or drainage of CSF by the lumbar route can invite ascending infection through a suction effect if the communication is not adequately sealed. Whenever the sinus is opened, but mucosal integrity is not affected, it is usually advisable to preserve the mucosa and cover the bone defect with bone chips or dust. In cases where the mucosa has been breached it is necessary to denude a large portion of mucosa or the entire mucosa up to the frontonasal duct from the sinus. The draining duct should ideally be denuded of mucosa. The mucosa may be removed with the help of a diamond drill, or may be stripped off the bone using periosteal elevators. Mucosal denuding helps not only to avoid collection of secretions but also provides a raw surface of bone for vascularization of the packing material. Ideally the sinus should be packed with a vascularized pedicled flap obtained either from the pericranium or galea. The sinus may be packed directing the pressure towards the draining duct. Bone dust, fat, meshed muscle and gel foam can be used.

Basal extension of a unilateral frontal craniotomy

Bicoronal scalp incision for performing basal extension of

the conventional frontal craniotomy needs to be slightly longer so that an exposure of the orbital rim may be obtained. If the circulation of the forehead is jeopardized for some reason, by procedures like radiation treatment or external carotid artery embolization, the incision should include the superficial temporal artery (by making the incision posterior to it) in the exposure. The superficial temporal vessels must also be preserved in situations where the lesion is in proximity to the internal carotid or middle cerebral arteries, which could be damaged during the surgery. These vessels may be preserved whilst taking the incision both anterior or posterior to the trunk of superficial temporal artery. Dissection in appropriate planes and mobilization of the artery can help in increasing the exposure while preserving the artery. The supraorbital nerves and vessels must be preserved. This can be performed by a subperiosteal dissection in the region of the supraorbital rim. Whenever a groove is encountered through which

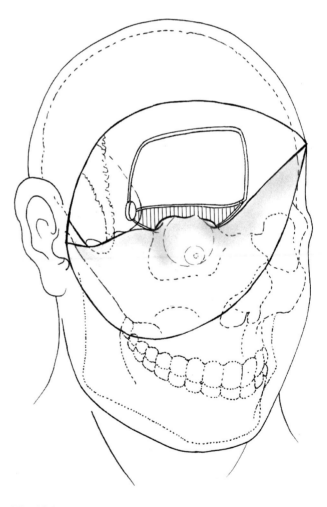

Fig. 13.4 Frontal scalp flap elevated anteriorly. Low frontal craniotomy is performed. The area depicted by shaded lines is the basal extension of the frontal craniotomy.

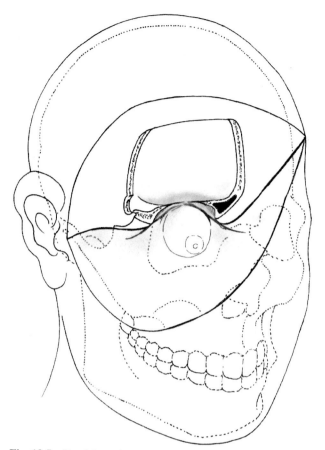

Fig. 13.5   Basal frontal craniotomy after the removal of the supraorbital rim with the help of an oscillating saw. The front air sinus is opened. The eyeball is exposed.

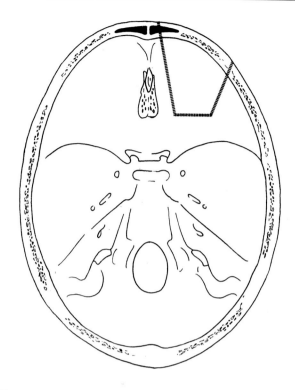

Fig. 13.6   Site of orbital roof cut.

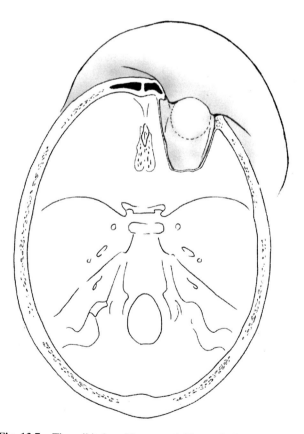

Fig. 13.7   The orbital roof is resected. The eyeball can be gently depressed inferiorly to gain additional exposure.

these nerves and vessels pass, a small osteotome may be used to open the groove. Subperiosteal dissection is continued and the eyeball is exposed, preserving the periorbita. Electric saws can be used to make cuts in the superior rim of the orbit (Figs 13.4, 13.5). During this procedure the orbital contents and frontal brain and dura are adequately protected. The orbital plate (roof of the orbit) should be cut as posterior as possible (Figs 13.6, 13.7). Either one can proceed and remove the entire orbital roof lateral to the cribriform plate or only a partial removal may be done, depending on the extent of the exposure that may be necessary. The cut along the medial end will essentially traverse through the frontal air sinus and adequate precautions need to be taken to pack it at the end of the operation. Such an additional bone cut provides a significantly improved basal exposure without disturbing the sense of smell. The eyeball can be depressed inferiorly to gain an additional exposure. The orbital roof can be removed posteriorly up to the optic canal. The optic nerve may be exposed by drilling the medial and superior wall of the canal. The nerve can even be mobilized whenever neces-

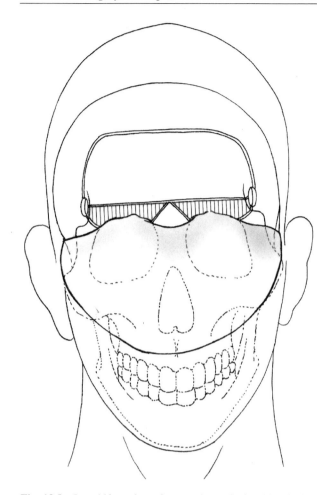

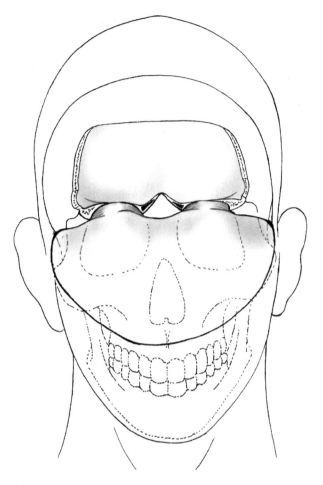

Fig. 13.8 Low bifrontal craniotomy. Areas depicted by shaded lines are the supraorbital rims which will be removed with the help of an oscillating saw. On some occasions the bifrontal craniotomy can be extended very low, a procedure that can avoid removal of the supraorbital bars.

Fig. 13.9 Basal bifrontal craniotomy exposure after the removal of supraorbital bars on both sides. The bone in the region of the nasion is not removed.

sary. The exposure can be used to limit the extent of frontal lobe retraction to a significant degree.

Basal extension of a bilateral frontal craniotomy (Goel 1994)

Various methods have been described for basal extension of a bifrontal craniotomy. Inclusion of the orbital roof in the craniotomy, or drilling of a supraorbital bar, and inclusion of the nasion in the craniotomy can improve the basal exposure (Figs 13.8–13.10). The more commonly employed method is to fashion an additional supraorbital bar osteotomy. This procedure provides a wide and extensive basal exposure. However, such an extent of exposure is seldom necessary and the procedure is tedious. The indications of fashioning a supraorbital bar osteotomy to have

a basal exposure for a tumor resection are extremely low in number.

A method is described which was used to extend a conventional bifrontal craniotomy basally, avoiding the cumbersome bone work through the frontal air sinuses. The procedure was seen to be quick to perform, avoided drilling through the frontal air sinuses, provided a wide and low basal exposure and was cosmetically superior. This method is now regularly used in our service whenever bifrontal craniotomy is performed to approach lesions in the parasellar region.

Technique

Three burr holes are drilled as shown in Figure 13.11. Holes 1 and 3 are lateral and hole 2 is superior to the

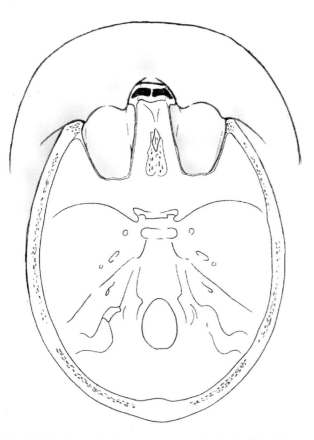

Fig. 13.10 The orbital roofs are removed on both sides. The area of bone in the region of the cribriform plate is preserved.

now made by using these two holes with a wide sweep of the saw directing the cut inferiorly, protecting the underlying dura with the help of small retractors introduced from holes 1–3. The basal extension of the cut through the tables of the frontal air sinus can be varied by altering the angle of cut of the Gigli saw and by varying the distance of burr holes 1 and 3. The bone cut could be extended down to the root of the nose and over the roof of the orbits after adequately protecting the eyeballs. The burr hole number 2 can even be avoided and the midline burr hole (number 4) of the superior edge of the craniotomy can be used instead of number 2 burr hole. Drilling of burr holes over the air sinuses, and the need for a supraorbital bar osteotomy, may be avoided (Figs 13.12–13.16).

Preservation of smell in anterior basal exposure

Unilateral frontal craniotomy, resection of the supraorbital bar, and a slight lateral perspective to the planum sphenoidale, without elevation of dura in the region of the cribriform plate, can lead to preservation of smell and provide an adequate exposure to the sphenoid sinus, sella and lower half of the superior and mid clivus in an extradural perspective. Intradural extensions of the lesion can be dealt with after opening of the dura and elevation of the frontal lobe off the orbital roof. Such a limited approach to midline lesions was found to be satisfactory in most cases with large parasellar lesions where transsphenoidal approaches were considered to be unsuitable. Bilateral exposure leaving both cribriform plates undisturbed can be performed (Figs 13.6–13.10). In cases with malignant tumor where radical en bloc resections are indicated a larger exposure may be required.

frontal air sinus. A Gigli saw guide followed by wire is first passed from hole 1 to 2. The saw guide is then removed from holes 1 to 2 and passed from hole 2 to 3. The Gigli saw wire is then passed from hole 2 to 3. We now have the wire passing from hole 1 to 3 (Fig. 13.11). The bone cut is

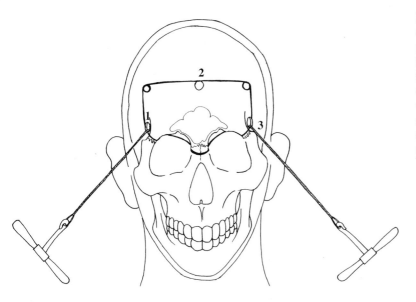

Fig. 13.11 Use of Gigli saw to basally extend a bifrontal craniotomy flap. The saw is passed from hole number 1 to 2 and then from 2 to 3. The drawing shows the wire after its final passage. The bone flap is elevated by directing the cut of the Gigli saw inferiorly while protecting the underlying brain and the superior sagittal sinus by introduction of small brain retractors from holes 1 to 2. The Gigli saw cut is in a wide sweeping motion.

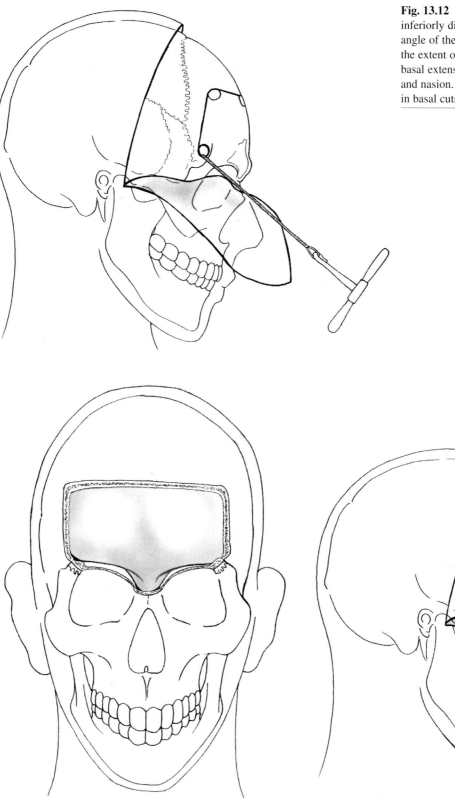

Fig. 13.12   Lateral view showing the inferiorly directed angle of the Gigli saw. The angle of the cut can be varied depending upon the extent of basal exposure required. The basal extension can include both orbital roofs and nasion. The eyeball needs to be protected in basal cuts extending over the orbital roof.

Fig. 13.13   The basal bone cut using the described technique. The medial part of both orbital roofs and the nasion are removed by the cut.

Fig. 13.14   Lateral view of the basal bone flap using the technique described.

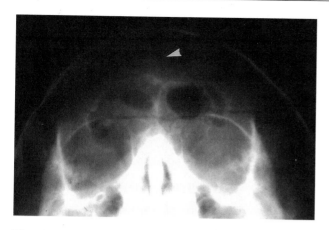

Fig. 13.15 Plain X-ray film showing anteroposterior view of the skull with arrowhead demonstrating the site of the midline burr hole. The bone cut passes through the root of the nose and medial half of the roof of the orbit. (From Goel 1994, with permission.)

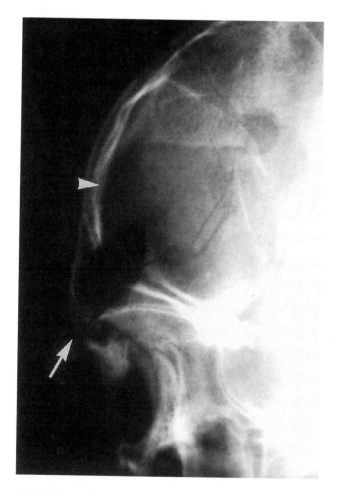

Fig. 13.16 Plain X-ray film showing the lateral view of the skull and the bone cut passing through the nasion (arrow). Arrowhead depicts the site of the midline burr-hole. (From Goel 1994, with permission.)

Transfrontal sinus approach

In this approach the anterior wall of the frontal air sinus is first removed with the help of an electric saw or small osteotomes. This can be removed in the form of a free (Fig 13.17) or an osteoplastic flap (Figs 13.18, 13.19). After this procedure the posterior wall of the sinus is removed. This provides a low approach to the sellar and parasellar region (Fig. 13.20). Both intra- and extradural approaches can be developed. Whether the cribriform plate should be removed or not is decided on the extent of surgical exposure that is necessary.

The advantage of a transcranial approach over a transsphenoidal approach in such cases is that the intracranial extension of the tumor can be removed, and dissection around the optic nerves and the carotid artery can be done under vision. The transcranial approach may be selectively extradural or a combined intra- and extradural approach. The bone of the planum sphenoidale can be drilled and the sphenoid sinus exposed.

In the transcranial route to skull base tumor wherein there is extensive manipulation of the basal dura or where elevation of the dura in the region of the cribriform plate is intended, adequate precautions and preparations have to be made for a firm reconstruction of the basal dura and, whenever indicated, the dural defect. Various reconstructive measures which may be useful in the reconstruction of the floor of the anterior cranial fossa are discussed in another chapter.

ANTERIOR SKULL BASE MENINGIOMAS

Meningiomas arising from the anterior skull base are usually detected after they have attained a large to massive size. Olfactory groove, planum sphenoidale, orbital roof and tuberculum sellae meningiomas are included in this category. The more posterior is the tumor, the more proximal it is to the vessels of the anterior circulation and visual apparatus and consequently the more difficult is surgical resection. Most of the meningiomas located in the anterior skull base are of firm consistency and are vascular, but are eminently resectable (Figs 13.21, 13.22).

More frequently these tumors are seen in middle-aged women. But men and the elderly are also commonly affected. The presentation is often in the form of symptoms of increased intracranial pressure. The mode of presentation varies with the site of origin of the tumor. Posteriorly situated meningiomas present frequently with visual deficits and are relatively smaller in size at the time of detection as compared to those arising from the olfactory groove. Memory and higher function disturbances and symptoms of increased intracranial pressure are often the

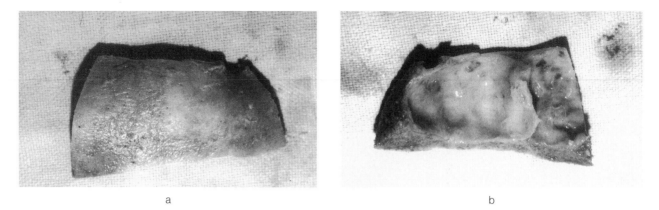

a   b

Fig. 13.17   a Intraoperative picture showing the anterior aspect of the removed anterior table of the frontal air sinus. This table will be replaced and stitched back at the end of the operation.**b** The posterior aspect of the anterior table of the frontal air sinus removed during the surgery.

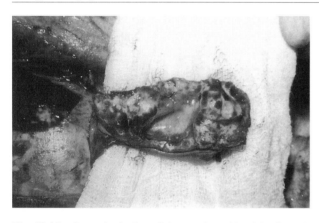

Fig. 13.18   Osteoplastic flap of the anterior table of the frontal air sinus. The flap is rotated laterally and is based on the pericranial flap.

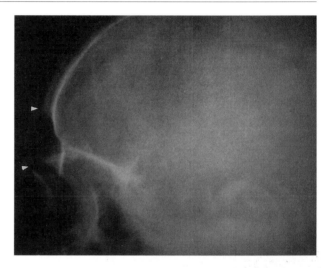

Fig. 13.19   Postoperative X-ray with arrowheads showing the site of the bone cut used for transfrontal air sinus approach.

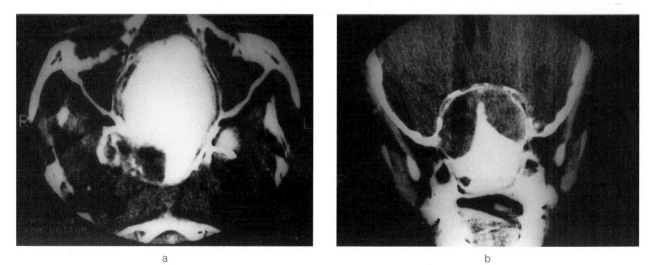

a   b

Fig. 13.20   a CT scan cut of the paranasal sinuses showing a massive bony tumor (histophathology: osteoblastic meningioma). **b** CT scan shows a massive bony tumor occupying the nasopharynx, sphenoid and posterior ethmoid sinuses and displacing the anterior cranial fossa floor including the sella, planum sphenoidale superiorly, sella, and stretching the optic nerves laterally.

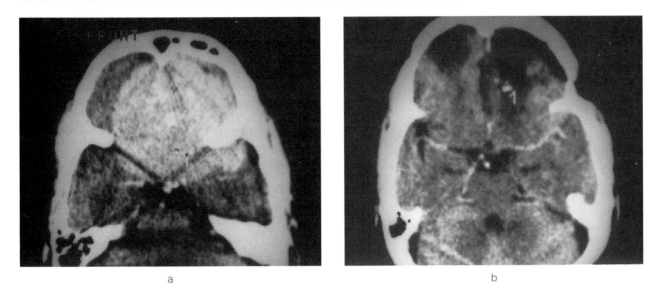

Fig. 13.21   **a** Transverse section of a hughe basal frontal meningioma. **b** Postoperative CT scan showing complete tumor resection.

initial presenting problems rather than anosmia and Foster Kennedy syndrome.

While CT scanning demonstrates the bony alterations, MRI is essential to delineate clearly the vascular and neural relationships and the tumor extensions. Most tumors have an extension in the superior direction, but some have extensions into the ethmoid and paranasal sinuses.

Surgical considerations

While planning surgery the exact site of origin, extent of dural and basal bone involvement, direction and nature of spread, vascular involvements, presence of arachnoidal plane of cleavage between the tumor and the brain and an estimate of the consistency of the tumor from clinical features and from radiological investigations should be made. Extent of frontal lobe edema should be noted. Angiography is helpful in evaluating the extent of vascularity of the lesion and the source of its blood supply. These features may help in assessing the need for tumor embolization and directing surgical strategy. Presence of evidence of sinusitis should also be looked into on the investigations and adequately treated. Most of the basal frontal meningiomas do not transgress the dural boundary and extension into the ethmoid sinuses is rare. The basal dura and the bone may be thickened to varying degrees. A rim of the frontal brain covers the anterior surface of the tumor in most cases. In adults at least partial resection of a part of the frontal air sinus is always required. Further basal and contralateral extension of the craniotomy will depend on the size of the lesion and its extensions. Frequently, a moderate-sized midline lesion with exten-

sions on either side of the midline can be resected by a unilateral frontal operation. The vascularity of the tumor arises principally from the basal meningeal channels and the initial attack has to be in the direction of the feeders in an attempt to devascularize the lesion. However, exposure of the base of the tumor in the initial phase of the operation is limited due to the presence of brain edema and the size of the tumor. To limit the need for retraction of the brain, the lesion is initially decored in the direction of the base, despite the bleeding which might occur during the procedure. Once a sizeable amount of tumor is excised, the base of the lesion towards its attachment can be attacked. In a relatively relaxed state of the brain the base can not only be exposed better, but also the bleeding can be controlled under vision. Frequently the basal attachment may be large. Decoring of the tumor can simultaneously proceed along with its basal disconnection. Often the major arteries are displaced posteriorly over the dome of the tumor. Sometimes these vessels are encased partially or completely within the lobulations of the tumor. The dissection of the vessel from the tumor has to be performed during the terminal part of the surgery. The success of the surgery usually depends on the extent that the normal vasculature and the perforators are preserved. Under no circumstance should a normal vessel be sacrificed for the sake of tumor resection. In case dissection of some part of the tumor from the vessel is not possible, it is advisable to leave that part of the residue behind rather than sacrifice the vessel.

Extent of resection

The radicality and totality of the resection of the tumor is

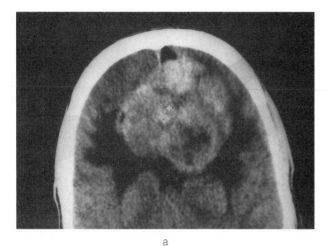

a

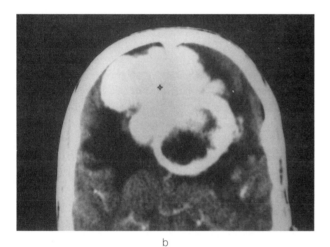

b

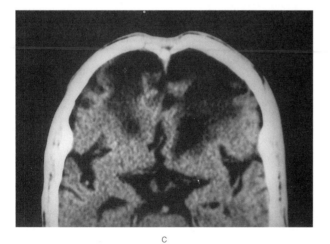

c

the principal objective of surgery as on this feature will depend the long-term outcome of the patient and the incidence of recurrence. In most meningiomas resection of not only the involved dura but also the adjoining bone is recommended. However, removal of the anterior cranial basal dura and the bone is dangerous as regards the exposure of the brain to nasal contamination and increases the possibility of CSF leakage. It is considered worthwhile to remove only the involved dura and leave the bone in situ. The involved dura can be coagulated instead of resected.

Some authors have recommended sectioning of the optic nerve to obtain an enhanced exposure of the tumor. In our series sectioning of the nerve was never required. In only extremely rare cases where the optic nerve is badly damaged by the tumor can this nerve be sectioned; in most other instances such a procedure should never be carried out. Various authors have reported recovery of vision in a blind eye after successful excision of large tumors.

Superior sagittal sinus section

As far as possible the superior sagittal sinus should be preserved. One can work alternately on both sides of the falx and avoid sectioning of the superior sagittal sinus.

REFERENCES

Goel A 1994 Supraorbital craniotomy. (Letter.) Journal of Neurosurgery 81: 642–643

Kobayashi S, Okudera H, Kyoshima K 1994 Surgical considerations on skull base meningiomas. In: Skull base surgery. First International Skull Base Congress, Hanover 1992. Karger, Basel, pp 173–174

Simpson D 1957 The recurrence of intracranial meningiomas after surgical treatment. Journal of Neurology Neurosurgery and Psychiatry 20: 22–39

Fig. 13.22   **a** Plain CT scan showing a massive hyperdense anterior skull base tumor. **b** Contrast infusion showing intense enhancement. **c**Postoperative scan showing complete tumor resection.

Anterior Skull Base Approaches
Chandranath Sen

A variety of benign and malignant tumors may be encountered in the anterior skull base region. In addition to these, the anterior skull base approaches may also be used for some selected extradural tumors of the middle and posterior skull base. The foremost issue in managing these tumors is the determination of its pathology and its exact anatomical extent. In many tumors the diagnosis can be strongly suspected on the basis of preoperative imaging work-up. In some cases, e.g. those arising from the paranasal sinuses and nasopharynx, a preoperative biopsy is necessary. Craniofacial resection for such tumors is performed in conjunction with an otolaryngologist.

The radiological assessment of these patients therefore consists of MRI, both before and after the administration of gadolinium. Tumors arising from the paranasal sinuses frequently will cause opacification of the sinus spaces. In a situation like this the exact determination of the tumor boundaries may pose a problem. The T1- and T2-weighted images are quite helpful in such differentiation since the secretions that build up due to obstruction present as a high-intensity signal on T2 whereas they are isointense on T1. Similar distinction is also helpful in the case of mucoceles of the frontal or sphenoid sinuses which can occasionally present as a large intracranial mass. Demarcation of the mass from the brain and cerebral arteries is also best performed with MRI as also from other soft tissues planes. The differentiation between vascular flow voids from fine calcifications is difficult on MRI. A high-resolution CT scan is complementary to MRI and is performed on all patients with skull base tumors because of the proximity to and involvement of the bony structures. The character of the bone destruction – smooth erosion or irregular destruction – is helpful in the differential diagnosis. Calcification, however minute, is seen in the CT scan which should also include bone algorithm. The most important aspects of this radiological evaluation is to determine the relation of the tumor to the orbit, orbital apex, the intracavernous internal carotid artery (ICA) and the brain. Angiography is rarely considered in purely anterior skull base tumors. Even in the case of large anterior skull base meningiomas, MRI angiography allows visualization of the anterior cerebral arteries. Tumors like large juvenile angiofibromas which extend into the middle fossa and sella may be considered for an anterior skull base approach in combination with some other approach. These lesions can usually be identified on the MRI scan by the presence of numerous vascular flow voids within the tumors. Angiography is performed for both diagnostic and preoperative embolization purposes in such tumors.

After the nature and anatomical extent of the lesion has been determined, the approach can thus be planned. There is a range of operative exposure that can be used in this area – from a standard bifrontal craniotomy to a craniofacial resection in which a craniotomy is combined with a transfacial approach. A bifrontal craniotomy with removal of the supraorbital rims is a versatile approach that can be used for all anterior skull base tumors and also some extradural tumors involving the sphenoid sinus and clivus. Malignancies arising from the nasopharynx or the paranasal sinuses often require a combined craniofacial resection in order to obtain an en bloc resection with tumor-free margins.

Incision and Scalp Dissection: The bicoronal scalp incision for craniotomy is preferably made posterior to the coronal suture rather than following the hairline. This is done so that a long pericranial flap may be available for reconstruction of the skull base. The pericranial or the galeopericranial flap is the mainstay of the reconstruction of the skull base. It is a sturdy flap and can cover a defect of almost any size in the anterior fossa. The vascular supply of the flap comes from the supraorbital, supratrochlear and the superficial temporal arteries, therefore these vessels must be carefully preserved. The pericranium is raised along with the scalp and not separately. It is separated from the scalp only at the time of reconstruction to avoid inadvertent damage, and also if for some reason the pericranium is not used at the operation it can be preserved for future use if it has not been violated unnecessarily. The scalp is brought down to the orbits and the nasion. Where the scalp turns into the orbit to continue as the periorbita, it is quite adherent to the orbital rim and must be carefully stripped. If removal of the supraorbital rims is to be performed, the periorbita is stripped in the roof, medial and lateral walls for a distance of 2–3 cm posteriorly from the rims.

Usually a single burr hole is made at the 'keyhole' after elevating the temporalis muscle from the anterior portion of the temporal fossa. In older patients more holes may be needed to separate the dura. A unilateral craniotomy is first made almost up to the midline, after which the sagittal sinus and the opposite dura are separated and a separate bone flap from the other side is raised. This technique avoids making a burr hole in the middle of the forehead.

Supraorbital Bar Osteotomy: Removing the supraorbital rims provides an additional 2 cm of room under the frontal lobes. It is performed when dealing with extradural tumors in the sphenoid sinus and clivus like chordomas and chondrosarcomas or for anterior skull base tumors where an additional low exposure may be desired. Even when the surgeon makes a bifrontal bone flap that is as low as possible on the roofs of the orbit, the configuration of the orbital roofs is such that performing the supraorbital osteotomy adds some more working room under the frontal lobes without increased retraction. The extent of the supraorbital osteotomy depends on where

treatment modalities for malignant tumors. It should also be emphasized that preoperative chemotherapy is very effective in certain tumors.

Primary Intracranial Tumors Arising from the Anterior Skull Base: Meningiomas arising from the olfactory groove, planum sphenoidale, sphenoid wing, and tuberculum sellae are common anterior skull base tumors. The basal invasion of meningiomas must be removed with the intradural part. Otherwise, it will recur usually several years after the intradural part has been removed. When meningiomas directly invade the sphenoid or ethmoid bone, bone resection is strongly recommended to prevent recurrence from the residual tumors in the complex bony structure. In cases of hyperostotic meningioma 'en plaque', hyperostosis which is pathological bone with meningioma cells must be resected.

Various bone tumors may arise from the anterior skull base and require surgical removal. Some are malignant such as sarcoma and usually inoperable. But benign bone tumors such as osteoma or osteoblastoma are resectable. Fibrous dysplasia must be discussed separately, because it is not a tumor. The disease begins in childhood and presents slow evolution and usually stops during the third decade. However, it is very difficult to predict the evolution of fibrous dysplasia. When the optic nerve or auditory nerve is compressed, removal of abnormal bone over the cranial nerves is sufficient to avoid further deterioration of neurological symptoms.

The Anterior Skull Base as a Route to Clival Tumors: Tumors of the clival area remain one of the most difficult tumors to remove. A variety of surgical approaches have been applied to these tumors, such as transoral, transmaxillary, petrosal and infratemporal. It is possible to reach clival tumors by the frontobasal approach. The approach to clival tumors depends on their pathology, consistency, attachment, direction of main extension, and relationship to the dura of the clivus. The frontobasal approach is especially effective to the clival tumors extending laterally. After the planum sphenoidale, tuberculum sellae, and sellar floor are removed, the whole clivus and the anterior margin of the foramen magnum can be approached. Laterally, with resection of the anterior clinoid process, the lesser sphenoid wing and the orbital roof, one can approach tumors located in the middle cranial base. The limit of this approach in the middle cranial base is the foramen rotundum, the foramen ovale, and the petrosal bone. Furthermore, this approach is limited by the optic nerves, the cavernous sinuses and the ICAs.

Cavernous sinus invasion of the tumors is a different problem which will be discussed elsewhere in this book.

Reconstruction: Our principle of anterior skull base reconstruction is multilayer reconstruction. The dura is closed tightly using continuous sutures and fibrin glue to maintain watertightness. The vascularized flap is an essential part of multilayer reconstruction. A pericranial flap, temporalis muscle flap, or vascularized free flap such as the rectus abdominis muscle is used depending on size, location, and dead space of the skull base defect. The pericranial flap and the temporalis muscle flap are reliable vascularized flaps, but often unavailable in cases of reoperation. Skull base bone reconstruction using cranial bone graft or cancellous iliac bone graft is done when the bone defect is large. Autologous bone grafts are recommended rather than any foreign material. A miniplate is useful to reconstruct the shape of the nasal bone and orbital rim. When the orbit, nasal cavity, and maxillary sinus are resected, vascularized bulky tissue is recommended to support the skull base. No dead space is left because any air-filled cavity in the face must be considered septic. Lumbar CSF drainage for about 5 postoperative days may be placed depending on the kind of surgery. Functioning lumbar spinal drainage is the first choice to prevent CSF leak. By this principle, we have not experienced CSF leak or breakdown of the reconstructed skull bases.

In the anterolateral craniofacial resection, the re-establishment of the lateral orbital and zygomatic contour is very important from a cosmetic point of view. We use a titanium miniplate to reconstruct the facial contour. Preoperative design of reconstruction by plastic surgeons is essential to obtain cosmetic satisfaction.

Surgery for acoustic neurinoma

Shigeaki Kobayashi   Kazuhiro Hongo
Yuichiro Tanaka   Atul Goel

14

Acoustic neurinomas are relatively common. They account for about 80% of the cerebellopontine angle tumors. Most of the acoustic neurinomas arise from the vestibular nerve. The length of the vestibular nerve in the subarachnoid space is about 25 mm, of which about 10 mm is in the internal auditory canal while 15 mm is in the cerebello-pontine angle (Lang 1991). The Obersteiner–Redlich zone, which is the border zone between the glial myelination and the Schwann cell myelination, is located in the internal auditory canal. Acoustic neurinomas usually arise from this zone distally in the canal.

Surgery on acoustic neurinomas can be divided into two broad categories: surgery on small lesions, and surgery on large lesions. The problems involved in the surgery of these two varieties of acoustic neurinomas are different. The main concern in small tumors is to adequately save the facial nerve and whenever applicable the hearing function, while the principal concern in large tumors is to protect the brain stem, lower cranial nerves and in the process pre-serve the function of the VIIth nerve.

The surgical result is influenced by the following factors:

1. size of the tumor;
2. consistency of the tumor, cystic or solid nature;
3. vascularity of the tumor;
4. direction of tumor growth;
5. degree of adhesion between the tumor and nerves;
6. surgeon's experience (Cohen et al 1986, Ebersold et al 1992, Fisher et al 1992, Glasscock et al 1993, Whittaker & Luetje 1992, Yoko et al 1993).

GENERAL CONSIDERATIONS

Surgery on acoustic neurinomas involves various contro-versial issues and some questions remain unanswered. The questions that sometimes arise in the case of small tumors may be as follows:

1. Should small tumors where hearing is preserved be

operated? The problem is that surgery involves risk to hearing and some but significant risk to facial nerve function. In the natural course of tumor growth an affect on hearing and possibly on facial nerve function could take many years.
2. Should surgical removal of the tumor give protection from tumor regrowth? The long-term natural history of these tumors is not convincingly known.
3. Is radiosurgery an effective mode of treatment in small tumors?
4. Should hearing preservation be attempted at all?
5. Is the preserved hearing serviceable? What is the long-term outcome of preserved hearing? (Goel et al 1992).
6. The appropriate surgical approach for these tumors is also a subject of debate.

The principal debatable issues in large tumors are:

1. Whether a subtotal and essentially intracapsular tumor excision would be adequate while minimizing the risk of facial nerve injury;
2. Whether a staged operation in massive-sized tumors is recommended;
3. The most suitable position of the patient during surgery;
4. Whether a middle fossa transtentorial approach has something to recommend it in large tumors?

Like most surgical units, our policy has been an attempt towards radical 'total' surgical resection of all sizes of tumors. An attempt is made to preserve hearing wherever it is preserved preoperatively. The issue of surgery on acoustic neurinomas has been discussed at length in the lit-erature. In this review we shall discuss some aspects of technical and technological issues which we have found useful while operating on acoustic neurinomas.

Acoustic neurinomas arise from the intracanalicular segment of the vestibular nerve. The inferior vestibular nerve is the more frequent site of origin. The tumor is benign and grows slowly and compresses the other nerves in its close proximity. The VIIth nerve, being more resilient, resists distortion and clinical manifestation for a significant period of time, while the cochlear nerve, being relatively weaker, becomes affected easily. The tumor in the cerebellopontine angle is entirely extra-arachnoidal. Preserving the arachnoid and dissection in the appropriate planes is critically important for successful resection of these lesions.

Historically, many noted neurosurgeons have performed surgery on these tumors, including pioneers such as Cushing, Dandy, and Olivecrona. Initially mortality was high but with the introduction of microsurgery results have markedly improved in terms of mortality, and also the incidence of facial and cochlear nerve preservation is now superior (Sugita & Kobayashi 1982, Samii & Ohlemutz 1981).

CLASSIFICATION OF ACOUSTIC NEURINOMAS

The tactics for surgery depends principally on two factors: tumor size and the extent of its extension into the canal. We have classified acoustic neurinomas into four types (Fig. 14.1a) according to these criteria (Tanaka & Kobayashi 1995). Type I is an intracanalicular tumor without extension of the tumor into the cerebellopontine angle. Type II is the most common type of tumor, which occupies the internal auditory canal and has an extracanalicular

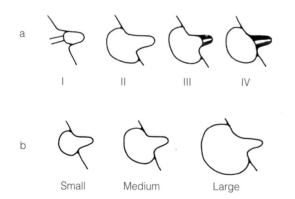

Fig. 14.1 **a** Classification of acoustic neurinoma according to its extension into the internal auditory canal. Type I: intracanalicular; Type II: intracanalicular tumor with extracanalicular extension; Type III: internal auditory canal is partially filled with tumor; Type IV: extracanalicular tumor. **b** Classification of acoustic neurinoma according to its size. Small: 0–15 mm; medium: 16–30 mm; large: 31 mm or larger.

extension. In type III tumors, the internal auditory canal is partially filled with tumor. In type IV, the tumor grows exclusively in the cerebellopontine angle cistern without significant extension into the internal auditory canal.

Types III and IV tumors have the following characteristics:

1. the tumor tends to reach a large size when diagnosed;
2. preoperative hearing level may be good;
3. preservation of hearing is difficult

We considered the size of the tumor as the maximum diameter of the extracanalicular portion of the tumor based on the preoperative computed tomography (CT) or magnetic resonance imaging (MRI) of an axial slice across the internal auditory canal. According to the size of the tumor the lesion was divided into three groups: *small* when the size was less than 15 mm, *medium* when the size was between 15 and 30 mm, and *large* when the size was more than 30 mm (Fig. 14.1b).

SURGICAL TECHNICAL CONSIDERATIONS

The most commonly used surgical route for acoustic neurinomas is the suboccipital retrosigmoid approach. The other often preferred routes are the translabyrinthine and subtemporal middle fossa approaches. As the suboccipital approach will be described in detail, some aspects of the other two approaches will be briefly described.

The translabyrinthine approach provides a clear visualization of the fundus of the internal auditory canal. With this approach hearing will be invariably lost as the labyrinth will be opened up and damaged during the approach. For this approach, which was intially used primarily by otolaryngologists, one needs to have a special skill in drilling the petrous bone with exact topographical anatomy in mind. Usually small neurinomas with substantial hearing loss are indications for this approach.

In the subtemporal approach, the intracanalicular anatomy will be seen better, and hence this approach is useful when the tumor is small, confined to the canal, and hearing preservation is intended. During surgery, however, opening the canal may be difficult when the tumor is small. During tumor removal procedures, the facial nerve courses between the tumor and surgeon. The chances for a mechanical injury will therefore be increased. It is possible to approach and remove the tumor entirely extradurally when the tumor is small. Possibilities of temporal lobe edema by retraction is one of the disadvantages of this procedure. Unlike the translabyrinthine approach the subtemporal approach has the disadvantage of difficulty in exposing the fundus of the canal without risking injury to the facial nerve.

Suboccipital approach

The most commonly used route is the suboccipital retro-sigmoid approach. With this approach it is difficult to see the fundus of the canal without damaging the semicircular canal or common crus. The facial nerve lies almost always in the depth of the field and away from the surgeon. This means that once the facial nerve is identified, the likelihood of its mechanical injury during surgery is less than when it is seen in the subtemporal approach. The cochlear nerve, on the other hand, lies in the way during the approach to the tumor.

Positioning

A sitting position used to be employed in many institutions, but in recent years either a lateral or supine lateral position is being increasingly used. The supine lateral position is easy but has the disadvantage that when the head is excessively rotated venous congestion can occur due to obstruction of blood flow to the jugular vein in the neck. We find a lateral position more suitable (Kobayashi & Sugita 1987, Sugita & Kobayashi 1982). While positioning an extra inferior angulation (lateral extension) is applied to the neck so that it falls away the ipsilateral shoulder, and the head is rotated contralaterally so that the posterior aspect of the petrous bone lies perpendicular to the floor. The neck is also flexed anteriorly (Fig. 14.2). These maneuvers provide extra space in the region and prevents to some degree obstruction to the hand movements by the shoulder. With this lateral position, venous drainage is good; however, one should be careful to maintain the head higher than the heart level of the patient to lower the venous pressure. In one of our experiments, we compared the jugular venous pressure and the axis of the patient's body with the floor of the room as reference. We found that the axis of the body is best when it is about 30° (Fig. 14.3). During surgical procedures in the cerebellopontine angle, the head can be rotated in either direction depending upon the part of the brain one wishes to see. When the head is rotated towards the floor one can see better the internal auditory canal, while when the head is rotated the other way one can see the brain stem side better (Fig. 14.4).

Monitoring

A facial nerve monitor consisting of a stimulator and tremogram to detect facial muscle movements via a speaker is routinely used. Auditory brain stem response (ABR) is recorded intraoperatively in cases with serviceable hearing.

Skin incision

Usually an S-shaped incision is made along the medial border of the mastoid process. The incision is about 12 cm

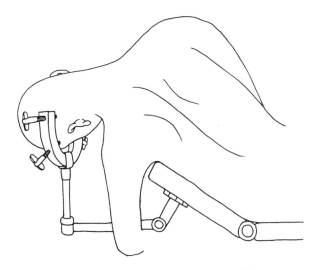

Fig. 14.2 Position of the patient. The top plate of the operating table is lifted. The neck is flexed anteriorly and bent contralaterally; the head is rotated about 30° contralaterally.

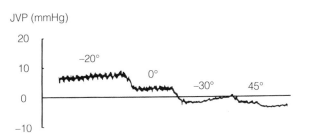

Fig. 14.3 Jugular venous pressure (JVP) monitored intraoperatively at various degrees of inclination of the operating table with a patient in the lateral position. A catheter with strain gauge at its tip was used. Note that in this case the venous pressure is about 0 torr at 30° of inclination. (From Kobayashi & Sugita 1989, with permission.)

long and is made 3–4 cm behind the hairline and 5 cm from the mastoid process. The muscle is divided in such a way that the attachment of the muscle to the bone remains for later approximation.

Bone opening

Instead of a craniectomy we routinely perform craniotomy. The craniotomy is designed preoperatively on the basis of the CT scan with the bone window. Formally, we had started employing a small bone opening, but now we use a larger opening. A larger bone opening helps in unrestricted movements in larger tumors and also helps in better visualization of the auditory canal in the region of its fundus by angulation of the microscope. Illumination of the mastoid air cell (Tanaka & Kobayashi 1995), in which an illuminating fiber cable (Nagashima Medical Instrument Co., 5–24–1 Hongo, Bunkyo-ku, Tokyo 113, Japan) is

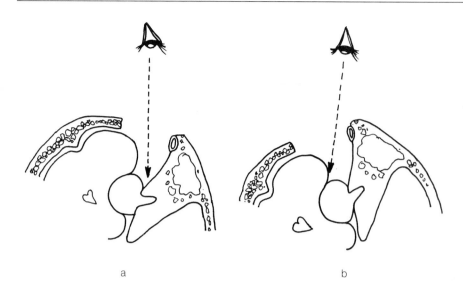

Fig. 14.4   Drawing showing how the rotation of the head alters the view. **a** Rotation to ipsilateral side to see the auditory canal side. **b** Rotation to the contralateral side to see the brain stem side.

a

b

placed inside the external ear canal, is helpful in estimating the position of the sigmoid sinus by illuminating the mastoid air sinuses (Fig. 14.5). In the majority of cases, the posterior margin of the illuminated air cells indicates the position of the sigmoid sinus. A gap between the posterior margin of the mastoid air cell and the position of the sigmoid sinus can be correlated with the help of CT scan images. During craniotomy the foramen magnum is not opened.

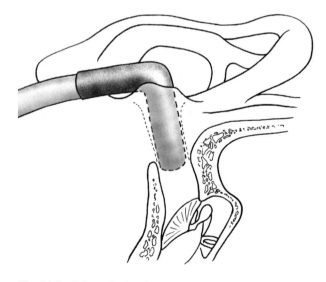

Fig. 14.5   Schematic drawing showing an earpiece of the illuminator in the right external auditory canal to estimate the sigmoid venous sinus. The size of the earpiece inside the external auditory canal is 22 mm, with a diameter of 6 mm.

Intradural procedures

During intradural removal of the tumor, two points are important:

1.   maintaining a bloodless field as much as possible; and
2.   intraoperative orientation with regard to individual nerves passing through the acoustic canal.

Some methods can help in keeping the operative field 'dry'. As described earlier, the head may be positioned at a higher level than the heart, thus reducing venous congestion. For continuous intraoperative suction, Bemsheet appears to be suitable. The tip of the sucker is placed on the Bemsheet, which absorbs blood in the field. If the Bemsheet is irrigated frequently with saline, clotting of blood and plugging of the Bemsheet can be avoided. The Bemsheet needs to be changed frequently. Irrigation with saline helps suctioning of blood through the Bemsheet. The Bemsheet also protects cranial nerves and small perforators from mechanical injury. The two-suction method (as described later) appears to be a good method for internal decompression or debulking of the tumor. The Bemsheet is helpful in removing pooling blood from the cerebellopontine angle continuously. We have recently developed a micro-ultrasound aspirator with a caliber as small as 1.9 mm. Suction power can be controlled by the tip of the index finger. This device has proved to be useful (Fig. 14.6). Meticulous manipulation to peel off the arachnoid fold covering the tumor from the side of the porus acousticus to the brain stem is the first step to preserve the vessels over the cerebellum. Identification of the facial nerve at the root entry zone is not difficult in small tumors. In medium or large-size tumors, internal decompression of the extracanalicular portion should be done before trying to find the facial and cochlear nerves at the junction of the brain stem. In cases with useful hearing, intraoperative identification of the cochlear nerve should be performed in the early stages of tumor dissection.

Intraoperative orientation

One should familiarize oneself with the topographical anatomy of the cerebellopontine angle with the patient in the lateral position. Experience of the normal anatomy of the region which one gains while performing Jannetta's microvascular decompression procedures is helpful. Initially one could become familiar with the anatomy on the right side and then convert the picture to the left side. After evacuating the cerebrospinal fluid (CSF) from the cisterna magna, the lower cranial nerves are identified first and protected by a silastic sheet. The tumor is then exposed in the cerebellopontine angle. The lower pole of the tumor is dissected. Here sometimes the anterior inferior cerebellar artery or its branches can be adherent to the tumor surface and have to be carefully dissected free (Goel & Sekhar 1990). In a relatively small tumor, the tentorial side of the tumor should then be observed carefully to determine the presence of individual nerves. For identifying the nerves, the normal anatomy or interrelation of the cranial nerves and the tumor is important to remember. The tumor usually originates in the canal and as it grows outside it usually maintains the interrelation of the nerves. It is important to become oriented to the anatomical relation of the individual nerves and their course while the patient is in the lateral position and the posterior lip of the acoustic canal is unroofed (Fig. 14.7). The transverse crest is vertically placed in this position. Superficially the superior and inferior vestibular nerves are located, and in the deeper space the facial nerve is located on the far side, with the cochlear nerve nearer to the surface. The interrelation between the facial and cochlear nerves outside the auditory canal is also important. The facial nerve crosses the cochlear nerve inferiorly as it enters the brain stem. The crossing point can be variable. It also varies in different cases and with different sizes of tumor. According to our intraoperative observations (Tanaka et al 1994), in 77% of tumors the crossing point was in the brain stem side between the equator of the tumor and the entry/exit zone of the facial nerve. When the nerves are represented by the clock at the internal auditory meatus, the cochlear nerve is positioned at 2 to 6 o'clock (mean 4.5 o'clock), while the facial nerve is at 4 to 8 o'clock (mean 6.3 o'clock) (Fig. 14.8). Considering the fact that the majority of tumors originate from the inferior vestibular nerve, one can get an idea of the location of the nerves by exploring the surface of the tumor. When the preoperative hearing is good, the cochlear nerve often appears relatively intact and as a bundle. If hearing is substantially impaired, the

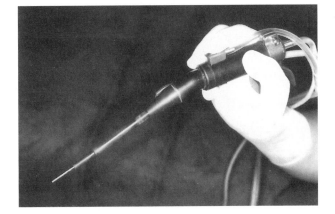

Fig. 14.6   Micro-SONOP.

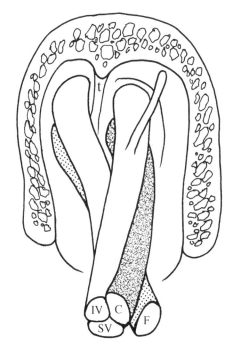

Fig. 14.7   Schematic drawing as seen from the right lateral suboccipital approach, showing the normal anatomy of the VIIth and VIIIth cranial nerves in the canal after drilling the posterior lip of the internal auditory canal. (C, cochlear nerve; F, facial nerve; IV, inferior vestibular nerve; SV, superior vestibular nerve; t, transverse crest.)

cochlear nerve can be found flattened over the surface of the tumor. The superior vestibular nerve can be relatively large. The facial nerve lying on the far side can be observed using a microsurgical mirror. The color of the facial nerve is characteristic in that it is darker than the components of the VIIIth nerve. It is usually easier to identify the individual nerves in small tumors than in large

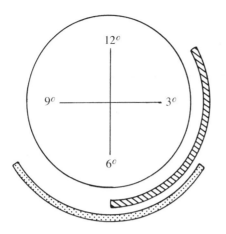

Fig. 14.8 Clock system for recording the position of the cochlear and facial nerves at the internal acoustic meatus as seen in the right side. The facial nerve (dotted range) was found at 4 to 8 o'clock (mean 6.3), while the cochlear nerve (hatched range) was at 2 to 6 o'clock (mean 4.5).

tumors. If the facial nerve cannot be identified, electric stimulation with sound monitoring is helpful as one can continue dissection by listening to the sound response. Identifying the cochlear nerve is sometimes difficult. We have tried cochlear evoked potential without much success. It may be because the cochlear nerve can be spread over a wider area so that the response is less constant. We therefore tend to depend more on the anatomical observations. Monitoring ABR is not helpful in finding the course of the cochlear nerve. After confirming the presence of facial electric stimulation, internal decompression of the tumor is carried out. Internal decompression can be done by an ultrasound aspirator such as CUSA or SONOP. An ultrasonic aspirator (SONOP, Aloka Co., 6–22–1, Mure, Mitaka-shi, Tokyo 181, Japan) with a lightweight hand piece is very helpful in removing the part of the tumor adherent to the nerves (Fig. 14.6). Compared to previous models, weight is reduced approximately to half, providing the surgeon with possibilities of quick and delicate movement. The recent model of our design enables one to change the tip to a small caliber (1.5 mm in outer diameter) for performing internal decompression for the larger extracanalicular portion. Excessive traction of the nerves can be avoided by use of the aspirator while removing an adherent portion of the tumor. We sometimes prefer a double suction method for tumor debulking. The larger sucker is held in the right hand and the smaller sucker in the left hand. After some internal decompression, the local situation is observed carefully prior to proceeding further. A rake retractor is helpful in keeping the tumor away from the nerves. We have developed several types of retractors, of which the most suitable type is chosen depending on tumor consistency, tumor size, and the direction of the

required retraction (Fig. 14.9). Several types of dissectors should be available and the most suitable one is selected depending on the situation during dissection of the nerves from the tumor. Silver dissectors of varying angles, shapes and sharpness should be available so that they can be remodeled during the operation if necessary (Fig. 14.10).

The first step is to observe the root exit zone of the facial nerve to identify the nerve; the second being exploring the tentorial side of the nerve and to dissect and expose the trigeminal nerve; thirdly one can use a rake retractor to retract the tumor from the brain stem side. Whichever method one uses, an attempt is made at least initially to preserve both cochlear and facial nerves. Our statistics show that if one attempts preservation of the cochlear nerve in addition to the facial nerve, the preservation rate of the facial nerve is increased. It is only that it takes some extra time in doing so. It is stressed again that the cochlear nerve requires extra care during dissection and direct touch or retraction should be avoided. After removing a substantial portion of the tumor in the cerebellopontine angle, the intracanalicular portion is then removed.

Drilling the auditory canal

Before drilling, the cerebellum, brain stem, blood vessels and the exposed cranial nerves should be protected (Hongo & Kobayashi 1995). All cotton pledgets should be removed from the wound. We usually use silastic sheet to protect the surface of the brain and hold it with one or two spatulas connected to self-retaining retractors (Shibuya et al 1991, Tanaka et al 1993). A rubber dam utilizing a surgical glove can be used instead of a silastic sheet, even though it is not entirely transparent. The extent of bone removal depends on the anatomy of the bone which can be assessed on the basis of preoperative CT scan using a bone window. Usually 7–8 mm of bone of the posterior lip of the canal can be removed safely, though one can drill the posterior lip up to 1 cm after adequate assessment of the preoperative CT scan. Opening up of the semi-circular canal and common crus should be avoided if hearing is to

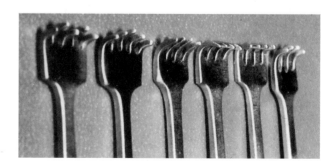

Fig. 14.9 Rake retractors.

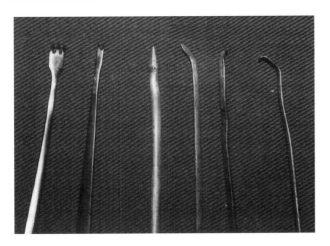

Fig. 14.10 Silver dissectors of various kinds and small rake retractors.

be preserved. Another important point is that in some cases the jugular bulb is so well developed that it lies close to the bone surface. In such a high-positioned jugular bulb it is best not to enter the jugular fossa, but if it is necessary to drill this portion extreme care should be taken not to injure the jugular bulb (Samii et al 1991). The jugular bulb can be retracted with a 2 mm spatula to further drill the bone. Drilling can be extended towards the petrous apex in the region of Kawase's triangle. Drilling over the canal for about 7–8 mm on both sides is usually safe. However, while drilling around the canal, care should be taken not to damage the dura of the canal as the facial and cochlear nerves course very close to the dura, the former in the tentorial side and the latter in the spinal side. We prefer to open the dura of the canal vertically in the midline and decompress the tumor to some extent so that the dura becomes slack and then we can retract the dura medially to drill the edge of the canal with a 1 mm bar. Bone resection of the posterior lip should be done as much as possible to accomplish total removal of the tumor in the canal. Staged drilling is recommended to remove the posterior lip effec-

tively without injuring the facial and cochlear nerves; removing the bone grossly with a 3 mm drill head first, incising the dura and removing tumor partially, and finally resecting the bone further with a 1 mm drill head using a tapered spatula or silastic sheet to protect the nerves (Fig. 14.11). Constant irrigation with saline is necessary while drilling to prevent heat damage to the nerves.

Removal of the intracanalicular portion of the tumor

Complete removal of the tumor cannot be achieved until the intracanalicular portion of the tumor is removed. In reviewing a small number of regrowth cases in our series, we observed that in the majority of cases the tumor regrew from the intracanalicular residual tumor. Another reason for total removal from the intracanalicular side is that during the first attempt of tumor removal the chances of preserving the VIIth and cochlear nerves are better as the nerves are relatively well demarcated in the canal. The tumor in the canal lies superficially and the VIIth nerve can be identified in the bottom of the canal on the tentorial side. The cochlear nerve lies on the spinal side, either as a flat spread-out bundle or a well-formed bundle. One should remember that the tumor originates from either the superior or inferior vestibular nerve. Naturally, therefore, if the tumor has originated from the inferior vestibular nerve, the superior vestibular nerve remains intact. The superior vestibular nerve can be mistaken for the facial nerve. However, the superior vestibular nerve courses superficially in the field while the facial nerve courses in the depth. Electric stimulation confirms the facial nerve. For removal of the intracanalicular portion of the tumor. SONOP is helpful. While using micro-SONOP here, the individual nerves have to be protected with a Silastic sheet or rubber dam or one can use a small piece of Bemsheet. As mentioned before, by the suboccipital approach the fundus of the canal is difficult to observe, especially when

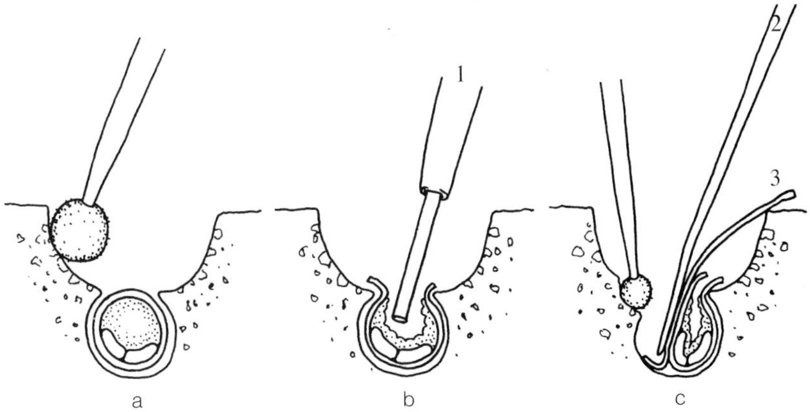

Fig. 14.11 Progressive drilling (**a** to **c**) of the lateral lips of the internal auditory meatus. The intracanalicular dura protects the cranial nerves during drilling. (1, micro-SONOP; 2, 2 mm spatula; 3, silastic sheet.)

a   b   c

one attempts to preserve hearing. The intracanalicular portion can be removed easily in some cases, but in other cases the tumor extends to the very bottom of the canal, continuing to the vestibular nerve. In such a case, complete removal is very difficult. The extent of tumor and the canal can be determined preoperatively with the help of MRI study. In order to visualize the fundus of the canal we can use either an endoscope or a microsurgical mirror. We prefer a microsurgical mirror because it is not only easier to handle but it can also be fixed by a self-retaining retractor so that the surgeon can continue the dissection with two free hands. To watch the fundus of the canal on the mirror is somewhat difficult as one has to convert the image of the fundus to the mirror (Fig. 14.12). When using mirror to reflect the fundus, the mirror is held in the deeper position to the meatus so that the images of the fundus are arranged unchanged in the horizontal plane but they are inverted on the vertical plane. It is important to remember the normal anatomy of the fundus of the right side and then convert images to the left side. We have recently designed a fibre-lighted mirror which can be used effectively to visualize the canal and its contents (Fig. 14.13).

Final removal of the tumor

The most difficult dissection of the tumor from the facial nerve is at the point just outside the meatus. The facial nerve can be very adherent to the tumor capsule and attenuated and flattened here. The tumor should be held gently, taking care not to pull excessively, and then gradually dis-

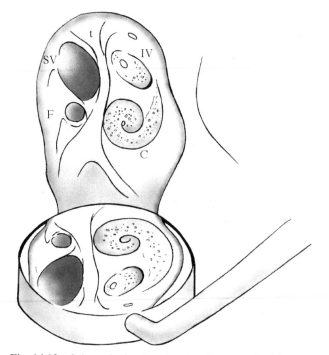

Fig. 14.12 Schematic drawing showing the reversal of the image of the fundus when seen through the microsurgical mirror. The upper part shows the fundus of the right acoustic canal seen from the brain stem side; the lower part shows the image of the above fundus reflected on the mirror. (Abbreviations are the same as in Fig. 14.7.)

sected using sharp instruments such as Rhoton's dissectors or the sharpened silver dissector of Sugita. Sugita's silver

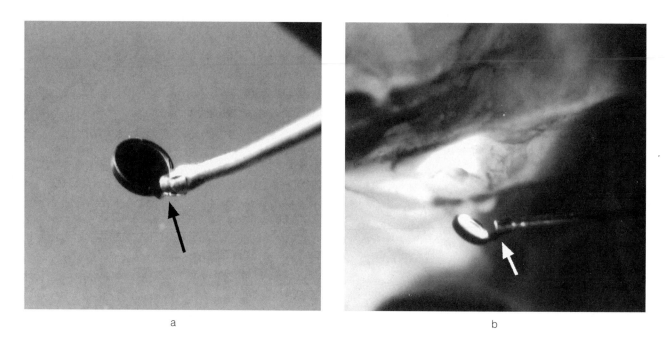

a

b

Fig. 14.13 Photograph showing the fiber-lighted mirror. **a** Light off. **b** Light on. Arrow shows the light source.

dissector is malleable and the tip of dissector can be bent in various directions. Different shapes are also available and each can be used according to the condition of the nerve in relation to the tumor (Fig. 14.11). The tumor can usually be dissected from the facial nerve by working in the subarachnoid plane.

Cranial nerves

Generally the VIIth nerve is stronger than the cochlear nerve. However, during dissection it is best not to pull or retract them. When one needs to touch or elevate them out of the way, they can be protected by silastic tubing or by a piece of Bemsheet covering the nerve.

After removal of the tumor

After removal of the tumor the wound is cleaned from blood and structures are identified. In removing the clots of blood from the field one should not use too strong a suction because it may injure fine vessels or cranial nerves which have often been shifted from the normal anatomy. Some clots can be left in the field if they are not too large in volume. Hemostasis can be confirmed by increasing the venous pressure by Valsalva maneuver. The dura is closed watertight with or without the use of homologous dural graft. The bone opening of the canal is filled by pieces of fat or muscle and treated with fibrin glue. The opened mastoid air cells are filled with muscle pieces and fibrin glue, and the skin is closed in layers. The bone flap is replaced with the gap filled with bone dust and fibrin glue.

Case 1

This 64-year-old male noticed left facial dysesthesia for about 1 month and a change of taste sensation at the left side of the tongue, with mild hearing difficulty in the left ear and gait ataxia. Preoperative studies showed almost normal hearing in both ears with 20 dB bilaterally. MRI showed a 3.0 cm mass in the cerebellopontine angle, with a laterally associated small multicystic component (Fig. 14.14). The cyst wall and the solid part of the tumor enhanced intensely on contrast administration.

With the patient in the lateral position, a left suboccipital craniotomy was performed (Fig. 14.15a). The dura was opened and the CSF was evacuated from the cisterna magna. Initially the arachnoid over the tumor was retracted towards the brain stem. Some of intratumoral cysts were opened and internal decompression was made. After further dissection and tumor removal a whitish band, the VIIIth nerve, was found on the spinal side and in the depth the VIIth nerve was also found and confirmed using electric stimulation (Fig. 14.15b). The trigeminal nerve was found in the tentorial side of the tumor. The tumor wall on the brain stem side was adherent to the brain

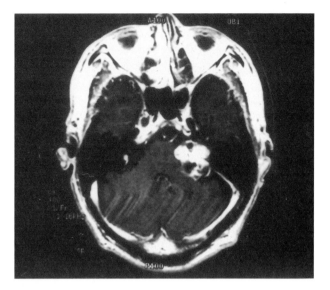

Fig. 14.14   MRI showing a 3 cm mass in the left cerebellopontine angle, with a laterally associated small multicystic component.

stem and to the cerebellum, and it took tedious dissection to dissect it off. The tumor had pushed the trigeminal nerve towards the tentorium (explaining the facial dysesthesia). After the tentorial and brain stem side of the tumor was removed, the remaining portion of the tumor was attached to the VIIth and cochlear nerves. Before removing the tumor from here, the intracanalicular portion of the tumor was approached. The internal auditory canal was drilled with 3 mm and 1 mm diamond burrs. Part of the jugular bulb was exposed but was not injured. The tumor from inside the canal was removed relatively easily (the tumor was of type 3 according to the Shinshu classification of acoustic tumors, Fig. 14.1). The cochlear nerve was located at the 8 o'clock position and the facial nerve at the 5 o'clock position in the canal. Finally, tumor residue between the VIIth and cochlear nerves was carefully removed (Fig. 14.15c). At the end of removal cranial nerves from V to XI were all identifiable and preserved except the vestibular nerves (Fig. 14.16). The wound was closed as usual. Postoperatively hearing was preserved with the same pure tone score.

Comments
1. Some tumors, particularly multicystic ones, can be very adherent to the brain stem and cranial nerves. In this case, it was adherent to the arachnoid on the brain stem side and also to the VIIth nerve.

2. The fiber-lighted mirror was useful in identifying the facial and cochlear nerves in the fundus of the canal. The transverse crest was observed in this case with the help of this instrument (Fig. 14.15d).

3. Postoperatively the facial function and hearing were preserved.

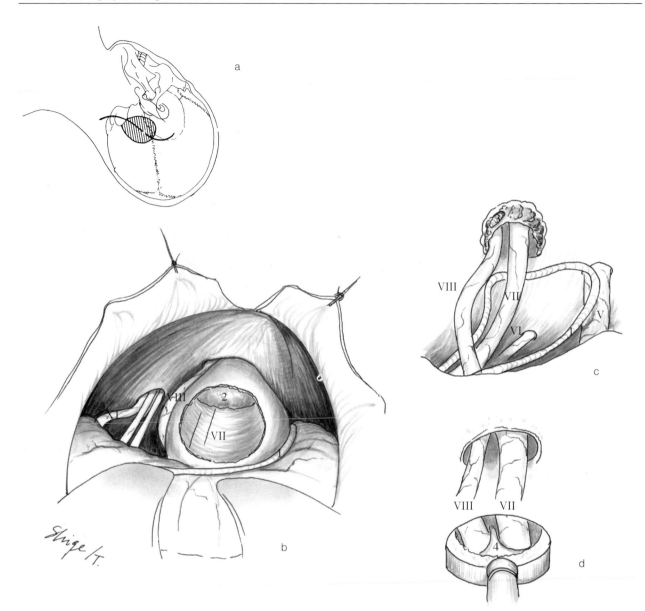

Fig. 14.15 **a** Left suboccipital craniotomy. **b** Exposure of the tumor, and the VIIth and VIIIth nerves. **c** Removal of tumor residue between the VIIth and cochlear nerves. **d** The transverse crest was observed using the fiber-lighted mirror. (1, anterior inferior cerebellar artery; 2, tumor nodule; 3, jugular bulb; 4, transverse crest.)

References

Cohen N K, Hammerschlag P, Berg H et al 1986 Acoustic neuroma surgery: an eclectic approach with emphasis on preservation of hearing. Annals of Otology, Rhinology and Laryngology 95: 21–27

Ebersold M J, Harner S G, Beatty C W et al 1992 Current results of the retrosigmoid approach to acoustic neurinoma. Journal of Neurosurgery 76: 901–909

Fisher G, Fisher C, Remond J 1992 Hearing preservation in acoustic neurinoma surgery. Jouranl of Neurosurgery 76: 910–917

Glasscock M E III, Hays J W, Minor L B et al 1993 Preservation of hearing in surgery for acoustic neuromas. Journal of Neurosurgery 78: 864–870

Goel A, Sekhar L N 1990 Anomalous subarcuate artery. Journal of Neurosurgery 75: 985–986

Goel A, Sekhar L N, Langhenrich W et al 1992 Late course of preserved hearing and tinnitus after acoustic neurilemmoma surgery. Journal of Neurosurgery 77: 685–689

Hongo K, Kobayashi S 1995 Drilling technique for the skull base surgery and for the cerebrovascular surgery: concept and technique. Advances in Clinical Neurosciences 5: 201–207

Kobayashi S, Sugita K 1987 Acoustic neurinoma surgery by lateral suboccipital craniectomy. Neurosurgeons (Jpn) 6: 192–198

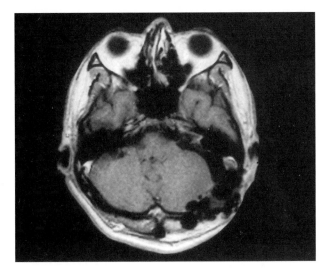

Fig. 14.16 MRI indicated that all nerves except the vestibular nerves were preserved.

Lang J 1991 Clinical anatomy of the posterior cranial fossa and its foramina. Thieme, Stuttgart, pp 83–91

Samii M, Ohlemutz A 1981 Preservation of eighth cranial nerve in cerebello-pontine angle tumors. In Samii M, Jannetta P J (eds) The Cranial nerves: anatomy, pathology, pathophysiology, diagnosis, Treatment. Springer-Verlag, Berlin, pp 586–590

Samii M, Matthies C, Tatagiba M 1991 Intracanalicular acoustic neurinomas. Neurosurgery 28: 189–199

Shibuya M, Sugita K, Kobayashi S 1991 Intraoperative protection of cranial nerves and perforating arteries by silicone rubber sheets. Technical note. Journal of Neurosurgery 74: 677–679

Sugita K, Kobayashi S 1982 Technical and instrumental improvements in the surgical treatment of acoustic neurinomas. Journal of Neurosurgery 57: 747–752

Tanaka Y, Kobayashi S 1995 Suboccipital approach to acoustic neuromas and the cerebellopontine angle. In: Torrens M J, Al-Mefty O, Kobayashi S (eds) Operative skull base surgery. Churchill Livingstone, Edinburgh in press

Tanaka Y, Kobayashi S, Hongo K, Oikawa S 1993 Intraoperative protection of cranial nerves and arteries by split silicone tube. Neurosurgery 33: 523–525

Tanaka Y, Kobayashi S, Toriyama T et al 1994 Acoustic neurinoma with special reference to anatomical correlation of the individual components of the 7th and 8th nerves. Skull Base Surgery, Samii, Karger, Basel, pp 825–828

Whittaker C K, Luetje C M 1992 Vestibular schwannomas. Journal of Neurosurgery 76: 897–900

Yokoh A, Kobayashi S, Tanaka Y et al 1993 Preservation of cochlear nerve function in acoustic neurinoma surgery. Acta Neurochirurgica 123: 8–13

Acoustic Neuromas
Albert L. Rhoton Jr

Microsurgical removal is recommended for most acoustic neuromas. Radiosurgical treatment is recommended if there are neurological or systemic factors which would increase the risk of removal and the tumor is of a suitable size. Elderly patients with mild neural compression can be followed with periodic MRI without treatment. Microsurgical removal remains the 'gold standard' of treatment.

The retrosigmoid approach is used for the removal of both small and large tumors because it offers the potential for the preservation of hearing. Auditory evoked potentials, if intact prior to surgery, and facial nerve monitoring plus the use of prophylactic antibiotics are routine. Decadron and mannitol are used with large, but not small, tumors. The exposure is done with the patient in the three-quarters prone position with the nasion to inion line parallel to the floor, and with the top of the head tilted slightly downward toward the patient's lower shoulder. The table is tilted so that the head is above the chest and abdomen.

The vertical lateral suboccipital scalp incision crosses the asterion. A free flap situated medial to the sigmoid sinus is elevated and the opening is enlarged as needed to expose the posterior margin of the sigmoid sinus. The dura is opened with the pedicle medially. The dural cuff bordering the transverse and sigmoid sinuses is tacked up to the adjacent muscles with sutures in order to minimize the need for cerebellar retraction. The cerebellum, which commonly bulges outward upon opening the dura, relaxes after opening the cisterna magna and allowing CSF to escape. Cerebellar resection or ventricular drainage is infrequently needed even when removing large tumors.

The surface of the cerebellum facing the posterior surface of the temporal bone is elevated to expose an acoustic neuroma. A tapered blade 15–25 mm wide at its base and 10–15 mm at its tip is commonly used. Care is taken to prevent the brain spatula from drifting inferiorly and damaging the glossopharyngeal and vagus nerves. No attempt is made to see the whole tumor upon initial retraction of the cerebellum. Only the posterior wall of the internal acoustic meatus and the lateral margin of the tumor are exposed with the initial elevation of the cerebellum.

The posterior wall of the internal auditory canal is removed with an irrigating drill as the initial step if the tumor is small. The intracapsular contents of the tumor are removed before opening the meatus if the tumor is large. The semi-circular canal and vestibule, situated just posterior to the lateral end of the meatus, should be preserved in drilling the meatal lip if there is the possibility of preserving hearing.

The facial nerve is identified near the origin of the facial canal at the anterior–superior quadrant of the meatus rather than in a more medial location where the direction of displacement is variable. The strokes of the fine dissecting instruments along the vestibulocochlear nerve are directed from medial to lateral rather than from lateral to medial when hearing can be preserved because traction medially may tear the tiny filaments of the cochlear nerve at the site where these filaments penetrate the lateral end of the meatus to reach the cochlea.

No attempt is made to see the whole posterior surface of a large tumor upon initially elevating the cerebellum. The operation is planned so that the tumor surface is allowed to settle away from the neural tissue rather than the neural structures being retracted away from the tumor. If the tumor is cystic, the intial step is aspiration with a needle. The surface of the tumor is then opened and biopsied and the intracapsular contents are removed. As the intracapsular contents are evacuated by means of a cup forceps and suction, the residual tumor folds inward, making it possible to remove more of it through the small exposure. In the final step, the last thin sheet of tumor capsule is removed from the side of the brain stem and the margins of the involved cranial nerve using fine dissecting instruments. The most common reason for tumor appearing to be tightly adherent to the neural structures is not adhesions between the capsule and surrounding tissue; rather, it is residual tumor within the capsule wedging the tumor into position. Prior to separating the capsule from the pia–arachnoid, it is important that all of the tumor within the capsule be

removed so that the capsule is so thin that it is almost transparent. Gentle irrigation directed in the plane between the neural structures and tumor capsule will help free the tumor from the neural structures.

There are a number of landmarks that are helpful in identifying the facial and vestibulocochlear nerves at the brain stem on the medial side of the tumor. These nerves, although distorted by tumor, can usually be identified on the brain stem side of the tumor at the lateral end of the pontomedullary sulcus, just rostral to the glossopharyngeal nerve, and just anterosuperior to the foramen of Luschka, flocculus, and choroid plexus protruding from the foramen of Luschka. After the facial and vestibulocochlear nerves are identified on the medial and lateral sides of the tumor, the final remnant of the tumor is separated from the intervening segment of the nerves. It is especially important that the segment of the cerebellar arteries adherent to the tumor capsule be preserved. The number of veins sacrificed should be kept to a minimum. Small acoustic neuromas can often be removed without sacrificing a petrosal vein.

The air cells that are opened in removing the posterior meatal lip are carefully closed with bone wax. A crushed patch of fat taken from a small transverse incision on the lower abdomen that will settle into the depression created by the drilling is then laid over the meatal margin. No CSF leaks have occurred in more than 100 consecutive operations in which we have closed the drilled meatus in this manner. The patient's own dura is carefully closed. The bone flap is held in place with silk suture brought through drill holes placed so as to avoid the mastoid air cells. Any remaining large defect in the bone is closed with methyl methacrylate. More than 95% of facial nerves have been preserved using this technique of removal and hearing has been preserved in one-half of the patients with tumors 1.5 cm or less in diameter with preoperative speech discriminations scores above 60%.

Summary of the Hannover Concept of Neurosurgical Management of Vestibular Schwannomas
Madjid Samii

The outcome in neurosurgical treatment of patients with vestibular schwannomas has changed dramatically within the last three decades. Nowadays, we expect a mortality of below 1%, except for neurofibromatosis patients, and an ongoing improvement with regard to cranial nerve morbidity. The refinement towards functional microsurgery has generated these achievements and still increasing expectations on the patient's side. Therefore, a neurosurgeon starting to deal with these lesions is confronted with the advantage of the experience gathered by his teachers and with the personal disadvantage that the standard is at a considerable higher level than before.

Completeness of resection with preservation of the

facial nerve are the major goals (Ramsay & Luxford 1993), as generally accepted and fulfilled at increasing rates. Any of the available approaches, such as the suboccipital, middle fossa, or translabyrinthine approach and their modifications, has its indications and, with training and experience, can be developed to a high standard with optimal patient safety regarding mortality and morbidity.

Still the only approach providing the opportunity to remove any size of tumor completely and the chance of functional nerve preservation is the suboccipital approach. Therefore, it should be part of the instruction on the management of these tumors.

Based on the experience of 2000 operations in the

cerebellopontine angle (CPA), including 1300 vestibular schwannomas, our standard of suboccipital tumor resection shall be presented.

The following aspects, some of which have already been stressed by the editor, will be focused upon:

- positioning;
- approach planning;
- drilling of the internal auditory canal;
- facial nerve;
- cochlear nerve.

Preparation for Surgery: All the patients are prepared by thorough clinical investigation, including ENT investigations, CT at bone windows, CT enhanced by contrast or gadolinium-enhanced MRI, and functional X-rays of the cervical spine. Neurofibromatosis patients receive preoperative MRI of the spine for diagnosis of tumors with spinal cord compression; then modified positioning with only slight flexion and rotation under neurophysiological control of somatosensory evoked potential is considered. In the case of additional craniocervical tumors, these are either operated before or during CPA surgery by extended exposure by opening of the foramen magnum and possibly by removal of C1 and C2 arches.

Tumor Removal by the Suboccipital Approach: In the semi-sitting position (Samii et al 1985, Samii 1989, von Goesseln et al 1991) with the patient's head tilted and rotated by 30° to the involved side, a suboccipital craniectomy is performed exposing the borders of the transverse and sigmoid sinuses. The dura is opened by a laterally convex dural incision and after CSF drainage by opening of the cerebellomedullary cistern the cerebellum is mildly retracted so that the posterior wall of the internal auditory canal (IAC), possibly a part of the tumor and the brain stem become visible. The dura from the posterior aspect of the IAC is removed, and the canal is drilled open by the use of decreasing sizes of diamond drills until the intrameatal tumor extension is exposed; the posterior and lateral semi-circular canals as well as the jugular bulb are respected (Shao et al 1993), and the distance to the fundus is intermittently measured by platelet-shaped knives of 2 mm diameter. If the tumor is of normal consistency, partial tumor mobilization inside the IAC is started and followed by extrameatal intracapsular tumor reduction with either the platelet-shaped knife or CUSA, thereby continuously decreasing compression of surrounding neural and vascular structures. If the tumor is of highly increased consistency, primary mobilization in the IAC might be impossible without severance of the cochlear nerve, then enucleation in the IAC or extrameatally has to be started. Under continuous saline irrigation by the 'third hand' – the neurosurgical assistant – precise bimanual nerve preparation is performed and bipolar coagulation is reduced to a minimum and left up to the end of surgery for final hemostasis. Thereby, maximum safety to brain stem and nerve vascular supply is guaranteed;

especially, early coagulation of tumor capsule vessels branching from nerve feeding vessels is prohibited and induction of vasospasm is prevented. As soon as the tumor mass is largely removed, the relation between tumor border and neural structures is relaxed. The final preparation and liberation of neural structures is performed by strictly gripping the arachnoid sheath with forceps and by limiting over-stretching in one direction (Jannetta et al 1984). The tightest junction between tumor and nerve–vessel bundle is encountered just before their entrance into the IAC (Samii 1989, Samii & Matthies 1995, Tos et al 1992), is prepared at the very end; here, sharp dissection might become necessary in order to prevent over-stretching of the facial nerve; its integrity is tested by continuous facial electromyography and by electrical stimulation at the end. Palpation with the platelet-shaped knife at the fundus, and, in very few cases, where drilling is very limited by labyrinthine structures (Jacob et al 1990), testing with a micro-mirror or the use of an angulated micro-endoscope (Tatagiba et al 1995) ensures completeness of intrameatal tumor removal. Jugular venous compression is performed by an anesthesiologist in order to make any opened or torn veins visible for final hemostasis. The opened mastoid cells at the IAC are carefully closed, for prevention of an intradural CSF otorhinological fistula, using some bone wax and a piece of muscle sealed with fibrin glue. A last careful inspection of the CPA and removal of the retractor are followed by continuous watertight dural closure.

Postoperative Care: This includes on average one night control in the intensive care unit, thereafter mobilization under physiotherapeutic guidance, control of audiometry and CT one week after surgery, with hospital discharge after 8–14 days. Clinical follow-up controls, ENT controls, MRI or contrast CT controls are scheduled for 1, 2 and 5 years postoperatively. Patients with facial nerve paresis and facial nerve reconstructions are controlled every 3–6 months. Patients with special hearing problems are also scheduled for 3–6-month controls.

Special Aspects
Positioning: The advantage of the semi-sitting position is based on the fact that any fluid from bleeding or irrigation will run out of the wound enabling a clear site, with little or no cauterization; the possibility of continuous irrigation guarantees the best possible overview to this critical area. Any disadvantages frequently discussed in relation to this positioning may be reduced to an absolute minimum by perfection of the positioning. It should be a semi-sitting or rather a semi-lying position, with the patient's feet being above the level of surgery. Thereby the danger of air embolism will be minimized. Moreover, based on our experience with somatosensory evoked potential monitoring during positioning, we may state that any further danger from positioning can occur in the semi-sitting as well as in the supine or prone positions, i.e. whenever some flexion, extension, or rotation of the neck is involved.

Approach Planning: Before surgery, analysis of the bone window will inform the surgeon of the position of the jugular bulb and of the labyrinthine structures in relation to the internal auditory canal. The danger of hearing impairment by surgical lesions to the labyrinth (despite nerve conservation) can be reliably calculated beforehand in order to modify surgical strategy and to reduce this risk. The so-called fundus–sinus line as the widest opening line bears a potential risk of labyrinth destruction of 33% and the ideal meatus–sinus line for a safe opening is delineated before surgery at the bone window CT; thereby, the minimal length of the posterior wall of the internal auditory canal that has to be preserved is calculated. On average, 3.4 mm of the posterior wall of the auditory canal has to be left intact to prevent a fenestration or opening of the vestibular system. Rare cases with an indication for intraoperative micro-endoscopy (Tatagiba et al 1995) or for a middle fossa approach are identified.

Drilling: If hearing preservation is the goal, opening of the internal auditory canal should be performed with a sharp diamond drill. The drilling will be safer, especially in large tumors, if it is performed before tumor reduction, when the brain stem is still covered by the tumor. With small nerve hooks of definite lengths the remaining part of the posterior wall is measured intermittently and compared to the calculated data.

The Facial Nerve: Identification of the facial nerve is to be well achieved at the intrameatal course where it must be expected at the anterior upper part and at the brain stem on light traction of the tumor away from it. At the latter, however, the nerve is usually spread into a thin broad layer of fascicles and displaced onto the upper and anterior tumor surface in large tumors. This part should only be exposed after considerable tumor enucleation in order to prevent any strong traction. The tightest junction will be found medial to the porus; this part must be approached from all directions and very carefully, instead of dissecting along the suspected tumor nerve border in one direction. As we do not use relaxation medication, we perform control of electromyographic responses to mechanic stimulation; only in pre-existing palsies with reduced response or very widespread nerve parts is direct electric stimulation used.

In cases of facial nerve interruption, immediate facial nerve reconstruction is performed by a sural nerve grafted, that is interposed, between the proximal and distal nerve stumps. This transplantation may be carried out within the cerebellopontine angle, or, in cases of distracted distal stump, towards the mastoid portion or, in cases of previous mastoiditis, towards the extracranial part at the stylomastoid foramen. If a facial nerve reanimation procedure becomes necessary, as in loss of the proximal stump or in degeneration of the nerve, the most reliable reinnervation will be produced by hypoglossal–facial combination (Samii & Matthies 1994).

The Cochlear Nerve: Early nerve identification is not the secret of functional cochlear nerve preservation; the early search for the nerve may be rather dangerous, leading to stretch, twisting and strangulation of the nerve or its feeders. The nerve must be expected at the lower anterior aspect of the tumor and this should be the area to avoid touching at the start. Enucleation must be performed until all the surrounding structures become relaxed. Dissection at the tumor nerve should then be performed during continuous monitoring of acoustic evoked potentials. Significant deterioration must be followed by a quick change of surgical activity; mostly light stretching in another direction or working at a different site will be followed by wave recovery. By this feedback, also the most difficult steps of intrameatal nerve preparation may be successfully performed. If despite change of action the waves do not recover, two considerations must be formulated: either the responsible action for wave deterioration had occurred some minutes earlier (like induction of microvascular spasm) or the most recent action was too vigorous.

Caudal Cranial Nerves: In a small number of large tumors these extend downwards towards the jugular foramen and its nerves. Whenever compression or displacement of these nerves is observed at surgery or even actual tumor attachment, special postoperative measures should be taken. At first the patient should not be extubated immediately in the operating theater. After regaining stable consciousness and cooperation the patient is tested clinically for sensation and reflexes of the caudal cranial nerves. Extubation is performed via fiber-optic endoscopic control and visualization of the vocal cords; thereby excessive mucus that could not be coughed up due to nerve compromise can be detected and removed. Depending on these findings, gastric tube feeding, restriction of oral and nutrition intake or stepwise physiotherapeutic exercises will be instituted. In this way, the rare but potentially disastrous sequelae of nerve dysfunction and aspiration pneumonia can be prevented.

References

Jacob U, Gerhardt H J, Staudt J, Dilba V 1990 Chirurgische Anatomie der Hoererhaltung bei der Operation von Akustikusneurinomen. [Surgical anatomy of the petrous canal and posterior cranial fossa in relation to hearing preservation in surgery of acoustic neurinoma.] HNO 38(3): 83–91

Jannetta P J, Moller A R, Moller M B 1984 Technique of hearing preservation in small acoustic neurinomas. Annals of Surgery 200: 513–522

Ramsay H A, Luxford W M 1993 Treatment of acoustic tumors in elderly patients: is surgery warranted? Journal of Laryngology and Otology 107(4): 295–297

Samii M 1989 Tumors of the internal auditory canal and cerebellopontine angle. I. Acoustic neuroma. In: Samii M, Draf W (eds) Surgery of the skull base: an interdisciplinary approach. Springer Verlag, Berlin, pp377–395

Samii M, Matthies C 1994 Indication, technique and results of facial nerve reconstruction. Acta Neurochirurgica 130: 125–139

Samii M, Matthies C 1995 Hearing preservation in acoustic tumour surgery. In: Symon L (ed) Advances and technical standards in neurosurgery (Vol 22). Springer-Verlag, Berlin, pp 343–373

Samii M, Turel K E, Penkert G 1985 Management of seventh and eighth nerve involvement by cerebellopontine tumors. Clinical Neurosurgery 32: 242–272

Shao K N, Tatagiba M, Samii M 1993 Surgical management of high jugular bulb in acoustic neurinoma via retromastoid approach. Neurosurgery 32(1): 32–36; discussion 36–37

Tatagiba M, Samii M, Matthies C 1995 The use of micro-endoscopy in acoustic neurinoma surgery. Presentation at the Annual Workshop on Microsurgery by the German Society of Neurosurgery, February

Tos M, Youssef M, Thomsen J, Turgut S 1992 Cause of facial nerve paresis after translabyrinthine surgery for acoustic neurinoma. Annals of Otology, Rhinology and Laryngology 101(10): 821–826

von Goesseln H H, Samii M, Bini W 1991 The lounging position for posterior fossa surgery: anaesthesiological considerations regarding air embolism. Chils Nervous System 7: 368–374

Removal of an Acoustic Neurinoma by the Lateral Suboccipital Approach
Masato Shibuya

It is important to set a primary target of an operation for the microsurgical removal of an acoustic neurinoma; (1) preservation of hearing; (2) facial function; (3) life. The aforementioned depends upon tumor size, preoperative hearing and the patient's age and occupation. The four main technically important points are summarized as follows.

Patient Positioning and Craniotomy: The patient is placed in a lateral recumbent position with the shoulder and head close to the operator's side of the table to prevent the operator's knee from hitting the table when the operating chair is in use. The head is fixed in the frame with chin, vertex and nose down in order to bring the mastoid eminence to the highest position. The patient's body should be comfortably held by the chest and sacral region in order that the table may be rotated axially, while the patient's legs are elastic-bandaged so as to avoid intraoperative hypotension. The key pin to fix the head in the frame is the one applied near the inion. This pin should be placed 1 cm contralaterally and caudally to the inion to allow enough space for the operator's hand on the tumor side. Care must be taken to avoid slipping of this pin toward the foramen magnum, especially in a patient with a steep occipital bone.

Craniotomy and dural opening are performed essentially as described by Yasargil et al (1977) and at a minimum, the edge of the transverse and sigmoid sinuses should be seen.

Tumor Removal: After retracting the cerebellum and the tumor becomes visible, it should be dissected from the surrounding tissues before these structures become stained with blood and lose their identity. A continuous suction tube is placed in the cisterna magna caudally to the vagus nerve. During surgery, this suction is very important as it keeps the operative field dry. After

checking the position of the facial nerve by electrical stimulation, a hole is made on the dorsal surface of the tumor and the content of the tumor is evacuated either with tumor forceps or suction tips used with both hands. Serrated suction tips (Shibuya et al 1988) are very useful for this purpose. The tumor is fixed with one suction tip held in one hand and gutted and suctioned with another suction tip held in the other hand. This reduces the time necessary for removal of the tumor and often is more convenient than using the ultrasonic suction system. After the tumor content has been removed, when the thickness of its wall is only a few millimeters and when the wall in its bottom starts to move, the position of the facial nerve is located by electrical stimulation from the inside of the tumor. Intratumoral hemostasis is accomplished by packing the empty cavity with a cotton ball soaked with hydrogen peroxide.

When the tumor wall becomes thin it can be retracted from the cerebellum by using the tumor hook attached to a self-retaining retractor. Usually the vein of the lateral recess of the fourth ventricle runs along the border between the cerebellum and the pons. This vein leads upward to the petrosal vein, which should be preserved as much as possible. The tumor should be dissected from the surrounding tissues: the petrosal vein and trigeminal nerve rostrally, and the lower cranial nerves caudally. Care must be taken to identify the origin of the VIIIth cranial nerve at the pons. Usually, an increased number of blood vessels are encountered here and the one that leads to the internal auditory artery should be protected if hearing is to be preserved. The facial nerve originates only a few millimeters ventral to the origin of the VIIIth nerve, and it can easily be identified by electrical stimulation.

Opening of the Internal Auditory Meatus: When the tumor mass is reduced by internal decompression, the posterior wall of the internal auditory meatus is drilled. The thickness of the posterior wall that is to be removed should be measured carefully by preoperative thin-sliced bone-level CT. Care must be taken to avoid injury to the semi-circular canal and the high jugular bulb. After opening the internal auditory canal the intracanalicular portion of the tumor is removed. Both the facial and cochlear nerves lie ventral to the vestibular nerves and usually remain uninjured when the tumor is removed. The tumor can usually be removed totally by blunt dissection, using a ball-point dissector or a ring curette; however, the bottom of the meatus should be checked carefully for any tumor that may still remain by use of a mirror or an endoscope.

Dissection from the Cochlear and Facial Nerve; monitoring: Either a sharp silver dissector or fine-tipped titanium forceps are useful for final dissection of the tumor from the cochlear and facial nerves. Facial nerve monitoring (Shibuya et al 1993) and monitoring of cochlear nerve function through the brain stem auditory evoked potential with a silver ball electrode in the region of the foramen Luschka (Moller et al 1994) are extremely useful for the preservation of function of these cranial nerves. To prevent heat injury to the nerves, bipolar coagulation should be avoided as much as possible. When unavoidable, the use of a 5% dextrose solution for irrigation instead of an ionic solution reduces heat injury by avoiding boiling between the bipolar forceps (Sakatani et al 1995).

Except for huge tumors, the facial nerve, in most cases, can be preserved. In patients with preoperative useful hearing or in patients with tumors less than 20 mm in diameter, the preservation of useful hearing has been 50%. Recently, the preservation of hearing has been improving further with the use of more sophisticated monitoring (Moller et al 1994) and more careful surgery. The problems left to be solved are: surgery of large and highly vascularized tumors, the preservation of visual function of those patients with marked papilledema, and the timing of surgery for bilateral acoustic tumors.

References

Moller A R, Jho H D, Jannetta P J 1994 Preservation of hearing in operations on acoustic tumors: an alternative to recording brain stem auditory evoked potentials. Neurosurgery 34: 688–693

Sakatani K, Morimoto S, Otaki M et al 1995 Measurement of local heat generation and effects of irrigation during electrical coagulation using bipolar diathermy forceps. Japanese Journal of Neurosurgery 4: 133–137

Shibuya M, Suzuki Y, Nakane T 1988 A serrated tip for tumor removal. Journal of Neurosurgery 69: 140–141

Shibuya M, Matsuga N, Suzuki Y et al 1993 A newly designed nerve monitor for microneurosurgery: bipolar constant current nerve stimulation and movement detector with a pressure sensor. Acta Neurochirurgica 125: 173–176

Yasargil M G, Smith R D, Gasser J C 1977 Microsurgical approach to acoustic neurinomas. In: Krayenbuhl H (ed) Advances and technical standards in neurosurgery (Vol 4). Springer-Verlag, Wein, pp 93–129

Anterior clinoidal meningioma

Atul Goel   Shigeaki Kobayashi

15

INTRODUCTION

The meningiomas originating in the region of the medial sphenoid wing are amongst the most challenging neuro-surgical problems. With the center of origin on and around the anterior clinoid process, these tumors vary in the extent of their dural attachment, size and extensions. Anterior clinoidal meningiomas frequently encase the carotid artery, involve the optic nerve and invade the cavernous sinus and other critical structures in the neighborhood, and thus constitute a challenging and formidable surgical problem. Various terminologies have been used to classify these meningiomas (Cushing & Eisenhardt 1938, Al-Mefty 1990). Relatively few large series have been reviewed in literature (Al-Mefty 1990, Ojemann 1980, Konovalov et al 1979, MacCarty & Taylor 1979).

DISCUSSION: PHILOSOPHY OF MANAGEMENT

The difficulty in surgically excising anterior clinoidal meningiomas stems from its relationship to the ipsilateral internal carotid artery and its branches which it frequently encases and/or displaces. The major concern during the surgery is preservation of these vessels as often dense hemispheric deficits or even death might result following the operation, which otherwise in the natural course of tumor growth would have never occurred or taken several years (Jefferson & Azzam 1979). From the usual mode of presentation, it is clear that most of these tumors are slow growing. If left alone the tumor 'might' grow in size and produce a rise in intracranial pressure, and in the long run 'may' affect the nerves of the cavernous sinus and optic nerve, and 'might' result in hemispheric deficits following carotid artery compromise. On the other hand, slow progression of the size of the tumor could result in crippling symptoms and neurological deficits. More importantly, the subsequent surgical excision of a larger tumor, with more complex arterial involvement, may be difficult. Any surgical endeavor must therefore weigh the natural history of these tumors, in the light of personal operative experience.

The extent of the surgical resection of the tumor determines the ultimate outcome of the patient, tumor recurrence and regrowth (Simpson 1957, Mirimanoff et al 1985, Skullerud & Lokn 1974).

CLINICAL PRESENTATION

A preponderance of anterior clinoidal meningiomas in females has been uniformly observed (Symon et al 1989). In our series of 24 patients seen in a 2-year period (1993–1994), 55% patients were females. The average age was 42 years. Like most other skull basal lesions, tumors arising from the anterior clinoid process have a relatively innocuous clinical presentation despite the commonly encountered large size. This feature was also seen in our series. The presentation of the tumor was primarily in the form of visual diminution in the ipsilateral eye, which was affected to varying degrees. Six patients in the presented series had complete blindness in the ipsilateral eye. The contralateral eye was affected in 12 patients. The extra-ocular nerves were not involved in any of the patients presented, and such involvement has been seen only as a rare feature (Al-Mefty 1990). Affect on pituitary function was also not encountered in our series, and has been reported infrequently (Symon et al 1989). Symptoms secondary to raised intracranial pressure were not seen, although have been reported by others. Progressive hemiparesis as a presenting symptom has also been reported (Ojemann 1980), but this was not observed in our series.

INVESTIGATIONS

Magnetic resonance imaging (MRI) scanning was found to be essential to clearly define the relationship of the tumor to the major blood vessels as regards their encasement and displacement. Angiography was helpful in delineating the extent of arterial compression and displacement, the vascularity of the tumor and in evaluating the collateral circulation. The information gained from angiograms and MRI was compiled and the exact tumor–artery relationship

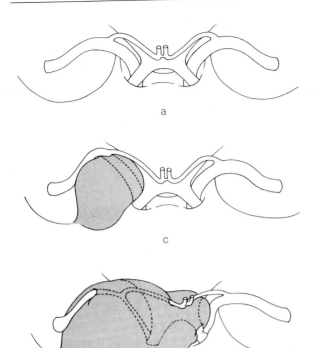

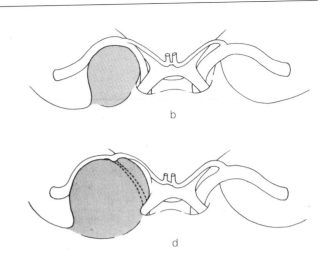

Fig. 15.1   **a** Schematic drawing showing the region of both anterior clinoid processes. Both optic nerves, chiasm, internal carotid arteries and their bifurcation into anterior cerebral artery and middle cerebral artery are seen. **b** Grade I tumor: the internal carotid artery is displaced by the tumor. **c** Grade II tumor: the internal carotid artery is encased by the tumor, but its lumen is not narrowed. **d** Grade III tumor: the internal carotid artery is encased within the tumor and its lumen is narrowed by it. **e** Grade IV tumor: the tumor extends to the contralateral side and displaces the opposite side carotid artery as well.

understood in each case. Computed tomographic (CT) scanning was of help in delineating the extent of bony involvement. Balloon occlusion test of the carotid artery (Sekhar et al 1989) was not found to be a necessity.

On the basis of the major arterial relationship to the tumor as seen on MRI scanning, these tumors were divided into four categories as shown below.

CLASSIFICATION 1 (Fig. 15.1)

I   displacement of ipsilateral internal carotid artery (ICA)
II   ICA encased but not narrowed
III   ICA encased and narrowed
IV   contralateral carotid and/or basilar displaced

This classification provided an idea of the nature of spread of the tumor and vascular relationships. This helped to some extent in planning the operative strategy, in anticipating the various problems involved in the surgical resection and in prognosticating the ultimate outcome.

The other important feature that affects the surgical procedure and its outcome is size of the tumor. The tumors are therefore divided into three groups on the basis of the size:

CLASSIFICATION 2

Type 1   size less than 3 cm (Figs 15.2, 15.3)
Type 2   size between 3 and 5 cm (Figs 15.4, 15.5)
Type 3   size above 5 cm (Figs 15.6–15.8)

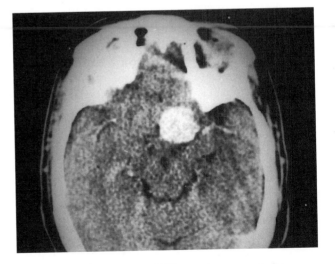

Fig. 15.2   Contrast-enhanced CT scan shows an anterior clinoid meningioma. The lesion is type 1 and measures less than 3 cm in diameter.

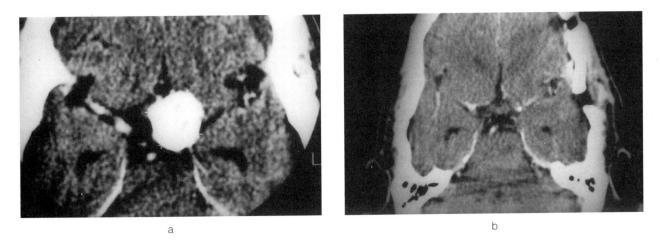

a   b

Fig. 15.3 **a** Contrast-enhanced scan showing a type 1 anterior clinoidal meningioma. **b** Postoperative scan showing resection of the tumor.

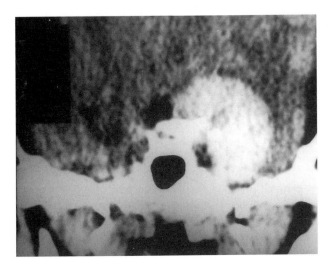

Fig. 15.4 Contrast-enhanced CT scan shows the type 2 meningioma, which measures in its maximum dimension 4.2 cm. The lesion has a wide attachment to the lateral wall of the cavernous sinus.

The extent of visual involvement was also an important factor that decided the course of the surgery. The more severe the visual involvement the firmer was the tumor and the more difficult was tumor resection. The tumors could therefore be divided according to visual involvement.

CLASSIFICATION 3

Grade 1   No visual loss
Grade 2   Partial visual loss
Grade 3a   Blindness in ipsilateral eye
Grade 3b   Partial or complete involvement of both eyes

It was seen that despite the large sizes of the tumor and their close relation to the superior and lateral wall of the cavernous sinus, invasion into it was identified to be only a tail-like extension via the dural cave of the IIIrd nerve and along the carotid artery. Gross invasion of the cavernous sinus was not encountered and appears to be a rare feature probably due to the barrier provided by the thick dura of the lateral wall. There was no invasion of the skull base and craniofacial cavities in any patient.

SURGICAL CONSIDERATIONS

No special anesthetic cerebral protection was utilized during the operative procedures. However, such measures have been advocated and could be of use in some situations. Preoperative spinal cerebrospinal fluid (CSF) drainage has been advocated by some (Al-Mefty 1990). This procedure was not found to be useful in our series. Considering the large size of the tumor a lumbar drainage of CSF was considered to be dangerous. The exposure for approach of these tumors was such that the entire tumor could be removed in one single operative field. Basal exposures which included orbitozygomatic osteotomies, removal of the roof and the lateral wall of the orbit, resection of the lesser wing of the sphenoid bone up to the clinoid process, in addition to the frontotemporal pterion-based craniotomy, was used in early cases. In the later part of the series it was observed that orbitozygomatic osteotomy could be avoided. Removal of the lesser wing of the sphenoid bone, posterior part of the roof and lateral wall of the orbit were found to provide a satisfactory and quicker exposure. Alternative approaches have been described (Brotchi & Bonnal 1991, Cushing & Eisenhardt 1938, Kempe 1968, MacCarty & Taylor 1979, Ojemann 1980).

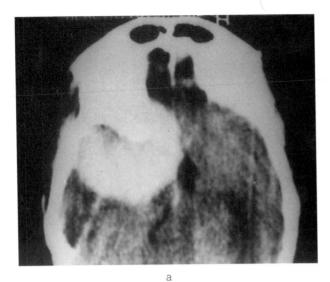

a

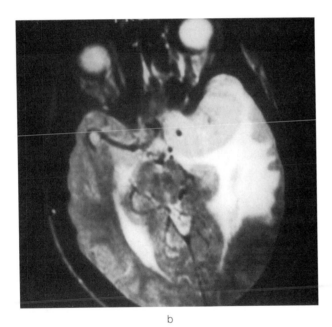

b

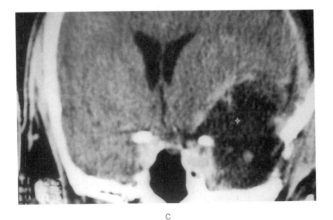

c

Fig. 15.5   a Contrast CT scan showing a large anterior clinoidal meningioma. The anterior clinoid process is thickened. **b** MRI showing the internal carotid artery encased by the tumor. **c** Postoperative scan showing complete resection of the tumor.

In none of our cases was it necessary to resect any part of the frontal or temporal lobe. Before the era of extensive usage of skull base approaches, some authors recommended temporal polar (Morley 1973) or inferolateral frontal lobe resection for safe tumor removal (Logue 1979). In one case proximal control of the internal carotid artery was obtained at the petrous apex. Although the neck was prepared for exposure of the carotid artery for proximal control in higher-grade tumors, this procedure was not necessary in any case.

A small or limited excision appears to have no significant effect on the long-term prognosis (Brotchi & Bonnal 1991). In one case with a Grade III lesion, the patient was referred after a very small excision had been performed. A decompressive craniectomy was done as the brain was found to be markedly tense. The patient worsened to hemiplegia following this operation. The exact cause of the hemiplegia could not be confirmed. However, it appears that the critical intracranial pressure balance was upset as a result of the craniectomy (Fig. 15.8). From the experience in the reported series, our opinion is that the planning of the operation has to be for a radical excision of the lesion with an adequate preparation for management of the involved arteries. We observed that if the arterial isolation is inadequate, a very limited resection is possible due to the constant fear of the approaching vessel. The initial surgical attack should be directed towards the anterior clinoid process, aiming to expose the internal carotid artery trunk and then to dissect it further. Although advocated by some authors (Symon et al 1989), others find tumor debulking followed by arterial isolation a better alternative (Brotchi & Bonnal 1991). It was seen that once this artery was free, rapid and relatively safe excision of the tumor could be achieved. Some surgeons have advised tracing of the internal carotid artery from distally (its middle cerebral artery branches) to its trunk (Al-Mefty 1990, Samii & Ammirati 1992, Ojemann 1980), but it was seen that this procedure was difficult and wrought with the danger of retraction injury to the brain. As the artery was exposed in the clinoidal area, there was no need to open the compressed sylvian fissure as advocated by some. While proceeding towards the anterior clinoid process the tumor was dissected free from its basal dural attachments and in the process devascularizing it. This dissection from the base and along the site of attachment of the tumor to the dura was relatively safe and as in any other meningioma an important preparatory step of the operation (Symon et al 1989).

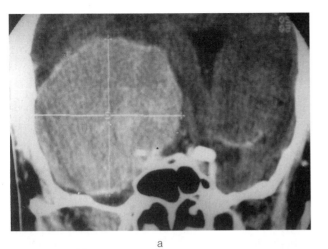

a

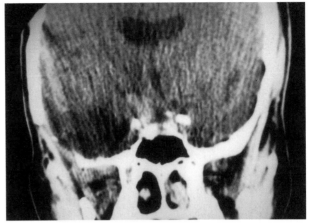

b

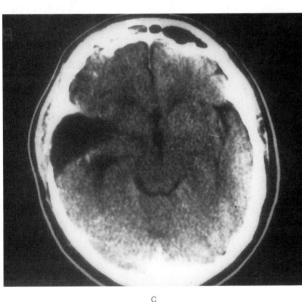

c

Fig. 15.6 **a** Contrast-enhanced CT scan shows a massive anterior clinoidal meningioma. The lesion is of type 3 variety measuring more than 5 cm in its maximum dimension. **b** Postoperative CT scan after resection of the large meningioma. **c** Axial cut showing complete resection of the tumor.

Drilling of the lesser wing of the sphenoid bone also helped to some extent in tumor devascularization.

From the experience in our series of cases, it appeared that the consistency of the tumor can usually be gauged by the extent and duration of visual impairment. The more severe the visual impairment and longer its duration, the firmer was the tumor, and the more difficult was tumor resection. The grading of these tumors according to the extent of visual impairment and the size helped in estimating the operative difficulties. Similar observations were made by Rosenstien & Symon (1984). The presence of calcific or ossified areas in the tumor on preoperative investigations was also an indicator of the consistency of the lesion. Grade 3 tumors (classification 1) were firmer than Grade 2 tumors and were consequently more difficult to resect. The arterial compression also appeared to be related to the consistency of the surrounding tumor, rather than invasion into the arachnoidal planes. In one Grade 1

patient we found that the internal carotid artery and its branches had made a groove for their passage on the surface of the tumor. Inability to recognize this was probably the cause of inadvertent injury to a branch of the middle cerebral artery in one case. In this case a severe hemispheric deficit resulted. It appears to us that an immediate reanastomosis or a bypass may have helped in such a situation. We found a well-defined arachnoid plane between the tumor and the artery in all cases despite the encasement in some cases. Al-Mefty divided these tumors into three groups according to the site of origin of the tumor and the presence of arachnoid plane around the artery (Al-Mefty 1990). It appears to us that if dense adhesions of the tumor with the artery are observed during the surgery, resulting in difficult dissection and isolation, there are two alternatives for the surgeon. Either one can satisfy oneself with a partial excision or do a superficial temporal artery–middle cerebral artery (STA–MCA), or external carotid

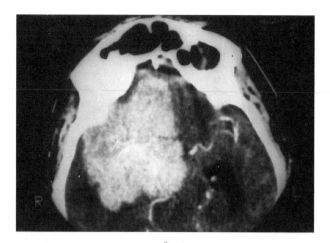

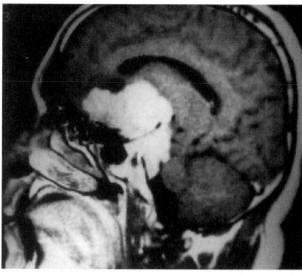

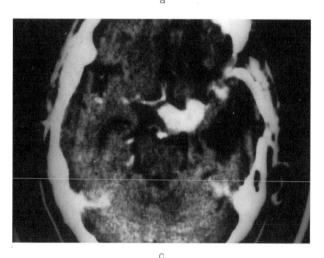

Fig. 15.7 **a** CT scan showing a massive (type 3) meningioma. **b** MRI scan showing the large tumor. The internal carotid artery is completely encased and narrowed by the tumor. **c** Postoperative CT scan shows a relatively small residual lesion.

artery–middle cerebral artery(ECA–MCA) bypass operation, leaving the arterial dissection and tumor resection for the subsequent stage. It is therefore necessary that the STA trunk be preserved intact during the exposure stage of the operation. However, the carotid artery could be dissected completely free in all our cases and there was no need to terminate the operation for this reason. In none of our cases was there a carotid arterial tear. However, in case there is an arterial injury (carotid or middle cerebral artery) during the course of dissection, the surgeon should be prepared for immediate arterial repair and reconstruction of the vessel. In case local reconstruction of the vessel is not possible then a long saphenous graft from the external carotid artery to the middle cerebral trunk is an alternative.

The optic nerve was compressed to varying degrees and displaced superomedially in most cases. In two cases the optic nerve was almost completely disrupted by the tumor and in one of these it was not even possible to clearly identify the nerve. In no other case was it necessary to section the optic nerve to enhance tumor exposure. In two cases

the tumor extended along the optic canal for a small distance and optic canal unroofing was necessary for tumor excision. In other cases a well-defined arachnoid sheath was found between the tumor and the optic nerve. The nerves entering the cavernous sinus were displaced inferiorly in all instances, with an intact arachnoid cover, which was subsequently reanastomosed and resulted in no adverse clinical effect, all cranial nerves were preserved intact during the operation. However, in cases where there is an inadvertent section of the nerve, neural reconstruction or repair might be considered, as useful function has been reported to have resulted following such a procedure (Sekhar et al 1989). The pituitary stalk was in close proximity to the tumor and markedly displaced in some cases but was never encased by it. None of the patients in the presented series developed postoperative pituitary dysfunction.

The operations were prolonged, as painstaking dissection of the blood vessels was necessary. The duration of the operation varied from 4 to 20 hours and was longer with

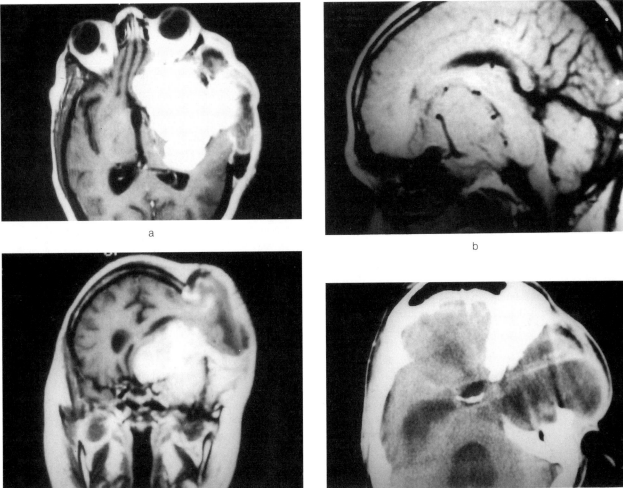

a

b

c

d

Fig. 15.8 **a** Contrast-enhanced MRI shows a massive anterior clinoidal meningioma. An attempt was made at a peripheral hospital to resect this tumor. However, on finding the tumor vascular the surgery was terminated. The bone flap was rejected to provide decompression. Following the decompression the patient worsened and developed hemiplegia. **b** MRI showed complete encasement of the internal carotid artery with narrowing of its caliber. **c** Coronal view showing herniation of the brain matter and the tumor through the craniectomy. **d** Postoperative scan showing complete tumor resection.

higher-grade tumors. With the avoidance of orbitozygomatic osteotomy the length of the operation was reduced. Vascularity of the tumors varied, most being of moderate vascularity. It was observed that adequate arrangement for replacement of blood should be made as large amounts may be lost during the exposure and resection and in the event of arterial catastrophe. Average loss of blood was about 1.5 liters. Laser and cavitron were not used in this series. In our opinion, whenever necessary the second-stage operation should be carried out at least 6–8 weeks after the first one as the brain may be 'angry' and edematous before this period, which may not permit adequate and safe retraction of the brain. In one case where

a reoperation was done 5 days after the first operation, the surgery had to be terminated for this reason.

Although there have been occasional reports showing visual improvement in a blind eye following surgery (Koos et al 1975, Rosenstien & Symon 1984), absence of recovery of vision is a more frequent observation (Ehlers & Malmros 1973, Jefferson & Azzam 1979). It has been observed that the duration of preoperative visual symptoms had a strong influence on visual outcome (Rosenstien & Symon 1984). Despite the shorter follow-up period in our series, we saw visual recovery in seven patients. In two cases visual recovery was observed in a blind eye. In no case did vision worsen after surgery.

artery, advancing the arachnoid ahead of it. This anatomic arrangement precludes dissecting the tumor from the carotid artery and middle cerebral artery branches. Group II meningiomas originate from the superior or lateral aspect of the anterior clinoid process above the segment of the carotid artery that is invested in the arachnoid of the carotid cistern, where the interfacing arachnoidal membrane continues. This membrane and, more distally, that of the sylvian cistern separate the tumor from the arterial adventitia, allowing the tumor to be dissected from the vessels even though they may be entirely engulfed. Because the optic chiasm and nerves of both Groups I and II tumors are wrapped in the arachnoidal membrane of the chiasmatic cistern, they can be microsurgically dissected. Group III meningiomas originate at the optic foramen and extend into the optic canal and to the tip of the anterior clinoid process. Generally small tumors, they appear early, with optic nerve compression and decreased visual acuity. The arachnoidal membrane is present, but because this tumor arises proximal to the chiasmatic cistern there may be no arachnoidal investment between the optic nerve and the tumor. Unfortunately, the type of tumor can be determined only during surgical dissection.

Group II accounts for approximately two-thirds of these meningiomas, which can be separated from the carotid artery, thereby allowing total removal without sacrificing the carotid artery; any tear that may occur in the artery can be repaired with sutures. For Group I tumors, I leave a small piece of tumor adhering to the artery to avoid the additional complications that stem from attempting a graft. The treatment of this residual tumor is predicated on its behavior and may include (a) merely observation; (b) stereotactic radiosurgery now that the tumor is no longer near the optic nerve and the brain stem; or (c) future surgery for carotid replacement with a graft. An unfortunate aspect of the last procedure is that the bypass requires 120 minutes to perform, and additional time may be required to remove and prepare the graft if this has not been done prior to the craniotomy. The benefits are limited to preserving ipsilateral vascularity and avoiding potential long-term effects of carotid occlusion; the procedure places patients at risk for induced complications related to establishing a graft that otherwise is not needed. Patients with absolute blood flow during test occlusion (<20 ml/100 g per minute) or strong cerebral blood flow (20–40 ml/100 g per minute) during occlusion require arterial reconstruction; the mechanisms available for cerebral protection may not compensate for this prolonged period of interrupted flow. In such patients, a preoperative prophylactic extracranial bypass is preferred if carotid sacrifice is planned or anticipated, even though it adds another operation. If a preoperative bypass was not performed and the carotid artery is injured beyond repair, then placement of a shunt should be considered (Al-Mefty et al 1990).

To avoid the risk of injury to the intracavernous carotid artery and ophthalmoplegia resulting from dissecting the cranial nerves in the cavernous sinus space, some authors advocate removal of the extracavernous portion of the tumor, with the intracavernous remnant left untouched. The reasoning is that the intracavernous portion can remain stable for years and that radiosurgery can be used to arrest progression of growth.

Admittedly, a risk of dissecting the cavernous carotid is cerebral ischemia, but the same risk arises if injury to branches of the middle cerebral artery and/or the supraclinoid carotid occurs. Because the risk of vascular injury is not eliminated by performing a procedure that stops short of dissecting the carotid, I believe that the potential of such risk is outweighed by the benefit gained by removing the tumor and the involved bone.

Although extensive radical surgery in the cavernous sinus carries a high risk of ophthalmoplegia, it is temporary, and in approximately 90% of patients preoperative function returns. Hence, if one is willing to accept immediate, but transitory, postoperative ophthalmoplegia, the prospect for preserving ocular muscle function through curative radical removal is warranted. Contrariwise, if ocular muscle function was deficient preoperatively, then, despite good surgical removal, the recovery is limited (DeMonte et al 1994).

In my experience and those of other neurosurgeons, tumor recurrence, including that of a skull base meningioma, is inversely correlated with the extent of tumor removal. Therefore, I advocate attempting to achieve Simpson Grade I or II removal during the first operation in the quest for cure and minimizing the chances of recurrence. Attaining these goals by a repeat operation is considerably less likely, and complications are much higher, especially if the patient has undergone radiation therapy.

In summary, I advocate an attempt at radical curative removal of the entire tumor and strongly believe in the value of preserving the carotid artery. If the tumor is of Goup I and its adherence to the carotid artery precludes dissection, I leave a small piece of tumor on the arterial wall for future treatment. If the carotid artery must be sacrificed, I recommend establishing a prophylactic preoperative bypass, or, if it is sacrificed beyond repair, an intraoperative interpositioned graft.

References

Al-Mefty O 1990 Clinoidal meningiomas. Journal of Neurosurgery 73: 840–849

Al-Mefty O, Khalil N, Elwany M N et al 1990 Shunt for bypass graft of the cavernous carotid artery: an anatomical and technical study. Neurosurgery 27: 721–728

DeMonte F, Smith H K, Al-Mefty O 1994 Outcome of aggressive removal of cavernous sinus meningiomas. Journal of Neurosurgery 81: 245–251

Anterior Clinoidal Meningiomas
Jacques Brotchi

Anterior clinoidal meningiomas still remain a challenge, even in the hands of very skillful neurosurgeons. These tumors must be differentiated from the sphenoid meningiomas. In 1980 (Bonnal et al), we proposed to classify sphenoid meningiomas in five groups, among which clinoidal meningiomas are the most difficult to remove. These tumors may extend upward into the cranial cavity from the dura of the cavernous sinus, the anterior clinoid process and from the internal part of the sphenoid wing. They are in close contact with the optic nerve and tract and with the carotid artery and its branches which may be shifted, stretched or encased. They may invade downward into the cavernous sinus (Brotchi & Bonnal 1991, Bonnal et al 1987).

Today, with MRI, diagnosis is rather easy. However, one should keep in mind that basal meningiomas are invasive, that hyperostotic bone means bone invaded by the tumor. That bone must be removed at operation. Therefore, a preoperative CT evaluation with bone windows remains imperative. Nevertheless, the main challenge in clinoidal meningiomas is the relationship between the tumor and carotid artery and branches. The angiogram is unable to differentiate between a stretched or an encased artery. When the carotid artery or its branches are shifted or stretched, great care must be taken in the surgical approach in order to avoid injury to the vessels whose dissection must be done from distal to proximal.

It is safer to go from middle cerebral artery, for example, to anterior clinoidal process rather than to try to find the carotid artery during separation of the tumor from its dural attachment. Al-Mefty (1990) has divided clinoidal meningiomas into three groups according to tumor–artery and tumor–optic tract relationships. He has nicely described in Groups II and III the arachnoid membrane of the carotid cistern and distally of the sylvian cistern which separates the tumor from the sylvian adventitia, making dissection possible, even with encased vessels. This is explained by the superior and lateral implantation of the tumor on the clinoid process. In Group I, the tumor grows from the inferior aspect of the anterior clinoid, enwrapping the carotid artery and adhering to the adventitia. There is no plane between the tumor and the artery. In Group I, radical removal without injury of the vessel is impossible. In that situation, morbidity and mortality are not low and the surgeon's aggressivity should be tempered. On the other hand, Al-Mefty's Group II and III tumors should be totally removed during the first surgical procedure. Previous surgery violates the arachnoid membrane, and makes finding of an adequate plane of dissection difficult. This explains why reoperation is so difficult in clinoid meningiomas, and why the dissection of vessels and nerve becomes harder with every new operation. Therefore, we propose that radical removal of the tumor be performed during the first surgical procedure. To us, total removal means resection of the tumor, dura and the involved bone (anterior clinoid process).

However, one should keep in mind the quality of the patient's life, which depends a great deal on the surgeon's experience (Brotchi et al 1991). Those who have a great mastery over skull base tumor surgery will be able to go further and be more radical in tumor resection and can perform the operation with less risk than others with less experience. Nevertheless, when the tumor enters the cavernous sinus, one should debate the justification of pursuing or to stopping surgery.

Sometimes, dissection and resection of a tumor bud may be possible from inside the cavernous sinus but usually a complete removal without injuring the cranial nerves is impossible. When there is no preoperative diplopia, we prefer to stop rather than induce one. We also prefer to stop when we do not find an adequate plane of cleavage between the carotid artery and tumor (Al-Mefty's type I). In that situation, we advocate radiosurgery on the small residual part of the tumor (when a security of 5 mm exists between optic tract and tumor) in order to respect the quality of life of the patient.

References

Al-Mefty O 1990 Clinoidal meningiomas. Journal of Neurosurgery 73: 840–849

Bonnal J, Thibaut A, Brotchi J et al 1980 Invading meningiomas of the sphenoid ridge. Journal of Neurosurgery 53: 587–599

Bonnal J, Brotchi J, Born J 1987 Meningiomas of the sphenoid wings. In: Sekhar L N, Schramm V L (eds) Tumors of the cranial base: diagnosis and treatment. Futura, Mount Kisco, NY, pp 373–392

Brotchi J, Bonnal J 1991 Lateral and middle sphenoid wing meningiomas. In: Al-Mefty O (ed) Meningiomas. Raven Press, New York, pp 413–425

Brotchi J, Levivier M, Raftopoulos C et al 1991 Invading meningiomas of sphenoid wings: what must we know before surgery? Acta Neurochirurgica (Suppl) 53: 98–100

Surgical management of giant pituitary tumors

16

Atul Goel Trimurti Nadkarni Shigeaki Kobayashi

Surgical treatment of giant pituitary tumors is amongst the most difficult and controversial neurosurgical subjects. While smaller tumors are relatively easily and completely excised, surgical therapy for massive tumors can be a difficult undertaking. We have treated 30 cases of giant pituitary tumors over a 5-year period and this experience is analyzed to bring out the complexities of management of these cases.

CLASSIFICATION (Goel & Nadkarni 1996)

Various classifications of pituitary tumors have been proposed on the basis of size, radiographic appearance, cytogenesis, staining properties and endocrine function. There is no consensus regarding the terminology to be used in describing these large pituitary tumors. The histological characters do not usually correlate well with the gross features (Landolt & Wilson 1982, Russell & Rubenstein 1977). Despite the huge size they are frequently histologically benign. Bailey classified them as malignant adenomas on the basis of rapid progression of symptoms and anatomic invasiveness (Bailey & Cutler 1940). Feiring et al (1953) preferred the term 'carcinoma'. Metastasis has been seen, but this does not generally match with the malignant potential of the cells and the size of the lesion (Kernohan & Sayre 1956, Lundberg et al 1977, Symon et al 1979, Wise et al 1955). Martins et al (1965) prefer to call those tumors which invade contiguous structures, but do not metastasize, invasive pituitary adenomas, the term carcinoma being reserved for tumors with blood-borne metastases. Hardy (1979) classified pituitary tumors on the basis of their biologic behavior. According to this classification grade III refers to tumors having localized invasion of the floor of the sella, grade IV indicates diffuse invasion and grade V indicates diffuse metastases. Some authors refer to pituitary tumors with a size in excess of 40 mm from the midpoint of the jugum sphenoidale, or those extending less than 6 mm from the foramen of Monroe, as 'giant' irrespective of their invasiveness (Fisher et al 1993). Jefferson

(1940) observed an incidence of invasive adenoma in about 6% of all cases.

In our series, those pituitary tumors have been considered as 'giant' which transgressed the sellar and diaphragma sellae boundaries and measured more than 5 cm in maximum diameter. These tumors were those which were considered to be unsuitable for or could not be satisfactorily resected by a transsphenoidal surgical route.

ANATOMICAL CONSIDERATIONS

The pituitary tumors are in general slow-growing tumors. Some pituitary tumors attain a giant size. Once the tumor emerges out of the pituitary capsule, it mushrooms out into the available crevices. As the sella turcica is a relatively compact and bony enclosure for the pituitary gland, the usual tendency for these tumors is to grow in a superior direction and elevate the diaphragma sellae (Fig. 16.1a). Supradiaphragmatic extension will probably depend on the size of the hiatus in the diaphragma sellae. Progressive intrasellar expansion may erode the walls of the sella turcica and undermine and later erode the clinoid processes by virtue of increasing pressure. Actual transgression of the tumor through the dura of the sellar floor is a relatively rare feature. Lateral expansion of the tumor, displacement of the thin medial dural wall of the cavernous sinus and later invasion (Fig. 16.1b) are relatively common (Ahmadi et al 1985, Fahlbusch & Buchfelder 1988, Nichols et al 1988). The medial wall of the cavernous sinus gives way relatively easily to the expanding tumor. The ease with which these tumors invade into the cavernous sinus may provide additional support to the hypothesis that the medial wall of the cavernous sinus is not actually 'dural'. The tumor invades into the available venous spaces in the cavernous sinus, surrounds the carotid artery and bloats up the cavernous sinus. The lateral dural wall of the cavernous sinus being thick and multilayered resists any lateral spread of the tumor. The lateral and superior walls of the cavernous sinus are frequently seen to be

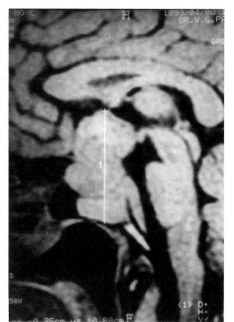

a

b

Fig. 16.1 **a** Sagittal view showing the large sellar tumor. The tumor has suprasellar extension which is infradiaphragmatic. **b** The large tumor has bilateral cavernous sinus and suprasellar infradiaphragmatic extension. The tumor has encased both the carotid arteries but the lumen is not narrowed.

bloated with tumor (Fig. 16.1b) but actual transgression of these dural walls was not seen in our series, nor has it been reported in the literature. Eccentric spread of the tumor and unilateral involvement of the cavernous sinus is more common (Scotti et al 1988). Some authors have reported infracavernous sinus spread of the tumor, wherein the medial and inferior wall of the cavernous sinus was displaced superiorly (Ahmadi et al 1985, Fahlbusch & Buchfelder 1988). Such an extension was not seen in this series.

Suprasellar extension of the tumor needs to be clearly differentiated from supradiaphragmatic extension as it has implications in planning the surgical approach. Frequently the diaphragma sellae is lifted superiorly by the tumor. The

remarkable stretchability and the resistance offered by the dural walls can be appreciated in this situation. The tumor escapes through the hiatus in the diaphragma sellae. Once in the suprasellar cistern the tumor displaces the chiasma and optic nerves superiorly and the enlarging tumor expands into the areas of least resistance. The pattern of expansion is usually under the chiasm and between the optic nerves, and through the corridors between the optic nerves and carotid artery and its branches the tumor either overflows into the middle fossa base or in the subfrontal region (Fig. 16.2). Posterior extension in the interpeduncular fossa and prepontine region is relatively rare. In our series such a posterior extension was seen in three cases (Fig. 16.3). The barrier provided by Lilequist's membrane

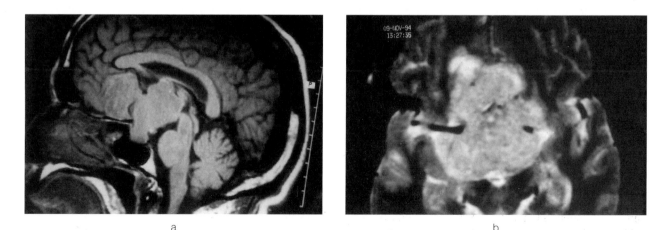

a

b

Fig. 16.2 **a** MRI shows a massive suprasellar and subfrontal extension of the tumor. The sellar part is relatively insignificant. **b** MRI shows encasement of bilateral supraclinoid internal carotid arteries and anterior cerebral artery complex by the tumor.

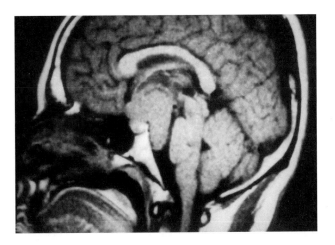

Fig. 16.3 The tumor has posterior fossa extension.

was not traversed by the tumor in any case. Intraparenchymal extension of the tumor is rare. Tumor invading through the sellar floor dura, sella turcica and the adjacent bones may extend into the nasopharynx or sphenoid and/or ethmoid sinuses (Fig. 16.4). Extension of tumor may occur posteroinferiorly in the retropharyngeal space by erosion of the clivus and petrous apices. Larger tumors may extend up to the foramen magnum (Fig. 16.4a). Some tumors preferentially spread through the hiatus in the diaphragma sellae into the suprasellar compartment, some invade into the cavernous sinuses, and some spread anteriorly through the sellar floor into the sphenoid sinus. The exact reason for the extension into a particular direction is not known: probably the site of origin of the tumor determined the nature of spread of these tumors. In this series only two tumors were hormonally active and

presented with gross acromegaly. In one of these acromegalic patients the tumor spread was predominantly in the sphenoid sinus and nasopharynx (Fig. 16.4). Considering the origin of the hormonally active tumors from the anterior pituitary, anterior spread of the tumor may have some correlation. Cystic changes within the tumor have been occasionally reported. However, in our cases the cyst formation was seen only at the periphery of the tumor in three cases. In all these cases it was believed that this was secondary to intraventricular extension of the tumor and loculation of a part of the ventricle (Fig. 16.5a,b). The soft nature of the tumors reflects on the infrequent cranial nerve deficits. The character of the tumor is like an epidermoid tumor, wherein the tumor spreads in the available spaces, engulfing or encircling the blood vessels and cranial nerves without actually invading these structures, rarely compromising the lumen of the artery and resulting in only moderate displacements. Invasion of pituitary adenomas into the walls of blood vessels has been reported, but such an infiltration extends no deeper than the adventitial layer. Considering the location of the VIth nerve in relation to the carotid artery, the complete encasement of this nerve appears to be as frequent as the encasement of the carotid artery. Cranial nerves III–V in the lateral dural wall of the cavernous sinus are displaced as the tumor occupies the available venous sinusoidal spaces and crevices in the cavernous sinus and distends them (Fig. 16.6). The pattern of invasion of the venous spaces of the cavernous sinus by the tumor is suggestive of a sinusoidal rather than a plexiform configuration of the veins of the cavernous sinus (Figs 16.7,16.8).

Preoperative diagnosis of the histological nature of the tumor on the basis of clinical parameters and radiological investigation is important to determine the extent of expo-

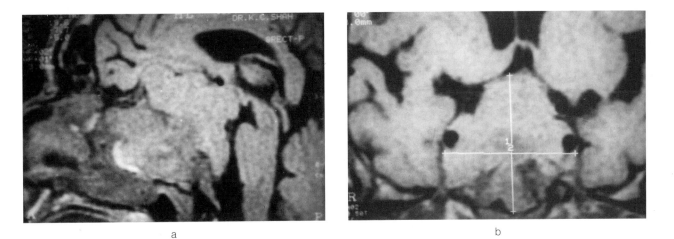

a   b

Fig. 16.4 **a** MRI showing the massive tumor with infrasellar and suprasellar extensions. **b** MRI (coronal view) shows the giant pituitary tumor. The internal carotid arteries in their course through the cavernous sinus are displaced laterally. The cavernous sinus is not invaded in this case.

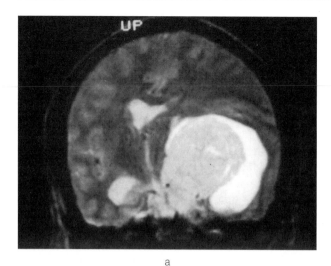

a

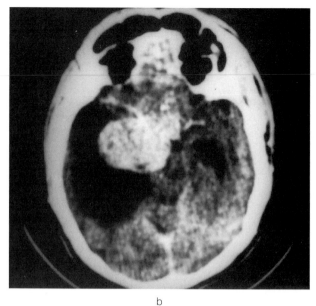

b

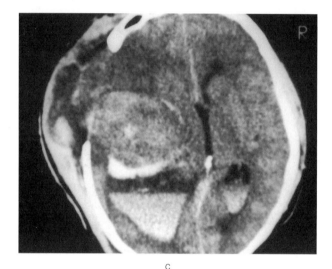

c

Fig. 16.5 a MRI (T2-weighted image) shows sellar tumor with large suprasellar extension. The tumor is seen to occupy and dilate the ipsilateral temporal horn. The hyperintensity of CSF in the 'loculated' ventricle is more marked when compared to contralateral normal ventricular fluid. **b** Contrast-enhanced CT scan showing the suprasellar part of the tumor and the loculated ventricle. **c** Postoperative non-enhanced CT scan showing the markedly dilated hyerdense tumor which now reaches the edge of the craniectomy. The posterior edge of the tumor shows blood clot. Blood level is seen in both occipital horns. The patient was re-explored within 45 minutes of wound closure. Craniectomy was necessary as large brain swelling did not permit dural closure and bone flap replacement.

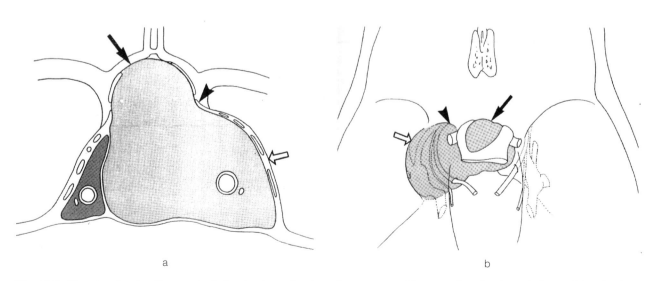

a

b

Fig. 16.6   Drawing showing the more typical extensions of a giant pituitary tumor. The tumor invades through the medial wall of the cavernous sinus and engulfs the carotid artery and the VIth nerve and displaces the lateral wall with its contained nerves. The white arrow shows that in a lateral approach to the cavernous sinus the markedly stretched cranial nerves are encountered early and possibilities of damage are greater. The black arrowhead shows an ipsilateral subfrontal approach. The tumor involving the cavernous sinus is difficult to approach due to the angulation necessary. Black long arrow shows a contralateral subfrontal approach. The angle of the approach provides a better opportunity to deal with intracavernous extension of the tumor.

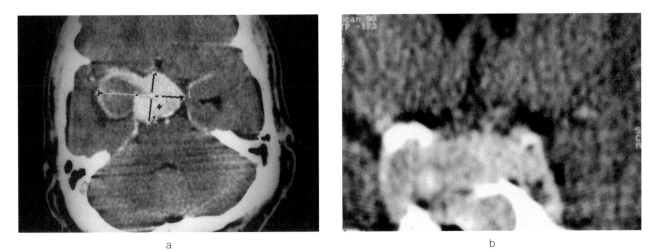

Fig. 16.7 **a** Contrast-enhanced CT scan shows a large pituitary tumor which has invaded into the cavernous sinus. The medial temporal extension is entirely intracavernous. A contralateral subfrontal approach was suitable to radically resect this tumor. **b** Coronal view showing the pituitary tumor with cavernous sinus invasion. The right cavernous sinus is definitely involved, while the involvement of the left cavernous sinus is not clear. MRI would clarify the invasion of the cavernous sinus by showing the relationship to the internal carotid artery.

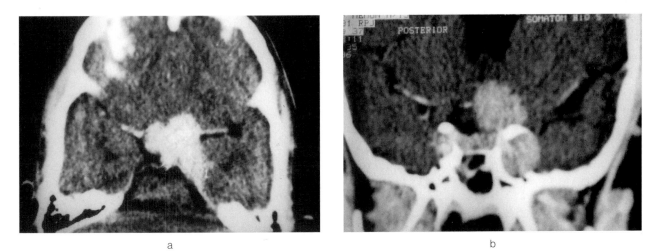

Fig. 16.8 **a** CT scan showing the pituitary tumor involving the cavernous sinus. **b** Coronal view of the scan shows unilateral involvement of the cavernous sinus. The suprasellar portion of the tumor is infradiaphragmatic.

sure that would be necessary, direction of the surgical approach, feasibility of radical resection of the tumor and prognosticating the ultimate outcome. Unfortunately both clinical and radiological investigations can be misleading and the impression about a pituitary tumor is more often presumptive (Feiring et al 1953).

CLINICAL FEATURES

The clinical features of our series of patients are summarized in Tables 16.1–16.3. There were 24 men (80%) and

six women (20%). The age range was 16–60 years (average age 33 years). The age distribution is shown in the Table 16.1.

Presenting symptoms and signs

Table 16.2 shows the principal presenting symptoms. The average duration of symptoms prior to admission was 21 months. The most common complaint on admission was impairment of vision (24 patients). There was no visual impairment in six patients. The visual impairment was

Table 16.1   Age distribution

Age (years)	Number
0–10	–
11–20	6
21–30	9
31–40	8
41–50	6
51–60	1
	30

Table 16.2   Principle presenting symptoms

Symptom	Number of patients
Loss of vision	24
Headaches	20
Vomiting	11
Behavioral disturbances	8
Diplopia	7
Urgency of micturition	4
Retrobulbar pain	6
Visual blackout	5
Convulsions	3
Altered sensorium	2
Fatigue, no desire to work	5

classified into mild and significant categories. By mild visual loss it is meant that the vision was at least 6/60 (in meters) and by significant visual loss it is meant that vision was limited to only finger counting. In six patients there was bilateral mild visual deficit. Sixteen patients had significant visual deficits. Nine had unilateral and seven had bilateral significant visual impairment. Two patients were blind in both eyes. Two patients had homonymous hemianopia while in all others a predominantly temporal field defect was observed. Fundoscopy showed mild to severe primary optic atrophy in all eyes with visual impairment. Diplopia, retro-orbital pain and visual blackouts were other vision-related symptoms (Table 16.2). At presentation three patients had a IIIrd cranial nerve paresis. One patient had both Vth and VIth nerve paresis. No other focal neurological deficit was observed. Four patients had irregular menstrual periods. Five patients had easy fatiguability and lack of desire to work. Behavioral alterations such as irritability, restlessness, mental slowing and irrelevance were noted in eight patients. Four patients had urgency of micturition, despite the normal volume of urine output.

Physical findings

Physical examination was done to rule out hormonal dysfunction. Two patients were acromegalic and thyrotoxic.

Table 16.3   Visual follow-up

Follow-up time (in months)		preop. vision R	L	postop. vision R	L	follow-up vision R	L
1.	3	2ft	PL	8ft	PL	6/60	PL
2.	48	6/6	6/6	6/6	6/6	6/6	6/6
3.	12	6/9	6/9	6/9	6/9	6/9	6/9
4.	36	10ft	6/9	10ft	6/9	10ft	6/9
5.	21	6/60	6ft	6/18	PL	6/9	PL
6.	12	3ft	6ft	3ft	6ft	6/9	6/12
7.	12	6/36	MB	6/60	MB	10ft	PL
8.	9	6/24	2ft	6/24	6ft	6/6	6/36
9.	1	6/60	6/18	6/36	6/18	6/24	6/18
10.	3	6/60	6/60	6/12	6/12	6/12	6/12
11.	–	6/12	6/18	6/12	6/18	–	–
12.	–	No PL	6/24	No PL	6/24	–	–
13.	36	No PL	No PL	No PL	No PL	No PL	No PL
14.	12	6/6	6/6	6/6	6/6	6/6	6/6
15.	20	6/60	6/12	6/36	6/12	6/36	6/12
16.	9	PL	6ft	2ft	8ft	6/60	6/36
17.	12	4ft	6ft	6/60	6/60	6/36	6/24
18.	2	6/6	6/6	6/6	6/6	6/6	6/6
19.	2	3ft	6/60	6ft	8ft	6/36	6/36
20.	12	MB	2ft	MB	2ft	MB	2ft
21.	44	6/6	6/6	6/6	6/6	6/9	6/9
22.	1	6/60	6/60	6/24	6/24	6/24	6/24
23.	2	6/36	6ft	6/60	3ft	8ft	MB
24.	4	No PL	2ft	No PL	2ft	No PL	6ft

Retarded physical growth, sparse secondary sexual characters and obesity were noted in five patients.

Discussion

Invasive pituitary adenomas tend to occur more frequently in a young age group and in males (Fraioli et al 1990). In our series 80% of cases were males. Various authors have commented upon lack of correlation between the size of the tumor and clinical manifestations (Feiring et al 1953, Martins et al 1965). In our series the average duration of symptoms was 21 months. Hormonally active tumors manfest clinically early, frequently by altering the endocrine status and sometimes due to pressure symptoms over the optic apparatus. The adrenocorticotropic hormone (ACTH)-producing tumors are usually detected when they are microadenomas due to the intensity of clinical manifestations (Rovit & Duane 1969). Growth hormone- and prolactin-producing tumors can sometimes become very large prior to their clinical and radiological detection. Decreased incidence of hypopituitarism in patients with invasive tumors may be due to the decompressive effect as a result of escape of the tumor from the sella turcica (Martins et al 1965).

Presentation with unilateral oculomotor palsy was seen in three patients. In these cases the involvement appeared to be due to distortion of the precavernous segment of the nerve rather than displacement in its course in the cavernous sinus. Although King stressed the importance of facial pain secondary to involvement of the branches of the trigeminal nerve as an important symptom in recognition of invasive pituitary adenomas (King 1951), this feature was observed in none of our cases wherein the cavernous sinus was involved. While the visual field defects have frequently been seen to be characteristic in non-invasive tumors, visual deficits in giant tumors have not been recorded to be consistent. Headaches, vomiting and behavioral disturbances were the other prominent presenting symptoms in our series.

DIAGNOSTIC STUDIES

In all our patients either computed tomography (CT) scan or magnetic resonance imaging (MRI) or both of these investigations were performed. CT scan showed an iso- to hyperdense, uniformly enhancing mass. Suprasellar extensions were noted to be either multinodular or irregular in outline. MRI showed vividly the optic nerve–chiasm apparatus compression and displacement, encasement of carotid artery, displacement of major vessels and cavernous sinus involvement. In one case there was no sellar involvement, the entire tumor being intracranial in the region of the lesser wing of the sphenoid bone (Goel et al 1990) (Fig. 16.9). All the other tumors had a sellar and

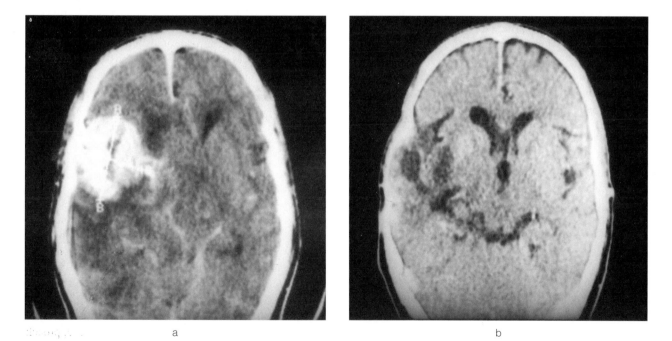

a   b

Fig. 16.9   a Contrast-enhanced scan showing the large tumor in the region of the lesser wing of the sphenoid bone. The tumor was extra-axial and the pattern of enhancement resembled a meningioma on scan. Tumor surrounding edema and the extensive mass effect is observed. **b** Postradiation therapy picture shows no evidence of the tumor. Postoperative changes are seen. Ipsilateral ventricle is mildly dilated.

parasellar extension. In six cases the sellar involvement by the tumor was relatively insignificant. In 24 cases the tumor extended superiorly and the floor of third ventricle was elevated. The obstruction at this level resulted in significant hydrocephalus in four cases. In eight patients the tumor extended into the middle fossa while in five patients there was a subfrontal spread (Fig. 16.2). In three cases there was a retrosellar posterior fossa extension (Fig. 16.3). Nine patients had a unilateral (Fig. 16.7) while four cases had bilateral cavernous sinus involvement (Fig. 16.8). In all these cases the internal carotid artery in the cavernous sinus was encased by the tumor. In three patients the tumor did not encase the intracavernous carotid, suggesting that the medial wall of the cavernous sinus was displaced laterally. The sellar floor was breached in four cases and the nasopharynx was involved in two (Fig. 16.4). Calcification was not seen in any tumor. A cyst on the superolateral surface of the tumor was seen in three cases (Fig. 16.5). The fluid content was xanthochromic in all cases and the protein content was high. In all these cases the cyst appeared to be secondary to loculation of the lateral ventricle. The supraclinoid internal carotid artery and its branches were at least partially engulfed in 14 cases (Fig. 16.2a,b). The diameter of the internal carotid artery was not compromised in any of these cases. In four cases the tumor had an hour-glass appearance with a constriction at the level of the diaphragm. In three cases the tumor invaded into the parenchyma of the brain. The invasion appeared to be through the choroidal fissure in two cases where the tumor invaded into the temporal horn (Fig. 16.5). In one case the exact site of frontal parenchymal invasion could not be clearly seen (only CT scan was done).

Twenty-three patients underwent preoperative evaluation of hormonal blood levels by estimation of serum triodothyronine (T3), thyroxine (T4) and thyroid stimulating hormone (TSH), cortisol, prolactin and growth hormone levels. In two patients the manifestations of hormonal hyperactivity in the form of acromegaly and thyrotoxicity tumor were seen. In five patients hormonal blood levels were estimated in the postoperative phase. In two patients such an assessment could not be made. Necessary correction by replacement therapy was done prior to and after the surgery.

Discussion

As the anatomical spread of the lesion is unpredictable, the radiological criterion for diagnosis of pituitary adenomas can sometimes be misleading. The usually encountered solid consistency, bright enhancement on contrast administration, irregular borders, encasement of arteries without compromise of their lumen (as seen on MRI) in the cav-

ernous sinus (Fig. 16.1) and in the suprasellar region (Fig. 16.2) can provide a reasonable clue in favor of pituitary tumors (Kaufman et al 1987, Nichols et al 1988, Scotti et al 1988, Stiener et al 1989). The sellar component of the tumor may sometimes be relatively small and insignificant (Fig. 16.2). However, extension of the lesion in the sella and its gross enlargement can help in differentiating these tumors. Prediction of the consistency of the tumor on CT scanning and MRI although very important in planning the surgical route can be difficult (Kaufman et al 1987). The presence of a large tumor, its vascular relationships and diffuse extensions with relatively subtle neurological signs can lead to a presumption of its soft nature. The involvement of the cavernous sinus can vary from displacement and compression of its medial wall to gross invasion into the sinus (Knosp et al 1991, Lundberg et al 1977, Martins et al 1965, Newton et al 1962, Scotti et al 1988). The encasement of the intracavernous carotid artery by the tumor as seen on MRI has been frequently reported to be a real indicator of cavernous sinus invasion.

MANAGEMENT

Giant pituitary tumors are relatively rare, histologically benign and slow-growing tumors. Due to the characteristic nature, frequently encountered soft consistency and invasive pattern of growth, the tumors are usually large when first diagnosed and have relatively innocuous presenting symptoms. The location of these tumors in proximity to vital neural and vascular structures and widespread extensions makes radical surgical removal difficult and the ultimate clinical course 'malignant'. Satisfactory surgical treatment of giant pituitary tumors continues to be difficult and the general outcome of such tumors has been observed to be dismal (Ahmadi et al 1965, Fahlbusch & Buchfelder 1988. Hashimoto & Kikuchi 1990, Knosp et al 1991, Symon et al 1979, Wilson 1979).

Surgical treatment

Patients underwent surgery by a frontal craniotomy (13 patients), bifrontal craniotomy (three patients), frontotemporal craniotomy (13 patients), and via a transfrontal air sinus approach (one patient). In three of these patients an initial attempt towards tumor resection was made by the transsphenoidal route. In the operations performed after 1992, basal frontal and basal pterional approaches were used. In two patients a contralateral subfrontal approach was adopted in an attempt to radically excise the cavernous sinus extension of the tumor. The aim of the surgery was radical resection of the tumor in all cases. Significant excision of the tumor was achieved ensuring decompression of the chiasm and optic nerves in all patients. In three patients additional transsphenoidal surgery was performed to excise the sellar part of the tumor. The tumor had a variegated consistency from soft and easily suckable to firm. 'Elastic' and relatively tough tumors with interlacing fibrous bands were encountered in four patients. Evidence of hemorrhage was seen within four tumors. In three patients a cerebrospinal fluid (CSF) diversionary shunt procedure for associated hydrocephalus was carried out (Goel 1995a).

Operative and postoperative management

During surgery, three patients developed an acute brain swelling. In these patients frontal polectomy in one and temporal polectomy in two respectively had to be done to check for clots in the operative fields. A swollen tumor secondary to its probable hemorrhagic infarction was noticed in these cases. The tumor was resected further. All these patients recovered well after the surgery.

In this series there were six deaths in the postoperative phase. Two patients deteriorated in sensorium after surgery. One worsened to deep unconsciousness about 45 minutes after surgery and in the other patient vision was noticed to have worsened 12 hours after surgery. Both these patients were re-explored. Huge tumor swelling secondary to their hemorrhagic infarction was observed (Goel 1995b). Both these patients had a stormy post-re-exploration course and eventually died (Fig. 16.5c). Two patients who developed contralateral hemiplegia and aphasia following surgery on the dominant side subsequently died. Postmortem examination revealed the presence of capsular and putaminal infarcts in these patients. One patient recovered from anesthesia in an unconscious state. Postoperative scanning showed only diffuse cerebral edema. He later developed bronchopneumonia and died. One patient with diabetes and hypertension developed postoperative CSF fistula and meningitis. In this patient a transfrontal sinus approach had been adopted. He was re-explored and the dural defect in the region of the planum sphenoidale and cribriform plate was repaired (Goel 1994, Goel & Gahankari 1995). However, he later developed convulsions and worsened in sensorium and ultimately died.

The other major postoperative complications in this series include IIIrd cranial nerve palsy in four and VIth nerve palsy in one patient. One of these patients had a combined IIIrd and VIth nerve deficit leading to total ophthalmoplegia. One patient had contralateral moderate hemiparesis. All these postoperative deficits have shown at least partial recovery over the period. Two patients developed diabetes insipidus which responded well to medical therapy, the patients requiring life-long replacement. The

internal carotid artery was accidentally lacerated in one patient. The rent was repaired uneventfully. Two patients developed CSF rhinorrhea, 2 months and 2 years after surgery and radiation therapy, both requiring a transethmoidal repair.

All tumors were confirmed on histological examination to be pituitary adenomas. There was no evidence of malignancy in any case.

Follow-up and results

Follow-up data were obtained in 22 patients by clinical review and notification at periodic intervals ranging from 1 to 48 months (mean 13 months). On postoperative MRI there was some tumor residue in all cases. One patient a year after surgery had status epilepticus, lapsed into coma and expired. In this patient vision progressively worsened and there was an increase in tumor size. One patient with a large residual tumor has been followed up for 3 years. He has been admitted for grand mal seizures three times. Other than this problem, he has remained stable, vision having improved when compared to the preoperative status. The postoperative and follow-up visual status is shown in Table 16.3. On follow-up assessment, as compared to the preoperative status, vision had worsened in four, remained unchanged in seven, and improved in 11 patients. There was bilateral improvement of vision in seven cases and unilateral improvement in four cases. Twenty-two patients completed radiation therapy. In three patients the residual tumor reduced significantly in size following radiotherapy. Two patients with irregular menses started getting regular periods. Preoperative hormone replacement therapy was continued in nine patients. Following surgery an additional two patients needed steroids, one needed thyroxine, and in three both steroid and thyroxine replacement was necessary. Two patients who developed diabetes insipidus needed life-long vasopressin. In four patients the hormonal status had improved during the follow-up assessment. In the relatively short duration of follow-up study, in two patients there was increase in the size of the residual tumor.

Discussion

As in most cases oculomotor function is preserved intact prior to surgery, the principal goal is to decompress the visual apparatus, maintain the oculomotor function and to reduce the tumor bulk as much as possible. In the presented series an attempt was made to radically excise all the tumors. However, despite the soft consistency, due to its invasive nature, extensions into various crevices, encasement of nerves and vessels, and high vascularity, radical

Lawson L J 1958 Intranasal chromophobe adenocarcinoma: report of a case. Archives of Otolaryngology (Chicago) 68: 704–709

Lundberg P O, Drettner B, Hemmingsson A et al 1977 The invasive pituitary adenoma: a prolactin-producing tumor. Archives of Neurology 34: 742–749

Martins A N, Hayes G J, Kempe L G 1965 Invasive pituitary adenomas. Journal of Neurosurgery 22: 268–276

Mohanty S, Tandon P N, Banerji A K et al 1977 Hemorrhage into pituitary adenomas. Journal of Neurology Neurosurgery and Psychiatry 40: 987–991

Newton T H, Burhenne H J, Palubinskas A J 1962 Primary carcinoma of the pituitary. American Journal of Roentgenology 87: 110–120

Nichols D A, Laws E R, Houser O W et al 1988 Comparison of MRI and computed tomography in the preoperative evaluation of pituitary adenomas. Neurosurgery 22: 380–385

Rothman L M, Sher J, Quencer R M et al 1976 Intracranial ectopic pituitary adenoma. Journal of Neurosurgery 44: 96–99

Rovit R L, Duane T D 1969 Cushing's syndrome and pituitary tumors: pathophysiology and ocular manifestations of ACTH-secreting pituitary adenomas. American Journal of Medicine 46: 416–427

Rovit R L, Fien J M 1972 Pituitary apoplexy: a review and reappraisal. Journal of Neurosurgery 37: 280–288

Russell D S, Rubenstein L J 1977 Tumors of adenohypophysis. In: Pathology of tumors of the nervous system (4th edn). Williams & Wilkins, Baltimore, pp 312–323

Scotti G, Yu CY, Dillon W P et al 1988 MR imaging of cavernous sinus involvement by pituitary adenomas. American Journal of Neuroradiology 9: 657–664

Sieck J O, Niles N L, Jinkins J R et al 1986 Extrasellar prolactinomas: successful management of 24 patients using bromocriptine. Hormone Research 23: 167–176

Stiener E, Imhof H, Knosp E 1989 GD-DTPA enhanced high resolution MR imaging of pituitary adenomas. RadioGraphics 4: 587–598

Symon L, Mohanty S 1982 Hemorrhage in pituitary tumors. Acta Neurochirurgica (Wien) 65: 41–49

Symon L, Jakubowski J, Kendall B 1979 Surgical treatment of giant pituitary adenomas. Journal of Neurology, Neurosurgery and Psychiatry 42: 973–982

Terry R D, Hayams V J, Davidoff L M 1959 Combined non-metastasizing fibrosarcoma and chromophobe tumor of the pituitary. Cancer 12: 791–798

Wilson C B 1979 Neurosurgical management of large and invasive pituitary tumors. In: Tindall G T, Collins W F (eds). Clinical management of pituitary disorders. Raven Press, New York, pp 335–342

Wise B L, Brown H A, Naffziger H C et al 1955 Pituitary adenomas, carcinomas, and craniopharyngiomas. Surgery, Gynecology and Obstetrics 101: 185–193

Surgery for Giant Pituitary Adenomas
Edward R. Laws

The authors have presented an outstanding review of the subject of giant pituitary adenoma and have presented a series with very good outcome. Most of the important points about the surgical management of these unusual lesions have been made, but several are worthy of re-emphasis.

We would agree completely with the definition of giant adenomas, that is, pituitary tumors that have at least one dimension 5 cm or more in length, and transgressing the boundaries of the sella. Although the size and apparent invasiveness of these tumors make them appear to be highly aggressive and dangerous lesions, the fact is that very few are actually malignant. In order to reach such a large size, these pituitary tumors must grow rather slowly so as not to produce symptoms that direct the patient toward early medical intervention. In most cases, there has been a significant delay in diagnosis because of the lack of active hormone secretion. For most of these tumors, the primary incidence is in men of a relatively older age. Occasionally, a giant adenoma will represent the rapid growth and expansion of a previously developed smaller-sized tumor undergoing a malignant degeneration. This is unusual, however, and most tumors have reached giant size simply by slow and steady, locally invasive growth. It is important to recognize that virtually all of these tumors are basically invasive lesions and involve the dura and bone at the base of the skull. For that reason, it is essentially impossible to achieve a 'total' surgical removal and this fact must be considered when planning the method and extent of surgical intervention. The basic invasiveness of giant pituitary adenomas tends to determine both the clinical symptoms at the time of presentation and the difficulties involved in the surgical removal of these lesions. When a giant tumor extends in a parasellar fashion to involve the cavernous sinus, it can produce cranial nerve involvement, most frequently numbness and occasionally pain from involvement of the trigeminal nerve. More commonly, patients present with evidence of suprasellar extension with involvement of the trigeminal nerve. More commonly, patients present with evidence of suprasellar extension with involvement of the optic tracts. A homonymous hemianopsia indicative of optic tract compression is frequently seen with giant adenomas and reflects the extent of intracranial involvement. Many giant tumors actually surround the cavernous portion of the carotid artery and may extend in the suprasellar space to surround branches of the circle of Willis. As mentioned, on rare occasions, there may be direct invasion of cranial nerves, the optic nerves or the adventitia of major arteries. The intimate involvement of the tumor with these vital structures makes surgical management particularly hazardous in giant adenomas. These same features also make it unlikely that surgery alone would provide a lasting cure of these tumors, and for that reason a combined program of management is usually recommended.

From the standpoint of immunocytochemical classification, most giant pituitary adenomas fall into the non-functioning group consisting of null cell adenomas, oncocytomas and gonadotropin adenomas. Occasionally, a silent ACTH adenoma can achieve giant size. Among the endocrine active tumors, prolactinomas are the ones most likely to achieve giant size. Very rarely giant adenomas may be seen in the setting of Nelson's syndrome. Cushing's disease or acromegaly, but these situations are extremely rare, as the endocrine disease usually alerts the physicians to the presence of the tumor before it reaches massive proportions.

From a technical standpoint, the choice of surgical management is guided by some of the principles mentioned above. Because virtually all of these tumors are surgically incurable, the goal of the operation should be thorough decompression of the intracranial and cavernous sinus structures that are involved, and a debulking of the tumor mass itself. Because 94% of pituitary tumors are soft in consistency, it is usually our practice to treat giant adenomas using a transsphenoidal approach as the initial surgical choice. This, of course, depends upon both the type of clinical presentation and the course of clinical symptoms. If a patient presents with rapidly failing vision and the major portion of the tumor is intracranial, then we would surely agree that a craniotomy designed to decompress the optic nerves and chiasm as quickly and efficiently as possible would be the procedure of choice. In other situations, where the pace of visual loss is slow, where the sella itself is grossly enlarged, and where a careful transsphenoidal approach might be acceptable, we would begin using transsphenoidal access with the hope of removing a large amount of soft tumor. Technical adjuncts to this type of transsphenoidal surgery include the use of an indwelling lumbar catheter so that air can be injected to increase intracranial pressure and push the tumor down and also to visualize the superior aspect of the tumor with intraoperative fluoroscopy. Occasionally, bilateral jugular compression during the operation can achieve the same goal of pushing the tumor down into the sphenoidal region. Careful suprasellar dissection can be guided by intraoperative fluoroscopy as well. If no intraoperative CSF leak develops, then the sella can be left decompressed so that the superior aspects of the tumor may ultimately descend into the region of the enlarged sella. On the other hand, if the tumor is firm or if a satisfactory removal of the intracranial portion cannot be carried out using the transsphenoidal approach, it is

necessary then to plan a subsequent or immediate craniotomy and, under these circumstances, a careful and compulsive repair of the sella is absolutely essential in order to prevent CSF leaks after the craniotomy. We usually accomplish this using fat taken from the right lower quadrant of the abdomen, carefully packed in the sella and secured in place with a large epidurally placed plate of nasal bone or cartilage to support the fat graft.

When a craniotomy is necessary, we ordinarily recommend either an extended subfrontal approach or a large frontotemporal approach, usually on the side of worse vision. The goal of surgery is to decompress the optic apparatus, the foramen of Monroe and the third ventricle, with an attempt at reversing visual loss, eliminating hydrocephalus and hypothalamic compression, and removal of tumor from around the vessels of the circle of Willis.

Regardless of approach, it is certainly true that if intracranial tumor is left behind, the risk of both postoperative hemorrhage and postoperative cerebral edema increase significantly. For those reasons, the removal of the tumor must be as thorough as possible.

Adjunctive therapy is desirable for most giant adenomas as the surgical removal of these lesions ordinarily is more or less incomplete and the risk of eventual recurrence is high. For prolactin adenomas, treatment with a dopamine agonist such as bromocriptine is certainly in order. Very occasionally, a giant prolactin adenoma can be satisfactorily treated with medical therapy alone, although the shrinkage of such a tumor usually occurs slowly over the course of many months and even years. Medical therapy for other types of giant adenomas ordinarily does not result in shrinkage of the tumor and will be of relatively lesser importance in the management of giant pituitary adenomas. Radiation therapy, if it has not previously been given, is generally recommended, with a maximum dose between 4500 and 5500 rads given in 180-rad daily fractions over a period of 4–5 weeks. Because of the large size of the interface with giant adenomas and the base of the skull, focused radiation therapy in the form of radiosurgery with a gamma knife or a focused linear accelerator usually is not helpful as initial management, although it can be added later for focal areas of recurrent tumor.

Despite the large size and imposing aspect of giant pituitary adenomas, the prognosis for patients can be surprisingly good if effective surgery is accomplished and the patient is followed carefully with appropriate adjunctive therapy and repeated monitoring using imaging studies. These cases represent a great challenge in decision making, surgical judgment and surgical technique, but in most cases the outcome justifies the effort involved.

Neurosurgical Management of Large Pituitary Adenomas
Yukitaka Ushio

One of the objectives of surgery for pituitary adenomas is to decompress the neural structures, particularly the visual pathways, which are almost always affected when the tumor is large. Another objective is to obtain complete and lasting restoration of normal hormone secretion. We make every attempt to achieve the former objective, especially to obtain restoration of normal visual function. The latter objective is often difficult to achieve if the tumor is invasive, regardless of size. However, even if the improvement is incomplete, reduction of tumor volume can enhance the effect of postoperative medical treatment.

As a rule, we attempt the radical excision of the tumor by the subnasal transsphenoidal approach. A catheter is inserted into the lumbar subarachnoid space so that air is injected as desired to outline the suprasellar dimension of the tumor during the operation. Under televised radiofluoroscopic control and the guide of dynamic pneumoencephalography we remove the tumor by curettage and aspiration, using various types of curettes. Usually the suprasellar expansion spontaneously collapses downward as the intrasellar part of the tumor is removed. Air injection for pneumoencephalography facilitates the collapse. If the suprasellar component does not descend sufficiently, we ask the anesthetist to increase the intrathoracic pressure briefly, so that increased intracranial pressure pushes the suprasellar tumor into the operative field. Occasionally the upper 'capsule', which consists of the thinned, stretched sellar diaphragm and thickened arachnoid, partially descends to the bottom of the excavated sella, obscuring the posterior extension of the tumor above and behind the dorsum sellae. In this situation, CSF is removed until the 'capsule' ascends, so that we can see any tumor remaining in a posterior–superior direction. We remove the tumor until the entire surface of the suprasellar 'capsule' is visualized. A mirror is useful to obtain an excellent view of otherwise inaccessible areas. The collapse of the suprasellar bulge is also verified by the free passage of air into the suprasellar cistern. After tumor removal fascia is placed underneath the upper 'capsule', much of the sella is packed with fat and the sellar opening is closed using cartilage or silicon plate slipped inside the dural edges.

Usually the pituitary adenoma is soft and relatively avascular, and using the subnasal transsphenoidal approach the majority of pituitary adenomas can be removed totally, or nearly so, even if they are large. However, on rare occasions, tumors are fibrous and firm in consistency. These tumors do not collapse into the operative field and it is difficult to achieve a radical removal. If visual improvement has not been obtained, we perform the transcranial approach 2 or 3 weeks later to remove the suprasellar tumor intracapsularly. We do not remove the 'capsule', because it does not belong to the tumor but to the patient.

When a substantial part of the tumor has extended into the subfrontal, retrochiasmatic, or middle fossa regions, we consider using a transcranial approach for the initial surgery. A transcranial approach is also indicated when the tumor is dumbbell shaped with a tight bottleneck constriction. We choose the paramedian subfrontal approach, pterional approach or subtemporal approach, depending on the direction of tumor growth. For tumors invading into the cavernous sinus we do not attempt to remove the tumor inside the sinus when the patient does not have cavernous sinus symptoms.

Treatment of Large Pituitary Tumors
Andrew H. Kaye

The treatment of large pituitary tumors presents special challenges for the neurosurgeon. The presenting clinical features of these tumors combine those of endocrine abnormality, including pituitary hypersecretion or hyposecretion and those attributable to the 'mass effect' of the tumor itself.

The amenorrhea–galactorrhea syndrome, involving hypersecretion of prolactin, is by far the commonest type of pituitary hypersecretion related to very large pituitary tumors. Less commonly, growth hormone-secreting tumors may present with large extrasellar extensions. Only rarely do patients with Cushing's disease (ACTH-secreting tumors) have large extrasellar extensions, except when associated with the Nelson–Salassa syndrome. This syndrome consists of an ACTH–secreting pituitary adenoma in a patient who has undergone bilateral subtotal adrenalectomy. An accelerated growth of an existing adenoma is induced by the loss of normal corticosteroid feedback, and unlike the adenomas of Cushing's disease, about half the patients with Nelson–Salassa syndrome have macroadenomas.

In at least half the patients presenting with pituitary tumors that have large extrasellar extensions, the tumor is a 'null cell' – that is, a clinically non-functioning adenoma. It is important to recognize that hyperprolactinemia is not always a feature specific to prolactin-producing adenomas. Moderate hyperprolactinemia can occur with any of a variety of structural lesions involving the sellar

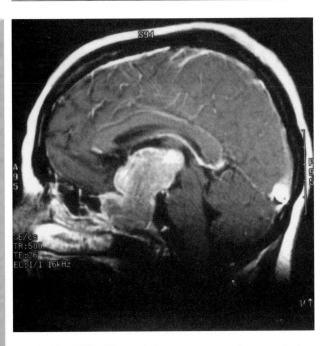

Fig. 16.10 MRI of large pituitary tumor extending superiorly into the third ventricle and inferiorly into the sphenoid sinus.

region. This phenomenon, frequently referred to as the 'stalk section effect', is a result of compressive lesions involving the hypothalamus or pituitary stalk.

The extrasellar growth of large pituitary tumors may involve a superior extension compressing the optic pathways and extension into the third ventricle with obstruction to CSF flow causing obstructive hydrocephalus. Alternatively, the tumor may extend laterally into the cavernous sinus, causing nerve palsies manifest by ptosis, facial pain or sensory changes and diplopia from involvement of the IIIrd, IVth and/or Vth cranial nerves. Occasionally, large pituitary adenomas can extend into the temporal fossa and patients present with complex partial seizures. Rarely, pituitary adenomas can become of such proportions that they extend into the anterior fossa and, occasionally, the posterior fossa. Large pituitary tumors may erode inferiorly into the sphenoid sinus and occasionally this extension manifests as CSF rhinorrhea.

Preoperative Assessment: The diagnosis and preoperative assessment involve:

1. Careful hormonal evaluation to ascertain the specific endocrinopathy. In most cases there were features of pituitary hyposecretion and appropriate therapy will need to be commenced promptly.
2. Radiological evaluation involves CT scanning, including direct coronal views with bone 'window' settings, so as to carefully ascertain the relationship between the tumor and the skull base.
3. MRI in sagittal, coronal and axial planes with

gadolinium enhancement has revolutionized the preoperative imaging to determine the exact extent of the tumor:

– superiorly, into the third ventricle;
– anteriorly, into the anterior cranial fossa;
– posteriorly, into the posterior cranial fossa;
– inferiorly, into the paranasal sinuses;
– laterally, into the cavernous sinus and temporal lobe.

The MRI will also show the relationship between the carotid arteries in the cavernous sinus and the tumor, and help exclude a giant aneurysm presenting as a pituitary tumor.

4. A complete ophthalmology evaluation is mandatory in all patients with large pituitary tumors. Visual field defects should be formally recorded on automated perimetry. This type of recording is particularly helpful to document the response to therapeutic intervention.

Treatment

Prolactin-secreting Tumors: In most cases of large prolactin-secreting adenomas, the initial treatment is bromocryptine therapy (Thapar & Laws 1995). Bromocryptine is a dopamine agonist and, by saturating dopamine receptors on the tumor cell surface, bromocryptine effectively inhibits prolactin secretion.

There is still some debate as to whether the most appropriate treatment for the large prolactin-secreting tumor is immediate surgery or bromocryptine therapy. In my opinion, provided the visual function is stable and not deteriorating and the other 'mass effect' features are not life threatening, it is appropriate to commence with bromocryptine therapy. If the therapy is tolerated by the patient (and a significant proportion of patients do not tolerate bromocryptine therapy due to its side effect) and provided there is a documented clinical and radiological response it is appropriate to continue bromocryptine therapy. Whilst bromocryptine therapy is effective in a significant percentage of cases, in many, the effect is limited and surgery will be necessary. Surgical management is mandatory if there is progressive visual loss and of course will be necessary for those patients who do not tolerate the bromocryptine therapy. Inevitably the treatment strategies for patients with large prolactin-secreting tumors will need to be individualized and will depend on the clinical presentation, and the effectiveness and tolerance of the patients to bromocryptine.

Surgical treatment: The transsphenoidal operation is almost always the most appropriate initial surgical procedure in the management of the large pituitary tumor. The development of the transseptal transsphenoidal microsurgical approach to the pituitary fossa has increased the safety of pituitary surgery and provides adequate access to the vast majority of large pituitary tumors.

The standard operative procedure involves an incision in the mucosa of the right nostril, separation of the mucosa away from the cartilaginous septum on the right side and from the body septum on both sides back to the anterior wall of sphenoid and a wide opening into the sphenoid sinus. With the aid of the operating microscope and the image intensifier, the floor of the often very thinned pituitary fossa is removed widely and the dura opened. The tumor within the pituitary fossa is excised with the aid of pituitary rongeurs, curettes and careful suction. The suprasellar extension of the tumor is then gently 'coaxed' down into the emptied pituitary fossa. Great care should be taken not to pull the tumor into the fossa, but rather let the normal pulsation of the brain, or valsalva maneuvers by the anesthetist, deliver the tumor into the fossa. Intraoperative pneumoencephalography through a lumbar catheter further aids the delivery of the pituitary tumor into the emptied pituitary fossa and at the same time helps to determine the extent of any suprasellar residual tumor. For this reason, we have preferred to inject filtered gas taken from the anesthetic machine, rather than saline as suggested by others. The excision of the tumor is only complete when the suprasellar membrane can be seen prolapsing down into the pituitary fossa. During the procedure, it can be difficult to control bleeding from the tumor, but hemostasis is quite easily obtained after the tumor has been completely removed.

If the suprasellar membrane has been opened and there is a CSF leak, fat together with the subdermis is taken from the abdomen and gently packed into the defect in the membrane. The suprasellar membrane is then lined by either a layer of subdermis or fascia lata and the fossa packed lightly with abdominal fat. The anterior wall of the fossa is reconstituted using either subdermis or fascia lata and nasal septum. In general, we do not pack the sphenoid sinus.

During the initial postoperative course, great care is taken to monitor vision and endocrine status, especially for the possibility of diabetes insipidus (Laws et al 1980).

Craniotomy for excision of large pituitary tumors is now only rarely necessary and is reserved for the following situations:

1. lateral extension of the pituitary tumor into the temporal lobe;
2. large pituitary tumors with a tough fibrous consistency which are not amenable to complete removal through the transsphenoidal route;
3. in the unusual case that the pituitary sella is 'closed' such that there is very little space between the anterior and posterior clinoid processes and so making access to the suprasellar extension difficult;
4. in the rare situation that access to the suprasellar extension is impeded by carotid arteries bulging into the sella bilaterally.

Radiation therapy: Radiation therapy has traditionally been an adjuvant postoperative therapy in the management of pituitary tumors. However, as surgical treatment has improved and postoperative evaluation with MRI has become more precise, the role of radiotherapy is less clear. In general, radiotherapy is used if the tumor is incompletely resected or if there is evidence of continuing hypersecretion by a tumor remnant that is refractory to medical management.

References

Laws E R, Abboud C F, Kern E B 1980 Perioperative management of patients with pituitary microadenomas. Neurosurgery 7: 566–570

Thapar K, Laws E R 1995 Pituitary tumors. In: Kaye A K, Laws E R (eds) Brain tumors. Churchill Livingstone, Edinburgh pp 759–773

Surgery of intra-axial brain stem tumors

17

Kazuhiko Kyoshima   Atul Goel
Shigeaki Kobayashi   Kazuhiro Hongo

The brain stem can be involved in a variety of neoplastic diseases. Whilst a large percentage of these lesions are malignant, a significant number are benign in nature. Surgical endeavor with lesions involving the brain stem can on various occasions crucially affect the management decisions. For benign lesions a successful surgery could be curative.

Surgery for intra-axial brain stem tumors is precise, difficult and hazardous. This is because the brain stem is densely endowed with vital neural structures such as nuclei and neural tracts. Surgery over brain stem lesions has mostly been limited to exophytic lesions or large tumors causing a significant bulge of the brain stem. Morbidity of varying degrees and mortality can result even following biopsies or partial removal (Villani et al 1975). Advances in magnetic resonance imaging (MRI) and microsurgery have made it possible to identify the exact location of a brain stem lesion and have renewed the interest in surgical approaches to the brain stem (Epstein & Wisoff 1987, Hacker & Fox 1980, Hoffman et al 1980, Kashiwagi et al 1990, Konovalov et al 1990, Pendl 1988, Yasargil 1988, Yoshimoto & Suzuki 1986). The main causes of morbidity relate to direct damage during the removal of the lesion, selection of an entry route into the brain stem, and the direction of brain stem retraction.

Some larger lesions result in a significant bulge in the brain stem. The bulge may point in a particular direction. It is crucially important to identify the exact site of the most prominent bulge on the surface of the brain stem from which site the tumor should be approached. Often the bulge is so large that the easiest and safest zone of entry into the brain stem is by making an incision through the most thinned out area of the brain stem. It is only in rare cases that the intra-axial lesion in the brain stem needs an elaborate incision over the surface of the brain stem. In cases of brain stem tumors where there is no significant bulge of the surface, the lesion itself is not causing a mass effect over the rest of the brain stem and in most cases does not need surgical attention.

After an anatomical review, we examined the possibility of making a medullary incision and retracting the brain stem, taking into account the symptomatology and surgical anatomy, and found two safe entry zones into the brain stem, while operating via the suboccipital route through the floor of the fourth ventricle (Kyoshima et al 1993). These safe entry zones are the areas where important neural structures are less prominent. One is the 'suprafacial triangle', which is bordered medially by the medial longitudinal fascicle, caudally by the facial nerve (which runs in the brain stem parenchyma), and laterally by cerebral peduncle. The second is the 'infrafacial triangle', which is bordered medially by the medial longitudinal fasciculus, caudally by the striae medullares, and laterally by the facial nerve. In order to minimize the the retraction-related damage to important brain stem structures, the brain stem should be retracted either laterally or rostrally in the suprafacial triangle and only laterally in the infrafacial triangle approach.

Although there are a few reports describing entry zones for intra-axial lesions of the brain stem, none consider retraction of the brain stem itself. Baghai et al (1982) reported a safe approach from the ventrolateral portion of the pons between the points of emergence of the Vth and VIIth cranial nerves, but this approach is useful only for biopsy and would be too narrow for direct surgery. Tapered brain retractors with a 2 mm wide tip connected with a light-weight, self-retaining titanium retractor for brain stem retraction and a two-pronged hook for tumor retraction are essential tools for direct brain stem surgery (Sugita 1985, Sugita & Kobayashi 1982).

SYMPTOMATOLOGICAL CONSIDERATIONS

If it is not possible to avoid impairment of brain stem function during surgery for a localized intra-axial brain stem lesion, it is important to know the kinds of impaired function that are relatively well tolerated by the patient in daily life. Severe disability caused by unilateral brain stem impairment includes hemiplegia, swallowing difficulty, and ataxia caused by impaired depth and position sens, and impairment of bilateral eye movement. At surgery, it is important not to damage the relevant structures: the corticospinal tract, lower cranial nerve nuclei, medial lemniscus, parapontine reticular formation or the corticonuclear tracts.

Motor impairment of the face or of unilateral eye movement including nystagmus may be tolerable. Of course it is better to preserve such relevant structures as the facial nerve or nucleus, the medial longitudinal fasciculus, the abducens nerve or nucleus, and oculomotor nerve or nuclei.

Tolerance or compensatable disability caused by unilateral brain stem impairment might include equilibrium impairment, cerebellar ataxia, unilateral hearing disorder, or impairment of face sensation. It might be acceptable at surgery, therefore, to damage the following relevant unilateral structures: vestibular nuclei, cerebellar peduncle, cochlear nuclei or lateral lemniscus, or trigeminal nuclei.

ANATOMICAL CONSIDERATIONS

The dorsal aspect of the fourth ventricle floor, after removal of the cerebellum, is referred to as the rhomboid fossa. It is 3 × 2 cm in size and is bordered rostrally by cerebellar peduncles and caudally by tubercles of gracilis

nucleus and cuneate nucleus, and tuberculum cinereum (Figs 17.1,17.2). Other external structures include the median sulcus in the midline, sulcus limitans, facial colliculus, and striae medullaris. The latter structures running across the floor of the fourth ventricle roughly indicate the border between the medulla oblongata and pons (Fig. 17.1). As for internal structures, the medial longitudinal fascicle runs just lateral to the median sulcus, the nucleus of the abducens nerve courses under the facial colliculus, and the facial nerve originates from its nucleus, which is located laterally deep under the striae medullares and runs up to and around the nucleus of the abducens nerve (Figs 17.1,17.2). The nuclei of the hypoglossal and vagus nerves are located just caudal to the striae medullares.

Important structures which cause severe disability, if damaged, are not densely distributed in the area between the cerebellar peduncle and facial colliculus, nor between the facial colliculus and the striae medullares. We have named the former area the 'suprafacial triangle' and the latter the 'infrafacial triangle'.

SAFE ENTRY ZONES INTO THE BRAIN STEM

Based on the symptomatology and surgical anatomy, we have analyzed the possibility of surgical incision and retraction of the brain stem and have identified two safe entry zones into the brain stem through the fourth ventric-

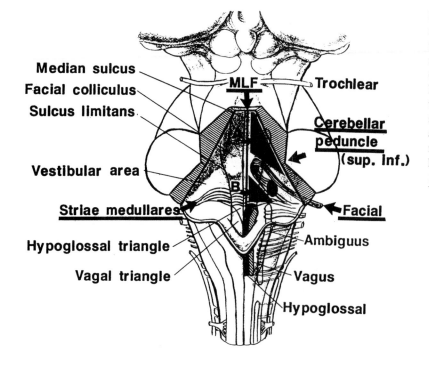

Fig. 17.1 Schematic drawing of the anatomy and safe entry zones to the brain stem via the floor of the fourth ventricle. Important neural structures are sparse in these safe entry zones. (A, suprafacial triangle; B, infrafacial triangle; MLF, medial longitudinal fascicle; trochlear, trochlear nerve; facial, facial nerve; sup. inf., superior and inferior; ambiguus, nucleus ambiguus; vagus, dorsal nucleus of the vagus nerve; hypoglossal, nucleus of the hypoglossal nerve.) (From Kyoshima et al 1993, with permission)

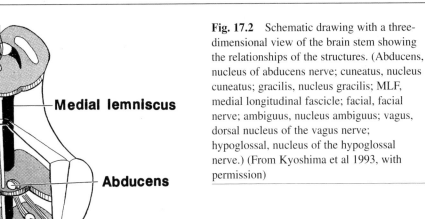

Pyramidal tract

MLF

Medial lemniscus

Abducens

Facial

Striae medullares

Cuneatus

Gracilis

Ambiguus

Vagus

Hypoglossal

Fig. 17.2 Schematic drawing with a three-dimensional view of the brain stem showing the relationships of the structures. (Abducens, nucleus of abducens nerve; cuneatus, nucleus cuneatus; gracilis, nucleus gracilis; MLF, medial longitudinal fascicle; facial, facial nerve; ambiguus, nucleus ambiguus; vagus, dorsal nucleus of the vagus nerve; hypoglossal, nucleus of the hypoglossal nerve.) (From Kyoshima et al 1993, with permission)

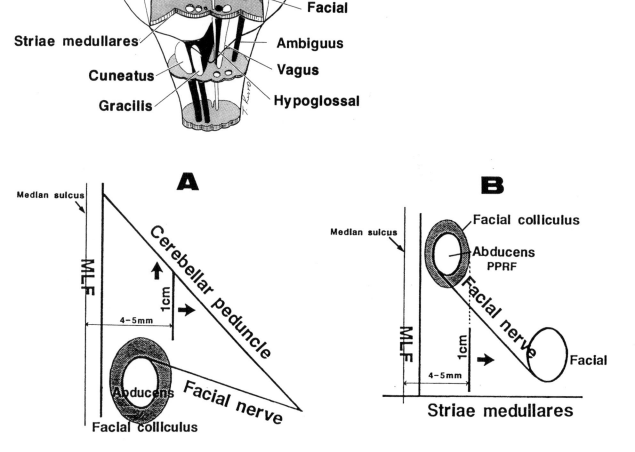

Fig. 17.3 **A** Suprafacial triangle approach to the brain stem. The triangle is bordered by the medial longitudinal fascicle (MLF) medially, the facial nerve caudally, and the superior and inferior cerebellar peduncles laterally. A 1 cm longitudinal medullary incision is made caudally from the edge of the superior cerebellar peduncle and 4–5 mm laterally from the median sulcus. The brain stem can be retracted either laterally or rostrally with relative ease (arrows). **B** Infrafacial triangle approach. The triangle is bordered by MLF medially, the striae medullares caudally, and the facial nerve laterally. A 1 cm longitudinal medullary incision is made rostrally from the caudal margin of the striae medullares and 4–5 mm laterally from the median sulcus. The brain stem can be retracted only laterally (arrow). (PPRF, parapontine reticular formation; abducens, nucleus of the abducens nerve; facial, nucleus of the facial nerve.) (From Kyoshima et al 1993, with permission)

ular floor via a suboccipital route. These safe entry zones are located where important neural structures are sparse (Figs 17.1, 17.2). One is the suprafacial triangle, which is bordered medially by the medial longitudinal fasciculus, caudally by the facial nerve (which runs in the brain stem parenchyma), and laterally by the cerebellar peduncles.

The second is the infrafacial triangle, which is bordered medially by the medial longitudinal fascicle, caudally by the striae medullares, and laterally by the facial nerve. At the bottom of these triangles are the medial lemniscus and corticospinal tract.

Structures potentially damaged by brain stem retraction or other surgical procedures approached via the suprafacial or infrafacial triangle are listed in Table 17.1, together with the symptoms related to them.

The brain stem parenchyma is vascularized by the perforating arteries coursing from the ventral or lateral aspect of the brain stem, but not from the surface of the fourth ventricular floor (Duvernoy 1978, Nakajima 1983). This means that on medullary incision from the fourth ventricular floor there is little possibility of causing brain stem dysfunction by damaging the perforating arteries. Furthermore, in parenchymal procedures approached from the fourth ventricular floor there is a low possibility of causing ischaemic brain stem damage to the remote area from the operative field. Thus, these two triangles can be designated safe entry zones in the brain stem for surgical treatment of a lesion located dorsal to the medial lemniscus.

Suprafacial approach

On the suprafacial triangle (Fig. 17.3A), the most feasible brain stem incision is made longitudinally, up to 1 cm in length, caudally from the edge of the cerebellar peduncle and about 5 mm lateral to the median sulcus. The length of the linear incision may be about 7 mm, because it is extended by brain stem retraction.

In order to minimize retraction-related damage to important brain stem structures, the brain stem should be retracted either laterally or rostrally. Retraction to the rostral side is possible because the oculomotor nuclei are located far from the triangle.

Infrafacial approach

The most feasible brain stem incision in the infrafacial triangle (Fig. 17.3B) is made longitudinally, rostrally from the caudal margin of the striae medullares and about 5 mm lateral to the median sulcus. The incision should be less than 1 cm in length. Brain stem retraction is possible only laterally, because the facial nucleus is located deeper and the facial nerve courses upward to the abducens nucleus. This triangle is narrow and is surrounded by more important structures compared to the suprafacial triangle. An initial medullary incision approximately 5 mm in length is suitable.

Table 17.1

Position relative to surgery	Structure	Symptom
Suprafacial triangle		
Lateral	Superior cerebellar peduncle	Hemiataxia
	Trigeminal nuclei	Sensorimotor impairment of the face
Medial Rostral	MLF	Gaze palsy, Nystagmus
	Superior cerebellar peduncle	Hemiataxia
	IIIrd and IVth nerves nuclei	Oculomotor and trochlear palsy
Caudal	Nucleus of VIth nerve	Abducens palsy
	Parapontine reticular formation	Lateral gaze palsy
	Facial nerve	Facial nerve palsy
Ventral	Medial lemniscus	Ataxia, depth perception impairment
	Lateral spinothalamic tract	Analgesia, thermanesthesia
	Corticspinal tract	Motor impairment
Infrafacial triangle		
Lateral	Facial nerve (deeper)	Facial nerve palsy
	Vestibular nuclei	Nystagmus
Medial Rostral	MLF	Nystagmus
	Nucleus of VIth nerve	Abducens palsy
	Parapontine reticular formation	Lateral gaze palsy
	Facial nerve	Facial nerve palsy
Caudal	Nuclei of lower cranial nerve	Swallowing impairment, dysarthria
Ventral	Medial lemniscus	Ataxia, depth perception impairment
	Lateral spinothalamic tract	Analgesia, thermanesthesia
	Corticspinal tract	Motor impairment

(From Kyoshima et al 1993, with permission)

Conclusions

Potential brain damage, including neurological dysfunction, caused by direct brain stem surgery may include: (1) damage caused by procedures for reaching the brain stem surface, such as injury of the bridging vein, incision of the brain, or brain retraction; (2) injury to the brain stem caused by attempts to reach a lesion, such as injury of the perforating artery or neural tissue by medullary incision of the brain stem; and (3) injury to the brain stem tissue around the lesion, caused by brain stem retraction or surgical procedures to remove a lesion.

It follows that a suboccipital approach by partially splitting the inferior part of the vermis is also a relatively safe procedure for reaching the brain stem surface because of the absence of bridging veins and minimum potential for retraction-related cerebellar damage. Therefore, the supra- or infrafacial approach is considered to be a relatively safe route to the brain stem.

The supra- or infrafacial approach is indicated for local-

ized intra-axial lesions located unilaterally and dorsal to the medial lemniscus in the lower midbrain to the pons. MRI is useful in selecting these approaches and intraoperative ultrasonography is helpful in confirming the exact location of a lesion before making a medullary incision. The safe entry zones can also be used as a route for aspiration of a brain stem hemorrhage as well as for biopsy of a tumor.

CASE 1

This 31-year-old man suffered a pontine hemorrhage on 24 August 1989, causing headache and numbness of the lips on the

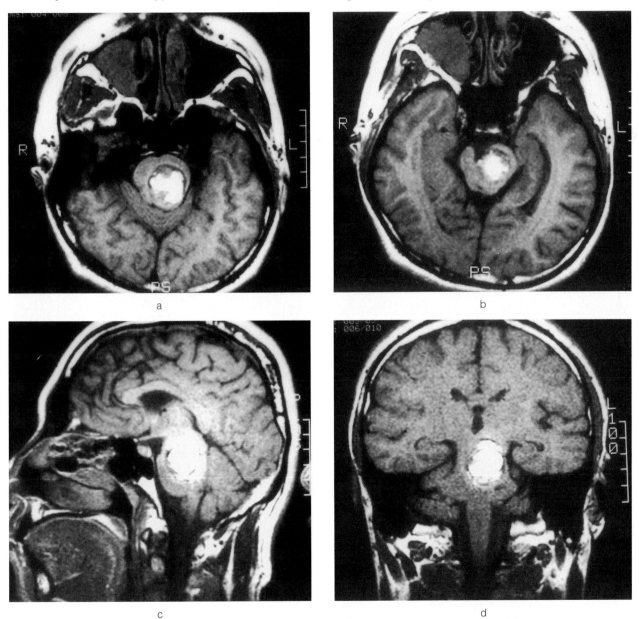

a

b

c

d

Fig. 17.4   This patient was treated by the suprafacial approach. The preoperative T1-weighted images of MRI show the localized intra-axial hematomatous lesion, which appears as an area of hyperintensity extending from the pons to the cerebral peduncle. (From Kyoshima et al 1993, with permission)

right side. The headache developed gradually and numbness extended over the right side of the face. A computed tomographic (CT) scan revealed a high-density mass in the brain stem and an MRI showed a mass in the left side of the pons measuring 15 mm in diameter. No abnormalities were detected on angiogram. The lesion was diagnosed clinically as a cavernous angioma and the patient treated conservatively. On 6 November he suffered another episode of headache. Neurological examination revealed left abducens paresis, nystagmus, numbness and hypalgesia of the right side of the face, right sensory disturbance for touch and pain, and cerebellar signs predominantly on the right side, with gait disturbance. CT revealed rebleeding in the brain stem, 28 mm in size, in the same area. A heterogeneous high-intensity mass with

a thin low-intensity rim was seen on T1-weighted MRI and a high-intensity mass with a thin low-intensity rim was visualized on T2-weighted MRI. The mass extended from the lower pons to the midbrain on the left side (Fig. 17.4).

With the patient in the prone position, a median suboccipital craniectomy was carried out. The upper floor of the fourth ventricle and the orifice of the aqueduct were exposed with an approximately 2 cm section of the inferior vermis. The surface of the fourth ventricle near the left superior cerebellar peduncle was yellowish and slightly protruding, and the median sulcus was shifted to the right side. After the location of the lesion was confirmed by ultrasonography, a 7 mm longitudinal medullary incision was made 5 mm lateral from the median sulcus. The hematoma was aspirated and a solid mass was completely

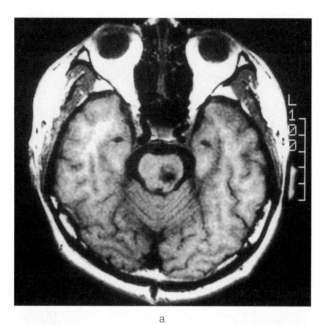

a

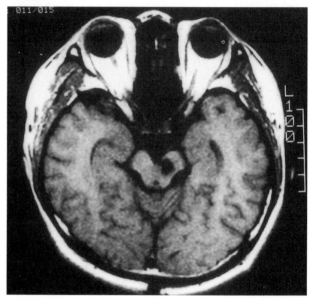

b

c

Fig. 17.5   Postoperative MRI showing complete removal of the lesion. (From Kyoshima et al 1993, with permission)

removed together with some veins and arteries observed in the bottom of the tumor cavity. The intraoperative diagnosis was an arteriovenous malformation rather than a cavernous angioma. During removal of the lesion, special care was taken not to retract the brain stem medially, caudally, or (as much as possible) rostrally.

The patient was alert immediately postoperatively and showed no further neurological deficits except increased gait ataxia, which improved gradually. Over the following several months, he became ambulatory without disability in daily life. The left abducens paresis and nystagmus improved gradually

and resolved completely over several weeks, and other symptoms almost entirely resolved. Postoperative MRI confirmed total removal of the lesion (Fig. 17.5). Histological examination of the surgical specimen demonstrated a vascular malformation.

CASE 2

This 42-year-old man, who had undergone nephrectomy for renal cell carcinoma 1 year earlier, suffered brain stem

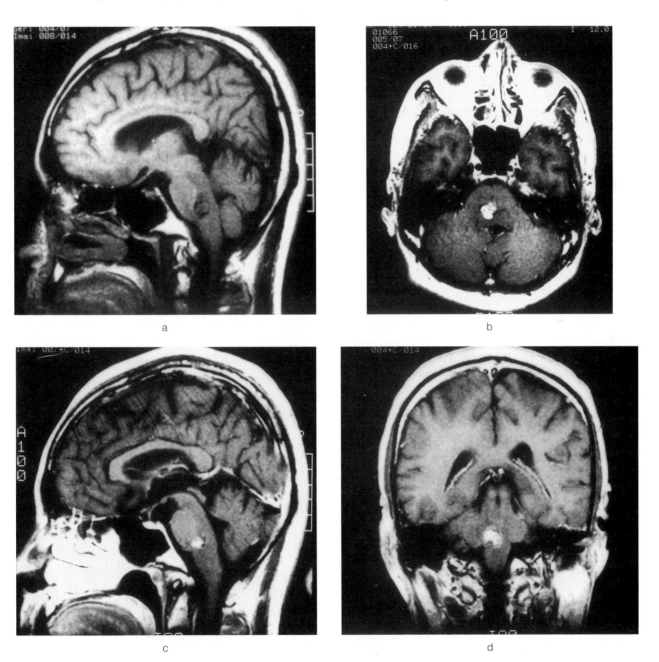

a

b

c

d

Fig. 17.6 This patient was treated by the infrafacial approach. Preoperative MRI shows an enhanced intra-axial tumor in the lower pons. The image **a** is unenhanced. (From Kyoshima et al 1993, with permission)

hemorrhage on 17 October 1989, with diplopia, numbness of the left extremities, and tinnitus on the left side. Neurological examination showed right abducens paralysis, bilateral hearing disturbance, slight left hemiparesis with mild hyperreflexia, a left sensory disturbance, and mild right cerebellar signs. A CT scan revealed a contrast-enhanced lesion in the brain stem and the right frontal lobe. MRI demonstrated an enhanced intra-axial mass in the lower pons located on the left side (Fig. 17.6).

One week after an uneventful removal of the metastatic tumor from the right frontal lobe, the tumor in the lower pons was removed with the patient in the prone position. A median suboccipital craniectomy was made and the floor of the fourth ventricle was exposed by minimally splitting the vermis. A longitudinal medullary incision was made on the floor of the fourth ventricle, about 5 mm rostrally from the caudal margin of the striae medullares and 4 mm laterally from the median sulcus, after confirming the location of the tumor with ultrasonography. The tumor was recognized 5 mm deep under the surface of the fourth ventricle and was well demarcated with a capsule. Some vessels were identified at the base of the tumor. The tumor was totally removed en bloc, with special care taken not to retract the brain stem medially or caudally. The final medullary incision measured 1 cm and the excised tumor was 1 cm in diameter. Postoperatively the neurological examination demonstrated moderate facial paresis, lateral right gaze disturbance, swallowing disturbance, and ataxic gait with loss of depth and position sense. The facial paresis and swallowing impairment resolved completely over several weeks. Pathological diagnosis was metastatic renal cell carcinoma. Postoperative MRI confirmed total excision of the lesion (Fig. 17.7). One year later the patient died of systemic metastasis.

CASE 3

This 65-year-old man became aware in February 1991 of sensory disturbance affecting his lips and cheek on the right side; right-sided hemiparesis gradually developed over the next 2 months. In April 1991 these symptoms worsened rapidly. Neurological examination revealed slight right-sided hemiparesis with sensory impairment for touch and position, hypesthesia and hypalgesia of the right side of the face, right conductive hearing impairment, and ataxia of the right side limbs. MRI revealed two well-enhancing lesions: a mass in the left pons to the midbrain and a lesion in the left occipital pole (Fig. 17.8).

With the patient in the prone position, a median suboccipital craniotomy was carried out. The rhomboid fossa was exposed via 2.5 cm section of the inferior cerebellar vermis. No remarkable structural change was observed on the fourth ventricular floor. A 7 mm longitudinal medullary incision was made 5 mm laterally from the median sulcus. The lower end of the incision was approximately 1 cm away from the cranial margin of striae medullares. The tumor was identified 2 mm beneath the brain stem surface. Tumor dissection was started first medially and then caudally. The tumor was relatively well demarcated and hard, but it was impossible to remove en bloc because the bottom of the tumor was vascular and did not have a clear border. The intraoperative diagnosis with biopsy was squamous cell carcinoma. Special attention was given not to retract the brain stem rostrally, but the medial side of the brain stem was nonetheless injured during the procedure. The right occipital lesion was not removed at this time. Postoperatively, neurological examination showed left abducens paresis and

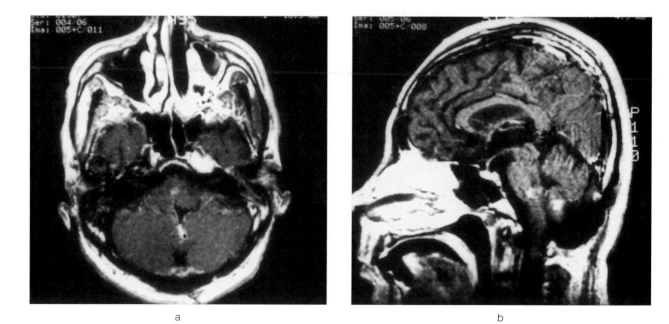

a   b

Fig. 17.7 a Postoperative contrast-enhanced MRI showing total removal of the tumor. **b** There is a high-intensity area around the route of approach and the tumor cavity. (From Kyoshima et al 1993, with permission)

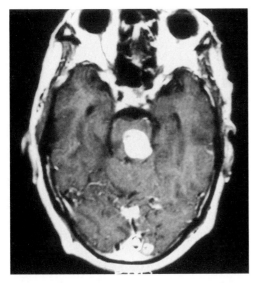

a

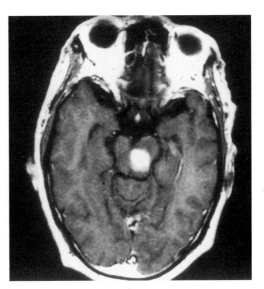

b

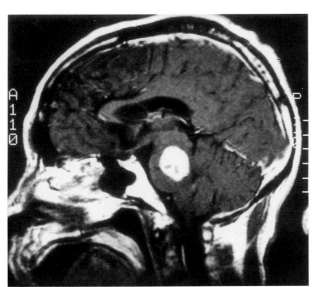

c

Fig. 17.8 This case was treated by the suprafacial approach. Preoperative MRI shows two well-enhanced lesions: one is in the pons to the midbrain in the left side and the other is in the occipital pole. (From Kyoshima et al 1993, with permission)

impairment of medial gaze with the left eye, both of which were improving. The cerebellar symptom had not worsened. Postoperative MRI revealed residual tumor in the rostral side of the tumor cavity (Fig. 17.9).

References

Baghai P, Vries J K, Bechtel P C 1982 Retromastoid approach for biopsy of brain stem tumors. Neurosurgery 10: 574–579

Duvernoy H M 1978 Human brain stem vessels. Springer-Verlag, Berlin

Epstein F, Wisoff J 1987 Intra-axial tumors of the cervico-medullary junction. Journal of Neurosurgery 67: 483–487

Hacker R J, Fox J L 1980 Surgical treatment of brain stem carcinoma: case report. Neurosurgery 6: 430–432

Hoffman H J, Becker L, Craven M A 1980 A clinically and pathologically distinct group of benign brain stem gliomas. Neurosurgery 7: 243–248

Kashiwagi S, van Loveran H R, Tew J M Jr et al 1990 Diagnosis and treatment of vascular brain-stem malformations. Journal of Neurosurgery 72: 27–34

Konovalov A N, Spallone A, Makhumudov U B et al 1990 Surgical management of hematomas of the brain stem. Journal of Neurosurgery 73: 181–186

Kyoshima K, Kobayashi S, Gibo H et al 1993 A study of safe entry zones via the floor of the fourth ventricle for brain-stem lesions. Journal of Neurosurgery 78: 987–993

Nakajima K 1983 Clinicopathological study of pontine hemorrhage. Stroke 14: 485–493

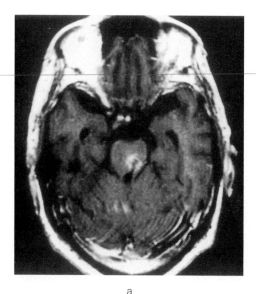

a

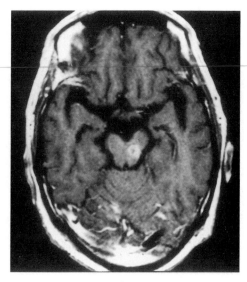

b

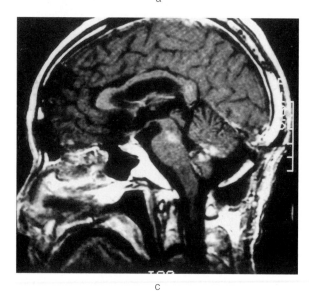

c

Fig. 17.9   Postoperative contrast-enhanced MRI obtained before discharge showing residual tumor in the rostral side of the tumor cavity in the pons. The area of high intensity around the route of approach is visible without contrast enhancement. (From Kyoshima et al 1993, with permission)

Pendl G, Vorkapic P 1988 Microsurgery of midbrain lesions. Acta Neurochirurgica Supplementum 42: 130–136

Sugita K 1985 Microsurgical atlas. Springer-Verlag, Berlin, pp 6–7

Sugita K, Kobayashi S 1982 Technical and instrumental improvements in the surgical treatment of acoustic neurinoma. Journal of Neurosurgery 57: 747–752

Villani R, Gaini S M, Tomei G 1975 Follow-up study of brain stem tumors in children. Child's Brain 1: 126–135

Yasargil M G 1988 Microsurgery, Vol IIIB. AVM of the brain, clinical conditions, general and specific operative techniques, surgical results, non-operated cases, cavernous and venous angiomas, neuroanaesthesia. Theime, New-York, pp 429–438

Yoshimoto T, Suzuki J 1986 Radical surgery on cavernous angioma of the brain stem. Surgical Neurology 26: 72–78

Surgery on Brain Stem Tumors
Fred Epstein

From my perspective, the most important 'message' that we must communicate to our colleagues in pediatric neurosurgery, neuro-oncology and neurology is that there is, in fact, no such thing as a 'brain stem tumor'. While this diagnosis was appropriate before the MRI era, it has become apparent that these tumors are, in fact, a heterogeneous collection of neoplasms that must be described according to their location and clinical presentation. It is only on this basis that one may make a conclusion as to the likely microscopic pathology and to then make a recommendation whether surgery should or should not be carried out.

The 'common denominator' to a successful surgical procedure is to operate on an indolent (i.e. low-grade) neoplasm. It does not do a great deal of good for a patient to partially, or even radically, excise a malignant tumor when the residual fragments will inevitably regrow in a finite period of time. However, in the presence of a slowly growing tumor, the residual fragments may become 'dormant' for an indefinite time period or only regrow after many years. In these circumstances, the surgery does make a major impact on the biology of the tumor as well as the functional survival of the patient. Therefore, it is incumbent on the pediatric neurosurgeon to identify those brain stem tumors which, by virtue of their location, clinical presentation and MRI appearance, are likely to be benefiting in a meaningful way by radical, though subtotal, surgical excision.

On the basis of a retrospective analysis of about 150 brain stem tumor surgical procedures that I have carried out, it has become very clear that a classification system which I first proposed in 1982 has remained appropriate with some additions. From my perspective, brain stem tumors may be divided into diffuse, focal and cervicomedullary. I am not including dorsal exophytic tumors in this classification, inasmuch as they are tumors that are growing posteriorly into the fourth ventricle and, while they clearly originate from the subependymal surface of the fourth ventricle, they are not truly brain stem tumors as we usually think about them. In addition, it has been very clear that after excising these tumors up to but not including the origin beneath the floor of the ventricle, patients often survive for long periods of time. I am also not including tectal tumors in this classification, inasmuch as they are by and large indolent, present with hydrocephalus and are well treated with a shunting procedure alone with adjunctive therapy only utilized for patients who develop evidence of radiologic or clinical progression.

The diffuse brain stem tumor is the 'stereotype' that we think of as these tumors were described in the past. There is invariably a relatively short history and clinical manifestations are ocular and lower cranial nerve dysfunction as well as ataxia, etc. The MRI scan discloses a very large tumor with the epicenter in the pons which extends both rostrally and caudally, generally involving both the midbrain and the medulla. Interestingly, contrast enhancement at the time of diagnosis is commonly absent.

The diffuse tumor is almost inevitably malignant and surgery has no place. In addition, there is no indication to carry out a stereotactic biopsy of these lesions, inasmuch as the microscopic pathology is obvious on the basis of the neurodiagnostic study.

Focal tumors, by 'definition' (my definition!), are circumscribed and are limited to one anatomic segment of the brain stem. They are either in the midbrain, the medulla or, rarely, in the pons. They do not extend to involve contiguous structures. In other words, unlike the diffuse tumor which infiltrates rostrally and caudally throughout the brain stem, the focal tumor remains confined to one area. It is of interest that about 50% of focal tumors are in the area of the cerebral peduncle, 40% in the medulla and only 10% in the pons. In addition, about 20% of the focal tumors have a cystic component and have the radiologic appearance quite similar to cystic astrocytoma of the cerebellum.

Inasmuch as focal tumors are almost invariably biologically indolent (i.e. low-grade astrocytomas, gangliogliomas, etc.), they are greatly benefited by radical surgical debulking. It is technically feasible to remove 50–90% of the volume of most of these neoplasms either through a subtemporal approach to the region of the midbrain or a posterior fossa approach to the medulla. Medullary tumors must be followed very closely after surgery, inasmuch as there is a tendency to hypoventilate with hypoxia and ultimately ischemia of the brain stem. We have found that if these patients are left intubated for 3–5 days, this complication does not occur and, in fact, respiratory dysfunction is minimal. It is, however, of the utmost importance to recognize that the major morbidity associated with medullary surgery, is lower cranial nerve dysfunction. Ten to fifteen per cent of patients undergoing radical removal of medullary tumors have required long-term tracheotomy and gastrostomy. Although in most of these patients these necessary support systems could ultimately be removed, there is an occasional patient in whom this is a permanent problem and it is very important that families be informed of this preoperatively.

In our experience of operating on about 75 focal tumors, we have noted that, in the presence of a low-grade astrocytoma or ganglioglioma, there has been no regrowth 5 years later in about 80% or 85% of the patients. We have not employed either radiation therapy or chemotherapy in these children. Therefore, the focal tumors of the brain stem are amenable to surgery and, although there may be inherent complications, the 5-year outlook is an excellent one if radical though subtotal removal is accomplished.

Cervicomedullary tumors are perhaps the most favorable of all 'brain stem' neoplasms. This is because, although the radiologic picture clearly discloses rostral extension of the neoplasm above the foramen magnum, the reality is that most of these tumors are, in fact, cervical spinal cord tumors which have grown rostrally and then posteriorly in the area of 'least resistance', which is the obex, at which location they become exophytic. If the MRI scan is looked at very carefully, in most cases it will be obvious that the medulla is in reality displaced rostrally, but is not infiltrated by tumor which is, in fact, growing posteriorly and might even be considered at least above the foramen magnum as dorsal exophytic the region of the obex.

Cervicomedullary tumors are, almost without exception, 'benign' and, following radical excision, about 85% or 90% remain asymptomatic for 5 years (we have not had the opportunity of studying our patient population that are farther out than this). As with the focal medullary tumors, radiation therapy and chemotherapy are not employed and the result with surgery has been excellent, with morbidity less than 5%.

In summary, brain stem tumors must be assessed as to both the clinical presentation as well as the neurodiagnostic morphology. Some tumors should never be operated on (diffuse), others should always be operated on (cervicomedullary), while medullary tumors are amenable to surgery but do have the potential of serious complications.

Developing a Strategy to Treat Patients with Brain Stem Tumors
Ahmed Ammar

Surgery for brain stem lesions historically passed through three distinct phases. In the first phase, traditionally brain stem tumors were considered inoperable with a poor survival rate, ranging from 4 to 15 months (Epstein & Farmer 1993). The second phase was the period of aggressive surgical attempts to remove the tumors. These attempts were greatly encouraged by the reports in the 1970s and early 1980s (Baghai et al 1982, Epstein & Murali 1982, Hoffman 1988, Pollack et al 1993). The overall survival rate of these patients was greatly improved up to 10 years or total cure in some cases of benign lesions. In the third phase, the accumulating results of the previous periods showed a remarkable difference in the survival rate and outcome of surgery for different brain stem lesions, therefore a more selective attitude towards these tumors became the rule, to remove benign lesions or lesions in the medulla or exophytic tumors. However, surgery may not be indicated in highly malignant lesions of diffuse intrinsic tumors of the brain stem (Epstein & Murali 1982, Hoffman 1988, Pierre-Kahn et al 1993, Pollack et al 1993). The incidence of brain stem tumor is believed to be nearly 1% (Yasargil 1994) of all central nervous system tumors or 5–15% of all intracranial tumors (Bouchard & Pierce 1960, Greenberger et al 1977, Konovalov & Atieh 1988); 25% of them are in children and young adolescents (Konovalov & Atieh 1988). Ten to twenty per cent of brain stem tumors in children are gliomas. A better understanding of the behavior of these tumors and the improvement in diagnostic procedures and surgical techniques have markedly improved the results, as has been reported by several authors (Epstein & Farmer 1993, Hoffman 1988, Isu et al 1994, Konovalov & Atieh 1988, Pierre-Kahn et al 1993, Pollack et al 1993, Sakai et al 1991, Stroink et al 1987, Villani et al 1975).

Surgery for brain stem lesions is highly challenging surgery. Because of the complicity of the brain stem structures and heterogeneity of the lesions a clear strategy should be made to achieve the best outcome in the form of favorable survival rate and reasonable quality of life. Many neurosurgeons were encouraged by the reports of Lassiter, Epstein and Hoffman (Epstein & Murali 1982, Hoffman 1988, Lassiter et al 1971) and started to operate these patients, and this challenge created a great debate and concern about the real value of some of these operations with regard to the quality of life of the patient following the surgery.

Therefore a realistic unbiased analysis should lead to the development of a strategy, to manage the unfortunate patients who harbor brain stem lesions, through answering the following questions:

1. What is the lesion and where is the lesion exactly?
2. What is the natural history of the lesion?
3. What is the indication for surgery or an alternative method of treatment?
4. In cases when surgery is indicated, which approach should be made?
5. What are the minimum facilities needed in the centers performing this surgery?
6. What is the optimal time for surgery?

The summation of the answers of these question may indicate the best methods for the treatment of such patients.

To answer these questions, many elements should be taken into consideration. From our experience of surgically treating 12 patients and reviewing the literature, we concluded that these factors should be considered in any decision about the management of these patients.

Management Strategy

I. Management plan and decision making: Several strategies have been described in the literature to help decide which avenue should be taken in the process of treating these tumors (Stroink et al 1987, Yasargil 1994).

The overall management plan, and the decision to choose the specific method of treatment, should be based on several factors such as:

A. The surgeon and the treating center

It is beyond any doubt that the facilities available in the treating center have an influence on the outcome of surgery of brain stem lesions. These factors can be summarized thus:

1. the surgeon's own experience, ethics and self-confidence and mastering microvascular techniques;
2. availability of modern diagnostic facilities; and radiotherapy or radiosurgery and chemotherapy;
3. operating room facilities, microscope, microsurgical instruments, laser and ultrasonic aspirator;
4. anesthesia technique and experienced anesthesiologist;
5. intraoperative special monitors, somatosensory evoked potential (SEP), ultrasound Doppler to detect air embolism in cases of surgery in sitting position;
6. postoperative well-equipped ICU and experienced ICU staff;
7. surgical alternative, radiosurgery, radiotherapy and chemotherapy.

B. The patient

1. Age.

The youngest patient successfully operated in our series was 21 months old. It seems that infants and children tolerate this kind of surgery better than old people. It has been proved that the reversibility of severe brain stem dysfunction in children is possible (Ammar et al 1993). However, malignant glioma comprises a considerable percentage of brain stem tumors in children. It is clearly seen by different reports that age plays an important role in determining the outcome of such lesions of the brain stem (Pierre-Kahn et al 1993, Pollack et al 1993).

2. General condition.

It is important to take into consideration from the beginning that the postoperative course can be very stormy and needs periods of intubation and rehabilitation. If the general condition of the patient is not encouraging, an alternative to open surgery should be considered.

3. Neurological condition, signs and symptoms and the course of the disease.

Most of the early clinical presentation of low-grade astrocytomas of the brain stem are either cranial nerve palsies or long tract signs, ataxia , spasticity or signs of high intracranial pressure caused by obstructed hydrocephalus. If the decision is made for stereotactic biopsy we recommend insertion of ventriculoatrial or ventriculoperitoneal shunt in the same session in cases of associated hydrocephalus. In some patients, especially in cases of brain stem cavernous angioma which bleeds into the brain stem, the deterioration of the patient's condition can be very rapid and serious, demanding immediate and urgent interference. We recommend urgent surgery to remove the cavernous angioma and evacuate the hematoma. The hematoma may help in finding the lesion and the approach is logically decided to be through the hematoma cavity to avoid additional defects.

4. Acceptance of the patient and his family to the surgery and the possible complications;

5. Patient's own environment, the existence of facilities for rehabilitation and adjusting to the possible postoperative complications.

C. The growth pattern, pathology and anatomical location of the tumor

These may be the most important factors for determining the outcome of these lesions and their method of treatment. The tumors can be either malignant by nature such as glioblastoma multiforme or malignant by location as in cases of diffuse mesencephalic pontine tumors. The tumors can be grouped into several subgroups according to these factors:

a. Intrinsic I. Mesencephalic midbrain
b. Exophytic II. Brain stem, pons, tegmentum
c. Diffuse III. Medulla, cervical peduncles
d. Extended from neighboring structures or metastasized

It has been noticed that the growth pattern of low-grade glioma differs greatly from highly malignant tumors; it seems that the growth of low-grade glioma in the brain stem is guided by anatomical structures of the brain stem such as fiber tracts and pial borders (Epstein & Farmer 1993). Therefore, surgery for focal medullary or medullary cervical junction or even dorsal midbrain or pons may be rewarding.

The location of the tumor is one of the most decisive factors for selecting the method of treatment. In general terms surgery in the medulla gives better results than surgery in the pons and the worst results are of the lesions in the midbrain. It is always possible to remove exophytic lesions successfully from any level, even the midbrain. The extended, diffuse, distracting lesions from neighboring structures, as in cases of medulloblastoma or ependymoma, in our experience were not successfully treated by surgery, and the final outcome was very poor. It is impossible to remove diffuse intrinsic tumor completely. So, in the case of solid diffuse tumors, stereotactic biopsy perhaps is enough or to be followed with radiotherapy or radiosurgery and chemotherapy (Edwards et al 1989, Hood et al 1986, Hood & McKeever 1989, Jenkin et al 1987, Pierre-Kahn et al 1993, Pollack et al 1993, Rusyniak et al 1992). However, in cases of cystic lesion attempts to evacuate the cyst and subtotal removal can be achieved successfully and then radiotherapy may have an effect.

Pathological lesions in the brain stem may be divided into:

a. High malignancy, such as glioma, medulloblastoma, ependymoma and metastatic tumors;
b. low malignancy, such as astrocytomas;
c. benign, such as cavernous angioma, abscesses and hematomas.

We believe every effort should be made to remove the benign lesion; however, the highly malignant lesion may be biopsied and alternative methods of treatment should be considered. In low-malignancy lesions surgery may be considered if the patient's condition permits. Therefore, the goal always should be to remove as much tumor as possible, as experience has shown significant improvement in the 5-year survival rate of total or subtotal removal, being 94% over partial removal, which is only 52% (18). The survival rate of surgically treated benign tumors in 3 years is 74%, however; it is only 22% in malignant tumors (Pierre-Kahn et al 1993).

It has been proven that radical excision of cavernous angioma is feasible and should be the first option of treatment (Fahlbusch et al 1990, Pierre-Kahn et al 1993, Yoshimoto & Suzuki 1986).

Surgery can sometimes be interrupted by cardiovascular upsets or functional or vital structure embers in the way of removing the lesion (Pierre-Kahn et al 1993). Twice we have had to stop the surgery after sudden dropping of the blood pressure; in one case the surgery could proceed after restabilizing the patient. In the second case the repeated dropping of the blood pressure forced us to stop the resection of the diffuse lesion.

Intraoperative monitoring the somatosensory evoked potentials is important besides the routine monitoring of blood pressure, and electrocardiogram to avoid devastating irreversible damage to brain structures (Rusyniak et al 1992).

Timing of surgery is still controversial especially as the period of symptoms greatly differs from a few days to several years. In cases of cavernous angioma early surgery soon after bleeding may be advisable (Fahlbusch et al 1990).

Different approaches have been described in the literature, such as subtemporal, midline with or without vermian incision via suboccipital craniotomy, or craniectomy with or without atlas laminectomy, retromastoid, parasigmoid, or via a relatively safe entry area in the floor of the fourth ventricle (Bahgai et al 1982, Kyoshima et al 1993, Pierre-Kahn et al 1993).

It is advisable to enter the tumor through the most apparent part in the surface and remain inside its cavity for debulking the tumors until normal tissue appears. The exceptions are cavernous angioma and cervical extension of medullary tumors which can be resected in the cleavage between the tumor and normal tissue.

The patient may be positioned in one of the following positions: sitting, prone or lateral. Acknowledging the advantages of the sitting position, I prefer the prone or lateral position in order to avoid the risk of air embolism (Cucchiara & Bowers 1982). The use of a laser may be of help (Seifert & Gaab 1989); however, we prefer using only bipolar coagulation and micro instruments. Monitoring the function of the brain stem is very important, so we recommend the use of SEP in such surgery (Wagner et al 1994). The ultrasonic aspirator has proved to be effective in brain stem surgery (Pierre-Kahn et al 1993).

Stereotactic biopsy remains a very good option to reach the diagnosis of the lesion as a step to a final plan for management (Hood et al 1986, Hood & McKeever 1989).

Hydrocephalus is rather commonly associated with brain stem tumors. In our small series, seven out of 12 patients suffered hydrocephalus. Therefore, VA or VP shunt may be essential to divert the course of obstructed CSF and subsequently to control ICP. However, surgeons should be alert to the possible hazards caused by shunt (Epstein & Murali 1982).

Survival rate of patients treated only with radiation is up to 20–30%; there are doubts about the optimal radiating dose, which ranges between 40 Gy and 72 Gy. Which is better: fractionated radiation or one dose of radiation as in the case of radiosurgery (Edwards et al 1989, Pierre-Kahn et al 1993)? This is a question which remains to be answered.

Radiotherapy of 45–50 Gy has been considered to improve the outcome, if associated with partial or subtotal removal (18,19). However, in pediatric patients, radiotherapy is still a subject of debate and concern because of the post-irradiation neurological and endocrinological complications of radiotherapy.

References

Ammar A, Awida A, Al Luwimi I 1993 Reversibility of severe brain stem dysfunction in children. Acta Neurochirurgica (Wien) 124: 2–4

Baghai P, Vries J K, Bechtel P C 1982 Retromastoid approach for biopsy of brain stem tumors. Neurosurgery 10: 574–579

Bouchard J, Pierce C B 1960 Radiation therapy in the management of neoplasms of the central nervous system with special note in regard to children: twenty years experience, 1938–1958. American Journal of Radiology 84: 610–622

Cucchiara R F, Bowers B 1982 Air embolism in children undergoing suboccipital craniotomy. Anesthesiology 57: 338–399

Edwards M S B, Wara W M, Urtasus R C et al 1989 Hyperfractionated radiation therapy for brain-stem glioma: a phase I–II trial. Journal of Neurosurgery 70: 691–700

Epstein F, Farmer J P 1993 Brain stem glioma growth patterns. Journal of Neurosurgery 78: 408–412

Epstein F, Murali R 1982 Pediatric posterior fossa tumors: hazards of the 'preoperative' shunt. Neurosurgery 3: 343–350

Fahlbusch R, Strauss C, Huk W et al 1990 Surgical removal of pontomesencephalic cavernous hemangiomas. Neurosurgery 26: 449–457

Greenberger J S, Cassady J R, Levene M B 1977 Radiation therapy of thalamic, midbrain and brain stem gliomas. Radiology 122: 463–468

Hoffman H J 1988 Tumors of the fourth ventricle technical considerations in tumor surgery. Clinical Neurosurgery 34: 523–545

Hood T W, Gebarski SS, McKeever P E et al 1986 Stereotaxic biopsy of intrinsic lesions of the brain stem. Journal of Neurosurgery 65: 172–176

Hood T W, McKeever P E 1989 Stereotactic management of cystic gliomas of the brain stem. Neurosurgery 24: 373–377

Isu T, Kamada K, Kobayashi N et al 1994 Focal brain-stem astrocytoma causing symptoms of involvement of facial nerve nuclei: long-term survival in six pediatric cases. Journal of Neurosurgery 80: 20–25

Jenkin R D T, Boesei C, Ertei et al 1987 Brain stem tumors in childhood: a prospective randomized trial of irradiation with and without adjuvant CCNU, VCR and prednisone. Journal of Neurosurgery 66: 227–233

Konovalov A, Atieh J 1988 The surgical treatment of primary brain stem tumors. In: Schmidek H H, Sweet W H (eds) Operative neurosurgical techniques: indications, methods and results, 2nd edn. Grune & Stratton/Harcourt-Brace-Jovanovich, pp 709–737

Kyoshima K, Kobayashi S, Gibo H et al 1993 A study of safe zones via the floor of the fourth ventricles for brain-stem lesions. Journal of Neurosurgery 79: 987–993

Lassiter K R L, Alexander E Jr, Davis C H Jr et al 1971 Surgical treatment of brain stem glioma. Journal of Neurosurgery 34: 719–725

Pierre-Kahn A, Hirsch J F, Vinchon M et al 1993 Surgical management of brain-stem tumors in children: results and statistical analysis of 75 cases. Journal of Neurosurgery 79: 845–852

Pollack I F, Hoffman H J, Humphreys R P 1993 The long outcome after surgical treatment of dorsally exophytic brain-stem gliomas. Journal of Neurosurgery 78: 859–863

Rusyniak W G, Ireland P D, Padlew M G et al 1992 Ultrasonographic and electrophysiological adjuncts to surgery within brain stem: technical note. Neurosurgery 31: 798–800

Sakai N, Tanigawara Y T, Andoh A T 1991 Surgical treatment of cavernous angioma involving the brain stem and review literature. Acta Neurochirurgica (Wien) 113: 138–143

Seifert V, Gaab M R 1989 Laser-assisted microsurgical extirpation of brain stem cavernoma: case report. Neurosurgery 25: 986–989

Stroink A R, Hoffman H J, Hendrick E B et al 1987 Transependymal benign dorsally exophytic brain stem gliomas in childhood: diagnosis and treatment recommendations. Neurosurgery 20: 439–443

Villani R, Gaini S M, Tomei G 1975 Follow-up study of brain stem tumors in children. Child's Brain 1: 126–135

Wagner W, Peghini-Halbig L, Maurer J C et al 1994 Intraoperative SEP monitoring in neurosurgery around the brain stem and cervical spinal cord: differential recording of subcortical components. Journal of Neurosurgery 81: 213–220

Yasargil M G 1994 The clinical decision making process. In: Yasargil M G (ed) Microneurosurgery IV. Thieme, New York, pp 319–322

Yoshimoto T, Suzuki J 1986 Radical surgery on cavernous angioma of the brainstem. Surgical Neurology 26: 72–78

Brain Stem Gliomas in Childhood
Harold J. Hoffman

Brain stem gliomas are a common tumor in childhood, making up approximately 10% of all pediatric brain tumors. The management of brain stem gliomas continues to be controversial. In the past, biopsy and radiotherapy or just radiotherapy alone was the usual standard of care. With the development of neuroimaging it has been possible to categorize brain stem gliomas and provide a rational method of management of these tumors.

The commonest brain stem tumor and the most difficult to manage is the diffuse intrinsic brain stem glioma. These tumors center in the pons and spread up into the midbrain and down into the medulla. Typically, the tumor expands the brain stem, produces cranial nerve palsies and long tract signs, and on imaging does not enhance

with gadolinium. Following radiotherapy, these tumors do shrink and the brain stem takes on a more normal appearance and the child's symptoms abate. However, the respite is relatively brief and, within 6 months to a year, the tumor is back and now enhances brightly with exophytic components coming out of the brain stem, frequently surrounding the basilar artery, and the child succumbs to this terrible disease.

The dorsally exophytic brain stem gliomas protrude from the floor of the fourth ventricle and typically fill the fourth ventricle, producing hydrocephalus. These patients with tumors arising from the floor of the fourth ventricle rarely have significant cranial nerve palsies. The tumors typically enhance and are usually low-grade astrocytomas and more rarely gangliogliomas.

These dorsally exophytic brain stem gliomas can be resected. It is not necessary to do a total resection because in order to do that one would have to get into the floor of the fourth ventricle and disturb the cranial nerve nuclei. However, with shaving off the tumor, the residual tumor frequently stabilizes and may indeed shrink. Some of these tumors do recur and if the recurrence occurs more than several years after the initial presentation, it is possible to go in and remove the recurrent tumor. The tumors that recur quickly may need adjunctive therapy. Such recurrences, however, are rare with this group of tumors.

The focal gliomas occur in localized sites in the brain stem. The commonest site for these focal tumors is the midbrain. Next in incidence is the medulla. Medullary tumors can spread down into the upper cervical cord. Rarely, a focal benign tumor can occur in the pons. These focal tumors can be resected. If the midbrain tumor is situated in the tegmentum laterally, it is possible to approach it subtemporally with splitting of the tentorium, which gives one a good view of the side of the brain stem and one can enter the brain stem and resect the tumor. The tectal midbrain tumors produce a block of the aqueduct resulting in hydrocephalus. Many of these tumors remain small and the only treatment necessary is a diversionary CSF drainage. Only when the tectal glioma is substantial in size is a surgical approach necessary. I prefer to approach these large tectal tumors through an occipital transtentorial approach, much like the approach to pineal tumor. Occasionally, the focal tegmental tumors of the midbrain are huge, with the child presenting with facial weakness and some Vth nerve involvement. It is possible to approach these tumors much like a cerebellopontine (CP) angle tumor. However, when the tumors are exceptionally large, it is sometimes difficult to get into the tumor through a CP angle approach, particularly without further injuring the VIIth and VIIIth cranial nerves. I have found that an approach through the cerebellar hemisphere has worked very well in dealing with these tumors, preferably utilizing a stereotactic navigational system.

The focal gliomas in the medulla and pons may be exophytic out the side of the brain stem and can be approached through a far lateral craniotomy which allows one to enter the medulla or the pons and carry out a subtotal resection of the tumor. Those tumors which are in the midline involving medulla and upper cord can be approached through a midline approach, much as one deals with an intramedullary spinal cord tumor.

Brain stem gliomas have been transformed from an inoperable hopeless situation in the past to a much more optimistic situation in the present. Half of the brain stem gliomas in childhood are low-grade astrocytomas or occasionally gangliogliomas which lend themselves to resection and frequently require no adjunctive therapy.

Chordomas: a clinical review

Atul Goel   Shigeaki Kobayashi

18

Cranial chordomas are rare, histologically benign but potentially malignant, slow-growing tumors that usually present between the third and fifth decades of life. Chordoma accounts for approximately 1–4% of all primary bone neoplasms. Although the sacrum is the most common site of origin, approximately 30% of these tumors occur in the region of the skull base. Male predominance has been recorded. They are thought to arise from remnants of the embryonic notochord along the spinal axis (Russell & Rubenstein 1989). The more frequent site of presumptive origin is the region of the junction of the basisphenoid with the basiocciput. These tumors arise usually in the midline, but often have an eccentric growth. After its origin from the clivus, the direction of predominant growth will determine the clinical presentation. Anterior growth will lead to the presentation as a nasopharyngeal mass. The usual pattern of growth is in the anterolateral direction towards the petrous apex. Falconer et al (1968) suggested three groups of chordomas: sellar, parasellar, and clival, each with corresponding clinical features. The clival origin is more frequent.

Clinical interest in cranial chordomas and chondrosarcomas has increased in the last few years. The reasons for this surge in interest are as follows:

1. High detection rate: better diagnosis of cases with the help of magnetic resonance imaging (MRI). Even with the help of computed tomography (CT) scanning it is difficult to detect some of these lesions as they are located in the base of the skull. Unclear delineation of the tumor due to bone artifacts may sometimes lead to difficulties in identification of the tumor. Higher detection rate of chordomas was clearly observed in the authors' series.

Years	Cases
1965–1970	1
1970–1980	3
1980–1990	9
1990–1995	28

2. Better evaluation: MRI not only helped in clearly defining the extensions of the tumor, but also clarified the relationships to adjoining neural and vascular structures. The relationship of the tumor to the internal carotid artery, which is crucial while planning and executing the surgical treatment, could be clearly seen on MRI.

3. Better treatment modalities: advancements in skull base surgical techniques in the last decade have increased the awareness and improved the management efficiency of these relatively difficult neurosurgical problems.

4. Parallel to the improved radiological and neurosurgical enthusiasm in the management of these cases, the pathology of these tumors is also a subject of renewed interest. Immunohistochemical and ultrastructural studies have also helped in differentiating and subclassifying these tumors.

These tumors arise from notochordal remnants, a tissue which is ordinarily found only in the early stage of the embryo. The tumor was first recognized by Virchow in 1857, who postulated that it was a cartilaginous entity. One year later, Muller proposed that this tumor had a notochordal origin. This theory has largely been accepted and later reaffirmed by others.

DIFFERENCES BETWEEN CHORDOMAS AND CHONDROSARCOMAS

The classification of these neoplasms is controversial. Chordoma and chondrosarcoma are frequently grouped together because of their clinical, radiological, surgical and histological similarity (Bahr & Gayler 1977, Grossman & Davis 1981, Morimoto et al 1992, Stapleton et al 1993). While chordoma has an epithelial origin, chondrosarcomas have a mesenchymal cell of origin.

These two varieties of tumors have similar sites of origin, nature of spread, radiological features, and therapeutic problems. In our study the nature and pattern of displacement of the carotid artery, cranial nerves and cavernous sinus by these lesions also matched. Chondrosarcomas have more cartilaginous content and are therefore more gritty in their feel. The introduction of immunohistochemical techniques have helped in differentiating these two varieties of tumor, but even this investigation is not fool-proof. Although both these varieties of tumors originate around the clivus, a tumor originating from the temporal bone or from an off-midline epicenter is more likely to be chondrosarcoma. Despite subtle differences, the surgical management has generally been reported to be similar (Sen et al 1989). With radical resection the ultimate outcome of chondrosarcomas matches that of chordomas.

CHONDROID CHORDOMA

Heffelfinger et al (1973) described a variety of chordoma which had some areas bearing a close resemblance to a chondrosarcoma and other areas with the features of a classical chordoma. He named such a tumor as 'chondroid chordoma'. This variety of chordoma is seen more frequently in relatively young individuals and has been recorded to have a better prognosis and longer survival than the classical chordoma.

The concept of 'chondroid chordoma' has been a subject of confusion and much debate. After the initial acceptance, several reports followed that challenged the concept. Brooks and colleagues (1987) in immunohistochemical studies found that these tumors failed to stain for epithelial markers and had an identical staining pattern with chondrosarcomas. They labeled them as 'low-grade chondrosarcomas'. Other investigators also found that chondroid chordoma was actually a low-grade chondrosarcoma.

More recent investigations based on electron microscopic and immunohistochemical analysis relate these tumors more to chordomas than to chondrosarcomas. Ultrastructural features of 'chondroid chordomas' resembled more closely those of classical chordoma (Cancilla et al 1964, Erlandson et al 1968) and were different from those described in chondrosarcomas. The presence of glycogen, prominent and dilated rough endoplasmic reticulum, and abundant fibrillogranular matrix is common to all three lesions. Well-formed tonofilament desmosome complexes and rough endoplasmic reticulum mitochondrial complexes are found only in chordoma and chondroid chordoma and not in cartilaginous tumors.

On light microscopy, chondroid chordoma revealed areas that resembled classical chordoma (chordoid areas) and areas that resembled low-grade chondrosarcoma (chondroid areas). 5-Nucleotidase, an enzyme that has been detected in chordoma but not in chondrosarcoma, was found in both the chordoid and chondroid areas of chondroid chordoma.

Even in immunohistochemical studies, the chondroid chordomas had more similarities to chordomas than to chondrosarcomas. Both the chordoid and chondroid areas of 'chondroid chordoma' had an epithelial phenotype and stained strongly for cytokeratin, EMA, S-100 and 5-nucleotidase. In contrast to chondroid chordoma, chondrosarcoma stained positive only for S-100 protein and was cytokeratin, EMA and 5-nucleotidase negative. These studies suggest that 'chondroid chordoma' is a variant of chordoma with histologic features that match chondrosarcoma.

CONTROVERSY OF BENIGN VERSUS MALIGNANT NATURE OF CHORDOMA

Some reports suggest that the chordomas are of benign nature while others suggest that chordomas are of malignant nature. There are still other reports which suggest that the tumor is of a low-grade malignancy.

Russell & Rubinstein (1989) mention that although these tumors are regionally invasive, and therefore of poor prognosis, most of these tumors are histologically benign.

According to Saeger et al (1983) chordomas are potentially malignant, whereas Derome and Guiot (Derome et al 1988) consider them histologically benign tumors. Heffelfinger et al (1973) opine that the main malignant potential of chordoma lies in its critical locations, its locally aggressive nature, and its extremely high recurrence rate; these account for the almost certain eventual death of the host.

Chordoma has been considered by most authors to be a slow-growing, locally aggressive and rarely metastasizing neoplasm with a high incidence of recurrence. Skull base chordomas are reported to metastasize in about 20% (Chambers & Schwinn 1979). In our literature survey no clear pattern of its tendency to metastasize emerges from some large series (Chambers & Schwinn 1979, Dahlin & MacCarty 1952, Higginbotham et al 1967) and several case reports.

Whether the different neoplastic potential is related to various degrees of tumor differentiation is difficult to establish. It seems equally difficult to identify those histologic features which may be indicative of local aggressiveness and of metastatic potential of chordoma. There appear to be very few reliable histologic features that aid in the prediction of the metastatic potential of this neoplasm. Further studies on this aspect of chordoma are still needed. However, in view of the potential of this neoplasm to recur and to metastasize, and the histologic unpredictability of its behavior, a wide local excision of the tumor would seem to be mandatory in the treatment.

Impressions on the basis of our study

An unusual location of a chordoma is more conducive to rapid growth and recurrence.

Unusual age is more conducive to rapid growth and recurrence. These tumors depict a clearly malignant clinical course.

Although the tumor presents more often in the third to fifth decades of life it is not clear when the tumor originates. Although the tumor arises from notochordal remnants the tumor cells may start dividing unusually only later in life. And when they start dividing the growth may be fairly rapid and symptomatic. The rapid progression of clinical symptoms, once they begin, suggests that the growth of the tumor begins late but progresses rapidly.

Symptoms

Due to the characteristic location and pattern of growth, the tumors are usually large when first diagnosed and have relatively innocuous presenting symptoms (Grossman & Davies 1981, Larson et al 1987, Morimoto et al 1992, Raffel et al 1985, Rich et al 1985, Russell and Rubenstein 1989, Sen et al 1989, Stapleton et al 1993). The most common symptom is pain secondary to destruction of bone and/or to pressure effects on nerves or adjacent organs. Due to the proximity of a clival chordoma to VIth nerve, unilateral or bilateral involvement of this nerve is commonly seen. Cranial nerves of the cavernous sinus are also frequently affected. In larger tumors multiple cranial nerves may be affected. Sellar or parasellar chordomas may present with visual deterioration, pituitary dysfunction, and a chiasmal or a cavernous sinus syndrome. Inferior clival chordomas may present with XIIth nerve palsy, dysphagia and dysphonia. As there is a high incidence of involvement of occipital condyle, occipital pain is also a frequent symptom. A craniocervical fixation procedure may be considered in such a case. The stability of the region is usually not affected in cases with unilateral condylar involvement.

Radiological features and growth characters

Chordomas and chondrosarcomas are often easily diagnosed radiologically due to the following features: their specific location; the frequently associated destructive and erosive bone changes; varying amounts of extracellular mucinous matrix; entrapped bony trabeculae; small dystrophic calcification; areas of necrosis; and recent and old hemorrhages (Grossman & Davis 1981, Meyers et al 1992, Oot et al 1988, Sen et al 1989, Utne & Pugh 1955).

Grossly, the chordomas are gelatinous, lobulated, semi-translucent grayish tumors. In soft tissues and cranial cavity, they appear 'encapsulated'. Such a demarcation from normal tissue was not present at the site of bone invasion.

Relationship to the carotid artery
(Goel 1995a)

In our series of these rare lesions, we observed that the tumor displaced the relatively immobile parts of the internal carotid artery in the petrous and precavernous segments along its anterolateral border (Figs 18.1–18.9). In some massive tumors, the entire intrapetrous segment of the artery was displaced (Figs 18.1–18.4). At the petrous apex, the Vth nerve was displaced superiorly while the carotid artery was displaced anteriorly (Fig. 18.8). The direction and the site of the displacement of the carotid artery provide additional evidence that the epicenter of origin of these tumors is the junction of basisphenoid and basiocciput. Complete encasement of the artery was not seen in any patient despite the massive size of the tumors. Narrowing of the lumen of the vessel was seen in one case and was apparently due to the severe stretch (Fig. 18.3). Myers et al noted vascular encasement by large tumors and observed that in spite of the complete encasement, the lumen of the vessel was not narrowed. Our observations and that of Myers et al (1992) suggest that these tumors are 'capsulated' and grow by expansion and bony destruction that displaces the soft tissues. As the tumor grows it pushes the internal carotid artery, making way for it by destroying the bone. Arterial encasement is a late feature and

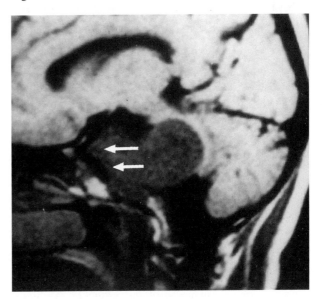

Fig. 18.1 T1-weighted MRI shows a massive petroclival chordoma. Arrows point to the anteriorly displaced internal carotid artery. (From Goel 1995a, with permission.)

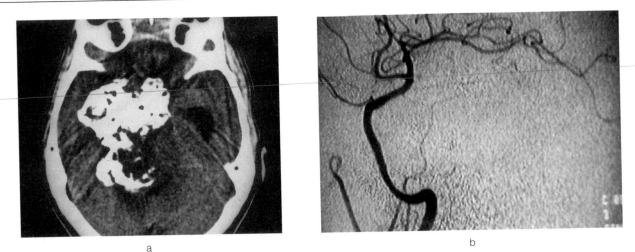

Fig. 18.2 **a** Plain CT scan shows a massive petroclival tumor (chondrosarcoma) with multiple calcific spots. **b** Internal carotid artery angiogram showing the displacement of the petrous and cavernous sinus segments of the artery along the anterior border of the tumor.

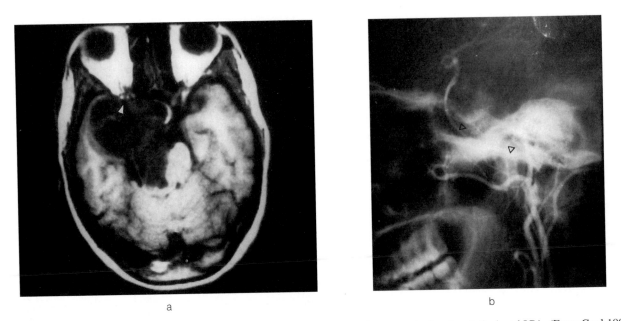

Fig. 18.3 **a** T1-weighted MRI showing the massive tumor. Arrowhead points towards the site of displaced ICA. (From Goel 1995, with permission.) **b** Common carotid angiogram shows a marked anterior displacement, stretching and thinning of the cavernous, horizontal and vertical intrapetrous segments of the ICA (arrowheads). (From Goel 1995a, with permission.)

appears to be secondary to the growth pattern of the tumor, wherein its lobulations surround the artery from its sides. Such a relationship to the carotid artery is not observed in the previously surgically treated or irradiated tumors.

In addition to other characteristic radiological features, a preoperative presumption of the nature of the tumor could be made on the basis of the arterial displacements. Such information can sometimes be critically important in planning the operative strategy in terms of the surgical exposure, need for arterial control, extent of resection, and prognosticating the ultimate outcome.

Relationship to cranial nerves and cavernous sinus (Goel 1995a)

Russell & Rubenstein (1989) mention that intracranial chordomas sometimes 'occupy' the cavernous sinus and

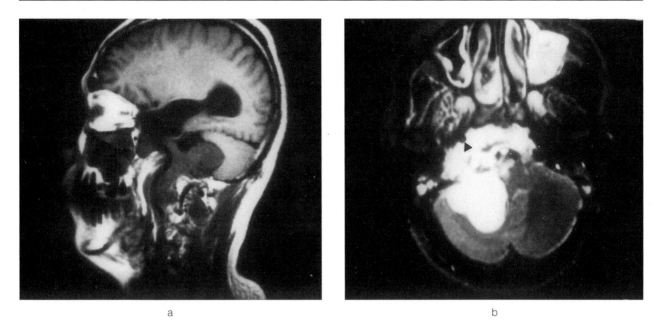

a   b

Fig. 18.4 **a** T1-weighted image shows the large chondrosarcoma displacing the petrous, precavernous, and cavernous segments of the ICA along its anterior border. (From Goel 1995a, with permission.) **b** T2-weighted axial image shows the partially encased ICA (arrowhead). (From Goel 1995a, with permission.)

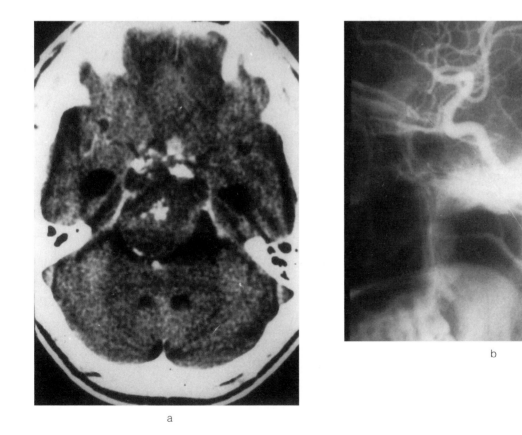

b

a

Fig. 18.5 **a** Contrast-enhanced CT scan shows the characteristic appearance of a chordoma with intratumoral specks of bone. (From Goel 1995a, with permission.) **b** Internal carotid artery angiogram showing the anteriorly displaced precavernous segments of ICA. (From Goel 1995a, with permission.)

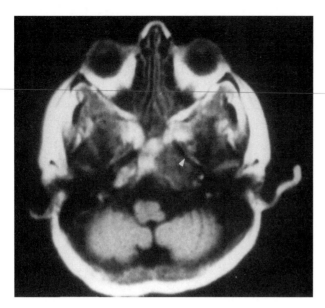

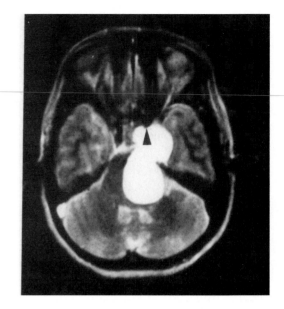

Fig. 18.6 T1-weighted MRI showing the anteriorly displaced horizontal intrapetrous and precavernous segments of the ICA (arrowhead). (From Goel 1995a, with permission.)

Fig. 18.7 T2-weighted MRI showing the large chordoma displacing the internal carotid artery (arrowhead) along its anterior suface. (From Goel 1995a, with permission.)

spread thence into the middle fossa. In our series we also observed that the cranial nerves and cavernous sinus were displaced on the dome of the tumor. The extension of the

chordomas is more frequently 'subcavernous' in nature. Despite the huge size of the tumors, actual invasion of the cavernous sinus was not seen (Fig. 18.8). Functional com-

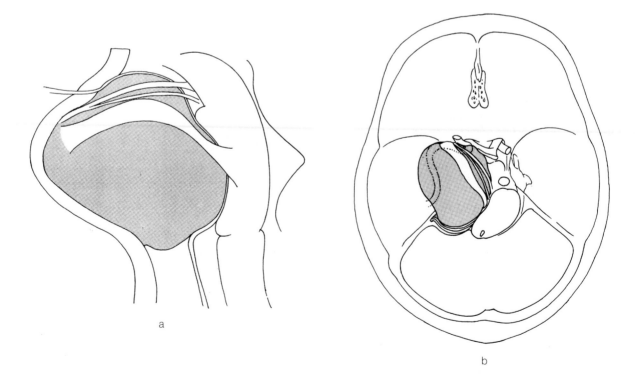

a

b

Fig. 18.8 Relationships of a typical petroclival chordoma. The large tumor spreads in the extradural plane in the subcavernous sinus region. The tumor displaces the soft tissues. The internal carotid artery is displaced anteriorly and the brain stem posteriorly.

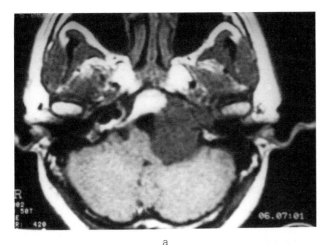

a

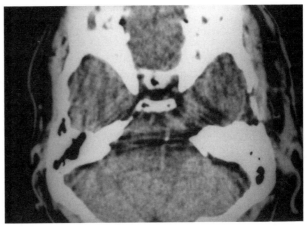

b

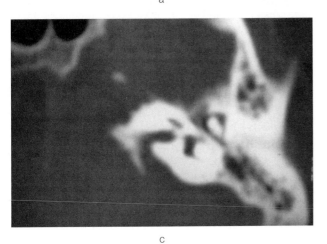

c

Fig. 18.9 **a** T1-weighted MRI image shows the large hypointense petroclival chordoma. Note the relationship with the clivus and petrous apex. (From Goel 1995c, with permission.) **b** Postoperative CT scan shows resection of the tumor. Part of the petrous apex is destroyed by the tumor and part was drilled during surgery. (From Goel 1995c, with permission.) **c** Bone window of the postoperative scan showing the petrous apex medial to the internal auditory meatus drilled during surgery. The part of petrous apex harboring the cochlea is left undisturbed. (From Goel 1995c, with permission.)

promise seemed to be related to the stretch on the cranial nerves, which are pushed towards the dome of the tumor.

The VIth nerve is maximally displaced due to the relation between the site of origin of the tumor and the course of

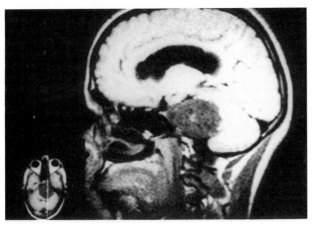

a

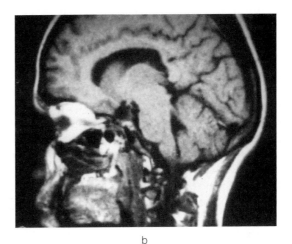

b

Fig. 18.10 **a** T1-weighted MRI shows the large clival chordoma displacing the internal carotid artery along its anterior surface. (From Goel 1995c, with permission.) **b** Postoperative scan showing complete tumor resection. (From Goel 1995c, with permission.)

the VIth nerve. In the cavernous sinus the VIth nerve is elevated superiorly, while the carotid is displaced anteriorly; thus the two are separated by the enlarging tumor. Both the VIth cranial nerves are likely to be affected by tumor growth. The Vth nerve root and the Gasserian ganglion are lifted superiorly by the tumor. The third and the second divisions of the Vth cranial nerve are also displaced anteriorly by the tumor. The Eustachian tube is preserved intact despite the destruction around it.

Relationship to the dura

In our series no tumor invaded through the dura. The dura of the posterior and middle cranial fossa and of the cavernous sinus was completely intact. Although on radiological investigations it appeared that some tumors had transgressed the dural border, during surgery the dura was always intact. The structures of the posterior fossa including the brain stem, arteries of the posterior circulation, and the cranial nerves of the cerebellopontine angle were displaced by the tumor, a thinned and stretched dura providing a firm tumor–brain barrier (Figs 18.1–18.5, 18.7–18.10). The carotid artery and cranial nerves were also seen to be separated from the tumor by a fibrous periosteal or dural sheath, thus providing a plane for dissection.

Relationship to the bone

The relationship of chordomas to the bone is unusual. It arises from the spheno-occipital synchondrosis. The tumor is primarily of bone-destructive character. More frequently encountered bone destruction is in one half of the clivus and the petrous apex. The tumor destroys the bone, and small bone pieces with normal bone trabeculae can be seen interspersed within the bulk of the tumor. Although the tumor destroys the bone the soft tissues are only displaced. The pattern of tumor expansion, wherein the bone is destroyed and the carotid artery is displaced along its anterior surface, is unclear. The theory that bone takes the shape defined by the underlying soft tissues appears to be clearly applicable in this situation. Tumor borders are slightly multilobulated and well defined except at sites of marrow invasion and bone destruction. The petrous apex destruction can spread laterally as far as the internal auditory canal, in which case the labyrinthine part of the facial nerve may be completely unroofed of its bony cover. The exact relationship of the cochlea to the growing tumor could not be adequately studied. The occipital condyle is frequently affected. The functional involvement of the XIIth cranial nerve is almost always confirmatory of condylar involvement.

Role of MRI

On short TR/TE images (T1-weighted images), chordoma usually has a low to intermediate signal (Figs 18.1,18.3a,18.4a,18.6,18.9a,18.10a). On long TR/long TE images (T2), chordomas often have a very high signal (Figs 18.4b,18.7). Signal intensity may be heterogeneous due to tumor characters. After Gd-DTPA administration most of the chordomas demonstrate some degree of contrast enhancement. MRI exactly delineates the location and extent of these neoplasms, the relationship of the tumor to neighboring structures such as the brain stem and the pituitary gland, and thus plays an important role in determining the optimal surgical approaches. The arterial relationships can be determined and, more importantly, displacement of large vessels by the tumor may be distinguished from encasement. Calcific areas in the tumor presenting as low-intensity signals can sometimes make identification of the course of the blood vessel (by its flow void) difficult. The information on MRI often renders angiography unnecessary or less useful.

Treatment

Although chordomas are soft, essentially extradural, and relatively avascular lesions, they are difficult to treat surgically because of their proximity to critical neural and vascular structures, depth from the surface and also widespread extension particularly into the adjacent structures such as cavernous sinus, sella, nasopharynx, and hypoglossal canal. These features make the ultimate clinical course 'malignant' and eventually fatal. These neoplasms have a locally aggressive and invasive nature, high recurrence rate and rarely metastasize (Brooks et al 1987, Derome et al 1988, Fisch et al 1984, Grossman & Davis 1981, Larson et al 1987, Meyer et al 1986). Effective outcome of these lesions has been reported to depend on the extent of the surgical resection of the tumor (Myers et al 1992, Morimoto et al 1992, Oot et al 1988, Raffel et al 1985, Rich et al 1985). The role of radiotherapy for chordomas is not established, but there are reports of successful outcome following this modality of treatment (Seifert & Laszig 1991, Sen et al 1989).

SURGERY

The following factors should be considered when one decides to operate on chordomas and chondrosarcomas.

1. Chordomas are usually soft, mucinous and suckable. There are interspersed bony spicules in the tumor which can usually be removed in large pieces. In situ-

ations where the bony part is difficult to remove, the soft tissue portion of the tumor around the bone should be removed. This procedure loosens the intratumoral bone, which can then be removed relatively easily and safely. Chondrosarcomas are relatively gritty and have a much larger cartilaginous content (Fig. 18.2a,18.4).

2. Most of the tumors are relatively avascular. Intratumoral coagulation is rarely necessary. Whenever significant bleeding occurs during tumor resection it is due to damage to a normal artery or decompression of a compressed venous channel.

3. The tumors are essentially extradural in nature.

4. The tumors grow by displacement of surrounding soft tissues and by destroying the bone. The carotid artery, which is in direct relationship with the tumor in its petrous, precavernous and cavernous segments, is displaced along the anterior border of the tumor (Goel 1995a). Sometimes this displacement may be as much as 3–3.5 cm. By working within the tumor the need to expose the carotid artery during the entire operation can be avoided in some cases.

5. Cavernous sinus involvement is in the nature of displacement rather than invasion. The tumor usually has a subcavernous sinus spread. The cranial nerves of the cavernous sinus are displaced on the superior surface of the tumor (Fig. 18.8). A thin sheet of dura separates the tumor from all neural and vascular structures.

6. Whenever the tumor extends posteriorly into the posterior cranial fossa, the brain tissue, vessels and nerves are displaced by the tumor. The tumor is separated from these structures by thinned and stretched-out dura.

7. The more frequent site of origin of these tumors is in the region of the spheno-occipital synchondrosis. From this site the tumor usually spreads eccentrically on one side. Midline spread is relatively uncommon (Fig. 18.11). Chordomas originating away from the more usual site of clivus with characteristic extensions are frequently more malignant in their nature and the outcome in these cases is generally poor (Fig. 18.12).

Operative strategy

Considering the nature of the tumor, its location and the arterial and neural displacements, an operative strategy has to be formulated. The exposure for the tumor should be such that all parts of the tumor can be approached in one field. The preparation should be for a radical surgical excision, which implies excision of the tumor and the involved bone. Sen et al (1989) suggest removal of about 1 cm of normal bone around the tumor involved bone. The direction of the approach should be such that the tumor bulk can be easily exposed. The extent of the exposure need not be extremely elaborate as the intratumoral debulking of this soft tumor results in additional exposure. The exposure should not deal with the internal carotid artery or the nerves of the cavernous sinus in the initial stages of the operation. These structures are stretched by the tumor and can be damaged during the process of mobilization or displacement. The tumor should be first debulked by intra-'capsular' removal. This procedure is safe, relatively easily performed and adds to the exposure. It results in release of stretch on the surrounding vessels and nerves which can

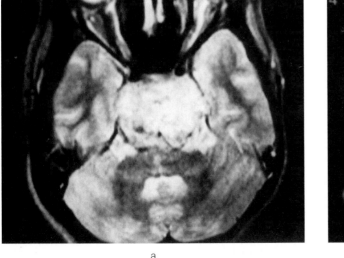

a

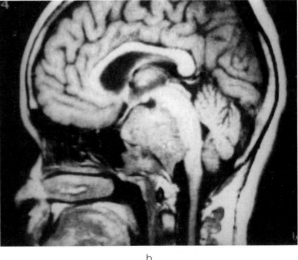

b

Fig. 18.11 **a** MRI shows a massive midline chordoma. The entire lesion was extradural. **b** Sagittal section of the midline chordoma with the pituitary stalk displaced anteriorly.

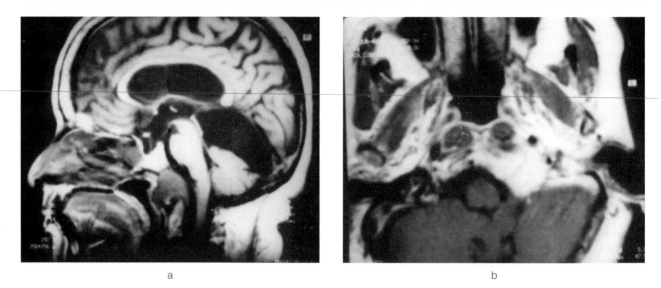

a   b

Fig. 18.12 **a** MRI shows a low clival chondrosarcoma. **b** Contrast-enhanced transverse view of MRI showing the tumor involving the condyle.

then be dissected off from the surface of the tumor. Sharp dissection in the tumor in the initial debulking stage should be avoided.

The approach selection depends on the site and direction of the growth of tumor. More frequently the growth is eccentric after it starts from the midline. Some tumors are strictly in the midline. Anterior surgical approaches (transoral, transmaxilla, transcervical) are sometimes suitable for midline lesions. However, for the more typical laterally extending lesions, midline approaches have the disadvantage of encountering the internal carotid artery early in the operation. An anterolateral approach through a pterional craniotomy has a similar disadvantage of early encounter with the carotid artery and should be avoided. Lateral approaches (subtemporal, infratemporal) appear to be more appropriate for internal carotid artery safety. Anterior approaches have the advantage that they are relatively simple approaches. In some predominantly midline lesions an anterior approach exposes the lesion on minimal tissue manipulation. In some tumors where the extension is in the retropharyngeal space a transoral or transmaxilla approach can expose the lesion after only a mucosal incision. The lateral extensions of the tumor may be difficult to reach by these routes and thus a radical or 'total' resection may be possible only in a minority of cases. Lateral approaches are usually better for radical excision of the more common form of tumor pattern with an eccentric growth, and also as regards the safety of the internal carotid artery. Lateral retrosigmoid and subsigmoid approaches are suitable for low clival lesions.

Radiotherapy

Some reports indicate the usefulness of radiation therapy for these tumors. In our opinion radiotherapy should not be given to these lesions. The incidence of recurrence in these tumors is high even with radical resections and radiotherapy. In cases where radiation therapy has been previously given, repeat surgery becomes difficult and dangerous. This makes further surgical resection or even palliation difficult. In case a significant residual tumor has been left behind at surgery, it is our opinion that radiotherapy should not follow such a procedure. Such tumors can either be reoperated or can be observed on serial investigations.

EFFECTS OF RADIOTHERAPY

Chordoma is considered a relatively radiation-resistant tumor. Total doses of radiation of 6000–7000 cGy, fractionated at 200 cGy per day, appears to be required for worthwhile palliation. Tumor eradication requires doses in excess of 6500–7000 cGy, but this can only be achieved in selected circumstances when treatment volumes are small and include minimal amounts of normal tissue. There are a few reports of rapid regression of the tumor following radiation treatment (Poppers & King 1952, Andrews 1942). High doses are needed to achieve these goals, indicating a relative radioresistance probably due to the slow growth of the tumor and limited mitotic activity. Since the tumors are slow growing, the effects of radiotherapy will be slower in appearing (Higinbotham et al 1967) but will last longer than the effects on faster-growing tumors.

Reoperations

Where definite evidence of growth of the tumor is observed a reoperation can be performed. Reoperations are relatively difficult as the tumor may spread intradurally through the rents in the dura made during the first operation. Such recurring tumors invade into the cavernous sinus. Some authors have noticed invasion of the chordomas into the cavernous sinus. However, most of these cases were the recurrent variety of tumor. Where radiotherapy has already been given, it makes dissection of the tumor from the surrounding vessels difficult and fraught with danger of injury to adjoining vessels, nerve and brain. In cases with recurrence despite surgery and radiation treatment, reoperation is the only effective mode of treatment and means of palliation.

MIDDLE FOSSA SUB-GASSERIAN GANGLION APPROACH TO CLIVUS CHORDOMAS (Goel 1995b)

Most of the lateral procedures described for resection of clival chordomas involve relatively complex and extensive skull basal dissection, exposure and mobilization of the carotid artery (Sen et al 1989, Sekhar et al 1987), facial nerve (Fisch et al 1984, House et al 1986, sigmoid sinus (Al-Mefty et al 1988) and temporomandibular joint (Fisch et al 1984, Sen et al 1989, Sekhar et al 1987).

A modified lateral subtemporal, transpetrous apex and sub-Gasserian ganglion approach was found to be most suitable for clival chordomas. The approach selection was based on typical anatomic relationship of chordomas in terms of site of origin, pattern of growth, bone destruction and neural and vascular displacements. The approach was suitable for dealing with tumor anterior and lateral to the brain stem, clival part of the tumor and its sub-cavernous sinus extensions. The carotid artery was under control. The approach had the advantage of being simple and relatively quick and its familiarity to general neurosurgeons. The tumor could be excised radically and extension of anterior, posterior and inferior exposure was possible.

Operative technique

The patient is placed in the lateral position and a continuous external drainage of cerebrospinal fluid (CSF) by lumbar subarachnoid catheter placement is set up. The approach is by a subtemporal route centered on the exter-

nal ear canal. A low temporal craniotomy is done. The temporalis muscle is displaced anteriorly after its adequate mobilization. The root of the zygomatic arch, roof of the condyle and external ear canal, and the base of the petrous pyramid are drilled to obtain a basal exposure along the anterior face of the petrous bone. The approach is in the direction of the external ear canal and zygomatic osteotomy is not necessary. In cases where a large middle fossa extension of the tumor is present, zygomatic arch osteotomy can be done to elevate the temporalis muscle out of the exposure (Goel 1996).

The approach is initially intradural where the temporal lobe is elevated off the middle fossa floor. By an intradural exposure and tentorial incision (Goel 1995d) the root of the trigeminal nerve and the Gasserian ganglion are unroofed of the dural cover and mobilized superiorly. Underneath the medial and inferior dural cover of the Gasserian ganglion is the most prominent bulge of the tumor. An incision is taken along the root of the Vth nerve over the dura of Meckel's cave. Vth nerve identification can sometimes be difficult. Identification of the nerve after an initial tumor debulking or following the nerve along its intradural segment are the alternatives available. The tumor is seen immediately underneath Meckel's cave. The petrous apex is drilled laterally as required, more frequently up to the medial end of the internal auditory meatus, taking care to preserve the cochlea. The internal carotid artery is identified in the petrous apex and is exposed and protected. The soft, relatively avascular and extradural nature of the tumor helps in expanding the exposure. The tumor is removed by an initial intratumoral debulking procedure which releases the stretch on the neural and vascular structures, which are then dissected free. Remaining intratumorally and debulking it is the safest way to preserve the adjoining critical structures. Anterior extension of the exposure by removal of the middle fossa base, condyle of the temporomandibular joint and mobilization of the petrous carotid artery, and lateral and inferior extension by additional drilling of the petrous bone and whenever necessary mobilization of labyrinthine and tympanic segments of the facial nerve (Goel 1995c) is possible. The clivus is directly in the line of the exposure and can be drilled widely.

It was observed that combined intra- and extradural exposure makes dissection of the tumor from the cranial nerves and brain stem relatively safe and under direct vision. A basal temporal exposure and lumbar drainage of CSF made temporal lobe elevation off the base relatively safe. The inclusion of the intradural route for the primarily extradural tumor, although against the principles of skull base surgery, was found to significantly increase the exposure which appeared critical for the safety of the patient and radical resection of the tumor. Direct lateral and basal exposure was the shortest surgical route to the tumor located in the clivus and adjacent areas. As the tumor adjoining segments of the internal carotid artery were displaced anteriorly by the tumor the direct lateral route was more appropriate for its safety. It was observed that the arteries and nerves were relatively easily dissected free from the tumor probably because their involvement was only compressive and not invasive in nature. The petrous apex and clival bone were eroded, precavernous and cavernous segments of the internal carotid artery were displaced anteriorly and the Gasserian ganglion was elevated on the dome of the tumor in all cases. These anatomical features were utilized in developing a sub-Gasserian ganglion exposure. The tumor, being soft and relatively avascular, could then be removed by debulking and blunt dissection (Figs 18.9, 18.10). The dura protects the brain stem and cranial nerves and an intact periosteal sheath protects the internal carotid artery. Reconstruction of the region is easy and safe.

The described middle fossa approach appeared to be ideal for dealing surgically with the more characteristic form of clival chordomas. This approach could be used and exposure widened depending upon the extensions of the tumor.

LATERAL SUBTEMPORAL TRANSPETROUS APEX TRANSCLIVAL APPROACH (Goel 1996)

The subtemporal, sub-Gasserian ganglion approach can be extended medially in the same direction to include the clivus which is already destroyed by the tumor. In most of the cases of clival chordomas, involvement of the ipsilateral condyle is frequently seen.

EXTENDED MIDDLE FOSSA APPROACH (Goel 1995b)

The lateral extension of the subtemporal sub-Gasserian

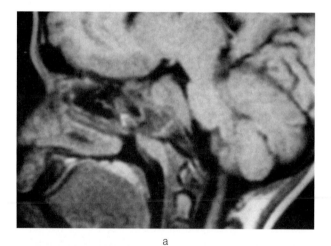

a

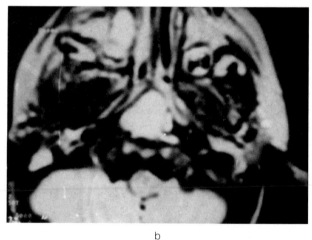

b

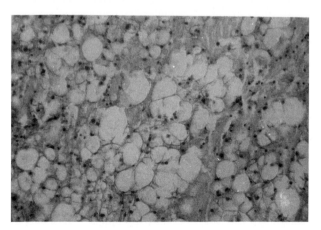

c

Fig. 18.13 **a** Sagittal view of the MRI showing the clival lesion in a 7-month-old child. **b** Transverse section of the MRI shows the clival chordoma. **c** Histology shows the classical features of chordoma with tissue composed of lobules of large clear physaliphora cells with small central or peripheral nuclei.

ganglion approach can be performed by additional drilling of the petrous bone. Facial nerve segments (tympanic and labyrinthine) can be mobilized to enable a lateral extension of the exposure. This approach is described in another chapter.

The above approaches are described for the more characteristic pattern of chordomas and chondrosarcomas, wherein, after their origin in the spheno-occipital synchondrosis, the tumor expands in an eccentric fashion. However, some tumors grow in the midline or in an unusual pattern and the approach should suitably be modified. Despite the unusual site of the growth of the tumors, they usually retain their character of extradural growth and displacement of soft tissues and destruction of the bone.

An unusual case

This boy developed noisy breathing, snoring and occasional apnea with cyanosis when placed in a horizontal position since 2 months of age. In an upright position he was asymptomatic but preferred a hyperextended neck posture. The frequency of apneic spells increased to three or four times a day as the child grew. When he was 7 months old, in a period of 10 days he developed three episodes of cyanosis followed by a 2–8-hour period of unconsciousness, and needed ventilatory assistance, arterial blood oxygen being grossly reduced each time. Magnetic resonance imaging (MRI) showed a large retropharyngeal and clival mass (Fig. 18.13a,b). Considering the age and the strict midline location of the tumor a relatively simple transoral surgical approach was considered to be safer in this patient. Radical debulking of the jelly-like tumor was done. Histology revealed the classical features of chordoma (Fig. 18.13c) with tissue composed of lobules of large clear physaliphora cells with small central or peripheral nuclei. The child had no further apneic episodes, breathing was comfortable and noiseless, and the neck posture returned to normal. Due to the patient's age, the tumor was not subjected to radiation treatment.

Discussion

The occurrence of chordomas in the pediatric age group is rare. Unlike the adult type, intracranial chordomas in children have been seen to run an acute clinical course and show frequent metastasis, more often in the lungs. In general, for chordomas the 5-year survival rate has been reported to be 30–50%. Combination of a 'radical debulking' operation followed by high-dose radiation therapy has been recommended as an effective mode of treatment in children. However, tolerance, effectiveness and long-term effects of radiation treatment in the pediatric age group are subject to great controversy.

Therapy and survival

Extensive surgery combined with radiation has been the management of choice for chordomas, particularly in recent years. The present series of patients were so treated, making it difficult to compare these modes of therapy when used singly. The major object of therapy appears to be to increase the patient's survival time and to make him productive and as comfortable as possible.

REFERENCES

Al-Mefty O, Fox J L, Smith R R 1988 Petrosal approach for petroclival meningiomas. Neurosurgery 22: 510–517

Andrews J R 1942 Spheno-occipital chordoma of unusual radiosensitivity. Radiology 39: 478–479

Bahr A L, Gayler B W 1977 Cranial chondrosarcomas: report of four cases and review of the literature. Radiology 124: 151–156

Brooks J J, LiVolsi V A, Trojanowski J Q 1987 Does chondroid chordoma exist? Acta Neuropathologica 72: 229–235

Cancilla P, Morecki R, Hurwitt E S 1964 Fine structure of recurrent chordoma. Archives of Neurology 11: 289–295

Chambers P W, Schwinn C P 1979 Chordoma: a clinico-pathologic study of metastasis. American Journal of Clinical Pathology 72: 765–776

Dahlin D C, MacCarty C S 1952 Chordoma: a study of fifty-nine cases. Cancer 5: 1170–1178

Derome P J 1988 The transbasal approach to tumors invading the skull base. In: Schmidek H H, Sweet W H (eds) Operative neurosurgical techniques, Vol 1, Grune & Stratton, New York, pp 619–633

Erlandson R A, Tandler B, Lieberman P H, Higinbotham N I 1968 Ultrastructure of human chordoma. Cancer Research 28: 2115–2125

Falconer M A, Bailey I C, Duchen L W 1968 Surgical treatment of chordoma and chondroma of the skull base. Journal of Neurosurgery 29: 261–275.

Fisch U, Pillisbury H C III, Sasaki C T 1984 Infratemporal approach to the skull base. In: Sasaki C T, McCabe B F, Kirchner J A (eds) Surgery of the skull base. Lippincott, Philadelphia

Goel A 1995a Chordoma and chondrosarcoma: internal carotid artery relationship. Acta Neurochirurgica (Wien) 133: 30–35

Goel A 1995b Extended middle fossa approach for petroclival tumors. Acta Neurochirurgica (Wien) 135: 78–83

Goel A 1995c Middle fossa sub-gasserian ganglion approach to clival chordoma. Acta Neurochirurgica (Wien) 136: 212–216

Goel A 1995d Tentorial dural flap for transtentorial surgery. British Journal of Neurosurgery 9: 785–786

Goel A 1996 Basal lateral subtemporal approach. British Journal of Neurosurgery (in press)

Grossman R I, Davis K R 1981 Cranial computed tomographic appearance of chondrosarcoma of the base of the skull. Radiology 141: 403–408

Heffelfinger M J, Dahlin D C, MacCarty C S, Beabout J W 1973 Chordomas and cartilaginous tumors of the base of the skull. Cancer 32: 410–420

Higinbotham N L, Philips R F, Farr H W, Hustu H O (1967) Chordoma: thirty five year study at memorial hospital. Cancer 20: 1841–1850

House W F, Hitselberger W E, Horn K L 1986 The middle fossa transpetrous approach to anterior–superior cerebellopontine angle. American Journal of Otology 7: 1–4

Larson T C III, Houser O W, Laws E R Jr 1987 Imaging of cranial chordomas. Mayo Clinic Proceedings 62: 886–893

Meyer J E, Oot R F, Lindfors K K 1986 CT appearance of clival chordomas. Journal of Computed Assisted Tomography 10: 34–38

Meyers S P, Hirsch W L, Curtin H D et al 1992 Chordomas of the skull base: MR features. American Journal of Neuroradiology 13: 1627–1636

Morimoto T, Sasaki T, Takakura K et al 1992 Chondrosarcoma of the skull base: report of six cases. Skull Base Surgery 2: 177–185

Oot R F, Melville G E, New P F J 1988 The role of MR and CT in evaluating clival chordomas and chondrosarcomas. American Journal of Radiology 151: 567–575

Popper J L, King A B 1952 Chordoma: experience with thirteen cases. Journal of Neurosurgery 9: 139–163

Raffel C, Wright D C, Gutin P H et al 1985 Cranial chordomas: clinical presentation and results of operative and radiation therapy in twenty-six patients. Neurosurgery 17: 703–710

Rich T A, Schiller A, Suit H D et al 1985 Clinical and pathologic review of 48 cases of chordoma. Cancer 56: 182–187

Russell D S, Rubinstein L J 1989 Chondrosarcomas and chordomas. In: Pathology of tumors of the nervous system. Williams & Wilkins, Baltimore, pp 819–821

Saeger W, Ludecke D K, Muller S et al 1983 Chordome des clivus. Histologie, Ultrastruktur und Klinik. Tumor Diagnostik Therapie 4: 74–79

Seifert V, Laszig R 1991 Transoral transpalatal removal of giant premesencephalic clivus chordoma. Acta Neurochirurgica (Wien) 112: 141–146

Sekhar L N, Schramm V L Jr, Jones N F 1987 Subtemporal–preauricular infratemporal fossa approach to large lateral and posterior cranial base neoplasms. Journal of Neurosurgery 67: 488

Sen C N, Sekhar L N, Schramm V L Jr et al 1989 Chordoma and chondrosarcoma of the cranial base: an 8-year experience. Neurosurgery 25: 931–941

Stapleton S R, Wilkins P R, Archer D J et al 1993 Chondrosarcoma of the skull base: a series of eight cases. Neurosurgery 32: 348–356

Utne J R, Pugh D G 1955 The roentgenologic aspects of chordoma. American Journal of Roentgenology 74: 593–608

Surgical Management of Chordomas and Chondrosarcomas of the Cranial Base

Laligam N. Sekhar   Donald C. Wright   William T. Monacci

Introduction: Chordomas and chondrosarcomas are rare tumors, constituting up to 0.2% of intracranial neoplasms. Surgical treatment has been difficult in the past because of their relative inaccessibility to conventional approaches. Refined cranial base techniques have resulted in significant advances in treatment and improved outcome.

Chordomas are thought to arise from remnants of the embryonal notochord and approximately 35% of tumors involve the skull base. They are predominantly midline tumors which may involve the following areas: sphenoid or ethmoid sinus, cavernous sinus, upper, mid, or lower clivus, petrous bone and the C1–2 area. Intradural invasion occurs late in the course of many tumors but some are intradural at their initial presentation. Signs and symptoms at presentation depend on the location of the tumor epicenter and the direction of growth. Tumors which arise from the base of the clivus produce lower cranial nerve dysfunction such as hoarseness or tongue atrophy. Ventral growth can result in presentation as a nasopharyngeal mass. Tumors arising from the mid-clivus compress the mid-pons ventrally and can produce VIth nerve paresis, often bilaterally. Tumors which can arise near the sella may produce visual field deficits or pituitary dysfunction. Their biology is of two types: most are of the slow-growing 'chondroid' variety. Their benign histologic appearance belies their locally invasive behavior which makes surgical removal difficult. A few are fast growing, as exemplified by the tumors which recur after radiotherapy. When the tumors contact the brain stem they may provoke a hemorrhagic reaction. In general these tumors are readily dissectable from cranial nerves, vessels and the brain; however, recurrent tumors and biologically aggressive variants may not display these characteristics.

Chondrosarcomas are of different histologic types. Tumors which involve the cranial base are usually a low-grade variant which have a slow growth pattern. These tumors usually start in the petrosphenoid junction and are often paremedian. Large or giant-sized tumors usually involve the same regions as chordomas but their spread into the C1–2 region has not been seen. Cranial base chondrosarcomas have a better prognosis than chordomas in both the senior author's series as well as the Massachusetts General series of proton beam radiotherapy (Arnold & Herrmann 1986).

Philosophy of treatment: The subject is quite controversial. Some surgeons prefer repeated partial resections, so-called 'wood-pecker' surgery (Arnold &

Herrmann 1986). Other surgeons perform subtotal tumor removals and then give radiotherapy (Austin et al 1993). Our philosophy has been to attempt to gross total resection of the tumor with removal of involved bone whenever possible. We reserve radiotherapy for those in whom a radical removal is not safely possible, and for recurrent tumors.

Reoperations are technically more difficult and increase the complication rate. When the patient has previously received radiation therapy the risk of surgery increases considerably due to increased risk of vascular and brain injury, compounded by poor wound healing.

The methods of radiotherapy are also controversial. External beam radiotherapy is still used but high doses (approximately 50–80 Gy) are needed because the tumors are relatively radio resistant. This increases the risk of radionecrosis of the brain. Proton beam therapy allows a higher dose to be administered to more precisely targeted neoplastic and margin areas. Radiosurgery utilizing the gamma knife or the linear accelerator is more precise in its ability to focus radiation; however, it is limited by the tumor volume that can be treated. Long-term tumor control rates have only been published for proton beam radiotherapy and are comparable to those of microsurgical series; however, only those patients in relatively good condition are being radiated whereas many patients in poor condition are operated on.

Preoperative Evaluation: MRI is the best modality for revealing the extent of tumor involvement in three dimensions. Bone windows available with CT demonstrate the detail of bony involvement. Three-dimensional bone-windowed CT scan shows the bone erosion most clearly. When arteries are encased by the tumor a cerebral arteriogram is performed. This will also demonstrate the venous anatomy, which is important for surgical planning. For patients who have recurrent or previously irradiated tumors with internal carotid artery encasement, a carotid occlusion test should be performed in order to prepare for the possibility of intraoperative arterial injury and the need for a bypass procedure.

It is important to assess preoperatively whether the tumor has an intradural extension. Triplaner MRI imaging is the best means for assessing this, particularly when the extension is large.

Operative Approaches: The following operative approaches are used for the removal of chordomas and chondrosarcomas: extended subfrontal (modified transbasal), frontotemporal orbitozygomatic, subtemporal–preauricular infratemporal, presigmoid petrosal, extreme lateral transcondylar, transmaxillary (facial translocation), and transoral. We will comment specifically about each of these approaches. Many large and giant-sized tumors require staged treatment utilizing more than one approach to obtain complete tumor resection.

The extended subfrontal approach is ideal for sphenoclival tumors located in the midline, predominantly extradurally. We have modified the original transbasal approach of Derome by adding a bilateral orbital and frontoethmoidal osteotomy, extensive ethmoid bone resection, and bilateral optic and orbital decompression. The approach can be extended even lower by removal of

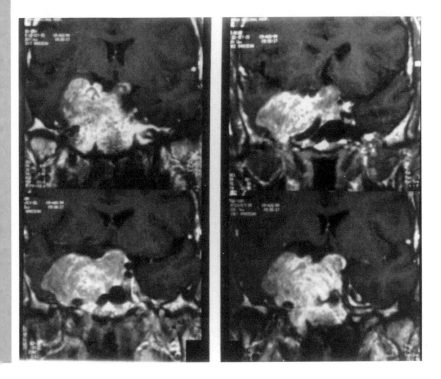

Fig. 18.14 T1-weighted MRI with gadolinium contrast of a patient with an extensive chondrosarcoma.

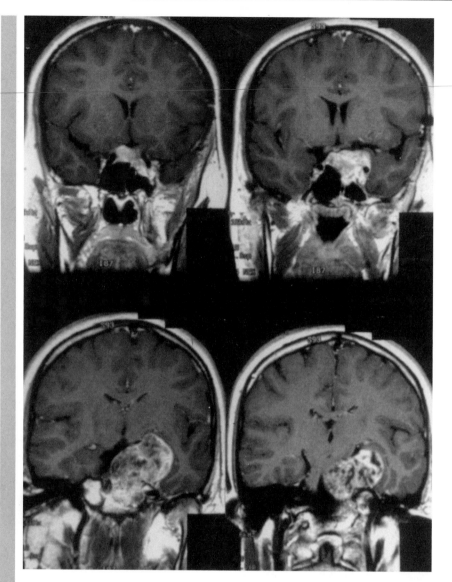

Fig. 18.15 T1-weighted MRI with contrast of a patient with a chondrosarcoma. Successful resection required stage 1 placement of an internal carotid to middle cerebral artery saphenous vein bypass.

the nasal bone. A modification described by Spetzler to preserve olfactory function has been used by us several times, but preserving smell has not been possible.

The extended subfrontal approach requires very limited brain retraction and affords a wide exposure. It has been described as X-shaped, because the surgeon can look across from one orbit to the contralateral petrous apex and hypoglossal area and from the other orbit to the ipsilateral side. Tumors can be removed from the sphenoid and ethmoid sinuses, the medial aspect of the cavernous sinus, the upper, mid and lower clivus with the exception of the dorsum sellae, and the medial aspect of the petrous apices, down to the foramen magnum area. The surgeon is limited laterally by the petrous and cavernous internal carotid artery (ICA), abducens nerves and the hypoglossal nerves. Small intradural extensions can be removed, but this approach is not recommended

for large intradural lesions. The dorsum sellae, the lateral aspect of the cavernous sinus, the petrous bone, and the occipital condyle cannot be reached by this approach. Reconstruction after this approach is readily performed with fascia lata (for dural defects), a vascularized pericranial flap, and autologous fat. Bone pieces are reattached with titanium mini-plates. Figure 18.14 is an MRI of a patient with an extensive chondrosarcoma which was approached with this technique. The bilateral extension of the tumor makes this method particularly effective in tumor removal.

The frontotemporal orbitozygomatic approach is generally used for tumors with significant intracavernous extension. Tumor can also be removed from the petrous apex and the lateral sphenoid extradural areas. The cavernous sinus is usually opened by intradural incision in its superior wall, or in its lateral wall between V1 and

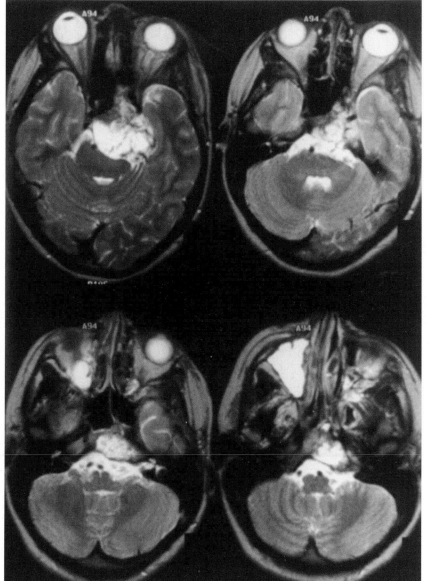

Fig. 18.16 T2-weighted MRI images of the same patient.

V2 or between cranial nerves IV and VI. We do not dissect the cranial nerves in the cavernous sinus extensively, to ensure a good functional result. The intracavernous ICA can usually be preserved easily but great care must be exercised with cranial nerve VI. Removal of tumor margins may be difficult because of extensive venous bleeding. The surgeon may unwaringly leave tumor behind. At the end of the resection, the cavernous sinus is packed with gel foam rather than Surgicel since it compresses the cranial nerves less. The dural incision must be closed meticulously in order to avoid a CSF leak. This approach can be combined with the extended subfrontal approach if the surgeon is prepared to perform an extra-long (> 12 hours) operation. Figures 15 and 16 are MRI images of a patient with a

chondrosarcoma which was approached with this method in combination with the extended subfrontal approach.

The subtemporal and preauricular infratemporal approach is ideal for tumors which involve the petrous apex and the ipsilateral half of the mid-clivus. This is the extradural approach which involves the exposure and anterior displacement of the petrous ICA. Loss of Eustachian tube function is a permanent disability as a result of this approach. The major potential risk with this operation, especially in inexperienced hands, is injury to the petrous ICA. This approach is easily combined with an extradural subfrontal approach or an intradural frontotemporal approach to the cavernous sinus or the petroclival area. Chondrosarcomas of the cranial base

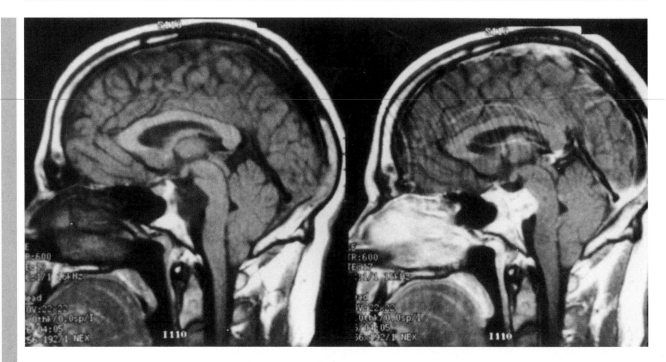

Fig. 18.17 T1-weighted MRI images with contrast of a patient with a chondrosarcoma.

are most commonly removed by this approach. After tumor resection, reconstruction is usually performed with autologous fat, and a portion of the temporalis muscle rotated as a flap.

The presigmoid petrosal approach is used for chordomas which extend extradurally and deeply indent the brain stem and/or encase the basilar artery. Additionally, chordomas arising from the upper clival (dorsum sellae) region are best accessed by this route, even if they are extradural. We prefer a presigmoid approach with partial labyrinthectomy, which enhances the exposure while preserving functional hearing. A zygomatic osteotomy is combined with this approach only if extreme middle cranial fossa work is necessary. At the end of the operation, the dural defect has to be closed meticulously with a graft (fascia lata or pericranial) to avoid a CSF fistula, especially when the extradural portion of the tumor is removed. Figure 18.17 and 18.18 are from a patient with a chondrosarcoma in whom a combination of approaches was effective in achieving tumor removal, including the petrosal and extended subfrontal techniques.

The extreme lateral transcondylar approach is used for tumors which involve the lower clivus, foramen magnum, occipital condyle, and the C1–C2 areas. This approach can be used both for extradural and intradural lesions. The advantage of this approach is that it does not transgress the oral cavity, and lesions which extend laterally towards the vertebral artery and the condyle can be resected. The potential risks include vertebral artery

and lower cranial nerve injury as well as CSF fistula. In previously operated cases, it is better to reflect the skin flap with the sternocleidomastoid muscle, to preserve its vascularity. If the occipital condyle is resected because of tumor invasion, an occiput-to-cervical fusion with titanium rods and bone graft is performed to avoid subsequent neck pain and instability. Figure 19 depicts MRI images from a patient with an extensive chordoma which was resected with a combination of approaches, including infratemporal and transcondylar routes.

The facial translocation or transmaxillary approaches are of two types. The first one (Ivo Janecka, Jon Robertson type) involves the unilateral dislocation of the maxilla and resection of the tumor (Janecka et al 1990, Cocke et al 1990). This is followed by reconstruction with fascia lata and temporalis muscle flaps. We have used this approach a number of times for other malignant tumors, but very few times for chordomas. We have also operated on patients previously treated by this approach. While the exposure of the clivus provided by this approach appears to be excellent, the reconstruction is potentially problematic. We are aware of an incidence of delayed carotid rupture after this approach by good surgeons, which presumably occurred because the artery was exposed to nasopharyngeal flora at the end of the operation. In late follow-up, some patients with chordoma operated by this approach appear to have significant jaw dysfunction and trismus due to secondary muscle scarring.

The second technique is via the Le Fort I maxillotomy

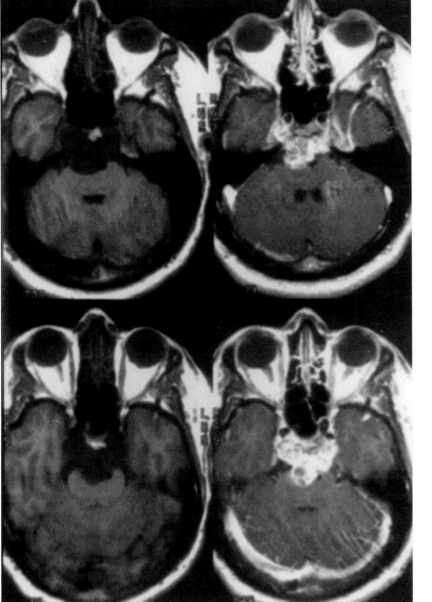

Fig. 18.18   T1-weighted MRI images with contrast of the same patient.

approach. While this method provides excellent exposure of the mid and lower clivus, there is no possibility of adequate reconstruction. Once this technique is used, future operations become more difficult because the pharyngeal mucosa is completely destroyed. We do not prefer this approach.

The transoral approach has been commonly used for the removal of lower clival and upper cervical chordomas. Variations of this approach include transmandibular (tongue-splitting) and transpalatal approaches. The transoral approach is good for debulking tumors, but not for their radical removal. As the tumor extends laterally, the removal of the lesion

becomes more difficult. If the occipital condyle or the vertebral artery is involved, or if the tumor extends intradurally, tumor removal may be fraught with serious complications, including arterial hemorrhage, CSF leakage, meningitis, and death. While we use the transoral approach for basilar invagination anomalies, we rarely use it for chordomas. At best it affords palliative tumor resection.

Surgical Technique: The core of a chordoma or a chondrosarcoma is usually soft and cartilaginous but may be mixed with areas of hard bone or hard cartilage. Removal of large pieces of hard tumor is made easier by

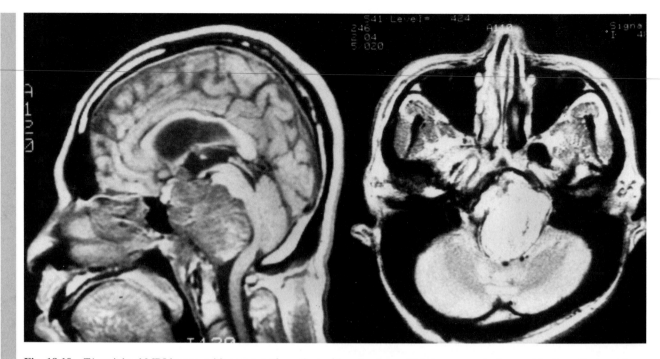

Fig. 18.19 T1-weighted MRI images with contrast of a patient with a chordoma. This tumor required a combination of approaches for resection.

removing soft components of the tumor first and then removing harder islands of tumor. Radical removal of the tumor remnants from the cavernous sinus is made difficult by bleeding from the venous plexus as the tumor margins are reached.

After most of the tumor is removed, the tumor margins in the surrounding bone must be drilled away. These tumors appear to infiltrate the cancellous bone more widely than the cortical bone. There may also be skip areas, i.e. apparent tumor invasion beyond what appears to be normal bone.

Arteries encased by these tumors can usually be dissected free, with some exceptions. In previously irradiated patients, the ICA may not be dissectable, resulting in vascular injury. This usually requires a vein graft bypass. When the basilar artery is encased by chordoma this may indicate a very invasive tumor, and the adventitia of the vessel may be violated, making intraoperative rupture likely. In these cases great caution must be exercised. In the case of basilar artery injury external carotid artery (ECA) to posterior cerebral artery (PCA) vein graft reconstruction may be necessary.

Cranial nerves involved by these tumors can usually be preserved except in previously operated or irradiated patients.

Results of surgery: The long-term results of 46 patients with chordoma and 14 patients with low-grade chondrosarcoma treated at the University of Pittsburgh have been recently published (Gay et al 1995). Briefly

summarizing the findings, 50% of patients had received prior treatment and surgical approaches varied depending on tumor location, as discussed previously; 6.7% of patients received a total or near total resection; 20% of patients went on to receive postoperative radiotherapy; 11 patients died during the 5-year follow-up period, including five as a result of tumor recurrence and two as a result of complications from radiotherapy. The recurrence-free survival for all tumors was 80% at 3 years and 76% at 5 years, with chondrosarcoma patients having a better prognosis, with a 5-year survival of 90% versus 65% for chordomas. Patients with prior surgery had a 5-year survival of 64%, while those patients without prior therapy had a 93% survival rate. Patients with a total or near total resection did not increase the complication rate.

An additional 37 patients have been operated on at the George Washington University Medical Center in the past 3 years (Cranial Base Surgery Data Bank, unpublished data). These include 11 chondrosarcomas and 26 chordomas. The prospective evaluation of their treatment is in progress and will be the subject of upcoming reports.

References

Arnold H, Herrmann H D 1986 Skull base chordoma with cavernous sinus involvement: partial or radical tumor removal? Acta Neurochirurgica 83: 31–37

Austin J P, Urie M M, Cardenosa G, Muzenrider J E 1993 The causes of recurrence in patients with chordoma and chondrosarcoma of the base of the skull and cervical spine. International Journal of Radiation Oncology, Biology, Physics 25: 439–444

Cocke E W, Robertson J T, Crook J P 1990 The extended maxillotomy and subtotal maxillectomy for excision of skull base tumors. Archives of Otolaryngology, Head and Neck Surgery 116: 92–98

Gay E, Sekhar L N, Rubinstein M A et al 1995 Chordomas and chondrosarcomas of the cranial base: results and follow-up of 60 patients. Neurosurgery 36: 887–897

Janecka I P, Sen C N, Sekhar L N, Arriaga M A 1990 Facial translocation: a new approach to the cranial base. Otolaryngology, Head and Neck Surgery 103: 413–419

Juvenile nasopharyngeal angiofibromas

Atul Goel   Kazuhiko Kyoshima
Shigeaki Kobayashi   Kazuhiro Hongo

As the name suggests, these tumors are seen in the 'juvenile' age group. There is an unusual male predominance. Occurrence in females and in the elderly is extremely unusual and in these instances the tumor has often more malignant potential. The tumors are slow growing and histologically benign. The tumor behaves in a malignant fashion due to the characters of local destruction, fatal hemorrhage and high recurrence rate after surgical resection. Nasopharyngeal angiofibromas are located in the posterolateral wall of the nasopharynx and spread locally in the submucosal plane. The usual site of origin is in the posterolateral wall of the nasal cavity in the region where the sphenoid process of the palatine bone meets the horizontal ala of the vomer and the roof of the pterygoid process. By direct spread the tumor can involve the nasopharynx, nasal cavity, pterygopalatine fossa, infratemporal fossa and intracranial cavity. The term 'intracranial extension' should be adequately understood as in most instances the tumor is essentially extradural and extracranial but pushes the basal dura and bone superiorly by the expansive pattern of growth which gives an impression on investigation that the tumor is intracranial. The basal bone may be eroded and thinned out by pressure. Cavernous sinus involvement also in most cases is in the form of displacement and compression rather than invasion. The entire cavernous sinus with its contained vascular and neural structures are displaced superiorly by the tumor (Fig. 19.1). Invasion into the cavernous sinus dura is rare. In our experience with massive tumors no cavernous sinus invasion has been encountered. The dura was always intact. This feature of the tumor assists in developing a plane between the tumor and the basal dura even with a blunt dissection. On CT scan it may appear that the entire cavernous sinus is involved by the tumor, but MRI and angiography usually clarify the picture.

Due to their location most tumors present when they are large in size despite their expansive growth characters. Larger tumors which present usually as mass lesions are often firm and fibrous in nature. Smaller and softer tumors present early with epistaxis. They have no true capsule. A

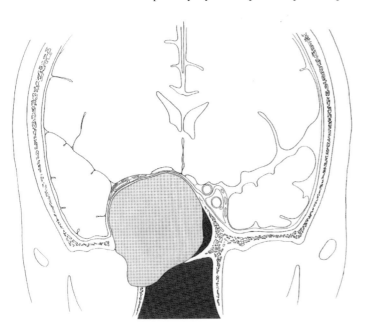

Fig. 19.1 Typical relationship of the nasopharyngeal angiofibroma to the base of the skull. The tumor is essentially extracranial and extradural. The cavernous sinus and its contained nerves and carotid artery are displaced on the dome of the tumor. (From Goel et al 1994, with permission.)

pseudocapsule of fibrous tissue is produced by compression of the normal tissues. The tumor is made up of a connective tissue stroma with a matrix of dilated vascular channels. The blood vessels lack a well-defined muscular layer, which may be responsible for the hemorrhagic tendencies of these tumors.

There have been reports of successful growth control by using radiotherapy as a primary modality of treatment (Cummings et al 1984). However, considering their histological benign nature, the general consensus favors a radical surgical excision (Jafek et al 1979, Ward et al 1974). Radiation treatment has been seen to induce malignant changes in the tumor. The long-term effect on cranial nerves and brain function are other factors which are against the use of radiotherapy as the principal mode of treatment. Preoperative hormone therapy has been tried to reduce tumor vascularity but has not met with adequate success. 'Intracranial' extension has been observed in 20–30% of patients with juvenile angiofibroma and such lesions are particularly difficult to treat surgically (Cummings et al 1984, Jafek et al 1979). In the past surgical excision was condemned due to intraoperative deaths (Cummings et al 1984, Krekorian 1977).

Nasopharyngeal angiofibromas are relatively difficult surgical lesions. The difficulty in resection of these lesions stems from their deep-seated location, wide extensions and intense vascularity. Most of these lesions are restricted to the nasopharyngeal areas and can be dealt with by an otolaryngologist. However, some tumors become large and have cranial extensions and such lesions warrant a combined neurosurgical and otolaryngological surgical approach.

Preoperative embolization of feeder blood vessels 1–3 days prior to surgery has been found to help considerably in reducing the extent of blood loss during surgery. Although these lesions appear vascular on angiography a bold operative effort is often fruitful. In situations where there is extensive bleeding during tumor excision, it is sometimes advisable to hurriedly resect the entire tumor and control the bleeding by pressure. Once the tumor is completely resected the bleeding is controlled spontaneously and as the major feeders come into view they can be adequately dealt with. Incomplete tumor resection is more prone to bleeding disasters and also has a high rate of recurrence. Smaller lesions can be removed en masse by gradual dissection from all around. In larger lesions rapid intra-'capsular' debulking and later excision under vision by blunt dissection of the 'capsule' from the sites of attachment can be performed after making adequate preparation for blood and volume replacement. Very large exposures for such lesions are only rarely necessary. Working space for tumor section and either large piecemeal or en masse removal is often necessary for resection. however, adequate preparation for control of major arteries should be made in rare cases with possibilities of uncontrollable bleeding. Most tumors receive their vascular supply from the internal maxillary branch of the external carotid artery. Occasionally small branches from internal carotid may also supply these tumors.

Various approaches providing wide exposure for massive lesions have been described recently, most of these being transfacial with or without the addition of the transcranial route (Krekorian 1977, Close et al 1989, English et al 1972, Moises et al 1991).

In most cases facial incision can be avoided. Mid-facial degloving procedures are appropriate in most of the large tumor cases. Even massive tumors may be removed by this approach and facial incision could be avoided. At least an attempt should always be made to avoid a facial incision. In cases with smaller tumors either a sublabial transnasal or an entirely transnasal approach may be suitable. In virgin cases, the tumor is not only extradural but also extracranial. In such cases, tumor resection is possible with only a limited exposure.

An extended transcranial approach is described here (Goel et al 1994). The approach was found to be effective in resection of massive angiofibromas in two patients. One case is described, discussing the technique and merits of the procedure. Such an approach is suitable only in selected cases of massive nasopharyngeal angiofibromas. The approach is more suitable in cases where the major bulk of the tumor is retrobulbar. It is also suitable in cases where there is tumor recurrence and where radiation therapy has already been given. In both these situations the dural divide between the tumor and the cranial cavity may not remain clearly defined. The arterial supply of the tumor also does not remain from the external carotid alone in these cases. In cases where external carotid artery embolization is done, or where the external carotid is blocked during an earlier surgery, the tumor extracts vascular supply from the internal carotid artery source. In this situation a large exposure with proximal control of the carotid artery is advisable.

Case

A 14-year-old boy was admitted with a 1-year history of progressive diminution of vision in the left eye. The vision had worsened to only perception of light in this eye. He recently observed mild proptosis in the same eye. The rest of the neurological examination did not reveal any abnormality. Magnetic resonance imaging (MRI) (Fig. 19.2) and computed tomographic (CT) scan (Fig. 19.3) showed a massive tumor occupying the nasopharynx, sphenoid, maxillary and ethmoid sinuses and extending into the infratemporal fossa, cavernous sinus and displacing the temporal lobe. Angiography showed the tumor to be very vascular. The external carotid feeding vessels were embolized. Large ophthalmic artery feeders were not embolized to avoid possible loss of vision as a consequence of the procedure.

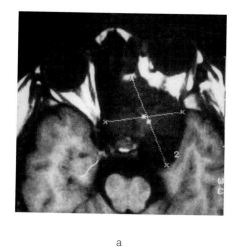

a

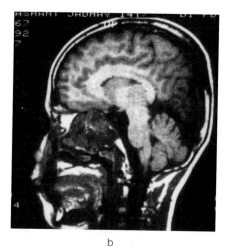

b

Fig. 19.2 **a** Axial MRI cut shows the large nasopharyngeal tumor. The tumor occupies the nasopharynx, involves the paranasal sinuses, pushes the eyeball anteriorly and optic nerve superiorly. The relationship with the cavernous sinus and the temporal brain is seen. Scale bar = 5 cm. (From Goel et al 1994, with permission.) **b** Sagittal cut of MRI shows the large nasopharyngeal tumor.

Surgical Technique

A bicoronal incision was extended to the preauricular region on the left side (Fig. 19.4). The scalp flap was reflected anteriorly, preserving the frontal branches of the facial nerve. The superficial temporal artery on the left and supraorbital arterial branches and nerves on both sides were preserved. Subperiosteal dissection was carried out to expose the zygomatic body, zygomatic arch and the maxillary bone from laterally up to the infraorbital foramen. The supraorbital rim, notch and the nasion were exposed (Fig. 19.5). A low, left frontotemporal craniotomy extending to the right side across the midline was carried out. This was followed by an orbitozygomatic osteotomy on the left which was extended to

the medial wall of the right orbit including the nasion (Fig. 19.6). The frontal and ethmoid sinuses were exposed widely. The infratemporal muscles were retracted off the greater wing, exposing the body of the maxillary sinus and the lateral pterygoid plate. The internal maxillary artery and its branches

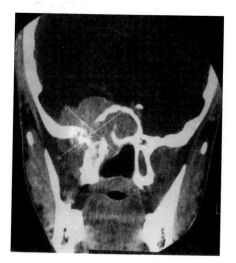

Fig. 19.3 CT scan shows the tumor extension into the maxillary sinus. The bony middle fossa is elevated superiorly. (From Goel et al 1994, with permission.)

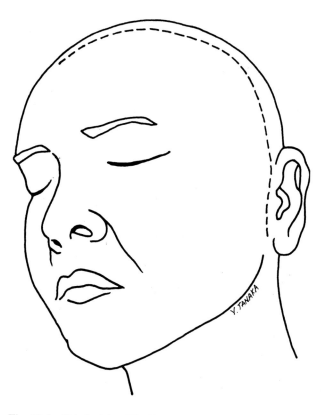

Fig. 19.4 Skin incision. The bicoronal incision extends to the preauricular region. (From Goel et al 1994, with permission.)

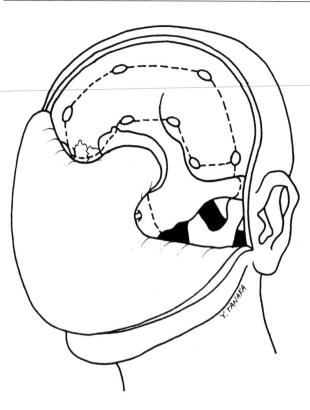

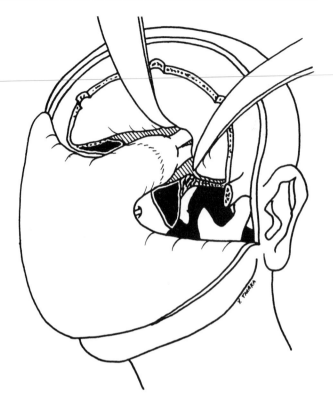

Fig. 19.5 The scalp flap is reflected anteriorly, exposing the infraorbital nerve anteriorly, zygomatic bone and nasion. The dashed lines indicate the site of bone cuts, resulting in a large frontotemporal bone flap and orbitozygomatic osteotomy. (From Goel et al 1994, with permission.)

Fig. 19.6 Exposure obtained after the bone work. The maxillary and ethmoid sinuses are widely opened up. The shaded area around the eyeball indicates the exposure obtained around it, the optic nerve and the superior orbital fissure. The temporal and frontal lobes are retracted. (From Goel et al 1994, with permission.)

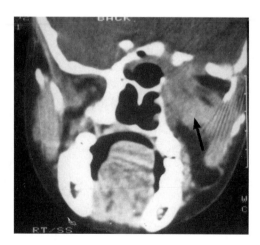

a

b

Fig. 19.7 **a** Postoperative CT scan shows the tumor resection. Arrowhead shows the rotated temporalis muscle in the posterior part of the orbit. (From Goel et al 1994, with permission.) **b** Axial cut of the CT scan showing the tumor resection.

were identified and coagulated close to the tumor. The dura was elevated exposing the crista galli from the left side. This maneuver permitted extradural retraction of the frontal and the temporal lobes (Fig. 19.7). The roof and the lateral wall of the left orbit were nibbled away up to the anterior clinoid process. The middle and posterior ethmoid sinuses were resected. A wide exposure to the tumor was now available from superior, anterior, medial and lateral directions (Fig. 19.8). The tumor was gradually excised piecemeal by a combination of intra- and extracapsular dissection, coagulating and cutting the feeding arteries close to the tumor capsule. The tumor in the presented case was mainly extradural with a small tail extending into the cavernous sinus. It had pushed the cavernous sinus superiorly and the temporal lobe laterally. The tumor extended into the maxillary sinus destroying the floor of the orbit. At the end of the operation the eyeball was devoid of bony support superiorly, inferiorly and laterally. Only part of the medial wall was preserved. The temporalis muscle was rotated underneath the eyeball in the form of a sling to hold the eyeball in place (Fig. 19.7). Small bone pieces and debris were used to reconstruct the walls. The bone flaps were sutured back. Postoperative scans showed complete resection (Fig. 19.7). At 6 months follow-up the child had marked improvement in vision in the left eye.

In the second case of massive nasopharyngeal angiofibroma with similar extensions the exposure obtained for the tumor excision was satisfactory. However, a small intracavernous extension of the tumor was inadvertently missed. This part was then subjected to radiotherapy.

Discussion

Basal extension of the conventional frontal craniotomy utilizing orbital rims and zygomatic arch (Al-Mefty 1987, Derome et al 1972, Jane et al 1982, Sekhar et al 1992) has been utilized for radical resection of cranial basal lesions. Ray and McLean were the first to describe a combined transcranial and transfacial approach for resection of a basal tumor (Ray & McLean 1943). Since then there have been many descriptions of the combined intracranial and extracranial approach for neoplasms involving the anterior cranial fossa floor (Ketcham & Van Buren 1988, Maran 1983, Panje et al 1989, Sisson et al 1976, Shah et al 1987, Smith et al 1954).

The approach described here was found to be suitable for the size of the tumor because it provided a large exposure circumferentially. It was particularly suitable for the part involving the cavernous sinus and that posterior to the eyeball. Additional facial incision could be taken if necessary. Exposure of the internal carotid artery at the petrous apex was possible in the same exposure (it was not done in the case described). This may be important when proximal control of this vessel is necessary while dealing with the part involving and invading the cavernous sinus. The internal maxillary artery, which is frequently the most predominant source of blood supply to these tumors, can be exposed and dealt with early. The vascularity of the scalp flap is preserved as all its major feeding vessels can be saved. Preservation of the vascularity of the flap is of great importance when the external carotid artery branches have been embolized in such tumors. The temporal and zygomatic branches of the facial nerve and the supraorbital

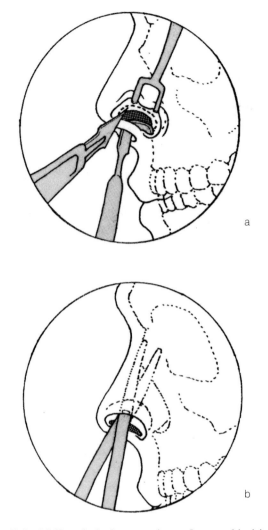

Fig. 19.8 Midface degloving procedure. **a** Intranasal incision is taken circumferentially over the mucosa in the nares. This is followed by a transfixion incision which is connected bilaterally with intercartilaginous, pyriform, and nasal floor incisions. **b** Intercartilaginous incision: the soft tissues of the nasal dorsum are separated from the upper lateral cartilage and nasal bone through the intercartilaginous incision in a subperiosteal plane.

nerves are preserved. No facial or eyelid incision is necessary and thus the operation is cosmetically superior. The nasal and oral mucosa are not traversed from an external direction and the operation is carried out in a relatively sterile field. This may be of critical importance while dealing with the cranial extension of the tumor. The anterior wall of the maxillary sinus is not disturbed surgically and thus the growth of the facial bones is not hampered. The temporalis muscle can be completely displaced and can be used for reconstruction.

However, the approach described is useful in only selected cases of massive nasopharyngeal angiofibromas, particularly those with large intracranial extension and cavernous sinus involvement. Fortunately such tumors are rare. For smaller tumors the lateral exposure provided by the approach discussed may not be necessary. As even large tumors often do not transgress the dural territory, most of these tumors can be excised by a simpler midfacial degloving, sublabial, maxillotomy or transfacial approach.

MODIFIED TRANSFACIAL APPROACH TO THE SKULL BASE WITH DEGLOVING PROCEDURE
(Kyoshima & Matsuo 1993)

A midfacial degloving approach is most suitable for most cases of large and massive nasopharyngeal angiofibromas. The advantages of this approach are as follows:

1. A large exposure can be obtained. The exposure is horizontally wide.
2. No facial incision is necessary. This is a crucial positive feature of this approach.

A modification of this approach as described by Kyoshima et al is discussed. The approach provides surgical access to lesions of the frontal base which extends from the region of the cribriform plate, sphenoid sinus, maxillary sinus, apices of both orbits, nasopharynx, clivus and upper cervical vertebrae.

The approaches to the central skull base are broadly classified into anterior and lateral approaches. There are some specific indications for an anterior approach (surgery for juvenile nasopharyngeal angiofibroma is one of them). The principal advantage of an anterior approach is that the major vessels and cranial nerves are not encountered early during the approach.

Various techniques of facial degloving procedure have been described and successfully used. We describe a transfacial approach which was combined with the midface degloving procedure.

Surgical technique

The operation is carried out under general anesthesia with orotracheal intubation. Preoperative tracheostomy is usually not necessary.

With the patient in the supine position, the head is fixed (in a head fixation system) with a chin-up tilt of about 15°. The surgeon may work from the frontal or the lateral side.

Midface degloving procedure
The medial palpebral ligaments are first dissected and wired after taking a small skin incision near the medial angle of the eye on each side. The wires are connected under the nasal skin at the end of the operation.

A nasal septal transfixion and intercartilaginous incision is taken which separates the nasal tip and dorsum from the

septum (Fig. 19.8). Extension of the mucosal incision circumferentially within the nasal vestibule at the skin–mucosal junction completes the release of nasal soft tissue at the pyriform aperture. Softe tissue of the nasal dorsum is widely elevated in the subperiosteal plane.

A sublabial incision is taken which extends much more laterally than the conventional incision for transsphenoidal surgery. It may extend up to or beyond the first molar on both sides. The skin and soft tissues of the face (superior to the upper lip) are then dissected in the subperiosteal plane over the maxilla, sparing each infraorbital nerve. Facial soft tissues including upper lip, cheeks, nasal tip and the alae, columella, and nasal skin are then reflected superiorly (Fig. 19.9). The elevation is wide and can be as high as the infraorbital rim and the glabella (Figs. 19.9, 19.10).

Osteotomies of facial bone
Nasomaxillary osteotomy
Nasomaxillary osteotomy is done as shown in Figures 19.11–19.13. An osteotomy is made in the maxillary bone medial to the inferior orbital foramen. The mucosa under the nasal bone is separated from it and an osteotomy of the nasal bone is performed near the frontonasal suture transversely, while taking precautions to preserve the nasolacrimal duct on both sides (Figs. 19.11, 19.12). the nasomaxillary bone is then removed.

Le Forte I osteotomy with cartilaginous septum
Le Forte I osteotomy with the cartilaginous septum is carried out with a power-driven bone saw and chisel and hammer.

The mucosa of the nasal dorsum is separated from the nasal cartilage and bone. The nasal septum is cut in its full thickness with scissors between the nasal cartilage and perpendicular plate of the ethmoidal bone. A sagittal mucosal incision is taken in the lateral wall of the pyriform aperture near the lateral margin of the nasal floor, preserving the greater palatine artery on both sides. After horizontal osteotomy of the maxilla, the lateral wall of the pyriform aperture is cut from anterior to posterior along the sagittal mucosal incision. Thus, the cartilaginous septum with mucosa continuing to the maxilla is obtained.

The maxillary segment is separated from the pterygoid plates with a curved chisel (Fig. 19.13). The maxilla can then be down fractured to gain full mobility and posterior exposure (Figs. 19.14, 19.15). Turbinectomy of the inferior and middle nasal conchae provides a wider lateral exposure.

Access to central skull base
The mucosa of the bony septum is divided on each side. Access to the central skull base is obtained by removal of the bony septum and retracting the mucosa laterally.

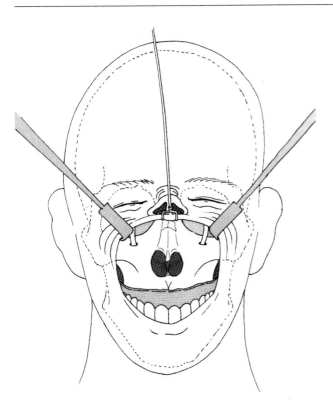

Fig. 19.9 Sublabial incision: the incision extends to the first molar tooth on each side. Labial mucosa remains on the gingival side to facilitate closure. The midfacial soft tissues are then elevated. The infraorbital nerves, orbital rims and glabella are seen.

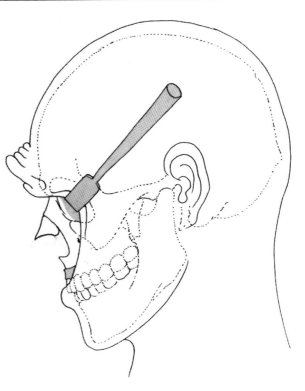

Fig. 19.10 Lateral view of elevation of midfacial soft tissues.

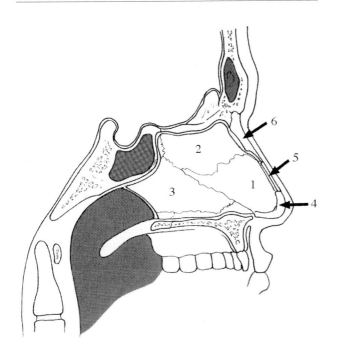

Fig. 19.11 Midfacial sagittal section. (1, cartilaginous septum; 2, perpendicular plate of the ethmoidal bone; 3, vomer; 4, nasolacrimal cartilage; 5, upper lateral cartilage; 6, nasal bone.)

Fig. 19.12 Dissection of the nasal septum. The cartilaginous septum is cut and freed from the bony septum in full thickness. The septal mucosa of the choana is also dissected. The nasal bone is removed and nasal skin including lower cartilage is reflected superiorly.

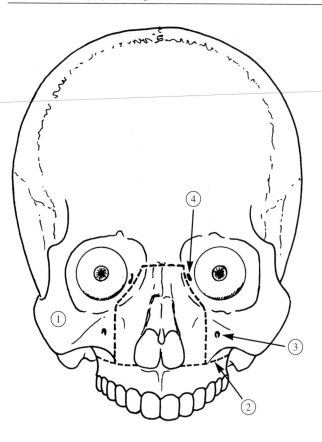

Fig. 19.13   Osteotomies of the facial bone. (1, nasomaxillary osteotomy; 2, Le Forte I osteotomy; 3, infraorbital foramen; 4, nasolacrimal canal; 5, horizontal osteotomy of maxilla.)

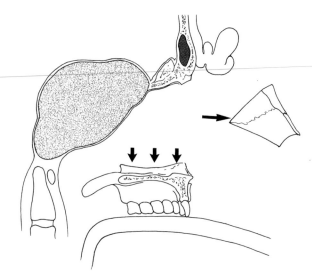

Fig. 19.14   Down fracture of maxilla with pediculated cartilaginous septum and access to the central skull base by the degloving transfacial approach. The lower clivus to upper cervical spine can be exposed under the mucosa of the pharyngeal wall. Superiorly the frontal base can be accessed. The cartilaginous septum is retracted laterally.

Nasomaxillary osteotomy provides access to the lower clivus up to the upper cervical spine under the mucosa of the posterior pharyngeal wall.

The downward displacement of the maxilla provides a direct line of vision to the clivus, the mucosa of the posterior pharyngeal wall and a wide view laterally. Le Forte I osteotomy affords wider exposure to the posterior aspect of the upper nasopharynx and central skull base area. Exposure from a selective transsphenoidal approach is limited by the lateral wall of the pyriform aperture.

Thus, by nasomaxillary and Le Forte I osteotomies, the central skull base is accessible from the frontal base to the foramen magnum. The lower clivus to C2 portion can also be exposed by further dissection under the pharyngeal mucosa.

Reconstruction and wound closure

The dead space remaining after tumor and bone removal is filled with autogenous material, such as abdominal fat or fascia lata strengthened by fibrin glue. The mucosa of the bony septum is closed without any tension of the wound and complete interception from the nasal cavity is obtained. This results in a defect in the bony septum.

Facial bone is stabilized with mini-plates. The cavity is packed with antibiotic-soaked petrolatum gauze which is brought out through the nares.

Limitations

The procedure does not provide a sufficient lateral exposure as it is limited by the pterygoid plates. In combination with another lateral approach a wider exposure can be obtained.

Extension of the operative field

The transmaxillary approach is easily combined with this technique, for tumors of the posterior sphenoid and clivus that have lateral extensions.

Transverse additional incisions of the mucosa at the choana also provide a more lateral exposure, and a longitudinal incision of the pharyngeal mucosa downward gains more inferior exposure. In such situations the mucosa of the bony septum may be used for suitable closure of the pharyngeal mucosa in case there is a defect in it.

If a tumor extends intradurally, opening the dura facilitates its exposure. Bifrontal craniotomy and a frontobasal interhemispheric approach can also be combined with this approach wherever necessary.

The pterygoid plates are the main obstructing factor in increasing the lateral exposure in the depth. Drilling the pterygoid process or mucous membrane near the choana provides a wider operative field laterally. The pterygoid plate can be fractured outwards or drilled off.

Advantages

1. The procedure is technically relatively simple.
2. This technique does not involve any external incisions over the face and hence the cosmetic result is excellent. There are no significant problems related to malocclusion. In our experience the postoperative discomfort is slight and settles quickly.
3. Le Forte osteotomy with cartilaginous septum with a vascularized pedicle fed by the greater palatine arteries limits the postoperative resorption of bone and thus deformity of the nasal dorsum.
4. Nasomaxillary osteotomy and Le Forte I osteotomy with down fracture provides access to the lower clivus and upper cervical region and the frontal base. These procedures also provide a wide working space, especially longitudinally. The technique allows good access to epidural lesions located in the midline, between the two carotid arteries.
5. The risk of wound breakdown and infection is minimal.
6. The approach can be expanded in superior, lateral and inferior directions by combination with other approaches.

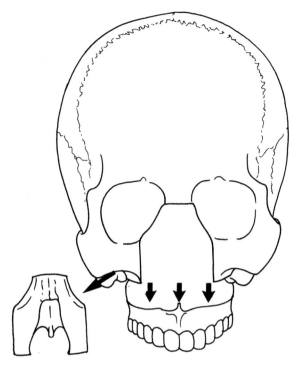

Fig. 19.15   Anteroposterior view after down fracture of maxilla.

REFERENCES

Al-Mefty O 1987 The supraorbital-pterional approach to skull base lesions. Neurosurgery 21: 474–477

Close L G, Schaefer S D, Mickey B E et al 1989 Surgical management of nasopharyngeal angiofibroma involving the cavernous sinus. Archives of Otolaryngology, Head and Neck Surgery 115: 1091–1095

Cummings B J, Blend R, Keane T et al 1984 Primary radiation therapy for juvenile nasopharyngeal angiofibroma. Laryngoscope 94: 1599–1605

Derome P, Akerman M, Anquez L et al 1972 Les tumeurs spheno-ethmoidales: possibilities d'exerese et de reparation chirurgicales. Neurochirurgie (Suppl) 18: 1–164

English G M, Hemenway W G, Cundy R L 1972 Surgical treatment of invasive angiofibroma. Archives of Otolaryngology, Head and Neck Surgery 96: 32–38

Goel A, Bhayani R, Sheode J 1994 Technique of extended transcranial approach for massive nasopharyngeal angiofibroma. British Journal of Neurosurgery 8: 593–597

Jafek B W, Krekorian E A, Kirsch W M 1979 Juvenile nasopharyngeal angiofibroma: management of intracranial extension. Head and Neck Surgery 2: 119–128

Jane J A, Park T S, Pobereskin L H et al 1982 The supraorbital approach: technical note. Neurosurgery 11: 537–542

Ketcham A S, Van Buren J M 1988 Tumors of the paranasal sinuses: a therapeutic challenge. American Journal of Surgery 150: 406–413

Krekorian E A 1977 Surgical management of nasopharyngeal angiofibroma with intracranial extension. Laryngoscope 87: 154–164

Kyoshima K, Matsuo K 1993 Modified transfacial degloving approach for central skull base lesions. Paper presented at the Japan National Congress, Tokyo.

Maran A G 1983 Surgical approaches to the nasopharynx. Clinical Otolaryngology 8: 417–429.

Moises A, Arriga, Janecka I P 1991 Facial translocation approach to the cranial base: the anatomic basis. Skull Base Surgery 1: 26–33

Panje W R, Dohrman G J, Pitcock J K et al 1989 The transfacial approach for combined anterior craniofacial tumor ablation. Archives of Otolaryngology, head and Neck Surgery 115: 301–307

Ray B S, McLean J M 1943 Combined intracranial and orbital operation for retinoblastoma. Archives of Ophthalmology 30: 437–445

Sekhar L N, Nanda A, Sen C N et al 1992 The extended frontal approach to tumors of anterior, middle and posterior cranial base. Journal of Neurosurgery 76: 198–206

Shah J P, Sunderesan N, Galicich J et al 1987 Craniofacial resection for tumors involving the base of the skull. American Journal of Surgery 154: 352–358

Sisson G A, Bytell D E, Beck S P et al 1976 Carcinoma of the paranasal sinuses and craniofacial resection. Journal of Laryngology and Otology 90: 59–68

Smith R R, Klopp C T, Williams J M 1954 Surgical treatment of cancer of frontal sinuses and adjacent area. Cancer 7: 991–994

Ward P H, Thompson R, Calcaterra T et al 1974 Juvenile angiofibroma: a more rational therapeutic approach based upon clinical and experimental evidence. Laryngoscope 84: 2181–2194

Approaches for trigeminal neurinomas

Atul Goel   Shigeaki Kobayashi   Kazuhiro Hongo

INTRODUCTION

Trigeminal neurinomas are relatively rare tumors and represent 0.2% of all intracranial tumors (Arseni et al 1975, Schisano & Olivocrona 1960). These tumors have characteristic clinical and radiological features (Goel et al 1994, Pollack et al 1989). Trigeminal neurinomas arise from the Schwann cells of the sensory root and can originate in any section of the Vth cranial nerve and correspondingly a variety of symptoms and signs may develop. The origin of these tumors is from a segment of the nerve and the rest of the nerve is involved by displacement by the growing mass. Hence the clinical presentation is usually in the form of pain and paresthesiae in a division of the nerve. Involvement of the motor division may be late and partial. It only implies that the part of the nerve involved due to pressure and displacement can be saved during surgery and can functionally recover. Dense motor and sensory involvement, including absence of corneal sensation, is uncommon and often suggests malignant changes in the tumor. More frequently they have a dumbbell shape with one portion in front of the brain stem in the posteror cranial fossa and the other in the layers of the dura of the petrous apex and lateral wall of the cavernous sinus. Larger tumors may present with involvement of nerves of cavernous sinus, VIIth–VIIIth nerve complex and pyramidal signs.

Various approaches have been described and successfully used to resect these lesions (Bordi et al 1989, Lesoin et al 1986). Their location between the layers of the dura in the middle fossa, frequently encountered large size, soft consistency and relative avascular nature can be advantageously used to limit the exposure. These tumors involve cranial nerves, blood vessels and brain only by displacement and not by invasion.

ANATOMICAL CONSIDERATIONS

The Vth cranial nerve after its exit from the medial aspect of the middle cerebellar peduncle traverses under the tentorium and later over the petrous apex, where it forms the Gasserian ganglion. The Gasserian ganglion then divides into three divisions, the first and second participating in forming the lateral wall of the cavernous sinus, while the third division exits from the cranial cavity via the foramen ovale and has a short intracranial course. As the Vth nerve travels over the petrous apex it is covered by a dural and arachnoid sheath forming Meckel's cave. There is a large subarachnoid space over the Gasserian ganglion in Meckel's cave containing cerebrospinal fluid (CSF) (Fig. 20.1). Apart from this dural and arachnoid envelope which are continuous with the corresponding layers in the posterior fossa, the Vth nerve is also covered by the two divisions of the middle fossa dura which divide at the lateral border of the Gasserian ganglion into two. The inner (cerebral) layer continues as the lateral wall of the

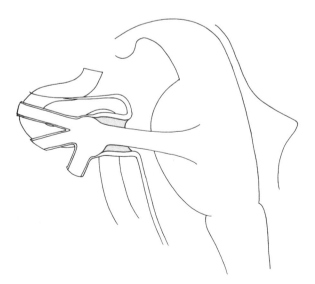

Fig. 20.1   Line drawing showing the Vth nerve and its dural relationship. The Gasserian ganglion is located in the dural Meckel's cave. Note that there is a large redundant space in Meckel's cave which is filled with CSF.

Gasserian ganglion and cavernous sinus while the outer layer (osteal layer) continues medially and forms the inferior dural layer of the Gasserian ganglion and the medial wall of the cavernous sinus. This sheath of the dura is closely approximated, but manually separable from the inner dural layers. The dural layers can be easily dissected from the Gasserian ganglion due to the large subarachnoid space. The dural layers merge with sheaths of the divisions of the nerve and dissection of the dura is relatively difficult from the neural tissue at this level. The superior petrosal sinus traverses in the layers of the dura superior and the inferior petrosal sinus traverses inferior to the root of the Vth nerve at its entry into Meckel's cave. The precavernous segment of the carotid artery lies posteromedial to the Gasserian ganglion and in approximately two-thirds of cases there is no bony divide, but a tough cartilaginous and dural layer provides a barrier between the two (Harris & Rhoton 1976). In the posterior fossa the trigeminal neurinomas are located intradurally. The middle fossa part of the tumor is in the dural sheaths and this location has sometimes been termed as 'interdural' (el Kalliny et al 1992, Goel 1995).

The tumor arises from a fiber of the trigeminal nerve in the region of the trigeminal Gasserian ganglion. The tumor then grows larger and spreads in the available spaces. Meckel's cave can accommodate a large amount of the tumor, which bloats up the cave (Figs. 20.2, 11.3) The tumor, being soft, is unable to open up the dural sheath beyond the ganglion into the roots. This may be the reason why in most cases the tumor does not extend beyond the dilated cave. The extra tumor spills over into the posterior fossa. The tumor presses the adjacent normal Vth nerve, most of which is clinically involved by direct pressure of the tumor. The tumor in proximity to the brain stem is not in continuity with the Vth nerve root which is not actually

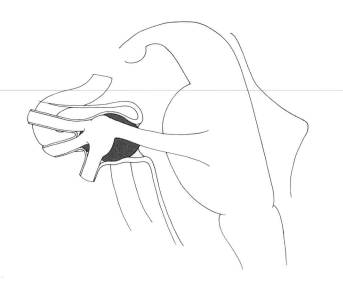

Fig. 20.2 Trigeminal neurinoma in Meckel's cave. The dural envelope of the cave is intact. The carotid artery traverses around the tumor, being separated from it by a firm dural layer.

tumorous. The part in proximity to the brain stem is in most cases like any other extra-axial tumor with a well-defined plane of cleavage.

SURGICAL CONSIDERATIONS

1. The trigeminal neurinomas are more frequently soft and suckable tumors. They are relatively avascular. These two features make the surgery on these lesions relatively easy. Occasional cases of highly vascular and tough tumor may also be encountered.

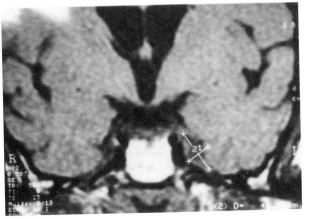

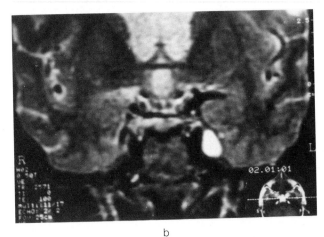

a   b

Fig. 20.3 a T1-weighted MRI shows a small hypointense trigeminal neurinoma in relationship to the cavernous sinus. **b** T2-weighted MRI image shows a markedly hyperintense trigeminal neurinoma.

2. The trigeminal neurinomas can frequently be diagnosed on the basis of the radiological features. The characteristic location at the petrous apex, dumbbell appearance and erosion and widening of Meckel's cave can frequently be seen. The most characteristic feature is the relationship of the precavernous and cavernous segments of the carotid artery. Due to the anatomical relationship of the carotid artery to the Gasserian ganglion, the precavernous carotid artery is located on the inferior surface of the tumor while the cavernous carotid is displaced medially.

3. Although the carotid artery is in close approximation to the tumor there is a well-defined dural sheath separating the two. If one remains in the confines of the tumor capsule there is little danger to the carotid artery. Due to this anatomical feature, there is seldom any need for perioperative control of the carotid artery.

4. The tumor, due to its location in the lateral wall of the cavernous sinus, displaces the venous plexuses and never invades into the venous spaces. If one remains in the tumor capsule one may seldom encounter venous bleeding.

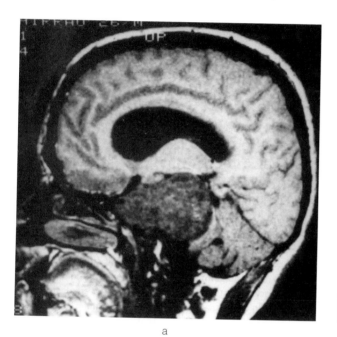

a

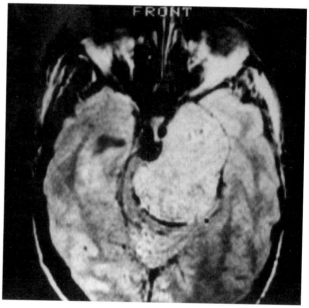

b

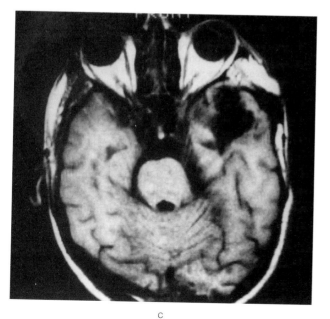

c

Fig. 20.4 **a** T1-weighted MRI shows a massive trigeminal neurinoma. **b** T2-weighted MRI shows the trigeminal neurinoma. A well-defined arachnoid plane separates the tumor from the brain stem. The lateral dural wall is seen to be bloated. The internal carotid artery forms the medial relation to the tumor. **c** Postoperative MRI shows complete resection of the large tumor. A largely infratemporal fossa interdural approach was adopted to resect the tumor.

exposed and safely excised. The head position and the surgeon's view of the tumor are modified to obtain a basal view. The craniectomy at this strategic site provides an avenue for control of the carotid artery at the petrous apex, avoids the need for brain retraction and permits safe and complete resection of the tumor. The approach appears to be ideal for selected cases of trigeminal neurinomas.

Operative technique

The patient is positioned so that the head is extended and turned to the contralateral side. The right-handed surgeon stands on the right side at the level of the chest of the patient irrespective of the side of the lesions and suitably alters the angle of the rotation of the head (Fig. 20.5g). A linear incision is taken over the zygomatic arch, which is completely resected (Fig. 20.5a–c). The temporalis muscle is either split in the direction of the incision (Fig. 20.5c), or can be reflected either superiorly or inferiorly. The mus-

cles of the infratemporal fossa are dissected from the bone by sharp subperiosteal dissection and the foramen ovale is exposed (Fig. 20.5d). With a microdrill a small craniectomy measuring approximately 3×3 cm is made in the infratemporal fossa, incorporating the foramen ovale (Figs 20.5e–g, 20.6). An incision is taken on the lateral surface of the dural sheath of the mandibular nerve at the level of the foramen ovale and extended posteriorly to the inferior and lateral surface of the dural sheaths covering the Gasserian ganglion. Usually the tumor is palpable in the region of the ganglion. The dura over the Gasserian ganglion and the lateral wall of the cavernous sinus is reflected, exposing the middle fossa part of the tumor (the temporal lobe exposure and middle fossa floor durotomy is avoided). The bulk of the tumor usually dilates the dural sheaths in each case and a large exposure can be obtained. After the debulking of the tumor the exposure can be further widened. The large tumor in the region of the Gasserian ganglion is seen to dilate Meckel's cave, thus providing sufficient exposure to the part anterior to the

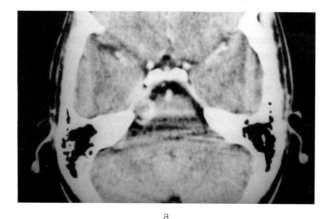

a

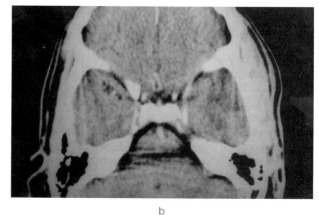

b

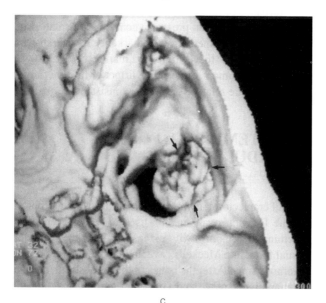

c

Fig. 20.6 **a** Relatively poor-quality CT scan shows the dumbbell trigeminal neurinoma. (From Goel 1995, with permission.) **b** Postoperative scan after complete tumor resection. (From Goel 1995, with permission.) **c** Postoperative three-dimensional CT scan with arrows showing the extent of craniectomy. Lateral two-thirds of the craniectomy is reconstructed using bone dust. (From Goel 1995, with permission.)

brain stem. The inner membranous dural layer separates the tumor from the venous channels of the cavernous sinus. The cavernous sinus part of the tumor can usually be resected by anterior angulation of the microscope. The tumor is followed in the posterior fossa along Meckel's cave. The operation is thus carried out in the infratentorial compartment. Tumor resection in the posterior cranial fossa can be carried out only if the tumor is small or is very soft and amenable to suction debulking and subsequent resection (Figs 20.4, 20.7).

A modification of the above-described interdural approach was suitable in some cases, particularly those with small tumors (Fig. 20.3). The patient is placed in the lateral position. A lumbar drainage of CSF is carried out. A limited subtemporal craniotomy in the line of the external ear canal is done. Zygomatic osteotomy is avoided. The temporalis muscle is displaced anteriorly. Extradural exposure of the foramen ovale is done. Dissection is done between the dural sleeves of the third division of the trigeminal nerve and the tumor is resected.

Various operative approaches have been described for the surgical resection of trigeminal neurinomas (Daspit et al 1991, Schisano & Olivocrona 1960, Wetmore et al 1986, Yasui et al 1989). Skull base techniques have recently been utilized (Al-Mefty & Anand 1990, Becker et al 1991, Fisch 1982, Goel 1995, Pollack et al 1989) to provide for a low and wide exposure and limiting the need for brain retraction. The approach described here utilizes an infratemporal fossa exposure after sectioning of the zygomatic arch. Such an infratemporal fossa approach has been described for petroclival area lesions (Al-Mefty & Anand 1990, Becker et al 1991, Fisch 1982, Souliere et al 1991). The

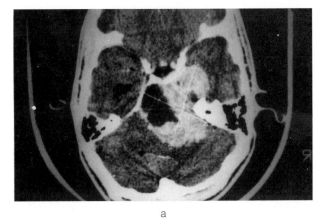

a

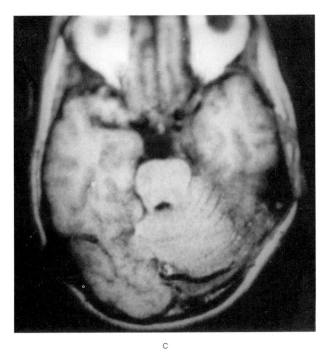

c

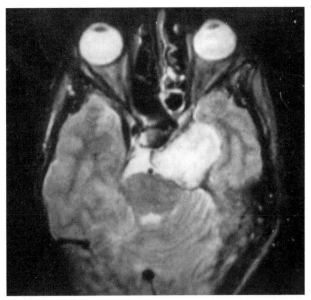

b

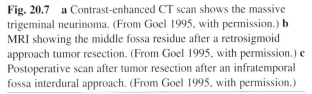

Fig. 20.7 **a** Contrast-enhanced CT scan shows the massive trigeminal neurinoma. (From Goel 1995, with permission.) **b** MRI showing the middle fossa residue after a retrosigmoid approach tumor resection. (From Goel 1995, with permission.) **c** Postoperative scan after tumor resection after an infratemporal fossa interdural approach. (From Goel 1995, with permission.)

association of atrophy of the temporalis and pterygoid muscles with trigeminal neurinomas makes the dissection in the infratemporal fossa relatively easy and exposure wider. Al-Mefty described section of the temporalis mus-

cle at its insertion at the coronoid process and superior displacement of the muscle (Al-Mefty & Anand 1990). The temporalis muscle can also be either split in the direction of its fibers or reflected inferiorly and later used for basal

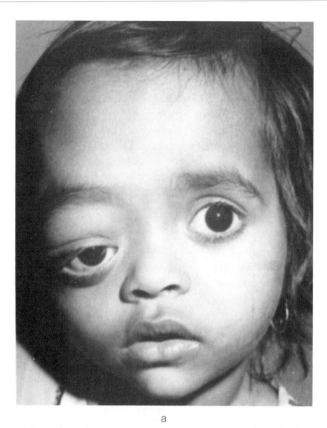

a

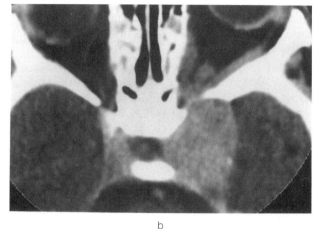

b

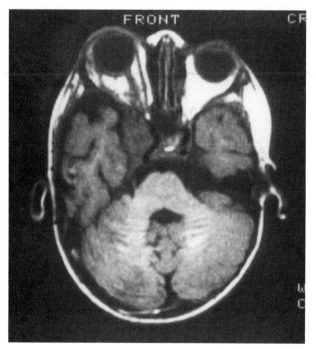

b

Fig. 20.8 **a** Photograph of the child showing proptosis. Enlargement of the supraorbital nerves can be seen. **b** CT scan showing the tumor in the region of the cavernous sinus. Enlargement of intraorbital nerves and muscles and the proptosis is seen. (From Goel et al 1994, with permission.) **c** MRI shows the intracavernous sinus with medially displaced internal carotid artery.

reconstruction (Goel 1994a, 1994b). The direction of approach and the surgeon's position in relation to the patient can be altered to provide a direct and low access to the lesion. The route of approach is interdural, avoiding the need to expose the temporal lobe and thus limiting the extent of temporal lobe retraction to the minimum. The possibility of anatomically dissecting the layers of the dura in cases of trigeminal neurinoma has been described earlier (el Kalliny et al 1992, Patouillard & Nanneuville 1972). Although the carotid artery at the petrous apex is not exposed as it is usually covered by a dural sheath (Harris & Rhoton 1976), it is close in the field and can be exposed relatively easily. The tumor bulk widens Meckel's cave and a large window can be obtained for resection of the posterior fossa portion of the tumor. The soft nature of the tumor can be used to circumvent the disadvantage of confronting the tumor prior to exposure of the brain stem. The approach to the tumor anterior to the brain stem is entirely infratentorial. In our series the exposure obtained by such an approach was seen to be adequate for safe and complete resection of the tumor. In none of the cases was there any need to extend the exposure for tumor removal. The entire procedure could be performed in significantly shorter time and was cosmetically appealing.

Case 1   An Unusual Trigeminal Neurinoma (Goel et al 1994)

An 18-month-old girl was brought with a complaint of progressive proptosis of the left eye for 14 months prior to her admission. Vision and extraocular movements were normal. There was no clinical evidence of trigeminal nerve dysfunction. The left-sided supraorbital nerves were thickened and this was obvious even visually (Fig. 20.8a). Computed tomography (CT) and magnetic resonance image (MRI) scans showed a large tumor occupying the lateral wall of the cavernous sinus displacing the intracavernous carotid artery medially (Fig. 20.8b). Intraorbital and infratemporal extension of the tumor was also noted. Angiography showed that the tumor was avascular. A radical excision was planned. The tumor involved the Gasserian ganglion completely, and also extended anteriorly along its three divisions. The tumor in the ophthalmic division extended into the orbit along the superior orbital fissure and involved the supraorbital nerve as well. The superior orbital fissure, foramen ovale and foramen rotundum were enlarged. A limited excision of the tumor was performed because of its firm consistency and due to the diffuse nature of its spread. It was felt that an attempt to excise the tumor totally would in all probability fail, and would also leave the child with extensive ocular morbidity. The patient was discharged with the proptosis unchanged. At the last follow-up 10 months after the surgery the proptosis remains unchanged. Later progression may force radical surgery. A strong family history of neurofibromatosis and evidence of café-au-lait spots on the child's torso were observed in retrospect.

Comments

Neurofibromatosis is rarely associated with a trigeminal nerve tumor. Only three cases of intracranial trigeminal neurinomas have been recorded in association with neurofibromatosis (Bonnal 1978, McCormick et al 1988, Paillas et al 1974). Though a plexiform nature of spread of an extracranial trigeminal neurinoma has been reported in one case (Biernacka & Zielinnska 1972) intracranial plexiform spread of a trigeminal neurinoma has never been reported. This is what we saw in our patient. The second unusual feature is the occurrence at such a young age (proptosis appeared at 4 months of age). These tumors usually occur in adults and have been only rarely reported below the age of 10 years. The previously recorded youngest patient was a 5-year-old girl (Ross et al 1984). Finally trigeminal neurinomas present with features of trigeminal nerve dysfunction, headache and diplopia. Proptosis as the only presenting feature of a trigeminal neurinoma has not been reported. All these were unusual features in this patient.

Case 2   Large Trigeminal Neurinoma Presenting as Pathological Laughter (Bhatjiwale et al 1996)

A 26-year-old male had uncontrollable explosive laughter during conversation for a year. The laughter lasted for a few seconds and stopped abruptly, whereafter the conversation would continue again. During these periods the patient lost track of his conversation and was unaware of this pathological emotional outburst. These episodes occurred at a frequency of four or five within half an hour of conversation. At the end of each spell he would pick up the broken stream of thoughts and continue his conversation once again. In addition he had paresthesias, numbness in the right half of face, giddiness and progressively worsening ataxia for about the same period. On examination his higher functions were normal. Both fundi showed papilledema. The right corneal reaction was sluggish and there was hypoesthesia in maxillary and mandibular divisions of the trigeminal nerve. The rest of the neurological examination was normal. MRI showed a large tumor extending from the left prepontine to the medial temporal region (Fig. 20.3). The midbrain, pons and the cerebellum were severely deformed by the tumor. The petrous apex was eroded. The ventricles were moderately dilated. An infratemporal fossa interdural approach (Goel 1995) was employed. The tumor was soft and only moderately vascular and could be removed with relative ease. A large number of fibers of the Vth cranial nerve could be preserved. The patient was relieved of his pathological laughter immediately after surgery. The histopathological report showed features consistent with the diagnosis of a neurinoma. On 1 year follow-up the paresthesias over the face had significantly reduced and ataxia had completely cleared. There was no recurrence of pathological laughter.

Comments

Pathological laughter is a sudden outburst of uncontrollable, spontaneous and inappropriate laughter. To our knowledge, only six cases of extra-axial brain stem tumors associated with inappropriate laughter have been documented in the literature (Cantu & Drew 1966, Ironside 1956, Isono et al 1979, Matsuoka et al 1977, Osumi et al 1976, Stevenson et al 1966). Of the six cases, there were two meningiomas, three chordomas and one case of bilateral acoustic nerve tumors. All these tumors were located ventral to the pontomesencephalic area. Trigeminal neurinomas have not been recorded to present with the symptom of pathological laughter.

REFERENCES

Al-Mefty O, Anand V K 1990 Zygomatic approach to skull-base lesions. Journal of Neurosurgery 73: 668–673

Arseni C, Dumitrescu L, Contantinescu A 1975 Neurinomas of the trigeminal nerve. Surgical Neurology 4: 497–503

Becker D, Ammirati M, Black K et al 1991 Transzygomatic approach to tumors of the parasellar region. Technical note. Acta Neurochirurgica (Suppl) (Wien) 53: 89–91

Bhatjiwale M G, Goel A, Desai K 1996 Pathological laughter as a presenting symptom of trigeminal neurinoma. Neurologia Medico. Chirurgica 36: 560–562

Biernacka M, Zielinnska H 1972 Pryzpadek neuroma plexiforme u 3-letneigo dziecka. Klinika Oczna 42: 1083–1085

Bonnal J 1978 Trigeminal tumors. In: EMC Neurologic Fasc 17376, A–10. Editions Techniques SA, Paris

Bordi L, Compton J, Symon L 1989 Trigeminal neurinoma: a report of eleven cases. Surgical Neurology 31: 272–276

Cantu R C, Drew J H 1966 Pathological laughing and crying associated with a tumor ventral to the pons: case report. Journal of Neurosurgery 24: 1024–1026

Daspit C P, Spetzler R F, Pappas C T 1991 Combined approach for lesions involving the cerebellopontine angle and skull base: experience with 20 cases – preliminary report. Otolaryngology, Head and Neck Surgery 105: 788–796

el Kalliny M, van Loveran H, Kellar J T, Tew J M Jr 1992 Tumors of the lateral wall of the cavernous sinus. Journal of Neurosurgery 77: 508–514

Fisch U 1982 Infratemporal fossa approach for glomus tumors of the temporal bone. Annals of Otology, Rhinology and Laryngology 91: 474–479

Goel A 1994a Vascularized osteomyoplastic flaps for skull base reconstruction. British Journal of Neurosurgery 8: 79–82

Goel A 1994b Extended vascularised temporalis muscle-fascia flap. British Journal of Neurosurgery 8: 731–733

Goel A 1995 Infratemporal fossa interdural approach for trigeminal neurinoma. Acta Neurochirurgica (Wien) 136: 99–102

Goel A, Ranade D, Nagpal R D 1994 An unusual trigeminal neurinoma. British Journal of Neurosurgery 8: 369–371

Harris F S, Rhoton A L Jr 1976 Anatomy of the cavernous sinus: a microsurgical study. Journal of Neurosurgery 45: 169–180

Ironside R 1956 Disorders of laughter due to brain lesions. Brain 79: 589–609

Isono G, Ishii R, Shgibata Y et al 1979 REM sleep without atonia in a case of bilateral acoustic tumor. Clinical Psychiatry 21: 1221–1228

Lesoin F, Rousseaux M, Villette L et al 1986 Neurinomas of the trigeminal nerve. Acta Neurochirurgica (Wien) 82: 118–122

Matsuoka S, Aragaki Y, Numaguchi K et al 1977 A case of angioblastic meningioma with pathological laughter – with special reference to laughter in brain tumor. Neurologia Medico-chirurgica 17: 195–201

McCormick P C, Bello J A, Post K D 1988 Trigeminal schwannoma. Journal of Neurosurgery 69: 850–860

Osumi Y, Yamadori A, Tamaki N 1976 A case of ventrally situated brain stem meningioma associated with forced laughter. Clinical Neurology 16: 715–720

Paillas J E, Grisoli F, Farnarier P 1974 Trigeminal nerve neurinomas: report of 8 cases. Neurochirurgie 20: 41–54

Patouillard P, Nanneuvile G 1972 Walls of the cavernous sinus. Neurochirurgie 20: 41–54

Pollack I F, Sekhar L N, Jannetta P J, Janecka I P 1989 Neurilemomas of the trigeminal nerve. Journal of Neurosurgery 70: 737–745

Ross D L, Tew J M, Benton C, Eisentrout C 1984 Trigeminal schwannoma in a child. Neurosurgery 15: 108–110

Schisano G, Olivocrona H 1960 Neurinomas of the Gasserian ganglion and trigeminal root. Journal of Neurosurgery 17: 306–322

Souliere C R Jr, Telian S A, Kemink J L 1991 The infratemporal fossa approach to skull base surgery. Ear Nose Throat 70: 620–636

Stevenson G C, Stony R J, Perkins R K et al 1966 A transcervical transclivus approach to the ventral surface of the brain stem for removal of a clivus chordoma. Journal of Neurosurgery 24: 544–551

Wetmore S J, Suen J Y, Snyderman N L 1986 Preauricular approach to infratemporal fossa. Head and Neck Surgery 9: 93–103

Yasui T, Hakuba A, Kim S H, Nishimura S 1989 Trigeminal neurinomas: operative approach in eight cases. Journal of Neurosurgery 71: 506–511

Surgical Treatment of the Trigeminal Neurinomas
Akira Hakuba   Kenji Ohata

General Considerations: Radical removal of the trigeminal neurinomas is important because recurrence is inevitable after incomplete removal (Pollack et al 1989, Visto et al 1992).

The surgical approach depends on the anatomical location of the trigeminal neurinoma. Accurate preoperative delineation of the tumor is essential in selecting the most appropriate surgical route (McCormick et al 1988). Thin-section axial bone density views on CT through the skull base shows the degree of bone involvement. The axial, coronal and sagittal sections with MRI demonstrate an accurate size and anatomical relationship of the tumor in both the middle and posterior fossa, and also precisely define the relationship of the tumor to the cavernous sinus and will identify extradural tumor extension into the pterygoid fossa or paranasal sinuses. A craniobasal approach such as an orbitozygomatic or oticocondylar transpetrosal approach (Ohata & Hakuba 1996) is the preferred route in most cases, because it offers excellent exposure of the middle fossa floor and also allows access into the posterior fossa. Lumbar CSF drainage and mannitol administration are also used to facilitate temporal lobe retraction while taking the epidural approach.

The suboccipital approach is appropriate only for those tumors entirely limited to the posterior fossa or with minimal extension into the cave. The sitting position is preferred for patients undergoing this procedure. Adequate illumination and adherence to microsurgical principles are essential prerequisites for successful removal of these tumors.

Surgical Anatomy of Meckel's Cave: The crescent-shaped trigeminal ganglion occupies Meckel's cave, which is an arachnoid–dural recess formed in a shallow bony impression on the anterior surface of the petrous apex. Its dorsal wall is composed of two layers: the outer dural layer and the dura propria of the trigeminal nerve and ganglion which continues as a dural sheath of the three branches of the trigeminal nerve, forming a part of the inner dural layer of the lateral wall of the cavernous sinus. The dura propria of the temporal lobe forming the outer dural layer of the dorsal wall of Meckel's cave continues across this border to become the outer dural layer of the lateral wall of the cavernous sinus. The ventral wall of the cave is also composed of two layers: the dura propria of the trigeminal nerve and ganglion, and the periosteum of the petrous tip. This periosteum continues across the border to become the inferior wall of the cavernous sinus (Hakuba et al 1989).

Surgical Strategy for Large Involvement of Meckel's Cave and Cavernous Sinus: A combined pre- and retroauricular transpetrosal approach (Hakuba et al 1988) with an oticocondylar osteotomy (Ohata & Hakuba 1996) is suitable for both root and ganglion types of trigeminal neurinoma involving largely Meckel's cave. Wide opening of the posterior margin of the enlarged cave is accomplished by dividing the temporal dura propria together with the dura propria of the trigeminal nerve and ganglion along the posterior wall of the tumor medially up to the trigeminal porus. The cleavage of the starting point of the dissection is readily found at the posterior margin of the foramen ovale. The posterior wall of the tumor within the cave is widely exposed by careful separation of the arachnoid membrane of the cave from the capsule of the exposed tumor. Initial subcapsular decompression

minimizes manipulation and protects the surrounding neurovascular structures. Care should be taken to avoid injuring the trigeminal nerve root. Tentoriotomy is accomplished, starting from the medial end of the dural incision along the posterior margin of the tumor in the cave which is located at the enlarged trigeminal porus, where the superior petrosal sinus has been ligated doubly and divided between the suture ligations, and then the dural incision is directed to the hiatus right behind the dural entrance of the IVth cranial nerve.

Because the tumor within the cave is covered by the arachnoid membrane and the dura propria of the trigeminal nerve and ganglion as well as the outer dural layer composed of the temporal dura propria dorsally and the periosteum of the petrous tip ventrally, the tumor growing into the cavernous sinus from the cave does not invade into its wall. The tumor extends into the cavernous sinus with displacement of the intracavernous structures by the enlarged Meckel's cave due to growth of the tumor. Therefore careful separation of the arachnoid membrane of the cave from the tumor capsule following the subcapsular decompression will relatively easily and safely deliver the tumor capsule from the cavernous sinus without opening its wall, and there is least possibility of injuring the internal carotid artery and cranial nerves passing through the cavernous sinus.

Via this combined pre- and retroauricular transpetrosal approach (Hakuba et al 1988), the tumor extending into the posterior fossa can also be relatively easily exposed and dissected out after its internal decompression. Because it is an epiarachnoidal growth, the cleavage of dissection can be identified almost entirely epiarachnoidally, and separation of the arachnoid membrane from the tumor capsule in order to leave this arachnoid membrane on the concaved cerebellum and brain stem will relatively easily deliver the tumor capsule from them. These surgical techniques are similar to those employed for acoustic neurinomas (Ohata et al 1996).

When the tumor originates from the trigeminal division, it will occupy the lateral wall of the cavernous sinus and extend extracranially with widening of bony canals of the divisions. Therefore, epidural separation of the temporal dura propria will easily expose the tumor via an orbitozygomatic infratemporal epidural approach (Hakuba et al 1989).

The trigeminal neurinomas, therefore, can be removed toally via the approach which is most suitable according to the origin of the tumors.

References

Hakuba A, Nishimura S, Jang B J 1988 A combined retro- and preauricular transpetrosal–transtentorial approach to clivus meningiomas. Surgical Neurology 30: 108–116

Hakuba A, Tanaka K, Suzuki T, Nishimura S 1989 A combined orbitozygomatic infratemporal epidural and subdural approach for lesions involving the entire cavernous sinus. Journal of Neurosurgery 71: 699–704

McCormick P C, Bello J A, Post K D 1988 Trigeminal schwannoma: surgical series of 14 cases with review of the literature. Journal of Neurosurgery 69: 850–860

Ohata K, Hakuba A 1996 Lateral extensive middle fossa approach. In: Torrens M, Al-Mefty O (eds) Operative skull base surgery. Churchill Livingstone, Edinburgh (in press)

Ohata K, Nagai K, Morino M et al 1996 Surgical technique for surgery of acoustic neurinoma. Neurosurgeons (in press)

Pollack I F, Sekhar L N, Jannetta P J et al 1989 Neurilemomas of the trigeminal nerve. Journal of Neurosurgery 70: 737–745

Visto A, Derome P, Masestro De Leon J L 1992 Sphenocavernous and infratemporal trigeminal neurinomas: surgical series of 15 cases. Skull Base Surgery 2: 142–148

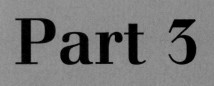

Miscellaneous

Craniovertebral and spinal stability 21

Atul Goel   Shigeaki Kobayashi

CRANIOVERTEBRAL ANOMALIES

Congenital craniovertebral anomalies present a challenging neurosurgical problem. A large array of complex bony and neural anomalies have been described in this region. The issues involved in the management include consideration for decompression of the region and provision of firm and stable fixation which is able to bear the stresses and strains of movements, distraction and compression. If correct and timely treatment is provided to these patients a satisfying long-term outcome can be obtained.

The craniovertebral junction is a funnel-shaped enclosure formed by the basiocciput, atlas and axis vertebrae. The craniovertebral region gains its importance from its contents – the cervicomedullary junction and the terminal segments of the vertebral arteries. Strictly speaking, craniovertebral anomalies include congenital bony abnormalities of the basiocciput, margins of the foramen magnum, atlas and axis. In most cases the neural compression at the craniovertebral junction is bony in nature. Soft tissue anomalies are often a consequence of the bony compression.

Chiari malformation and syringomyelia are other major groups in craniovertebral junction anomalies.

Clinical features

Most of the patients with congenital craniovertebral anomalies present at a young age. Males are more frequently affected. The symptoms result from involvement of upper cervical spinal cord, medulla, lower cranial nerves and vertebral arteries. When mild, such lesions may cause pain in the neck, torticollis, spasticity of limbs and quadriparesis. When severe, and especially if onset is acute, quadriplegia, respiratory arrest and death ensue.

For a proper understanding of these anomalies it is important to recapitulate some embryology. The base of the skull and occipital bone develops by ossification of membrane. The occipital bone is formed from four sclerotomes. The atlas is formed by fusion of the caudal (densely staining) half of the last occipital sclerotome with the clear, cephalic portion of the first cervical sclerotome (failure of separation of the caudal half of the last occipital sclerotome leads to the 'occipitalized atlas' where we see no distinct first cervical vertebra). The tip of the odontoid also develops from the last occipital sclerotome but the body of the odontoid is formed from the first cervical sclerotome. It later fuses with the body of the axis, formed from the second cervical sclerotome.

Classification of clinically important anomalies

Bony abnormalities
1. Malformation of the skull base: basilar invagination. (Platybasia – a flattening of the base of the skull – may not manifest clinically.)
2. Atlantoaxial anomalies: occipitalization of atlas, atlantoaxial dislocations with the following types of odontoid processes:
   (a) well formed, fused odontoid;
   (b) well formed, separate odontoid;
   (c) hypoplastic or aplastic odontoid.

(Occipitalization of the atlas, by itself, is of no clinical significance.)

Basilar invagination
This term refers to invagination of the base of the skull and the upper cervical spine into the posterior cranial fossa. Whilst the invagination is commonly congenital, it also follows diseases which weaken the bone around the foramen magnum. Padget's disease, osteomalacia, hypothyroidism, rickets, hyperparathyroidism, injury and destructive inflammatory and neoplastic diseases are some such causes.

Basilar invagination has been generally divided into anterior, posterior and lateral invagination. In anterior basilar invagination the odontoid process invaginates into the foramen magnum. In posterior basilar invagination the posterior rim of the foramen magnum projects superiorly, indenting the neural structures. In lateral invagination the occipital condyle or the lateral masses of the atlas project excessively into the foramen magnum. From our experience we note that basilar invagination is a more complex group of anomalies. A combination of all three varieties of basilar invagination is commonly encountered. Anterior basilar invagination is frequently associated with lateral basilar invagination.

Basilar invagination reduces the space available in the posterior fossa and the foramen magnum. Crowding and compression of neural structures in this region result in paresis of lower cranial nerves, involvement of pyramidal tracts, and signs due to lower brain stem and cerebellar dysfunction. Low hairline and short neck provide clues to the diagnosis. Basilar invagination is frequently associated with other complex bony and soft tissue anomalies. A fixed atlantoaxial dislocation is commonly associated. In the presence of basilar invagination mobile atlantoaxial dislocation is rare.

Pain in the neck in association with craniovertebral anomaly is suggestive of an element of instability of the region. Pain is usually due to an excessive effort imposed on the muscles to maintain stability of the region. Whenever there is pain, subtle dislocation can be expected and on the basis of this symptom alone a fixation of the craniovertebral region may be planned. In cases with significant preoperative pain, during operation the positioning of the patient should be delicate and guarded as under anesthesia the muscle support is reduced and there is an enhanced possibility of dislocation. Whenever flexion of the head and neck provoke transient electric shock-like sensations in the limbs and trunk (Lhermitte's sign), investigations are required to rule out atlantoaxial dislocation.

Investigations

As the anomalies are complex and bony abnormalities are frequently associated with neural and vascular anomalies, all cases should be investigated elaborately. Computed tomographic (CT) scan with emphasis on bone windows and magnetic resonance imaging (MRI) scanning clarify the bony and soft tissue anomalies respectively. Previously X-rays and tomograms formed the thrust of investigations. On X-ray films and tomograms the base of the skull is evaluated using Chamberlain's line (joining the dorsal lip of the foramen magnum to the posterior end of the hard palate). In anterior basilar invagination more than the cephalic third of the odontoid process projects above this line.

Treatment

In most cases the basilar invagination is principally a bony anomaly and bony decompression of the medullospinal junction is the treatment. Whenever the compression is predominantly from the anterior aspect, an anterior operation is advocated. Transoral surgery and decompression of the bony elements is the most preferred route of anterior surgery. Whenever the compression is posterior, bony decompression by removal of the posterior rim of the foramen magnum is necessary. During posterior decompression only a thin rim of the foramen magnum should be removed. Whenever possible foramen magnotomy (as described later in treatment of Chiari malformation) may be carried out. Metal and bone fixation of the craniovertebral region should preferably be simultaneously carried out even when only a fixed atlantoaxial dislocation is present. Sometimes the basilar invagination is predominantly lateral. In this situation the projecting edge of the joint has to be resected. Whenever by a transoral route, the joint capsule of the atlantoaxial or occipitoaxial facet joints are opened up, or partial fectectomy is done to provide an additional decompression, a bony fusion is usually necessary. The lateral basilar invagination is difficult to diagnose on conventional imaging. High-quality three-dimensional CT scanning and MRI are necessary to delineate the exact site of lateral compression.

Prior to surgical treatment of anterior basilar invagination the patient is placed in skeletal traction in an attempt to bring down the odontoid. In cases where the symptoms are at least partially relieved by traction, results of surgery are generally seen to be good. Traction also helps during surgery by the transoral route as the odontoid process is pulled down, resulting in easier access.

Atlantoaxial dislocation (AAD)

In the more common form of AAD, the atlas dislocates over the axis. In cases with occipitalization of atlas, the head and atlas form one unit and the axis forms the other unit. The odontoid process of the axis is normally in close approximation with the anterior arch of the atlas. In AAD, the head and atlas dislocate ventrally on the axis on flexion of the head, markedly widening the atlantodental interval and reducing the diameter of the spinal canal, with consequent pressure on the cervicomedullary junction. The dislocation increases on flexion of the head and reduces in extension in the mobile variety of AAD. In a few patients, hyperextension of the head produces posterior dislocation of the atlas. In the fixed variety, the dislocation persists even on extension of the head.

Pain in the upper part of the neck and restriction of rotary movements of the head and neck are the common early warning symptoms. The patient may give a history of an injury that flexed the head and neck (as when he is hit on the back of the head) as the precipitating factor. Weakness and spasticity of all limbs follow. Hemiparesis may precede quadriparesis. Slippers fly off the feet. There is difficulty in moving in the dark. Loss of appreciation of joint position and vibration is obvious. All the deep reflexes are exaggerated and the plantar responses are extensor. Wasting of the intrinsic muscles of the hands is a frequent accompaniment. This may follow damage of the anterior spinal artery or an associated syringomyelia. Acute worsening of the dislocation (as by an injury causing flexion of the head) may produce respiratory paralysis, coma and even death. Uncommonly, such injury may damage the vertebral artery to produce a stroke along its distribution.

Radiographs showing the lateral views of the atlantoaxial region with head and neck flexed and extended confirm the diagnosis. Tomograms in the coronal and sagittal planes clarify the exact nature of the anomaly. Careful radiology yields all the information needed for diagnosis and treatment. CT with three-dimensional images clarifies the bony configuration and provides information which is crucial in planning and executing the surgical treatment. MRI provides information about displacements of the medullospinal axis. This investigation is also invaluable if associated syringomyelia is suspected.

Where the dislocation is mobile, it is reduced to its normal position by extension of the head and neck and if necessary by the use of skull traction. The region is then fused in a reduced position by one of several techniques available.

Where the atlas is fixed in the dislocated position, an attempt is made to reduce the dislocation with the help of traction. Traction is continued for about 2 weeks and the situation of the craniovertebral region is checked with the help of serial X-rays. By traction over the period the neck muscles relax, providing an opportunity for the displaced bony structures to return to normal alignment. Where the alignment becomes normal or significantly reduced, fixation may be carried out in that position. In cases where no reduction is possible the cervicomedullary junction is relieved by excising the bone causing compression. More often in fixed atlantoaxial dislocation the compression to the neural structures is from the anterior direction and such patients need anterior transoral surgery. If anterior compression is relatively insignificant a posterior decompression by means of resection of the rim of the foramen magnum and posterior arch of the atlas may be carried out.

Surgical considerations in atlantoaxial dislocation

The aim of surgery in general is to restore normal or the best possible alignment and to achieve stability of the atlantoaxial joint. As the region is biomechanically complex a clear understanding of the pathophysiology of the lesion and site and the direction of the compression should be analyzed on the basis of radiology and clinical features.

Various methods for fixation and fusion for atlantoaxial dislocation have been described, accepted and successfully used (Alexander & Davis 1969, Aprin & Harf 1988, Cybulski et al 1988, Dickman et al 1991, Dove 1986, Fang & Ong 1962, Flint et al 1987, Gallie 1939, Goel & Laheri

1994, Heywood et al 1988, Holness et al 1984, Kelly et al 1972, Luque 1982, Magerl & Seeman 1986, McGraw & Rusch 1973, Mixter & Osgood 1910, Newman & Sweetnam 1969, Ransford et al 1986, Simmons 1982). Such methods employ autologous bone graft, acrylic, sublaminar wires, metal loupes and rectangles. However, the search for the biomechanically most appropriate method of fixation for this clinically vexing problem continues.

The ideal method of surgical fusion of the atlantoaxial dislocation should satisfy the following criteria: it should

1. provide a firm fixation of the region and permit absolutely no movement. This provides an opportunity for the bone graft to fuse with the parent bone and ultimately result in bony fusion. In the presence of even slight movement bony fusion will not occur;
2. provide an extensive area for bone graft placement;
3. permit immediate mobilization of the patient;
4. whenever required permit decompression of the region without affecting the fusion procedure;
5. provide an opportunity to reduce fixed dislocation;
6. permit CT scanning and MRI;
7. be technically simple.

The search for an ideal method of fusion continues.

Metal implants provide an initial period of fixation of the region facilitating bony fusion. Bony fusion takes about 3 months and the metal implants should be strong enough to hold the region for that period. It ultimately depends on the bony fusion to provide stability to the region.

Lateral mass plate and screw fixation for atlantoaxial subluxation

We have described a method of fixation of the lateral masses of atlas and axis by using a 'radius–ulna' internal-fixation stainless-steel plate and screws (Goel & Laheri 1994) and a summary of this fixation method is given here (Fig. 21.1a). This method of fixation was successfully used in 45 cases of congenital atlantoaxial dislocation (Fig. 21.1b, c). A 100% union rate was achieved, with no morbidity or mortality, and no instrument fatigue or failure. The technique provided immediate rigid segmental internal fixation, permitting early mobilization with minimal external support. Onlay and interfacetal bone grafts subsequently produced bony fusion. Direct application of screws to the atlas and axis, thus utilizing the firm purchase in their thick and large corticocancellous lateral mass, provides a biomechanically strong fixation of the region. Occipitocervical fusion could be done in selected cases by modification of the method (Fig. 21.2a, b).

Fusion of the lateral masses for atlantoaxial dislocation has been performed previously. Barbour (1971) described a method of fusion by transarticular screws. Subsequently, various groups have attempted fusion of the lateral masses

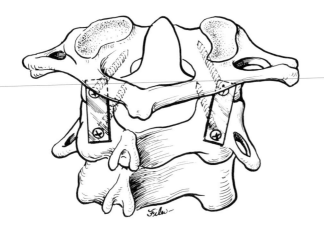

a

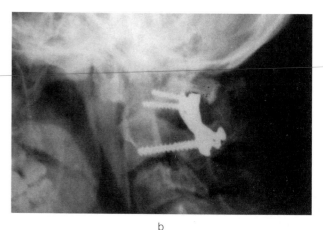

b

c

Fig. 21.1 **a** Small plates and screws demonstrating the procedure of fusion. Note the site of placement of plates and the direction of the screws in the lateral masses. (From Goel & Laheri 1994, with permission.) **b** Lateral X-ray of a 34-year-old man taken 9 months after surgery. The plate and screw fixation and the osseous fusion between atlas and axis are seen. **c** Lateral X-ray of a 10-year-old boy showing plate and screw fixation. Note the fusion between the spinous process of axis and arch of atlas.

by screws and by bone grafts (Du Toit 1976, Fang et al 1964, Grob & Magerl 1987, Lesoin et al 1987, Magerl & Seeman 1986, Roy Camille et al 1982).

The described method of fixation is particularly useful in some complex congenital or traumatic craniovertebral region instabilities where conventional methods have failed or are not suitable. The method can be used in a regular case of atlantoaxial dislocation as well, as it provides firm and rigid fixation and permits absolutely no movement in the region – a factor which is crucial for bony union. After a 3-month period it seems that the fixation provided by the plates and screws is no longer required and the bony union holds the region and the metal implant in situ. Titanium plates and screws (commercially available) can be used to provide MRI compatibility (Aldrich et al 1991). Occipitoatlantoaxial fusion can be achieved by modification of the method (Fig. 21.2a, b). The occipital bone also provides a firm ground for fixation of the plate

with screws or wire (Bryan et al 1982, Heywood et al 1988). The only apparent problem with this method of fixation is that the surgical procedure is technically difficult and demanding. Precise anatomical understanding of the region is necessary when one contemplates performing this operation (Figs 21.3–21.5).

Operative technique and relevant anatomy

The patient is operated under general anesthesia in the prone position. A cervical Gardner–Wells traction is applied to hold the region in reduced position and to partially immobilize and stabilize the area, thus assisting during the operative procedure. A 15–30° head-high position provides counter traction and helps reduction of venous engorgement, which is an important factor considering the large venous plexuses around the joint (Fig. 21.6). Care should be taken such that there is no rotational element during positioning as this could adversely affect the surgi-

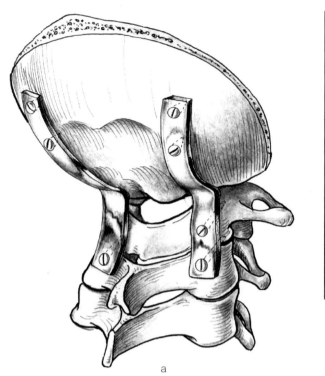

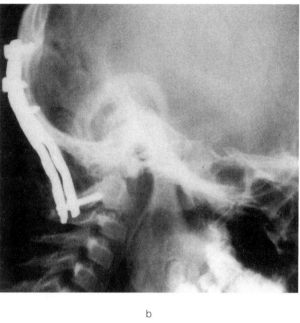

b

Fig. 21.2   a Occipitoatlantoaxial fixation using longer plates and screws. On the left side occipitoaxial fixation and on the right occipitoatlantoaxial fixation with screws are shown. (From Goel & Laheri 1994, with permission.) **b** Lateral X-ray of a 9-year-old girl taken 7 months after operation showing occipitoaxial plate and screw fixation. Occipitalized atlas is seen. Also note that the bone graft has been well accepted. (From Goel & Laheri 1994, with permission.)

cal procedure. Even mild twisting of the neck can alter the location of the vertebral artery and thus place the entire operation in danger. After the positioning a lateral radiograph of the craniovertebral region is obtained to confirm reduction of the dislocation. The suboccipital region and the upper cervical spine are exposed through a longitudinal midline incision. The lateral masses of the atlas and axis and their facet joints are bilaterally exposed by retracting the paravertebral muscles by sharp subperiosteal dissection. In our series the vertebral artery, during its course from the transverse foramen of the atlas to its position posterior to the lateral mass and then over the groove on the upper surface of the posterior arch of atlas (Kowada et al 1973, Newton & Mani 1974, Takahashi et al 1970, Teal et al 1973), had to be dissected away from the field for application of screws on one occasion. In other cases there was no need to identify or dissect any part of the vertebral artery. However, the presumed pathway of the artery was adequately protected and isolated during the surgery (anomalies of the vertebral artery in this area are rare; Newton & Mani 1974). Large extradural veins frequently cause troublesome bleeding. The second cervical root ganglion, which lies over the posterior aspect of the atlantoaxial joint, is sacrificed and cut to expose the posterior aspect

of the joint space adequately. On some occasions a relatively large intervertebral artery traverses along with the cervical root. During the sectioning of the ganglion this artery has to be sectioned. Thick capsule overlying the joint space is sharply cut and the facet joint opened widely. The adjacent synovial surfaces of the atlantoaxial joint are roughened and decorticated widely by micro-drill, thus providing a large recipient area for bony fusion. Pieces of harvested bone from the iliac crest are stuffed into the joint space. Under direct vision and after carefully studying the local anatomy, guide holes are drilled into the lateral masses through the pedicle of the axis and directly into the lateral mass of the atlas as shown in the Figure 21.1a. The direction of the holes and screws has to be sharply anteromedial to avoid the vertebral artery. The angle of screw implantation is varied according to the requirements of the particular case (Fig. 21.7). A two- or three-hole (about 2–3 cm long) radius–ulna internal fixation plate (or any other commercially available metal plate) is placed in position over the exposed lateral mass of the atlas and pedicle of the axis (Figs 21.1, 21.8–21.14), whenever necessary cut and molded into shape, and the screws are screwed in. Adjacent surfaces of the posterior arch of the atlas and lamina of the axis are drilled with a high-speed drill to pro-

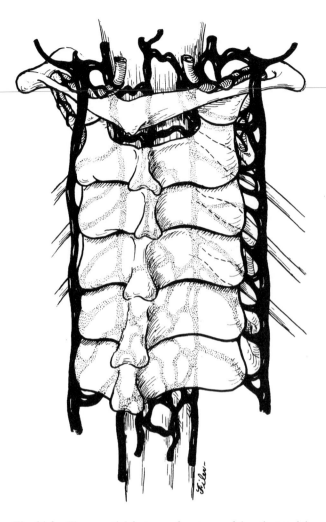

Fig. 21.3   The essential features of anatomy of the atlantoaxial region. The relationship of the vertebral artery and venous plexuses to the atlantoaxial joint is seen.

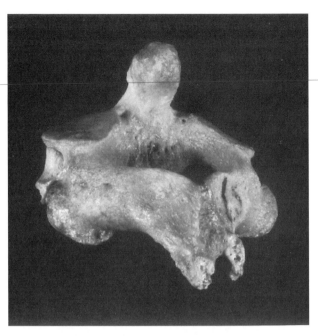

Fig. 21.4   Axis vertebra. Note the large size of its lateral mass available for implantation of the screw.

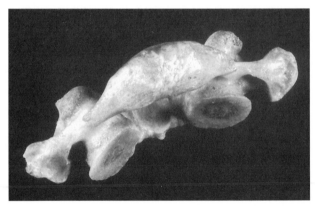

Fig. 21.5   Atlas vertebra. Note the large size of its lateral mass available for implantation of the screw.

vide additional space for placement of the plate. In an adult, screws of 2.5–2.9 mm diameter and 18–24 mm length are required. Smaller screws are used in children. Large pieces of corticocancellous bone graft from the iliac bone are then placed in the adequately prepared receptor area of the arch of the atlas and lamina of the axis. In cases where there is an occipitalization of the atlas the suboccipital region is prepared for graft placement. After closure of the wound the cervical traction is removed. For occipitoaxial fixation, longer, multi-holed plates (Figs 21.2, 21.17, 21.18) are used. The occipital end of the plate is fixed either with the help of screws (Fig 21.2) or with wires (Figs. 21.17, 21.18). The occipital screws are of 3–3.5 mm diameter and of 8–10 mm length. The length of the screw is altered so that it engages both the cortices of the occipital bone for a firm fixation. A thick muscle layer

is sutured over the plate. Wire fixation of the plate to the occipital bone is a stronger, easier and safer method.

Donor bone graft is taken from iliac crest.

Material and results

Surgical indications: Of the 45 cases treated during the period 1988–1995 (4 years 10 months), 38 patients had congenital and seven post-traumatic instability of the atlantoaxial region. The ages of the patients ranged from 5 to 74 years. Fifteen of these patients were females. The patients presented with symptoms of varying degree of high cervical cord compression and lower cranial nerve

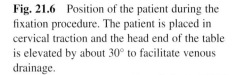

Fig. 21.6 Position of the patient during the fixation procedure. The patient is placed in cervical traction and the head end of the table is elevated by about 30° to facilitate venous drainage.

involvement. In the early part of the experience the described procedure was performed only in selected cases where midline procedures had failed, were not possible or where foramen magnum decompression or midline surgical procedures were also necessary. However, with more satisfactory results and familiarity with the anatomy, in the latter phase the procedure was employed as the primary method of fixation. As the majority of the patients in the presented series belonged to the group of congenital instability, they harbored various combinations of anatomical complexities posing a therapeutic challenge.

In the 38 cases in the congenital group, the indications of the operation varied. In two children the posterior arch of the atlas was cartilaginous and the sublaminar wiring procedure was not considered. In four cases sublaminar wiring and in one case the metal loop fixation procedure had failed and the described procedure was performed as a secondary method of fixation. Five patients had Arnold–Chiari malformation and syringomyelia with atlantoaxial instability (Figs 21.11, 21.19, 21.20). Foramen magnum decompression and syringosubarachnoid shunt was done in addition to lateral mass plate and screw fixation in these cases (Figs 21.17, 21.18). In eight cases the atlantoaxial dislocation was only partially reducible. It was considered that foramen magnum decompression was necessary in addition to fixation of the region in these cases (Fig. 21.12). In the rest of the patients with congenital instability of the region, where the conventional methods of fixation could have been used, the plate and screw method of fixation was selected.

In the congenital category 26 patients underwent atlantoaxial fixation and 10 patients underwent occipitoax-

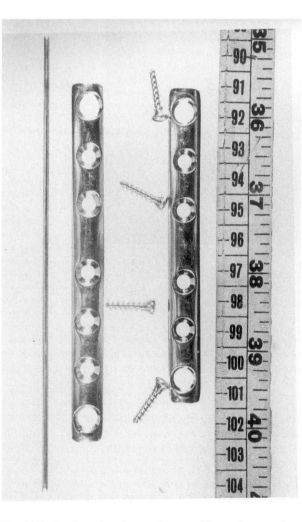

Fig. 21.7 Radius–ulna plates and screws. These plates can be molded and cut into shape. Various sizes are commercially available. (From Goel & Lanheri 1994, with permission.)

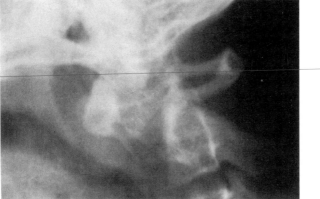

a

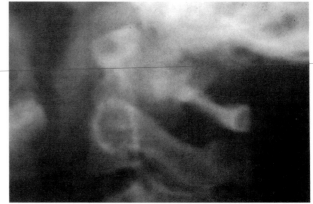

b

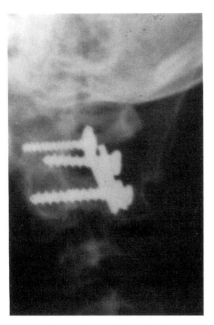

c

Fig. 21.8 **a** Lateral X-ray in flexion of a 40-year-old man showing atlantoaxial dislocation. (From Goel & Laheri 1994, with permission.) **b** Lateral X-ray in extension showing complete reduction of the dislocation. (From Goel & Laheri 1994, with permission.) **c** Lateral X-ray 10 months following atlantoaxial fixation with plate and screws.

ial fixation. In two patients atlantoaxial fixation was carried out on one side and occipitoaxial fixation was done on the other due to technical problems during surgery, as discussed later (Fig. 21.10). In general, occipitoaxial fixation was preferred in cases with occipitalization of the atlas (Figs 21.19, 21.20). In two cases atlantoaxial fixation was carried out even in the presence of occipitalized atlas (Fig. 21.11). One patient, in addition to lateral mass atlantoaxial fixation, also underwent sublaminar wire fixation (Fig. 21.9). This was done in the initial phase of our experience. Foramen magnum decompression was carried out in 15 patients after fixation. Occipital fixation was done with screws in two (Fig. 21.2), and with wires in eight patients (Figs 21.19, 21.20). Seven patients had post-traumatic reducible atlantoaxial dislocation; in four there was frac-

ture of the odontoid process. All these patients underwent atlantoaxial fixation.

In general, the format for treatment was followed as per guidelines suggested in various reviews on this subject (Dickman et al 1991, Jackson 1950, VanGilder et al 1987, White & Panjabi 1983).

Perioperative problems: In the initial part of the experience, in one patient plate and screw fixation was carried out only on one side as profuse venous bleeding prevented adequate exposure on the contralateral side. The fixation, however, has remained satisfactory and after 16 months of follow-up a strong bony union has been observed.

In one case with partially reducible atlantoaxial dislocation, occipitalized atlas and basilar invagination, after transoral decompression posterior fixation was performed.

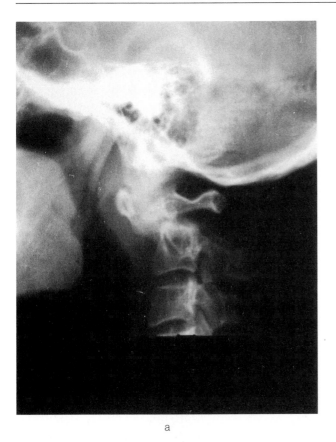

a

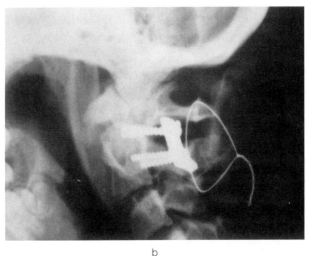

b

Fig. 21.9 **a** X-ray of a 14-year-old girl in flexion showing atlantoaxial dislocation. A separate odontoid process is seen. (From Goel & Laheri 1994, with permission.) **b** X-ray in flexion 16 months after the operation, showing plate and screw fixation. Sublaminer wire has been passed. Note the acceptance of the bone graft. (From Goel & Laheri 1994, with permission.)

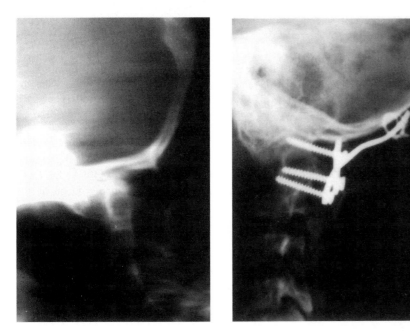

Fig. 21.10 **a** Lateral X-ray of a 14-year-old girl in flexion. X-ray shows occipitalized atlas, congenital fusion between axis and third cervical vertebra and compromised canal at craniovertebral junction. The X-ray in extension did not exhibit reducibility. (From Goel & Laheri 1994, with permission.) **b** Fixation and foramen magnum decompression was done after transoral surgery. Occipitoaxial fixation on one side and atlantoaxial fixation on the other side was done. The occipital fixation is done with metal wires.

However, lateral mass fixation could be carried out only on one side due to twisting of the neck and distortion of the anatomy following inadvertent wrong positioning of the traction tongs. Occipitoaxial fixation had to be performed on the contralateral side (Fig. 21.10).

In two patients the fixation was done in a partially dis-

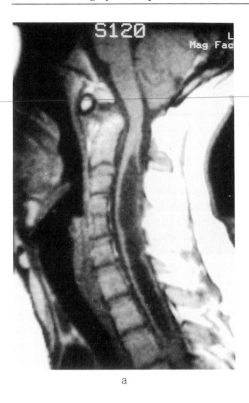

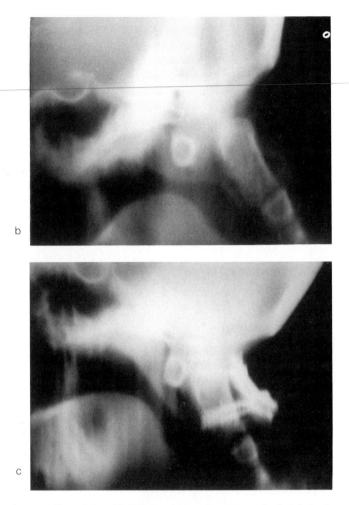

Fig. 21.11   a MRI scanning in extension shows the extensive syringomyelia and Arnold-Chiari malformation. (From Goel & Laheri 1994, with permission.) **b** Tomogram with the head in flexion showing the fused axis and third cervical vertebra, with severely compromised canal at the atlas. (From Goel & Laheri 1994, with permission.) **c** Foramen magnum decompression, excision of the arch of the atlas, syringostomy and plate and screw fixation of the atlas with the axis. (From Goel & Laheri 1994, with permission.)

located position. However, there was no neurological complication.

Results:

All patients had improvement or stabilization of neurological status. Although bony fusion could not be confirmed in all cases due to inadequate visualization of the bone graft on X-rays, with the average follow-up of 30 months, no patient has developed recurrent instability of the joint needing reoperation. There has been no evidence of screw loosening, instrument failure or fatigue. No patient in this series complained of any numbness or pain in the second cervical dermatome in spite of the sectioning of the root.

Discussion

The technique of fusion described here appears to be biomechanically stable and firm with the ability to with-

stand strains of flexion and extension and of compression and distraction (Goel & Winterbottom 1990). As the fixation procedure directly applies to the articular facets of the synovial capsule-denuded joint, the construct, with its mechanical advantage, has more tensile strength. The lateral masses of the atlas and axis, being large and strong with little cancellous bone, allow good placement of the plate and purchase by screws (Magerl & Seeman 1986). The procedure can be performed in all cases of atlantoaxial dislocations where the lateral masses are normal. As described in other methods of lateral fixation (Barbour 1971, DuToit 1976, Grob & Magerl 1987, Lesoin et al 1987, Roy Camille et al 1982) midline operative procedures can be done without affecting the fixation process. Whenever necessary foramen magnum decompression can be carried out to provide for additional space in the region. Unlike fusions incorporating occipital bone and lower cer-

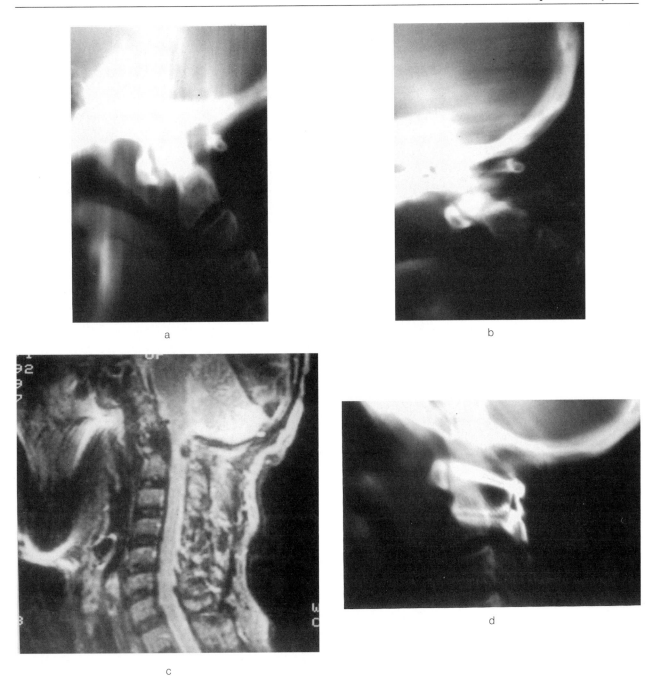

a

b

c

d

Fig. 21.12 **a** Lateral X-ray in flexion of a 70-year-old man showing atlantoaxial dislocation. (From Goel & Laheri 1994, with permission.) **b** X-ray in extension showing complete reduction. (From Goel & Laheri 1994, with permission.) **c** MRI scanning in the position of reduction shows the compression of the craniospinal canal by the posterior arch of the atlas. (From Goel & Laheri 1994, with permission.) **d** Excision of the posterior arch of the atlas and fixation. (From Goel & Laheri 1994, with permission.)

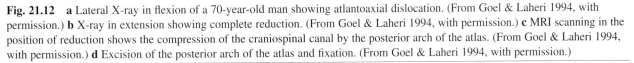

vical levels required in most metal loop and acrylic fixation methods, cervical mobility and growth are preserved. Sublaminar introduction and complications following over-tightening and breakage of metal wires (Clark & White 1985, Geremia et al 1985, McCarron & Robertson 1988) is avoided. A large area of the facet joint can be

used for bony fusion in addition to the ground provided by the occipital squama, posterior arch of the atlas and lamina of the axis (Dickman et al 1991). Rigid external immobilization with Halo brace/cervical traction has been advocated to maximize bone formation (Sonntag & Hadley 1988) following the fixation. However, in the described

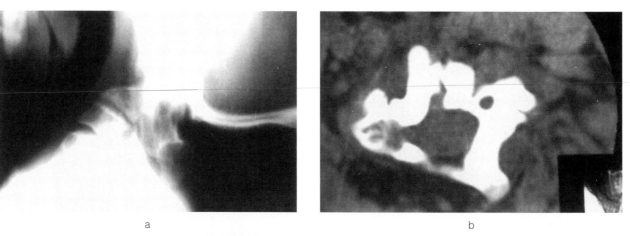

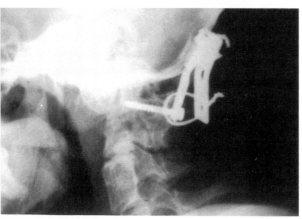

Fig. 21.13 **a** Lateral X-ray of cervical spine showing occipitalized atlas and basilar invagination. **b** Post-transoral decompression CT scan at the lower border of resection of the body of the axis shows its marked rotation. On the right side the vertebral artery canal is directly in line with the screw implantation. **c** Postoperative X-rays show occipitoaxial fixation. On the left side plate and screw fixation, while on the right side plate and wire fixation is carried out. On the right side screw implantation was considered to be dangerous due to the twisting of the axis.

procedure, the internal fixation appeared to be firm, permitting no movements, and only minimal or no external immobilization was found to be necessary. This could have

a bearing in some children and elderly who tolerate screw implantation for Halo brace/traction poorly.

Lateral mass fusion is ideal and is sometimes the only

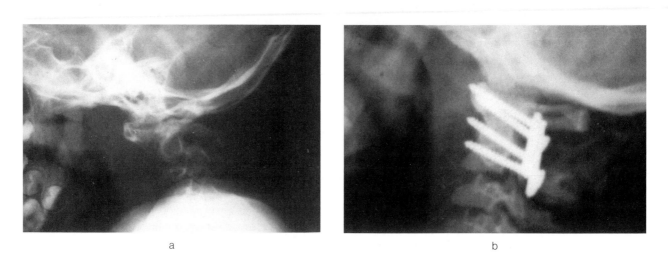

Fig. 21.14 **a** X-ray in flexion of a 7-year-old child shows marked atlantoaxial dislocation. **b** Postoperative X-ray showing atlantoaxial fixation with plates and screws.

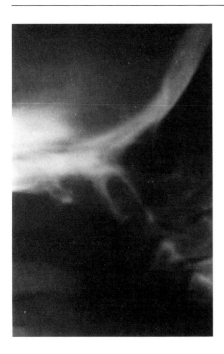

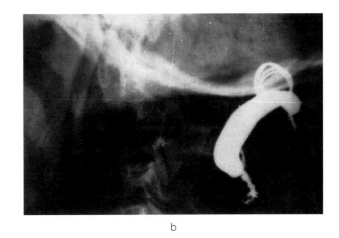

Fig. 21.15 **a** Lateral X-ray showing altantoaxial dislocation, occipitalization of the atlas and basilar invagination. The atlantoaxial dislocation was of a fixed variety. **b** Metal loop used for fixation of the occipital bone to the spinous process of the second cervical vertebra. The procedure was performed after transoral decompression.

available alternative in situations where the posterior arch of the atlas is either congenitally absent, hypoplastic (Lipson & Hammerschlag 1984, VanGilder et al 1987), cartilaginous or broken following trauma or sublaminar wire tightening. Foramen magnum decompression and wide C1 and C2 laminectomies have been advocated for acute brain stem and spinal cord decompression in patients with craniovertebral problems presenting as neurosurgical emergencies (Bertrand 1982). Lateral mass fusion can be done simultaneously if there is instability. In cases of unstable traumatic spine with fractures of laminae and odontoid process wire-tightening procedures may not be possible. Plate and screw fixation can be performed if the lateral masses are normal. Failure of an attempted fusion by metal rectangles or sublaminar wire present a difficult situation. Lateral mass fusion is ideally suited in such cases. Finally, compression plates and screws are less expensive when compared to preformed loupes and clamps.

Other methods of fixation for atlantoaxial dislocation

- Multiholed plate and wire fixation (Fig. 21.15).
- Hartshill rectangle and wire fixation.
- Sublaminar wire fixation (Fig. 21.16).
- Transarticular screw fixation.

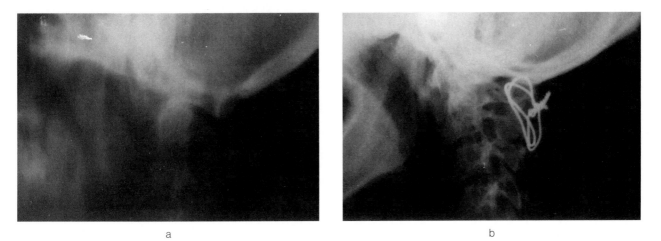

Fig. 21.16 **a** Lateral X-ray showing atlantoaxial dislocation. **b** Atlantoaxial fixation using sublaminar wire fixation.

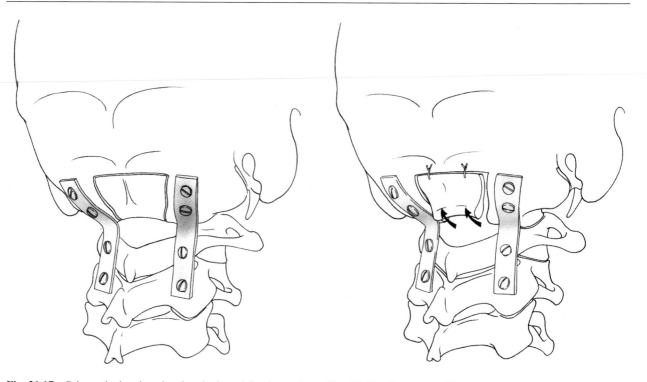

Fig. 21.17 Schematic drawing showing the lateral fixation and site of cut for foramen magnotomy.

Fig. 21.18 Procedure of foramen magnotomy. The bone flap is reversed. The superior edge of the reversed flap is stitched to the occipital bone while the inferior edge swings away from the neural structures.

Chiari malformation associated with atlantoaxial dislocation

Surgical treatment of Chiari malformation and atlantoaxial dislocation has been extensively described in the literature (Gardner 1965, Hoffman et al 1990). We encountered a rare situation in five cases where Chiari malformation was associated with atlantoaxial dislocation. Such a clinical situation is rare, but when seen may be difficult to treat as these cases require a posterior decompression in addition to a fixation procedure. The conventional fixation methods using the occipital bone and upper cervical laminae for fixation may not be possible in such a situation due to the non-availability of bone following decompression. A lateral mass plate and screw fixation as described earlier was successfully used and the midline decompressive surgery did not affect the fixation procedure. Reversal foramen magnotomy was performed in these cases. Such a procedure provided additional area for bone fusion after adequate bony decompression.

In our cases with atlantoaxial dislocation and Chiari malformation, which are generally relatively discrete pathological conditions, they were present jointly in association with other anomalies. Two patients had occipitalized atlas, two had basilar invagination, three had fused axis and third cervical vertebra and three had syringomyelia. Three patients underwent atlantoaxial fixa-

tion (Fig. 21.11) while in the other two occipitoaxial fixation (Figs 21.19, 21.20) was carried out. In three patients reversal foramen magnotomy (Figs 21.19, 21.20), and in two the conventional bony and dural foramen magnum decompression was done. Successful bony union and fixation and adequate foramen magnum decompression were achieved in all cases.

Patient data
Age at admission ranged from 22 to 54 years (mean 36 years). The duration of preoperative symptoms ranged from 10 months to 4 years. All patients presented with varying degrees of symptoms and signs of cervicomedullary compression. The patients with syringomyelia had additional lower motor neuron signs in the upper limbs and reduction in pain and temperature sensations.

Operative technique for foramen magnotomy
With the help of a micro-drill a flap of foramen magnum was drilled as shown in Figures 21.17 and 21.18. Durotomy and dural decompression were then carried out. No attempt was made to lyse adhesions around the herniating tonsils. The occipital bone flap was reversed, denuded of pericranium and roughened. The upper end of the reversed bone flap was sutured to the bone defect as shown in Figures 21.17 and 21.18. The convex outward surface of

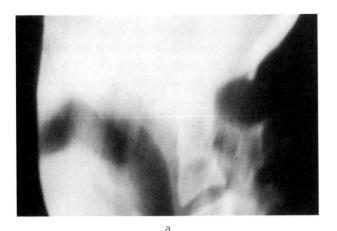

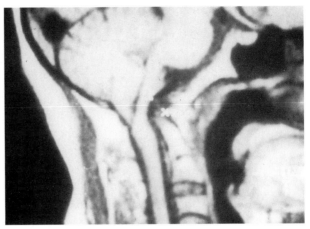

a

b

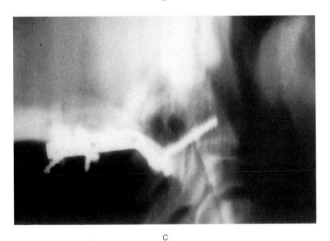

c

Fig. 21.19 **a** Lateral X-ray in flexion shows the atlantoaxial dislocation, occipitalized atlas and fusion of the second and third cervical vertebra. (From Goel & Achawal 1995, with permission.) **b** MRI shows the Chiari malformation and atlantoaxial dislocation. (From Goel & Achawal 1995, with permission.) **c** Postoperative X-ray showing the occipitoaxial plate and screw fixation. Foramen magnotomy was performed.

the occipital bone with the edge of the foramen magnum was now concave outwards. Bone graft taken from the iliac crest was stuffed into the articular cavity of the facet joints and longer pieces placed in the midline over the foramen magnotomy flap.

Posterior fossa craniectomy with or without upper cervical laminectomy (foramen magnum decompression) is the most frequently performed surgical procedure for Chiari malformation (Gardner 1965, Hoffman et al 1990). The need for dural decompression and shearing of adhesions around the herniating tonsils is controversial (Isu et al 1993). Foramen magnotomy, as described, utilizes the curvature of the occipital bone for providing adequate and safe decompression of the craniocervical region while preserving the bone in the midline. The superior edge of the magnotomy bone flap is a tight fit due to the nature of cuts, and can be sutured in place while the rest of the flap swings away from the neural structures with little chance of recurrent compression by the bone flap. The large bone surface available is utilized for the placement of onlay bone graft, which may be critically important for the bony fusion and the ultimate stability of the region. Such an expansive foramen magnotomy procedure can be performed in the case

of Chiari malformation without atlantoaxial dislocation as the procedure provides an adequate decompression by resulting in an increase in the diameter and volume of the foramen magnum. However, this may not be as important or even necessary in such cases. Occasional cases have been reported wherein instability of the cervical spine developed following posterior fossa decompression in cases of Chiari malformation (Aronson et al 1991). A reversal foramen magnotomy operation can be considered if instability of the region is feared. Fusion of the region was observed in all our cases, including those where the conventional foramen magnum bony decompression was performed. On these grounds, the exact utility of a reversal foramen magnotomy procedure cannot be ascertained. However, the additional area provided for midline bony fusion could be important in some of these complex and challenging clinical problems.

TRANSORAL SURGICAL APPROACH

The transoral route is a well-accepted surgical approach for bony decompression in cases with basilar invagination,

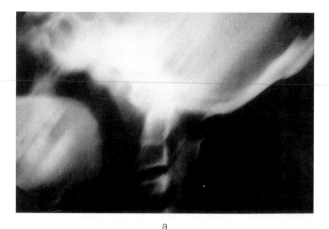

a

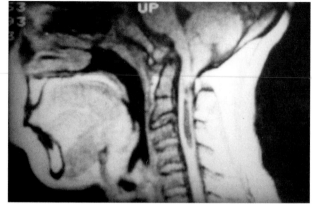

b

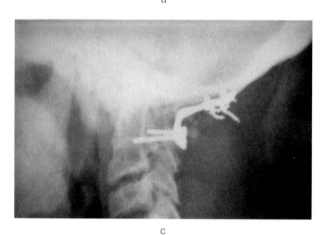

c

Fig. 21.20   a Lateral X-ray in flexion showing the atlantoaxial dislocation. Occipitalized atlas and the fused second and third cervical vertebra are seen. (From Goel & Achawal 1995, with permission.) **b** MRI shows the Chiari malformation and the syrinx. (From Goel & Achawal 1995, with permission.) **c** Postoperative X-ray showing the occipitoaxial fixation in reduced position. (From Goel & Achawal 1995, with permission.)

fixed and irreducible atlantoaxial dislocation where there is anterior compression and distortion of the cervicomedullary region. The compression may be from the tip of the odontoid process and in some rarer cases from other parts of the second or third cervical vertebra. Although the operation is simple and technically easy in submucosal tumors or in atlantoaxial dislocation following rheumatoid arthritis or other such disease process, wherein the craniovertebral region is only diseased but not abnormal or deformed in structure and location, the transoral approach for congenital atlantoaxial dislocation can be a difficult and technically challenging operation on some occasions. Soft palatal incision was always necessary in the authors' cases of congenital basilar invagination. This was due to superior anatomical position of the odontoid process. This surgical route is also useful in cases with extradural tumors located in the retropharyngeal area and interior to the cervicomedullary region.

Except in extremely rare situations, this approach is contraindicated for intradural lesions. The problems in this approach for intradural dural lesions are the following (Goel 1991):

1. There are dangers of life-threatening infections. This is because oral contamination with the operative field cannot be avoided. Such communication persists during the entire operation of tumor removal. Such an infection can be fulminant and resistant to antibiotics.
2. A relatively long mucosal and muscular layer incision in the retropharyngeal wall has to be taken to adequately expose the area. Such a long incision may lead to velopharyngeal insufficiency. This could be a disabling condition.
3. The clival venous plexus is large and any incision in the clival dura can lead to excessive hemorrhage which can be difficult to control.
4. The dura is difficult to close at the termination of the operation. Despite various suggested methods of closure and sealing of the posterior pharyngeal wall, the possibility of CSF fistula remains high. Drainage of CSF via a lumbar external drainage has been recommended. The suction effect of lumbar drainage of CSF enhances the possibilities of transmission of oral flora intradurally.
5. There is no avenue for proximal control of major ves-

sels in cases with operative disasters. The surgeon encounters the tumor first and the tumor–brain stem interface at the termination of the operation. This could have a bearing on the operation and its outcome.

Technical issues:

The instruments designed by Crockard have made transoral surgery relatively easy (Crockard et al 1986). The lateral operating position as suggested by him is also a useful surgical method. The entire operation can be performed whilst the surgeon remains comfortably seated and the microscope positioned as for most other neurosurgical procedures. Micro-drills have made the procedure safe. Intraoperative traction was found to be important. It helped in pulling the odontoid process inferiorly and resulted in its easier access. Traction also stabilized the position of the head during the operation. This stabilization is important when one is operating with the patient in the lateral position. Any inadvertent twist in the neck and body can result in directing the operation towards the vertebral artery. Oral endotracheal tube placement was found to be suitable for most cases of basilar invagination. However, in cases where the body of the C2–3 region was also required to be drilled nasal intubation was found to be useful. Although soft palatal retractors can be useful, in our series it was seen that soft palatal incision and retraction of the two flaps away from the midline was easier and provided an added superior exposure which was found to be always necessary in cases with congenital anomalies. The excision of the odontoid process en masse is rarely possible in cases with fixed atlantoaxial dislocation and basilar invagination. The entire odontoid process has to be tediously drilled. The tip of the odontoid is firmly adherent to the apical ligament and dissecting it from this ligament can be a difficult task.

Instability after transoral odontoidectomy:

Various authors have opined on the issue of instability after transoral odontoidectomy in cases with basilar invagination in fixed atlantoaxial dislocation. The general consensus is that transoral odontoidectomy primarily does not destabilize the craniovertebral region. However, the surgery may exacerbate potential instability of the region. It appears to the present author that after a transoral decompression wherein only selective odontoidectomy is performed the possibility of instability is less likely. In any case there is usually no urgent need for a fixation procedure and the patient can be observed. In cases where there is persistent pain in the occipitocervical region after trans-

oral surgery a fixation procedure should be employed as this finding suggests excessive strain on muscles secondary to instability of the region. In two cases the author performed anterior transoral plate and screw fixation after odontoidectomy. This procedure is described here.

Transoral plate and screw fixation of the craniovertebral region
(Goel & Karapurkar 1994)

Instability of the craniovertebral region and development of delayed kyphus after odontoidectomy in an otherwise stable joint has been reported (Menezes & VanGilder 1988, Dickman et al 1992) and also has been seen in our series of cases. Most authors describe posterior fixation of the atlantoaxial region after transoral odontoidectomy. Satisfactory results have been obtained by such twin procedures (Crockard et al 1986, Menezes et al 1980). Anterior transoral fixation with the help of bone grafts and metal implants has been used for the fixation of the fractured bones and dislocations of the region (Barbour 1971, Geisler et al 1989, Penteleyni et al 1988, Sakou T et al 1984, Strelli 1983). However, various authors have cautioned against the use of foreign material by this route for fear of infection.

Case 1:

A 12-year-old boy was admitted with complaints of weakness of the left side of the body for 2 months. The weakness was progressive and on admission he could stand or walk only with support. He had marked torticollis and short neck since birth. Parents noticed hoarse speech for about a fortnight before admission. On examination he had mild palatal weakness on the right side. There was spastic quadriparesis, the left side being weaker than the right. There was mild impairment of the posterior column sensation on the left limbs. Investigations showed severe basilar invagination. The odontoid process was pointing posteriorly and severely compressed the spinomedullary junction (Fig. 21.21). X-rays of the region in flexion and extension did not reveal any instability of the region. Transoral odontoidectomy and excision of part of the bodies of upper cervical vertebrae was done as considered necessary. The lower part of the clivus had to be drilled to expose the top of the odontoid process. A double compression stainless-steel radius–ulna fixation plate (a titanium plate, which is commercially available, can be used to provide MRI compatibility) with multiple holes was molded to fit into the region. The length of the required screws was measured on serial tomographs of the region. Iliac crest bone graft pieces were placed posterior to the plate and the screws were applied. The cervical screws were fixed into the body of the third cervical vertebra. The mucosa over the superior end of the plate could not be adequately sutured over it. This was most probably due to the more than necessary coagulation. Relaxing incisions were taken in the nasopharyngeal wall to help in the closure, but this was also unsuccessful. Later, part of the muscle from

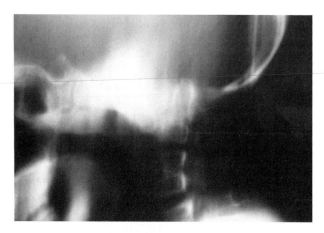

a

Fig. 21.21   **a** X-ray of the craniovertebral region showing basilar invagination. (From Goel & Karapurkar 1994, with permission.) **b** MRI with head flexed, showing severe indentation of the odontoid process over the medulla. (From Goel & Karapurkar 1994, with permission.) **c** X-rays of the craniovertebral region showing the plate and screw fixation of the clivus with the body of the third cervical vertebra. (From Goel & Karapurkar 1994, with permission.)

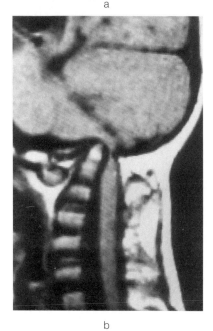

b

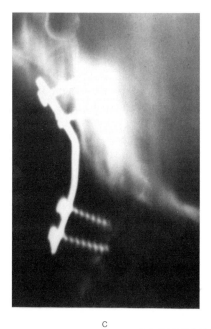

c

the region of the iliac crest was sutured at the site of the exposed plate. Endotracheal intubation was retained in situ in the postoperative phase to help in ventilation. The patient was mobilized with the help of a hard collar as soon as the endotracheal tube was removed. There was a great doubt about the acceptance of the implant, considering the poor nutritional status of the patient and bad general oral hygiene, and also that there was difficulty in covering the mucosa over the plate. However, there were no wound or infection problems. The patient was mobilized with the help of a hard collar. At 4 months follow-up he had shown marked improvement of the power in his limbs. X-rays at this time, although not showing the harvested bone graft clearly, confirmed the firm fixation of the region (Fig. 21.21).

Discussion

The patient presented was a poor-risk case, as the nutritional status and oral hygiene were far from satisfactory. In spite of these factors the wound healed well and the plate was accepted. This only suggests that the highly vascular nasopharyngeal wall has an excellent healing potential and can accept grafts.

Although the described procedure is technically challenging and precise and fraught with the dangers of infection and rejection of the implant, it can be useful in a rare case, particularly in a well-nourished patient with good oral hygiene. The fixation appears to be excellent, with clivus and the cervical body forming a strong ground for screws. Provision of complete immobility of the region is crucial for bony fusion, which would ultimately stabilize the region, and is the main purpose of the operation. With the plate in situ the possibility of shifting of the harvested bone graft is minimized. The patient can be mobilized early with minimal external support. This may be of particular importance in children and in the elderly, who tolerate prolonged traction and Halo fixation poorly. A second operation of posterior fixation is avoided. In cases of basilar invagination, after decompressive surgery, further settling of the vertebrae has been reported (Harkey et al 1990). This can be avoided by this method of fixation. Dislocations and injuries of the craniovertebral region can sometimes be very difficult to treat and fix. The described procedure can be useful in some of these cases. However, until further experience with such metal implants is gained, the authors would advise the use of such a method of fixation only in a situation when the easier and safer methods of posterior fixation are unsuccessful or are not possible. It is suggested that the described fixation procedure with plate and screws can be performed by transcervical or retropharyngeal surgery, circumventing the risk of infection (Lesoin et al 1987, McAfee et al 1987). Although the implant appears to be biomechanically suited to withstand strains of flexion and extension and of compression and distraction, its ability to sustain the rotatory stress is debatable. In this regard the dens transfixation plate as described by Strelli (1983), utilizing more than one screw at the base to prevent the plate torquing out, may be useful.

TRANSORAL FUSION WITH BONE GRAFT

After adequate anterior decompression, a bone graft may be placed extending between the lower end of the decompression to the clivus (Fig. 21.22). Complete immobilization of the region with the help of external braces or Halo fixation is mandatory for successful fusion. However, such an immobilization is difficult and bony fusion is only rarely seen.

SPINAL STABILITY

Posterior inter-body fusion after spinal tumor resection (Goel 1996)

Laminotomy and minimal bone resection have been advocated for tumor resection instead of wide laminectomies and facetectomies to prevent complications related to instability (Allen et al 1987, Cusick et al 1988, Katsumi et al 1989). Various anterior and posterior same-stage or delayed fixation techniques have been reported following spinal tumor resection (Di-Lorenzo et al 1985, Hohmann & Leibig 1987, McAfee & Bohlman 1989, Simpson et al 1993). Direct posterior inter-body fixation technique as described can be useful in some cases where a spinal tumor results in significant bony destruction and instability is feared following the tumor resection.

Case 2

A 32-year-old woman was operated elsewhere for a large dumbbell neurofibroma diagnosed on myelography. X-rays of the cervical spine showed a large bone defect caused by the lesion (Fig. 21.23c). Excision of the intradural portion of the tumor was performed using the conventional wide laminectomy procedure at three levels. The sixth cervical root was completely destroyed by the lesion and was sectioned to assist tumor removal. A large residual extradural and extraspinal lesion was demonstrated on MRI (Fig. 21.23b). Complete encasement of the vertebral artery was noted (Fig. 21.23c). Considering the benign nature of the tumor it was decided to resect the residual tumor as radically as possible. A gross total tumor excision was performed. The tumor-involved vertebral artery was dissected free. The tumor resection involved additional lateral bone removal and facetectomy at two levels. At the end of the tumor resection and during the two operative procedures it was considered that the extensive bone destruction by the tumor and the sacrifice of the involved nerve root could lead to an immediate or delayed instability of the spine. Plates were placed directly over the posterolateral surface of the adjoining vertebral bodies after adequately preparing the bed, and screw implantation was carried out (Fig. 21.23d–f). Discoidectomy was done and the intervertebral space was stuffed with bone graft taken from the iliac crest. The procedure of fixation was seen to be easy and safe due to the already displaced dural tube and the cord medially and the vertebral artery laterally. The purchase for the screws of the corticocancellous bone of the bodies of the vertebrae was found

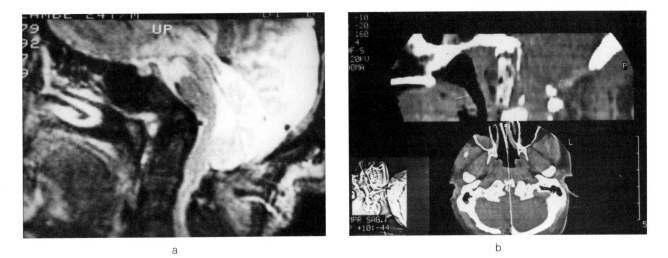

a   b

Fig. 21.22   **a** MRI showing marked platybasia and basilar invagination. **b** Postoperative film showing placement of bone flap extending from the lower end of the clivus to the body of the axis. The procedure was performed after transoral bony decompression.

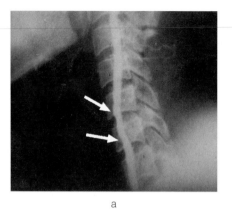

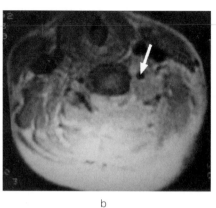

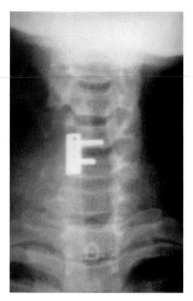

a

b

c

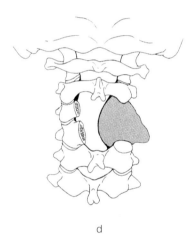

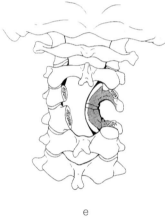

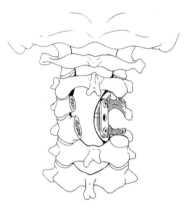

d

e

f

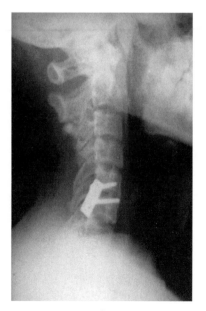

g

Fig. 21.23   a Angiogram showing the vertebral artery. Arrows indicate the site and extent of involvement of the vertebral artery. **b** MRI with arrow showing the left vertebral artery completely encased by the tumor. **c** Anteroposterior X-ray of the cervical spine showing the implanted plate and screws. Note the area of bone destruction. **d** Shaded area depicts the site and extent of bone involvement by the tumor. **e** The situation after tumor resection. Note the extent of bone destruction. The displaced dural tube is seen, exposing widely the site of plate and screw implantation. **f** The implanted plate and screws on the posterolateral surface of the vertebral bodies. **g** Lateral view showing the plate and screws. Good alignment of the cervical spine is seen.

to be adequate. In the postoperative phase a hard collar was prescribed. X-rays done when the patient was seen 6 months after surgery showed good alignment of the cervical spine (Fig. 21.23a, g). Bone fusion could not be demonstrated on X-ray.

Discussion

Occasionally, there arises the need for wide laminae removal and facetectomies to obtain an adequate exposure for safe and complete spinal tumor resection. There have been multiple reports of immediate or delayed instability following such a procedure (Allen et al 1987, Cusick et al 1988, Katsumi et al 1989, Goel et al 1985, Lonstein 1977, Raynor et al 1985, Sim et al 1974, White et al 1975, Yasuoka et al 1981). Some authors feel that a simple laminectomy does not adversely affect the stability of the region. However, addition of partial or complete facetectomy and sacrifice of a root is considered by most to result in an unstable spinal segment. The chronic presence of a neurological deficit in association with vertebral deficiency are the principal predisposing factors in the development of a deformed spine (Alexander 1985). Laminotomy, instead of laminectomy, has been advocated in an attempt to prevent such an eventuality. Some authors advocate stabilization procedures like multiple-level Harrington's rod fixation, sublaminar, facet to facet, facet to spinous process wire fixation and anterior inter-body bone, acrylic or plate fixation (Cusick et al 1988, McAfee & Bohlman 1989, Simpson et al 1993, Alexander 1985).

A spinal fixation was considered to be necessary in the presented case due to the previously performed multiple level laminectomy, near complete facetectomy at two levels, and sectioning of the tumor-involved nerve root. A lateral exposure was necessary for the radical resection of the lesion. The tumor had displaced the vertebral artery laterally and the cord medially. After tumor resection, there was a large space available for the application of plate and screws directly over the posterior surface of the adjoining vertebral bodies. Sacrifice of the root at this level added to the ease and safety of the procedure. The corticocancellous bone of the vertebral bodies provided a strong ground for the purchase of the screws. The fixation appeared to be adequate for temporary segmental immobilization of the region until bony fusion occurred. In the reported case no bony fusion could be demonstrated on the X-rays, but the alignment and curvature of the spine remained satisfactory when the patient was seen 6 months after surgery. Long-term follow-up and larger experience with such a method of fusion is necessary to assess the capability of the plate and screws to sustain the stress of movements and compression and distraction in the cervical spine.

VASCULARIZED PEDICLE LAMINOPLASTY

Laminoplasty instead of a laminectomy procedure is finding favor with some surgeons. Various methods of laminoplasty have been described and successfully used.

A simple method of vascularized pedicled laminoplasty is described. Such a method of laminoplasty has been described in the pediatric age group but not in adults. The laminae were pedicled on supraspinous, interspinous and interlaminar ligaments. The procedure was carried out in eight cases and in an average observation period of 14

months no significant resorption of the bone was observed in any case. Laminoplasty using a vascularized pedicle as described provides a better opportunity to retain its bone matter and the segment is more resistant to infection and radiotherapy. It is a simple, safe and stable alternative to the previously described procedures of laminoplasty. No sophisticated instrumentation, prosthetic material or technically complex maneuvers are required.

Technique:

The essential elements of the technique are shown in Figures 21.24 and 21.25. After a midline incision, the paraspinal muscles are sharply dissected off the lateral aspect of the spinous processes, preferably using scissors, preserving the strong and fibrous supraspinous (homologous with the ligamentum nuchae in the cervical spine) and the relatively thin interspinous ligaments. Cautery is avoided. The paraspinal muscles are separated off the spinous processes and the laminae, taking precautions to avoid a subperiosteal elevation. The procedure retains the thin layer of periosteum covering the spinous processes and laminae. Care is taken to avoid damage to the interlaminar (ligamentum flava) ligaments. The laminae are cut

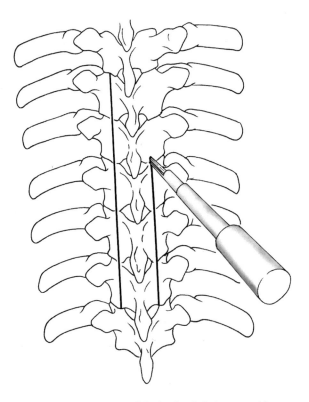

Fig. 21.24 Lateral aspect of the lamina is being cut with a power-driven drill. A five-level laminoplasty is planned.

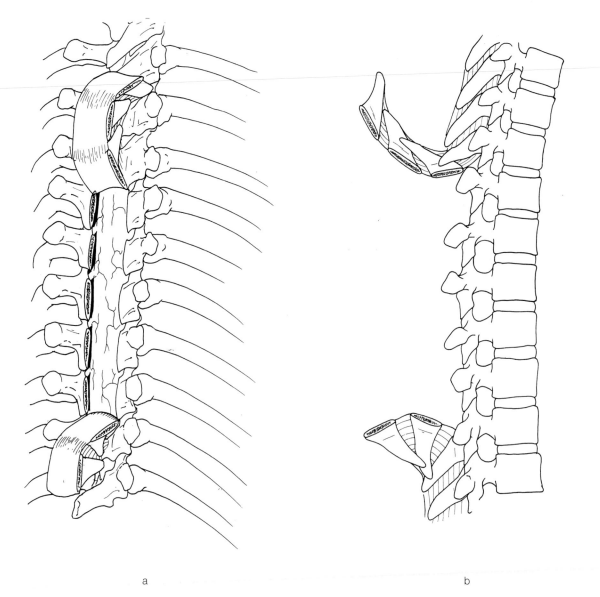

a   b

Fig. 21.25 **a** An angled view to the vascularized pedicled laminoplasty. Two flaps are everted. The superior laminoplasty flap contains three laminar segments while the inferiorly displaced flap contains two segments. **b** Lateral view showing the laminoplasty flaps.

either by using power-driven drills or small rongeurs in their lateral aspect. The flap of laminae attached to each other with supraspinous, interspinous and interlaminar ligaments is everted on the same ligaments attached to the normal laminae and spinous processes (Figs 21.25, 21.26). In cases with multilevel laminectomy (more than three levels), two flaps carrying two to three laminae could be simultaneously everted both superiorly and inferiorly to facilitate vascularization from both sides. After termination of the operation, the laminar flap is replaced to the original site and fixed either with silk or wire sutures. In

our series only silk sutures were used, primarily to facilitate radiography.

Material and methods:

Vascularized pedicled laminoplasty was done in eight patients. Six of these patients were operated for tumors while two underwent syringostomy. In five patients cervical and in three dorsal laminoplasty was carried out. Six of these patients were males and two were females. The ages

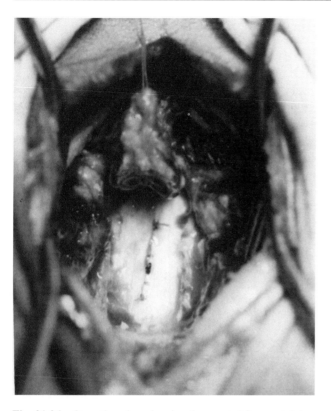

Fig. 21.26 Operative view showing the everted flap containing two laminar segments. The dural suturing has been completed.

of these patients ranged from 21 to 48 years. The laminoplasty was done for two vertebral levels in three cases, three vertebral levels in four cases and five vertebral levels in one case. In the patient where a five-level laminoplasty was carried out two flaps were everted, one containing three laminae being rotated superiorly, and the other containing two laminae inferiorly. None of these patients were re-explored to assess the status of laminoplasty flap. In the average follow-up period of 8 months (range 1–16 months) in none of the patients was any significant bone resorption seen on plain radiographs. None of the patients complained of any discomfort secondary to the procedure.

Results:

The follow-up period in these patients ranged from 3 to 14 months. Persistence of spinous process and laminar segments could be demonstrated in all cases on plain radiography.

Discussion:

Laminoplasty is usually advocated to prevent postopera-

tive instability and deformity and to avoid local scarring. Although the precise usefulness of such a procedure has occasionally been challenged, it is recently finding increasing favor. Whenever laminoplasty is performed with free bone tissues, the principal problem is that in the highly vascularized area in the vicinity the bone becomes partially absorbed and irregular, resulting in the subsequent surgery in the area whenever necessary being relatively more difficult and cumbersome.

Various groups have conducted experimental studies independently on the evolution of free compared with vascularized pedicled bone flaps. The studies confirmed that vascularized bone flaps remain viable and are characterized by normal evolution, while the free bone grafts show typical signs of necrosis and resorption. The interlaminar and interspinous ligaments have an extensive blood supply to the spinous processes and the laminae through multiple small vertical perforators which traverse into the bone directly and through the periosteal layer. Elevation of the laminar flap with wide attachment to these ligaments results in a well-vascularized flap. The periosteal layer covering the laminae and spinous processes comprises an outer layer of loose aereolar tissue and an inner layer of osteoblasts, and contains extensive vascular network. The ligaments and the periosteal layer derive their blood supply from intervertebral arteries and muscular branches of the paravertebral muscle and have multiple anastomoses with arteries above and below and with the opposite side arteries. In the described procedure the lateral feeders at the site of the laminoplasty will be sectioned. In this event vascularization of the laminae occurs from the vertical feeders. In cases where multiple-level laminectomy is performed, the laminae remote from the site of attached ligaments will be more prone to reduced vascularization. In such cases, the laminar flaps based on the vascularized pedicles can be simultaneously rotated both superiorly and inferiorly, saving vascular feeders from both ends. The ease of harvesting the described laminar flap is an important consideration. It avoids the need for shaping and cutting of the bone pieces to suit the local environment as is necessary in some of the described procedures. As the laminae are cut vertically, the bone segments are a relatively perfect fit and can be firmly secured, avoiding dislocation and compression of the spinal cord. The procedure of bony fusion is segmental, and thus avoids the need for immobilization of the spine for fusion. There is no compromise of the diameter of the spinal canal or its asymmetry as a result of the procedure. It may even be possible that the ligaments may retain their function, affecting the mobility and stability of the column. The local availability of the vascularized pedicle can be used without any major additional maneuver. Such a vascularized laminoplasty flap appears to be more resistant to infection, tolerates radiation therapy better, is mechanically stronger, retains its shape and size better, contracts less and survives better when compared to free bone grafts. Additional surgical procedure, as is necessary when autologus bone grafts from iliac crest or tibia is used, is avoided. There is no added postoperative morbidity and discomfort for the patient. No metal implants, acrylic or other similar foreign material are necessary.

THORACIC LAMINOPLASTY USING SPINOUS PROCESSES
(Goel & Deogaonkar 1996)

A simple method of thoracic laminoplasty using spinous processes is described. The procedure involves refashioning the spinous processes which have been removed during laminectomy and suturing these back into position to provide at least partial cover for the dura. The procedure was carried out in four cases. Laminoplasty using spinous processes appears to be a safe and stable alternative to the previously described procedures. No sophisticated instrumentation, prosthetic material or technically complex maneuvers were required.

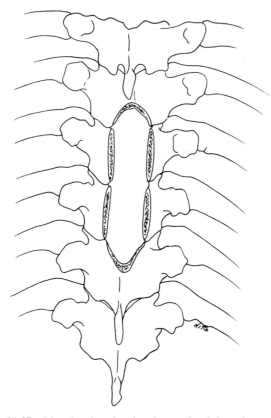

Fig. 21.27 Line drawing showing the two-level thoracic laminectomy.

Technique

The described procedure is clearly shown in Figures 21.27 and 21.28. The spinous processes were cut at the base using the regular laminectomy bone-cutting instrument. After the termination of the operation, the spinous processes at two levels were placed side by side, after adequate shaping with the help of a micro-drill. These were then stitched to one another and to the edges of the laminectomy with silk sutures. For four-level laminoplasty the spinous processes were fixed in two blocks.

Patient material

Thoracic laminoplasty was done using spinous processes in four patients. Two of these patients were operated for syringostomy operation and the other two had spinal tumors. Two of these patients were males and two were females. The ages of these patients ranged from 23 to 34 years. The laminoplasty was done for two vertebral levels in three cases and for four levels in one patient.

Results

The follow-up period in these patients ranged from 3 to 14 months. Persistence of spinous process segments could be demonstrated in all cases on plain radiography.

Discussion

Indications of laminoplasty in the thoracic spine are further limited as the rib cage plays a major role in stabilization, and laminectomy will not create instability unless it is coupled with a destructive process in the vertebral bone or pedicle.

The dimensions of spinous processes and laminae as calculated from dry bone specimens and averaged with the data available from the literature were studied. It was observed that the alignment of spinous processes as described is suitably broad and long to form a flat posterior element. After adequate molding of the spinous processes, similar laminoplasty could be performed in the lumbar spine as well. The principal advantage of the procedure is that it is technically simple, safe and quick to perform. Moreover the procedure involves use of tissue which is otherwise disposed of.

REFERENCES

Aldrich E F, Crow W N, Weber P B et al 1991 Use of MR imaging-compatible Halifax interlaminar clamps for posterior cervical fusion. Journal of Neurosurgery 74: 185–189

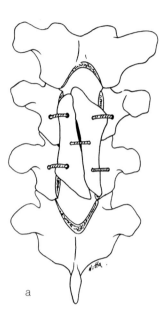

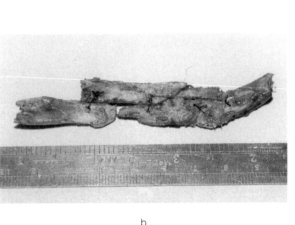

b

Fig. 21.28 a Drawing showing the two spinous processes placed to the sides and in a reversed manner, and sutured to each other and to the adjacent cut end of lamina. It is adequately shaped using a micro-drill. **b** Intraoperative photograph showing the placement of four spinous processes to the sides of each other. These will be used for re-formation of the site of laminectomy.

Alexander E, Jr. 1985 Postlaminectomy kyphosis. In: Wilkins R H, Rengachary S S (eds) Neurosurgery. McGraw-Hill, New York, pp 2293–2297

Alexander E Jr, Davis C H Jr 1969 Reduction and fusion of fracture of the odontoid process. Journal of Neurosurgery 31: 580–582

Allen B L, Tencer A F, Ferguson R L 1987 The biomechanics of decompressive laminectomy. Spine 12: 803–808

Aprin H, Harf R 1988 Stabilization of atlantoaxial instability. Orthopedics 11: 1687–1693

Aronson D D, Kahn R H, Canady A et al 1991 Instability of the cervical spine after decompression in patients with Arnold–Chiari malformation. Journal of Bone and Joint Surgery 73: 898–906

Barbour J R 1971 Screw fixation and fractures of the odontoid process. South Australian Clinics 5: 20–24

Bertrand G 1982 Anomalies of the craniovertebral junction. In: Youmans J R (ed) Neurological surgery: a comprehensive reference guide to the diagnosis and management of neurosurgical problems, 2nd edn (Vol 3). Saunders, Philadelphia, p 1496

Bryan W J, Inglis A E, Sculo T P et al 1982 Methylmethacrylate stabilization for enhancement of posterior cervical arthrodesis in rheumatoid arthritis. Journal of Bone and Joint Surgery (Am) 64(A): 1045–1050

Clark C R, White A A III 1985 Fractures of the dens. A multicenter study. Journal of Bone and Joint Surgery (Am) 67: 1340–1348

Crockard H A, Pozo J L, Ransford A O et al 1986 Transoral decompression and posterior fusion for rheumatoid atlanto-axial subluxation. Journal of Bone and Joint Surgery (Br) 68: 350–356

Cusick J F, Yoganandan N, Pintar F et al 1988 Biomechanics of cervical spine facetectomy and fixation techniques. Spine 13: 808–812

Cybulski G R, Stone J L, Crowell R M et al 1988 Use of Halifax interlaminar clamps for posterior C1–C2 arthrodesis. Neurosurgery 22: 429–431

Dickman C A, Sonntag V K, Papadopolous S M 1991 The interspinous method of posterior atlantoaxial arthrodesis. Journal of Neurosurgery 74: 190–198

Dickman C A, Locantro J, Fessler R G 1992 The influence of transoral odontoid resection on stability of the craniovertebral junction. Journal of Neurosurgery 77: 525–530

Di-Lorenzo N, Nardi P, Fortuna A 1985 Benign tumors and tumor-like conditions of the spine: radiological features, treatment, and results. Surgical Neurology 25: 449–456

Dove J 1986 Internal fixation of the lumbar spine: the Hartshill rectangle. Clinical Orthopaedics 203: 135–140

Du Toit G 1976 Lateral atlanto-axial arthrodesis: a screw fixation technique. South African Journal of Surgery 14: 9–12

Fang H S Y, Ong G B 1962 Direct anterior approach to the upper cervical spine. Journal of Bone and Joint Surgery (Am) 44A: 1588–1604

Fang H S Y, Ong G B, Hodgson A R 1964 Anterior spinal fusion: the operative approaches. Clinical Orthopaedics 35: 16–33

Flint G A, Hockley A D, McMillan J J et al 1987 A new method of occipitocervical fusion using internal fixation. Neurosurgery, 21: 947–950

Gallie W E 21939 Fractures and dislocations of the upper cervical spine. American Journal of Surgery 46: 495–499

Gardner W J 1965 Hydrodynamic mechanism of syringomyelia. Journal of Neurology, Neurosurgery and Psychiatry 28: 247–259

Geisler F H, Cheng C, Poka A 1989 Anterior screw fixation of posteriorly displaced type II odontoid fractures. Neurosurgery 25: 30–37

Geremia G K, Kim K S, Cerullo L et al 1985 Complications of sublaminar wiring. Surgical Neurology 23: 629–634

Goel A 1991 Transoral approach for removal of intradural lesions at the craniocervical junction. Letter. Neurosurgery 29: 155–156

Goel A 1996 Interbody fixation following spinal tumor resection. British Journal of Neurosurgery 10: 201–203

Goel A, Achawal S 1995 The surgical treatment of Chiari malformation associated with atlantoaxial dislocation. British Journal of Neurosurgery 9: 67–72

Goel A, Deogaonkar M 1996 Thoracic laminoplasty using spinous processes. Neurologia Medico-chirurgia (Tokyo) 36: 552–553

Goel A, Karapurkar A P 1994 Transoral plate and screw fixation of the craniocervical region: a preliminary report. British Journal of Neurosurgery 8: 743–745

Goel A, Laheri V 1994 Plate and screw fixation for atlantoaxial subluxation. Acta Neurochirurgica (Wien) 129: 47–53

Goel V K, Winterbottom J M 1990 Ligamentous laxity across C0–C1–C2 complex. Spine 15: 339–342

Goel V K, Clark C R, Harris K G et al 1985 Kinematics of the cervical spine: effect of multiple total laminectomy and facet wiring. Presented at the 13th Annual meeting of the cervical spine research society, Boston, MA, 5 December

Grob D, Magerl F 1987 Operative stabilisierung bei fraketuren von C1 and C2: Orthopade 16: 46–54

Harkey H L, Crockard H A, Stevens J M et al 1990 The operative management of basilar impression in osteogenesis imperfecta. Neurosurgery 27: 782–786

Heywood A W B, Learmonth I D, Thomas M 1988 Internal fixation for occipito–cervical fusion. Journal of Bone and Joint Surgery (Br) 70(B): 708–711

Hoffman H J, Neill J, Crone K P et al 1990 Hydrosyringomyelia and its management in childhood and adolescence. Neurosurgery 26: 591–597

Hohmann D, Liebig K 1987 Technik der ventralen spondylodese an der unteren Halswirbeelsaule. Orthopade 16: 62–69

Holness R O, Heustis W S, Howes W J et al 1984 Posterior stabilization with an interlaminar clamp in cervical injuries: technical note. Review of the long term experience with the method. Neurosurgery 14: 318–322

Isu T, Sasaki H, Takamura H et al 1993 Foramen magnum decompression with removal of the outer layer of the dura as treatment for syringomyelia occurring with Chiari I malformation. Neurosurgery 33: 845–850

Jackson H 1950 The diagnosis of minimal atlanto-axial subluxation. British Journal of Radiology 23: 672–674

Katsumi Y, Honma T, Nakamura T 1989 Analysis of cervical instability resulting from laminectomies for removal of spinal cord tumor. Spine 14: 1171–1176

Kelly D L, Alexander E, Davis C H et al 1972 Acrylic fixation of atlantoaxial dislocation. Journal of Neurosurgery 36: 366–371

Kowada M, Takahashi M, Gito Y et al 1973 Fenestration of the vertebral artery: report of 2 angiographically demonstrated cases. Neuroradiology 6: 110–112

Lesoin F, Autricque A, Franz K et al 1987 Transcervical approach and screw fixation for upper cervical spine pathology. Surgical Neurology 27: 459–465

Lonstien J E 1977 Post-laminectomy kyphosis. Clinical Orthopaedics 128: 93–100

Lipson S J, Hammerschlag S B 1984 Atlantoaxial arthrodesis in the presence of posterior spondyloschisis (bifid arch) of the atlas: a report of three cases and an evaluation of alternative wiring techniques by computerized tomography. Spine 9: 65–69

Luque E R 1982 The anatomic basis and development of segmental spinal instrumentation. Spine 7: 256–259

Magerl F, Seeman P 1986 Stable fusion at atlas and axis by transarticular screw fixation. In Kehr P, Weidner A (eds) Cervical spine. Springer, Wien

McAfee P C, Bohlman H H 1989 One stage anterior cervical decompression and posterior stabilization with circumferential arthrodesis. A study of twenty-four patients who had traumatic or a neoplastic lesion. Journal of Bone and Joint Surgery (Am) 71: 78–88

McAfee P C, Bohlman H H, Riley L H Jr 1987 The anterior retropharyngeal approach to the upper part of the cervical spine. Journal of Bone and Joint Surgery (Am) 69: 1371–1383

McCarron R F, Robertson W W 1988 Brooks fusion for atlantoaxial instability in rheumatoid arthritis. Southern Medical Journal 81: 474–476

McGraw R W, Rusch R M 1973 Atlanto-axial arthrodesis. Journal of Bone and Joint Surgery (Br) 55B: 482–489

Menezes A H, VanGilder J C, Graf C J et al 1980 Craniovertebral abnormalities: a comprehensive surgical approach. Journal of Neurosurgery 53: 444–455

Mixter S J, Osgood R B 1910 Traumatic lesions of the atlas and axis. Annals of Surgery 51: 193–207

Newman P, Sweetnam R 1969 Occipito-cervical fusion: an operative technique and its indications. Journal of Bone and Joint Surgery (Br) 51B: 423–431

Newton T H, Mani R L 1974 The vertebral artery. In: Newton T H, Potts D G (eds) Radiology of the skull and brain. Mosby, St Louis, pp 1659–1709

Pentelenyi T, Szarvas I, Bodrogi L 1988 Screw fixation of odontoid fractures: preliminary report. Injury 19: 139–142

Ransford A O, Crockard H A, Pozo J L 1986 Cervical instability treated by contoured loop fixation: Journal of Bone and Joint Surgery (Br) 68: 173–177

Raynor R B, Pugh J, Shapiro I 1985 Cervical facetectomy and its effects on spine strength. Journal of Neurosurgery 63: 278–282

Roy Camille R, Saillant G, Judet T et al 1982 Lateral atlantoaxial arthrodesis. Revue De Chirurgie Orthopedique et Reparatrice de l'Appareil Moteur 68: 139–142

Sakou T, Morizono Y, Morimoto N 1984 Transoral atlantoaxial anterior decompression and fusion. Clinical Orthopaedics 27: 134–138

Sim F H, Svien H J, Bickel W H et al 1974 Swan-neck deformity following extensive cervical laminectomy: a review of twenty-one cases. Journal of Bone and Joint Surgery (Am) 56: 564–580

Simmons E H 1982 Alternatives in the surgical stabilization of the upper cervical spine injuries. In Tator C H (ed) Early management of acute spinal cord injury. Raven Press, New York, pp 393–433

Simpson J M, Ebraheim N A, Jackson W T et al 1993 Internal fixation of the thoracic and lumbar spine using Roy Camille plates. Orthopedics 16: 663–672

Sonntag V K H, Hadley M N 1988 Non-operative management of cervical spine injuries. Clinical Neurosurgery 34: 630–649

Streli R 1983 Neue denstransfixationsplatte. Hefte zur Unfallheikunde 165: 280

Takahashi M, Kawanami H, Watanabe N et al 1970 Fenestration of the extracranial vertebral artery. Radiology 96: 359–360

Teal J S, Rambaugh C L, Bergeron R T et al 1973 Angiographic demonstration of fenestrations of intradural intracranial arteries. Radiology 106: 123–126

VanGilder J C, Menezes A H, Dolan K D 1987 The craniovertebral junction and its abnormalities In: VanGilder J C, Menezes A H, Dolan K D (eds) Radiology of asymptomatic craniovertebral anomalies. Futura, New York, pp 69–98

White A A, Panjabi M M 1983 Clinical biomechnicas of the spine. Lippincott, Philadelphia pp 54–61

White A A III, Johnson R M, Panjabi M M et al 1975 Biomechanical analysis of clinical instability in the cervical spine. Clinical Orthopaedics 109: 85–96

Yasuoka S, Peterson H A, Laes E R Jr 1981 Pathogenesis and prophylaxis of post-laminectomy deformity of the spine after multiple level laminectomy: difference between children and adults. Neurosurgery 9: 145–152

Craniovertebral Anomalies: A Perspective
U.S. Vengsarkar

The bony and soft tissue anomalies at the craniovertebral junction are myriad. Occurring singly or in combination, they produce disturbances at the cervicomedullary junction and of the cerebellum, to produce a host of clinical symptoms and signs.

I became involved in these anomalies, after reading the lucid description by Spillane (1957), during my residential years. His description included the details of their structural defects, radiological features and clinical syndromes. Surprisingly, the surgical management was outlined in an ending paragraph with a note of caution, to perform decompression only in patients undergoing progressive clinical deterioration.

Basilar Invagination: Basilar invagination, with or without occipitalization of the atlas, is the most frequent among the anomalies and needs proper evaluation from the viewpoint of surgery. Spillane (1957), even in those early days, had stressed that the compression of the neuraxis in this anomaly could occur from front or behind by the incurving rims of the stenosed foramen magnum, the displaced dens and the assimilated anterior or posterior arches of the atlas.

Despite this awareness, posterior craniovertebral decompression continued to remain the surgery of choice for nearly 25 years. Sudden deaths and increased morbidity were reported in some patients and were attributed to disturbances because of sudden decompression and intra-axial hemorrages. To minimize such events, we started performing decompressions in the prone position (avoiding the sitting position with the head maintained in flexion) with a skeletal head traction applied preoperatively. The purpose of the skeletal traction was to dis-impact the upwardly displaced odontoid and to reduce the posterior displacement of the neuraxis, during decompression. With these precautions I personally, did not encounter sudden deaths, though clinical deterioration did occur in some cases following surgery. A few patients, after preoperative application of traction, did show immediate respiratory distress, and the traction in such cases had to be discontinued. Dural decompression was carried out in cases where myelography had suggested Arnold–Chiari malformation or syringomyelia. While decompressing the foramen magnum, I always extended the excision of the posterior rim as laterally as possible to free the inferior cerebellar peduncles. The inferior cerebellar peduncles contain the proprioceptive and spinovestibular–cerebellar fibers. Their decompression appears to be mandatory to relieve vertigo and ataxia.

In some cases of basilar invagination with occipitalized atlas, I had observed a certain degree of instability between the atlanto-occipital complex and the axis. This was measured by noting the distance between the odontoid and the fused rims of the atlas in flexion and extension. I used to refer to this instability as 'rocker-bottom' instability. In such cases, in addition to the decompression I have performed occipitocervical fusion using rib grafts.

The necessity for anterior transoral transpharyngeal decompression of the craniovertebral junction became clear to us after the advent of MRI in Bombay in 1988. The anterior indentation of the cervicomedullary junction by the displaced and tilted odontoid could be seen, beyond doubt, in the lateral mid-sagittal cuts. Routine use of the operating microscope and the introduction of power-driven micro-drills in neurosurgical instrumentation permitted a safe transoral excision of the odontoid peg. Posterior occipitocervical stabilization which follows the decompression also became easier because of the availability of a variety of metal loops and wires. The chapter of craniovertebral decompression and fusion thus became complete.

Chronic atlantoaxial dislocation: Chronic atlantoaxial dislocation forms the next common most anomaly and is diagnosed easily by plain X-rays, tomography and by MRI.

The dislocation is either reducible or irreducible. When reducible, atlantoaxial fusion is performed, as is done in the traumatic variety. Various techniques have been used for this fusion. I personally preferred the one described by Alexander & Courtland (1969), wherein the atlas is approximated and anchored to the spinous process of the axis by a central wire loop and rib struts are fixed, by wires, to the laminae laterally. Even though the fusion appeared sound on the operating table and during the immediate postoperative period, the atlas slipped forwards to a variable extent in later follow-up X-rays in nearly 30% of cases. Currently, I prefer metal loop and wire fixation and place bone graft in the occipitocervical region for fusion.

When the dislocation is irreducible, transoral excision of the anterior arch and the odontoid is followed by occipitocervical fusion.

Arnold–Chiari Malformation and Syringomyelia:
Arnold–Chiari malformation and syringomyelia are commonly associated soft tissue anomalies at the craniovertebral junction and may coexist with other bony anomalies. Each one, however, has a distinctive clinical presentation. When these anomalies coexist with the bony anomalies, their treatment forms a part of the total surgical management.

Arnold–Chiari malformation, of a large size, produces intermittent or constant occipitonuchal pain with or without vomiting, vertigo and ataxia. It may produce difficulty in swallowing, nasal regurgitation, hoarseness of voice or a nasal twang, when it compresses on the lower cranial nerves. A downbeat nystagmus is commonly observed. Posterior craniovertebral decompression and duroplasty is the surgical treatment of choice.

Syringomyelia, which very often coexists with Chiari malformation, usually presents as a progressive myelopathy with the characteristic dissociated sensory loss.

Initially it was believed to result from a pulsatile CSF flow from the fourth ventricle into the central canal of the cervical cord as a result of the outlet obstruction to the fourth ventricle by the Chiari malformation. MRI studies, however, have failed to demonstrate a continuity between the fourth ventricle and the syrinx. The more likely mechanism seems to be a pulsatile rise of CSF pressure within the cervical subarachnoid space because of the projecting cerebellar tonsils, which in itself gets transmitted to the central canal through the cord

parenchyma. This mechanism receives support from the fact that the CSF pressure reduced either by a craniovertebral decompression or a lumboperitoneal shunt results in the collapse of the syrinx in a large number of cases (Oldfield et al 1994).

I propagated percutaneous thecoperitoneal shunt as a treatment for syringomyelia, because it was a simple, safe and effective technique, as compared to conventional craniovertebral decompression (Vengsarkar et al 1991); however, many feel that as a primary procedure it runs the risk of further herniation of the cerebellar tonsils and cervicomedullary compression (6). I now prefer to perform conventional craniovertebral decompression as the primary procedure and reserve the lumboperitoneal shunt only for those cases where the cyst persists despite the decompression.

Thus, with the recent advances in radiological imaging and the surgical technique, the management of craniovertebral anomalies has become more meaningful. It should, however, be remembered that in order to achieve the best clinical benefits, every patient needs careful clinical and radiological evaluation and an appropriate surgical therapy which will answer the pathology responsible for symptoms.

References

Alexander E, Courtland H D 1969 Reduction and fusion of fracture of the odontoid process. Journal of Neurosurgery 31: 580–882

Menezes A H, Van Gilder Jr 1988 Transoral transpharyngeal approach to anterior cranio-cervical junction. Journal of Neurosurgery 69: 895–903

Oldfield E H, Muraszko K, Shawker T H et al 1994 Pathophysiology of syringomyelia associated with Chiari I malformation of the cerebellar tonsils. Journal of Neurosurgery 80: 3–15

Spillane J D 1957 Developmental anomalies in the region of the foramen magnum. In: Williams D (ed) Modern trends in neurology (Second series). Butterworth, London, pp 240–258

Vengsarkar U S, Panchal V G, Tripathi P D et al 1991 Percutaneous thecoperitoneal shunt for syringomyelia. Journal of Neurosurgery 74: 827–831

Technical Issues and Management of Craniovertebral Abnormalities
Arnold H. Menezes

The craniovertebral region describes the area of the occipital bone that surrounds the foramen magnum, the atlas and the axis vertebrae. This houses the medulla, cervicomedullary junction and upper cervical spinal cord,

cerebellum, lower cranial nerves as well as the vascular supply and drainage to the region. The CSF pathways play a major role in this junctional area of the nervous system. A constellation of symptoms and signs referable to this region may be invoked by abnormalities or tumors of this location.

The first systematic evaluation of foramen magnum tumors was performed by Elsberg and Strauss in 1926. The classic radiographic studies on basilar invagination by Chamberlain in 1939 opened the region to study and thus abnormalities of the craniovertebral junction emerged from the realm of anatomic and pathologic curiosity to the clinical field of practical neuroscience. Surgical treatment of conditions affecting the craniovertebral junction usually consisted of a posterior decompression by enlargement of the foramen magnum and removal of the posterior arch of the atlas vertebra. However, the mortality and morbidity associated with such treatment was high for patients with irreducible lesions with cervicomedullary compression. Both Scoville and Klaus in the early 1950s felt that this mortality and morbidity could be severely reduced if a ventral approach was possible to this area. Over the next decade, surgical approaches to this region in a ventral or ventrolateral manner were proposed by Fang and Ong, Gutkelch, Stevenson and Adams, Greenberg, DeAndrade and MacNab; with an improving outcome. The problems that one faces with lesions in this location are compounded by the complex anatomy that includes the nervous system above, the spinal canal below, the head and face with the ororespiratory tract anteriorly and the strong cervical musculature posteriorly. The proximity of the carotid and vertebral vessels, their coursing from an extracranial to an intracranial location intertwined with cranial nerves and the crowding makes the problem enormous. To add to this, one has to be able to cross the midline. A host of congenital, developmental and acquired abnormalities affect this region. The situation is further compounded by a developing individual. CSF dynamics and the biomechanics of the region must be taken into consideration. Osseous pathology that effects this region is usually benign and thus a radical resection is essential since neither chemotherapy nor radiosurgery is the answer.

Thus, it is evident that one has to have a thorough knowledge of the anatomy, embryology and development, and biomechanics and the disease process affecting this complex transitional area. In 1977, the author proposed a surgical physiological approach to this region based on:

1. the type of lesion affecting the region, be it bony, tumor or soft tissue;

2. the reducibility;
3. the manner of encroachment of the lesion;
4. the associated craniovertebral bony and neural abnormalities, e.g. Chiari or syrinx; and
5. the growth potential

Reducible lesions required craniovertebral stabilization. This was best achieved in a dorsal manner. In the rare situations of Grisel's syndrome (craniovertebral instability secondary to an inflammatory process in the upper respiratory tract), immobilization in an external brace allowed for ligamentous reconstitution. Irreducible lesions mandated decompression in the manner in which encroachment occurred. If a ventral encroachment was present, a transoropharyngeal decompression was made. A dorsal decompression was made in the face of dorsal compression. In either circumstance, if instability resulted, a fusion procedure was necessary.

Improvement in neurodiagnostic imaging, microsurgical technique and instrumentation for stabilization have increased the neurosurgical armamentarium such that whole new vistas have been added to our field. The ventral approach to the foramen magnum includes the transbasal, the transsphenoethmoidal, transpalatal, the Le Forte I drop-down maxillotomy with an extended maxillotomy, the transpalatopharyngeal approach, the labiomandibular split with median glossotomy approach and the lateral extrapharyngeal route to the ventral and ventrolateral aspect of the clivus, foramen magnum and upper cervical canal. Lateral approaches to the foramen magnum are also possible via the preauricular and retroauricular infratemporal fossa route going either in front of or behind the carotid artery. These techniques have been improved with rerouting of the facial nerve to provide for a shorter working distance and greater safety. The transcondylar and extended far lateral approaches to the foramen magnum may be combined with the previously mentioned lateral approaches or likewise combined with a posterior fossa route. Thus, the blending of skull base approaches to the foramen magnum have only strengthened the early treatment algorithm that was proposed by the author. Likewise, the menu for craniovertebral stabilization is vast but only a few have stood the test of time and management outcome. The original treatment algorithm has held for the subsequent 2200 patients with symptomatic craniovertebral abnormalities evaluated by this author.

Surgical Tactics in Craniovertebral Lesions
Hiroshi Nakagawa

Lesions of the craniovertebral junction may cause a variety of symptoms due to involvement of the medullocervical junction. CT and MRI in addition to dynamic study have greatly improved the accuracy of the diagnosis of the craniovertebral lesions and provide

sufficient information to select the optimal surgical method.

Aside from lower posterior fossa lesions such as aneurysms and tumors in which the transcondylar approach can be employed, atlantoaxial dislocation

(AAD) is the surgical challenge and a subject of controversy.

The main causes of AAD are trauma, congenital anomalies, rheumatoid arthritis and tumors. In traumatic AAD, odontoid fracture (Anderson type II) is most frequently encountered and needs surgical fixation after reduction. Posterior fusion with bone graft and newly devised titanium wires and clamps are the standard procedure, although anterior screw fixation of the fractured odontoid process itself or posterior screw fixation of C1 and C2 facets or pedicles can be utilized.

Hangman fracture in which fracture of C2 pedicles is often associated with subluxation at C2–C3 is treated with anterior plate fixation with intervertebral graft. In congenital AAD which is often irreducible with cord compression by odontoid process or os odontoideum, one-stage surgery is a safe and effective method.

In supine–prone position or lateral–rotatory position, transoral decompression and posterior fusion with bone graft wires, clamps or loops are carried out under the same anesthesia.

In AAD and basilar invagination due to chronic rheumatoid arthritis, posterior fixation including the occiput by using a metallic loop is preferable.

With the advent of MRI-compatible devices, spinal instrumentation can be utilized in surgical management of unstable craniovertebral lesions for early ambulation without Halo brace and subsequently early reinstatement.

Craniovertebral Junction Lesions: Approach and Reconstruction
Michael J. Torrens

When planning the surgical approach and reconstruction for lesions at the craniovertebral junction it is not only necessary to assess the stability of the region but also to take into account three particular factors which influence the management. These are:

1. the intrinsic quality of the tissues you are operating on;
2. the prognosis of the condition;
3. whether the lesion is extradural or intra/transdural.

These factors may be considered in relation the etiology of the problem, which usually falls into one of four categories:

1. congenital (basilar impression, subluxation);
2. traumatic (C1/2 fractures);
3. neoplastic; and
4. degenerative (especially rheumatoid disease).

Occasional low-placed vertebrobasilar aneurysms may excite the neurosurgeon, but it is likely these will in future be treated by endovascular methods.

Quality of Bone and Soft Tissues: Degenerative disease is an important cause of instability and neural compression in the craniocervical region. The patients are older and the bone and joints may be destroyed locally. The disease and the potential instability may extend lower down the spine. The quality of bone for autografting may be poor. The bone may not hold screws or wires and external fixation may be more necessary. The general healing potential may be lower and the need for rehabilitation greater.

The optimal management may be relatively conservative. For example, a rheumatoid atlantoaxial instability with moderate neural compression and quadriparesis may improve after immobilization in a Halo jacket. Then a simple fusion in situ may be all that is needed.

The greater the number of motion segments included in any fusion the more the chance of iatrogenic instability at the adjacent mobile levels. Also an immobile neck is a serious handicap for any patient.

Prognosis: The techniques of operation and reconstruction vary greatly between non-neoplastic or benign lesions and malignant tumors. In the latter the best and most rapid palliation, without unnecessary mutilation, must be achieved. The reconstruction may be with artificial materials only and not bone grafts. The need for follow-up MRI or CT imaging will affect the choice of reconstructive materials. The possibility of requiring access for multiple reoperations (e.g. chordoma) must be considered when reconstructing.

All the other cases with a normal expectation of life must be managed in such a way as to maintain maximum mobility (a minimum of fused segments) and to use bone as a fusion agent as much as possible.

Relation to the Dura: In general the rule for decompression of the medulla and spinal cord is that any anterior compression should be removed by the anterior approach and any posterior compression from posteriorly. Anterior central lesions should thus require a transoral approach. This rule is modified for intradural or transdural lesions because of the difficulty in making a watertight dural repair by this route, and because lesions that are not strictly midline may not be fully accessed by the transoral route. It is fair to say that even surgeons with great experience of the transoral route prefer to approach such intradural lesions by a far lateral, retro/transcondylar route if possible.

Indications for Reconstruction: Reconstructive procedures are necessary at the craniovertebral junction either when the lesion itself has caused instability or when the operative approach destabilizes the spine. In the former case the instability should be obvious on the preoperative investigations (flexion/extension MRT is often useful). Potential instability produced by surgery will be discussed in relation to the respective approaches.

Extensive posterior decompression can produce late instability in patients with neurological deficits, especially in children. All such patients should be followed up indefinitely. Prophylactic fusion is seldom appropriate, however, because of the disability it produces. An exception to this is any case where facet joints have been damaged on both sides.

The far lateral approach to the foramen magnum region (with mobilization of the vertebral artery) does not destabilize unless it involves removal of the major part of the occipital condyle/lateral mass of atlas and/or the C1/2 articulation. Fixation may be with a titanium plate (bent to shape) screwed and wired between the occiput and C3, or with a bone strut fixed with titanium mini-plates and surrounded by bone chips. The latter requires Halo body immobilization postoperatively but creates a more permanent fusion.

Reconstruction and stabilization are usually needed after a transoral approach because of the nature of the underlying disease, but the operation itself does not contribute much to instability. The division of the anterior arch of the atlas may allow the lateral masses to be 'sprung apart' (pushed laterally) creating subluxation at the atlanto-occipital joint as well as at C1/2. Therefore surgical technique may be modified to keep intact some of the anterior arch, even when removing the odontoid process. It is not my policy routinely to fuse cases who have been decompressed anteriorly for basilar impression. Should C1/2 fusion be necessary then any anterior bone graft is probably best inserted laterally into both the C1/2 joints. This has the advantage of locating the graft away from the pharyngeal incision. Otherwise, although successful clivus to C2/3 anterior grafting has been described, most surgeons rely on a concurrent posterior occipitocervical fusion with plates or a specially designed system such as the Ransford–Hartshill loop (which is now available in titanium).

Surgery of Intramedullary Spinal Cord Tumor: An Evolving Strategy
Phyo Kim

Introduction: Recent advances in imaging technology and the methods of microsurgery radically changed concepts and treatment of intramedullary spinal cord tumors. In fact, a new strategy is evolving currently as experiences of extensive microsurgical resection and MRI data are cumulating. Until the 1980s, the intramedullary tumors were generally considered not amenable to radical resection, although there had been earlier sporadic reports and descriptions of total removal of the tumors (Elsberg 1925, Greenwood 1963, Guidetti 1967). Experiences were cumulated with total and subtotal resection of ependymoma where the tumor is well circumscribed (McCormick et al 1990, Epstein et al 1993). It appears that a notion is shared among a majority of neurosurgeons that if the biopsy of the tumor yields ependymoma, total resection should be attempted but in cases of astrocytoma extensive resection should be withheld and auxiliary treatments have to be planned. However, a series of experiences of total resection of astrocytomas has been reported, indicating that many of the tumors, especially those histologically classified as grade 2, are also amenable to radical resection (Cooper & Epstein 1985). It has been the author's contemporaneous experience that total resection can be achieved in the majority of grade 2 astrocytomas. Even in cases of tumors which were histologically classified as grade 3 astrocytoma due to the presence of a component of high cellularity, radical resection could be achieved with no evidence of recurrence up to 18 months. Reciprocally, the role of auxiliary therapies in the treatment strategy of the intramedullary tumor may

possibly be revised when the long-term outcome of radical resection is established in the near future.

Surgical Techniques: Techniques employed in the present series of intramedullary spinal cord tumor includes routine exposure of the posterior component of the vertebrae, a laminoplastic opening by midline splitting ('french door' laminotomy) of the laminae, opening and tucking-up of the dura and the arachnoid together. Myelotomy is made at the dorsal median fissure at the levels caudal or cephalad to the bulk of the tumor. Usually the median fissure is distorted at the level of the mass, and it is very difficult to identify and separate. The fissure is retracted open applying traction to the pia at the edge of the fissure using sutures of 8–0 nylon. Blunt separation of the fissure should be avoided to prevent trauma to the dorsal column and to minimize the disturbance of limb position sense. The substance of the cord is sharply divided until the surface of capsulation or the gliosis surrounding the tumor is encountered. Once the plane of gliosis is identified, maximum concentration should be paid to maintaining the cleavage, and removing the tumor totally. Internal decompression is warranted to minimize trauma to the surrounding cord substance, and YAG or KTP laser with a contact probe is useful for the purpose. Care is taken not to damage the anterior spinal artery; at the end of the removal procedure, the remaining ventral cord substance is usually very thin. A 0.1 mm GoreTex sheet employed for pericardial closure is used for reconstruction of the arachnoid and prevention of adhesion. The dura is

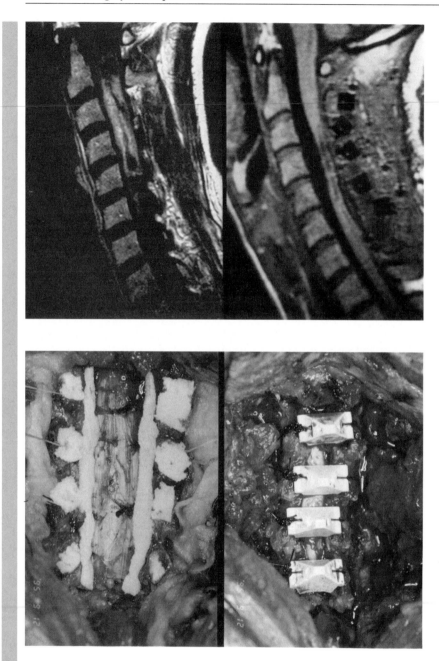

Fig. 21.29   Properative (left) and postoperative (right, 1 year following total resection) MRI of T1W1 with contrast enhancement, in a 34-year-old female with grade 3 astrocytoma. Note the result of laminoplastic reconstruction using hydroxyapatite, and restoration of normal lordotic curve of the vertebrae.

Fig. 21.30   Intraoperative photographs showing midline splitting of the cervical laminae (left) and reconstruction (right) of the posterior elements using hydroxyapatite grafts (original design).

closed with or without a dural substitute. The laminae are reconstructed by bridging the laminal flaps with a graft made of hydroxyapatite.

Somatosensory evoked potential (SEP) is monitored during surgery but often the baseline potential is not reliably recorded, and the potential deteriorates once the resection of the intramedullary mass is started. Since restoration and recovery of motor and dorsal column function are observed postoperatively despite impairment in the potentials, we do monitor SEP but do not depend on it as a warning to limit extent of resection.

Results: Efficacy of Resection and Functional Outcome: Table 21.1 summarizes the histological

subtype, extent of removal, and functional outcome in the follow-up period. In this series, no patient underwent radiation or other auxiliary treatments. To date, in the mean follow-up period of 19.8 (5–66) months, no local recurrence was detected in repeated MRI examinations.

Regarding functional alterations, transient loss of joint position sense, dysesthesia and paresthesia were invariably observed immediately after surgery. In a long-term follow-up, improvement of function status was seen except in those who had been paralyzed prior to surgery. As has been pointed out, the most significant factor to predict the severity of postoperative dysfunction is the preoperative status (McCormick et al 1990, Epstein et al 1993).

Table 21.1 Histological diagnosis, location, extent of removal and functional outcome

No.	Age	Sex	Histological type	Location	Extent of removal	Karnofsky score		Follow-up
1	45	m	Ependymoma	Th1–4	Total	↑ 60	→ 80	66 months
2	30	f	Ependymoma	C3–6	Total	↑ 80	→ 90	24 months
3	53	f	Astro. Gr2	Th2–5	Total	↓ 50	→ 40	20 months
4	47	m	Astro. Gr2	C4–5	Total	→ 60	→ 60	20 months
5	51	m	Ependymoma and pilocytic astro	C5–7	Total	↑ 70	→ 80	17 months
6	41	m	Astro. Gr3	Th1–4	Total	↑ 80	→ 90	17 months
7	34	f	Astro. Gr3	C2–7	Total	↑ 70	→ 80	13 months
8	63	f	Ependymoma	C2–4	Total	↑ 50	→ 70	9 months
9	46	f	Astro. Gr2	C7–Th3	Total	→ 40	→ 40	7 months
10	39	m	Astro. Gr2	C1–6	Partial	↓ 70	→ 60	5 months

Roles of Auxiliary Treatments: In general, relative incidence of malignant subtype of the glial tumors is smaller in the spinal cord than in the brain. The proportion of grade 3 and 4 tumors among the intramedullary astrocytomas is reported to be 7.5% and much less than that of 36% in the brain (Cohen et al 1989). In the case of low-grade tumors, unlike in the situation of the classical series (Greenwood 1963, Guidetti et al 1981, Malis 1978), the advent of MRI made it possible to diagnose at earlier stages when the deficits are not yet severe, and these tumors are increasingly being treated with radical resection.

In the past, survival rate of the group undergoing radiation after partial resection has been reported to be comparable to that seen in the group of total resection (Hulshof et al 1993). A recent study done at the Mayo Clinic, reported that pilocytic astrocytoma has a definitely better prognosis than the diffuse fibrillary type. In their series most of the cases were treated with radiation following partial resection, but the 10-year survival is reported to be 81% in the former and 15% in the latter (Minehan et al 1995). However, in most of the studies in the past, including these two studies, comparison of functional status in the long term was not elaborated.

In our present series, radiation therapy is reserved for future possible recurrence. Especially for patients with astrocytomas classified as grade 3 due to the finding of high cellularity, a thorough discussion was made with the patient and the family regarding therapeutic options. Studies done by Hulshof et al failed to prove difference in the recurrence rate between the group treated with partial resection/radiation and those treated with total resection only (Hulshof et al 1993). Surveillance with MRI allows early detection of local recurrence, and once the option is agreed upon there seems to be no compelling evidence to reject the policy of reserving radiation for future possible recurrence, if that should occur. The possibility of radiation induced myelopathy, and especially in the situation of traumatized cord, also favors withholding radiation until it becomes the last resort.

Primary intramedullary glioblastomas, which are not included in the present series, have a very different clinical characteristic and course; these tumors have a very poor prognosis with rapid progression with diffuse seeding in the subarachnoid space, and typically presents with hydrocephalus (Cohen et al 1989). Chemotherapy using agents such as vincristine, CCNU, 5FU, hydroxyurea, 6MP, VP16, BCNU, thiotepa or a combination of these have been used but efficacy of the treatment is not proven, failing to alter the dismal survival of the high-grade astrocytoma (Finlay et al 1990, Pons et al 1992, Rodriguez et al 1988).

Conclusion: Advanced techniques in microsurgery and postoperative close surveillance with MRI allow treatment of most of the intramedullary tumors with radical resection, including astrocytomas. In fact a high rate of total resection has been achieved in our series, with no local recurrence to date, without using auxiliary therapies. If the surgery is done before weakness and disability become severe, risks of deficits due to surgical removal are reasonably small and functional improvement in the long-term follow-up can be expected.

References

Cohen A R, Wisoff J H, Allen J C, Epstein F 1989 Malignant astrocytomas of the spinal cord. Journal of Neurosurgery 70: 50–54

Cooper P R, Epstein F 1985 Radical resection of intramedullary spinal cord tumors in adults: recent experiences in 29 patients. Journal of Neurosurgery 63: 492–499

Elsberg C A 1925 Tumors of the spinal cord. Hoebner, New York, Hoeber, pp 206–239

Epstein F J, Farmer J P, Freed D 1993 Adult intramedullary spinal cord ependymomas: the result of surgery in 38 patients. Journal of Neurosurgery 79: 204–209

Finlay J L, August C, Packer R et al 1990 High dose multiagent chemotherapy followed by bone marrow rescue for malignant astrocytomas of childhood and adolescence. Journal of Neurooncology 9: 239–248

Greenwood J Jr 1963 Intramedullary tumors of spinal cord: a follow-up study after total surgical removal. Journal of Neurosurgery 20: 665–668

Guidetti B 1967 Intramedullary tumors of the spinal cord. Acta Neurochirugica 17: 7

Guidetti B, Mercuri S, Vagnozzi R 1981 Long-term results of the surgical treatment of 129 intramedullary spinal gliomas. Journal of Neurosurgery 54: 323–330

Hulshof M C C M, Menten J, Dito J J, Dreiseen J J R, von der Bergh R, Gonzalez D G 1993 Treatment results on primary intraspinal gliomas. Radiotherapy Oncology: 29: 294–300

Malis L I 1978 Intramedullary spinal cord tumors. Clinical Neurosurgery 25: 512–539

McCormick P C, Torres R, Post K D, Stein B M 1990 Intramedullary ependymomas of the spinal cord. Journal of Neurosurgery 72: 523–532

Minehan K J, Shaw E G, Scheithauer B W, Davis D L, Onofrio B M 1995 Spinal cord astrocytoma: pathological and treatment considerations. Journal of Neurosurgery 83: 590–595

Pons M A, Finlay J L, Walker R W et al 1992 Chemotherapy with vincristine and etoposide in children with low-grade astrocytoma. Journal of Neurooncology 14: 151–158

Rodriguez L A, Prados M, Fulton D et al 1988 Treatment of recurrent brain stem gliomas and other central nervous system tumors with 5-fluorouracil, CCNU, hydroxyurea and 6-mercaptopurine. Neurosurgery 22: 691–693

Tumor-obstructive hydrocephalus: a natural defense mechanism

22

Atul Goel   Junpei Nitta   Shigeaki Kobayashi

The ventricular and subarachnoid cerebrospinal fluid (CSF) is the principal buffer system of the brain assisting in accommodating the mass lesion. An intra-axial tumor and its associated brain reaction in the form of cerebral edema result in flattening of the gyri, obliteration of the subarachnoid cisterns and narrowing and displacement of ventricles. In situations where the tumor obstructs the pathway of CSF flow 'obstructive hydrocephalus' is a result. Preoperative shunt surgery, temporary drainage of CSF or diverting its flow have been advised in various situations. This procedure is done in an attempt to reduce the raised intracranial pressure and relieve the patient's symptoms, to normalize the altered cerebral blood flow and to 'relax' the brain, which would assist the surgeon in the definitive surgical procedure on the tumor. Although complications following the insertion of a shunt in supra- and infratentorial tumors have been occasionally reported, this issue has not been adequately discussed in the literature.

In this section we present our experience with some specific regional tumors where preoperative shunt surgery was carried out. The insertion of a shunt was usually guided by the severity of the hydrocephalus, size and nature of the tumor, clinical status of the patient and the extent of presumed tumor resectability. The various problems related to the shunting procedure are described. Some complications were related to mechanical problems related to the shunt assembly, while others appeared to be secondary to alterations in the delicately adjusted intracranial pressure mechanisms. In our opinion tumor-obstructive hydrocephalus is a protective response of the brain. The increase in supratumoral intracranial pressure is an attempt by the body to push the tumor away from vital neural structures like the brain stem and hypothalamus. The use of ventricular drainage or any artificial alteration in CSF pressure prior to surgical resection of the tumor appears to be an irrational strategy of management.

POSTERIOR FOSSA VERMIAN TUMORS

Some degree of hydrocephalus is present in almost all cases of medium to large posterior fossa tumors. The initial symptoms in such cases are usually due to the hydrocephalus and the increased supratentorial pressure. These symptoms more often precede those primarily due to local tumor invasion and compression of the brain stem by a significant length of time. It has been recognized that hydrocephalus and consequent raised intracranial pressure make surgery for these tumors difficult. Initially ventricular taps were employed to deal with hydrocephalus prior to surgery on the tumor. This was then replaced by external ventricular drains and later by shunts. The initial enthusiasm for the routine use of a preoperative shunt procedure has gradually waned with the passage of time. There have been various reports in favor of a preoperative shunt and also against its use.

Material

Sixty-two cases of large posterior fossa tumors were treated surgically from January 1987 to April 1989. Benign cerebellopontine angle tumors were not included in the study. The histopathology of these tumors is shown in Table 22.1 and symptoms and signs at the time of presentation are shown in Table 22.2. There was clinical evidence of increased intracranial pressure (in the form of headache, vomiting, and worsened vision with papilledema) in 59 of these cases. Mild to severe hydrocephalus was present in all cases irrespective of the tumor size and the duration of symptoms. In 26 patients preoperative shunt surgery was

Table 22.1 Histopathology of the posterior fossa tumors

Medulloblastoma	21
Astrocytoma	21
Ependymoma	8
Hemangioblastoma	7
Metastasis	4
Choroid plexus papilloma	1

Table 22.2 Signs and symptoms at the time of presentation in posterior fossa tumors

Major symptoms	Number of cases	Average duration of symptoms
Headache	59	4 months
Vomiting	55	3 months
Ataxia (trunkal and limb)	51	25 days
Lower cranial nerve involvement	12	20 days

performed. In 10 patients a silastic tube was placed during surgery for the tumor from the aqueduct to the cisterna magna as has been described by Lapra. Two of these patients had also undergone a preoperative shunt operation.

Results

Radical surgical resection of the tumor was performed in all 62 cases. Two of these patients died in the postoperative phase (within 7 days of operation) and four patients suffered varying degrees of morbidity. Of the 26 patients where a preoperative shunt was performed, five developed shunt infection and the shunt had to be removed. Two patients developed blockage of the shunt which had to be revised. In six patients it was seen that following the shunt, despite relief from headache and vomiting, the patients worsened as regards their level of consciousness and ataxia of the limbs, with additional involvement of the lower cranial nerves. Two patients developed an increase in the frequency of vomiting following the shunt. The other patients where a shunt operation was performed fared well after the procedure. However, the author observed operative difficulty in the resection of the tumor due to the closer proximity of the tumor to the brain stem following shunt surgery in at least six patients. In two patients where a preoperative shunt was performed tension pneumocephalus developed in the postoperative phase and air had to be drained through a burr hole.

Discussion

The concept of preoperative shunts for posterior fossa tumors was introduced by Abraham & Chandy (1963). Cushing (1931) considered hydrocephalus as the major cause of problems in posterior fossa surgery and advised ventricular taps and drainage of CSF prior to surgery. Ingraham & Campbell (1941) initiated the use of external

ventricular drains. Over the years surgery for posterior fossa tumors has developed remarkably. How far any credit can be given to preoperative shunting in this improvement is debatable.

It is well known that ventricular tapping and shunt insertion in the presence of a large posterior fossa tumor may result in upward or reverse tentorial herniation. It is apparent that movement occurs in the tumor due to change in pressure dynamics following drainage of CSF from the lateral ventricles. Such movements may be the cause of haemorrhage in some tumors (Epstien & Rajgopalan 1978, Vaquero et al 1981). Following gentler movements of the tumor, the space between the tumor and the floor of the fourth ventricle is reduced to a varying degree, and the tumor may compress the brain stem, with resultant symptoms. Although there is recovery from symptoms secondary to hydrocephalus and raised intracranial pressure following the shunt, those due to brain stem compression may worsen. In this series we noted worsening in the consciousness level, incoordination and ataxia, and involvement of the lower cranial nerves in six of our patients after the shunt was introduced (Fig. 22.1). It was seen that in two patients with posterior fossa ependymomas the severity of vomiting increased following insertion of the shunt (Goel 1993).

German (1961) considered that surgery on a slack brain following shunt surgery makes the lives of the surgeons more 'tranquil'. This is the opinion of many advocates of preoperative shunts. It was observed in the present series of cases that following the preoperative shunt there was in some cases increased space between the bone and the dura, and between the dura and the cerebellum even in the presence of massive tumors. This made the initial part of the surgery easier and trauma to the cerebellum was minimized. However, it appeared that there was movement of the tumor and the cerebellum away from the dura towards the brain stem. This made the later part of the surgery near the brain stem more difficult. Radical surgical excision of the lesion, which is the most acceptable form of treatment, can be difficult and on occasion hazardous owing to the proximity of the tumor to the brain stem. A posterior parietal burr hole and drainage of CSF during the operation may help in avoiding the rare situation of severe cerebellar herniation after the dura is opened. Present-day anesthetic and decongestive measures have helped greatly in avoiding such a situation.

There is mild to severe hydrocephalus in at least 80–90% of moderate to large posterior fossa tumors (Albright 1982). In the presented series, hydrocephalus was seen in all the cases. Even though the tumor is responsible for blockage in the pathway of CSF it is only very rarely that the CSF pathways are totally blocked or that there are no alternative pathways for CSF outflow available. In this situation of total blockage of CSF pathways or

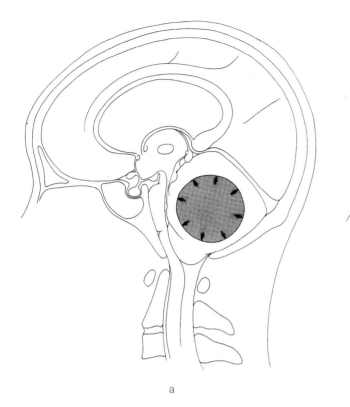

a

b

c

Fig. 22.1 **a** Schematic drawing showing the midline vermian
large tumor. The arrows show how the tumor is exerting
pressure circumferentially. The most dangerous area of pressure
exertion is anteriorly towards the brain stem. The posterior part
is the squeezed vermis which pushes against the occipital
squama. The pressure exerted posteriorly against the bone is
reflected back towards the tumor. **b** The response of the body in
an attempt to neutralize some of the pressure over the brain
stem. The large arrowheads show increase in intraventricular
pressure. The small arrowheads show how the rise in
intraventricular pressure is pushing the tumor away form the
brain stem. **c** Drainage of CSF through a ventricular cannula.
The tumor now has no resistance from the anterior side and is
pushed anteriorly by the negative effect superiorly and from the
occipital squama posteriorly. The brain stem thus becomes
compressed by the tumor.

inadequacy of drainage channels the intraventricular pressure will rise very rapidly and there is risk of transtentorial herniation due to hydrocephalus. In such an emergency situation, to tide over the crisis a ventricular tap may be done at the risk of problems that may occur due to the tumor.

Surgery for shunts is not always simple or quick. Shunt dependency often results and delayed complications may occur due to blockage. No patient in the present series who did not undergo preoperative shunt surgery required a delayed insertion of a shunt.

In most of the cases with medulloblastomas, after an adequate tumor decompression the aqueduct is usually seen widely open. It was observed that a gush of CSF indicating the opening of the aqueduct was an important warning sign for the surgeon of the approaching brain stem. In cases where shunts are done preoperatively, CSF drainage was limited and this indicator to the surgeon was lost.

Trans-shunt systemic metastases have been reported and is a major contraindication for preoperative shunting. However, no patient in the present series developed trans-shunt metastasis.

It was also observed that the period of hospital stay increased in cases where a preoperative shunt was performed. There was delay in the surgery on the tumor and in the radiotherapy that was given subsequently. It is possible that this delay might affect the long-term prognosis.

The amount of CSF lost after the shunt, and from the aqueduct after its decompression by tumor excision, appears to result in an increased postoperative incidence of intracranial air and its resultant complications. Two cases of tension pneumocranium were encountered in this series. Both patients had preoperative shunts. Cases of pneumocephalus after ventriculoperitoneal shunt placement in posterior fossa tumors have been reported previously (Pitts et al 1975). However, an increased incidence of tension pneumocephalus following surgery in posterior fossa tumors secondary to prior placement of shunt has not been reported.

A relatively raised pressure situation in the intracranial cavity without the placement of shunt might even help in prevention of air embolism in cases operated in a sitting position.

SUPRASELLAR TUMORS

A mild to severe degree of hydrocephalus is present in most cases of large suprasellar tumors. Symptoms of increased intracranial pressure are usually dominant and frequently precede the symptoms primarily due to tumor invasion and compression. Preoperative shunts or some form of ventricular drainage have been advocated, and frequently employed since the early 1950s, delaying a defini-

tive procedure until the ventricles have decompressed and the patient has stabilized. The principal aim is to reduce the intracranial pressure, facilitating adequate and safe retraction and handling of the brain during surgery on the tumor. Bilateral shunting has been suggested if the tumor has obstructed both foramina of Munro (Carmel 1985). With the availability of modern anesthetic agents and decongestive measures, the use of a preoperative ventricular CSF diversion procedure has gradually waned.

Material

Twenty-two cases of large suprasellar tumors underwent a preoperative shunt prior to definitive surgery on the tumor. These cases were treated between 1990 and 1993 at our Institute. The histopathology of these tumors is shown in Table 22.3. The average diameter of the tumor as calculated from the computed tomography (CT) scan picture was 55 mm. There was clinical evidence of increased intracranial pressure in all these cases. In cases where the effect on vision was secondary to optic nerve compression by the tumor other corroborative evidence of raised intracranial pressure was studied. Moderate to severe hydrocephalus was present in all cases. In six cases bi-ventriculoperitoneal, while in the rest one-sided ventriculoperitoneal shunt, was performed.

Results

In 22 patients a preoperative shunt was performed. Ventricular CSF pressure was found to be 'very high' in all cases (manumetric pressure measurements were not made). No patient had shunt infection or developed immediate or delayed blockage. Twelve patients fared well and were relieved of the raised intracranial pressure symptoms.

In seven cases it was observed that the patients had become abnormally drowsy after the insertion of the shunt, despite the relief from headache and vomiting. Two of these patients became incontinent of urine. In six cases the increased drowsiness was noticed within 8–10 hours, while in one patient drowsiness was noticed 2 days after the insertion of the shunt. In three of these patients a blocked shunt was considered to be the cause of the increased drowsiness and ventricular tapping was done through an additional burr hole. CSF pressure was seen to be low, suggesting ade-

Table 22.3 Histopathology of suprasellar tumors

Craniopharyngioma	13
Pituitary tumor	4
Optic nerve glioma	4
Suprasellar germinoma	1

quate functioning of the shunt. Three patients recovered from their drowsiness in 36 hours, 72 hours and 5–6 days respectively. The remainder of the patients were operated for the tumor in the drowsy state.

The eighth patient who worsened was a 5-year-old girl who had a large optic chiasm/hypothalamic glioma with a large cyst extending from it to the right frontotemporal region. The superior end of the tumor extended up to the foramen of Munro. She developed left hemiparesis and worsening of vision in both eyes following right ventriculoperitoneal shunt surgery. A repeat scan showed reduction in the size of the ventricles with no evidence of injury to the hemisphere caused by the passage of the shunt tube.

The ninth patient was a 36-year-old male patient with a large craniopharyngioma who was severely drowsy prior to shunt, with feeble limb movements. He became almost akinetic and mute following surgery. This state continued until the operation on the tumor. Despite a radical tumor resection he did not improve. He later developed pneumonia and ultimately died.

One patient was drowsy prior to the shunt and this state persisted after the surgery in this case.

Radical surgical excision was attempted by the subfrontal or subfrontotemporal route in cases with pituitary tumors and craniopharyngiomas. A relatively conservative approach was adopted in cases with large optic nerve/chiasmal/hypothalamic gliomas. The author observed operative difficulty in radical resection of the tumor in cases where a preoperative shunt had been performed. This was due to the apparent closer proximity of the tumor to the base of the brain.

Discussion

In the present series, seven patients developed marked drowsiness following the shunt. One patient became akinetic and mute and one patient developed worsening of vision and hemiparesis. In the absence of other definite reason, these major problems are presumed to be related to superior migration of the tumor and increased pressure over the hypothalamus and other structures in the vicinity following the release of ventricular CSF (Fig. 22.2). In effect, it is postulated that the ventricular dilatation and the consequent increase in intraventicular pressure could be a natural protective mechanism of the brain, whereby pressure is exerted over the dome of the tumor so that it remains away from the hypothalamus and other critical basal forebrain areas (Goel 1995a). It is possible that there is a balance between the tumor pressure and the ventricular pressure. As soon as the pressure is reduced by draining the ventricular CSF, the tumor directly presses over the neural structures by a 'sump effect'. The centers more frequently affected appear to be those which influence the

state of wakefulness. Such a migration of tumor was not demonstrated in the present series by actual shift of the tumor on radiological imaging and is thus only an assumption.

In cases where our patients worsened following the shunt it was observed that the tumors were of massive size and the symptoms of increased intracranial pressure were of significantly long duration. Patients with relatively small tumors fared well after the shunt surgery. This suggests that the natural protective mechanisms of the brain are stretched to their limit in large lesions and any alteration in CSF pressure levels could critically upset the balance.

It was observed that in cases where a preoperative shunt was not done, once intratumoral decompression or evacuation of the cystic component of the tumor was achieved the brain relaxed and was maneuverable. In none of these cases was it found necessary to drain ventricular CSF to relax the brain. The author observed marked difficulty in resection of the tumor in cases where a preoperative shunt was performed, probably due to the increased proximity and 'impaction' of the tumor into the basal brain. This affected the ease of resection, made it relatively unsafe and probably affected the ultimate outcome. The emergence of better-quality anesthetic and decongestive agents and the advent of microsurgical and basal surgical approaches have added to the ease of exposure of the suprasellar tumors and lessened the extent of brain retraction, and consequently the need for a preoperative CSF diversionary procedure.

THALAMIC TUMORS

Of the 60 patients with thalamic gliomas treated between 1987 and 1994 at our Institute, 31 underwent a preoperative shunt operation, and these cases were analyzed. There were 15 male and 16 female patients in this series and their ages ranged from 7 to 60 years (average 28 years). There was clinical evidence of increased intracranial pressure in all these cases. The clinical features at the time of presentation and their duration are shown in Table 22.4. The shunt was performed on the side contralateral to the tumor to avoid interference from the tube during surgery on the tumor. Moderate to severe hydrocephalus was present in all cases. In two cases bi-ventriculoperitoneal shunt, while in the rest one-sided ventriculoatrial (26 cases) or ventriculoperitoneal (three cases) shunt, was performed.

Results

In 31 patients a preoperative shunt was performed. Manumetric intraventricular pressure recordings were not made. In 22 cases 'very high' ventricular CSF pressure

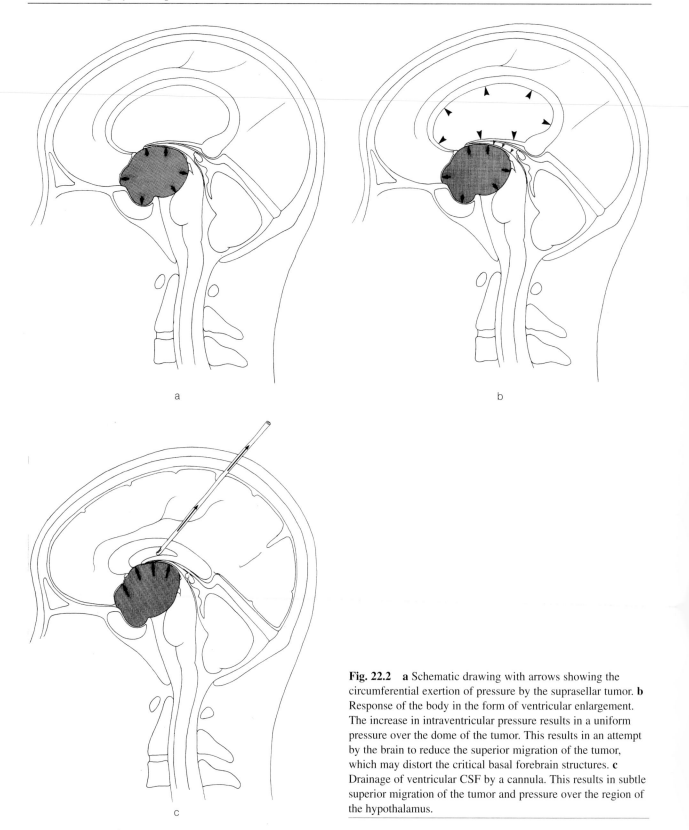

Fig. 22.2 **a** Schematic drawing with arrows showing the circumferential exertion of pressure by the suprasellar tumor. **b** Response of the body in the form of ventricular enlargement. The increase in intraventricular pressure results in a uniform pressure over the dome of the tumor. This results in an attempt by the brain to reduce the superior migration of the tumor, which may distort the critical basal forebrain structures. **c** Drainage of ventricular CSF by a cannula. This results in subtle superior migration of the tumor and pressure over the region of the hypothalamus.

was recorded. In other cases this information was not available from the hospital records. In one patient the shunt had to be revised due to the peri-catheter CSF leak.

One patient developed shunt infection and the shunt assembly was removed. No patient developed clinical evidence of immediate or delayed blockage. Twenty-one

Table 22.4   Symptoms in thalamic tumors

Symptoms	Number	Average duration
Headache	31	4 months
Vomiting	28	3 months
Visual disturbance	28	3 months
Paresthesia	3	20 days
Limb weakness	5	15 days
Ataxia	5	15 days
Altered behaviour	7	15 days
Worsened sensorium	3	5 days
Convulsions	4	2 months
Tinnitus	3	2 months
Diplopia	3	15 days

patients underwent the procedure uneventfully and were relieved of the raised intracranial pressure symptoms to varying degrees.

Eight patients worsened in neurological condition after the shunt. These cases have been summarized in Table 22.5.

Seven patients worsened in sensorium. Of these four were recorded to have become abnormally drowsy and three unconscious after the insertion of the shunt. In all cases the altered state of sensorium was noticed within 8–10 hours after the insertion of the shunt. Four patients recovered from the worsened level of sensorium in about 36 hours. The remainder of the patients were operated for the tumor in the altered state of consciousness. One patient developed persistent vomiting and incontinence of urine, both of which lasted for 2 days. Three patients developed hemiparesis on the side contralateral to the tumor. In two patients hemiparesis recovered within 36 hours. In the third patient hemiparesis progressed to hemiplegia in 24 hours. In three patients extraocular movement was affected. In one patient there was right VIth nerve weakness, one had restriction of upward gaze and one non-paralytic squint with restriction of vertical movement. In two patients the pupils were noted to be sluggish in reaction and in one there was pupillary inequality. In three of these patients a blocked shunt was considered to be the cause of the worsening in sensorium. In two cases ventricular tapping was done through an additional burr hole and in the other case the shunt was revised. The CSF pressure was seen to be low in all of these cases, suggesting an adequate functioning of the shunt. In four cases a CT scan was repeated to analyze the cause of clinical worsening. There was significant reduction in the ventricular size in all these cases, with no evidence of cortical injury. No tumor movement could be radiologically demonstrated.

Table 22.5   Clinical feature of thalamic tumor patients who worsened after the shunt

No.	Age/sex	Preoperative symptoms	Duration of symptoms	Post-shunt complications
1	10/M	H, Vo, Vi	1 month	Unconsciousness Hemiparesis VIth nerve palsy
2	17/M	H, Vo, Vi	1 month	Drowsiness Non-paralytic squint Sluggish pupils
3	10/F	H, Vi	2 months	Drowsiness Restricted upward gaze
4	40/F	H, Vo, Vi, ataxia	20 days	Drowsiness
5	15/M	H, Vo, Vi, paraesthesia	6 months	Unconsciousness
6	F/19	H, Vi, Vo	1 year	Unconsciousness Hemiparesis worsened Unequal pupils Sluggish pupils
7	M/10	H, Vo, Vi, ataxia, altered behavior	25 days	Persistent vomiting Incontinence
8	F/23	H, Vo, Vi	3–4 months	Drowsiness Hemiparesis

H, headache; Vo, vomiting; Vi, visual disturbance.

Discussion

In the presented series of thalamic tumors eight patients worsened in their neurological state following a shunt procedure. Seven patients worsened in sensorium, from excessive drowsiness to unconsciousness. One patient developed persistent vomiting and incontinence of urine. Four patients developed abnormal eye signs. Three patients developed hemiparesis. In the absence of any other explanation for the development of these major neurological complications, it is apparent that an abnormal stretch or pressure on the hypothalamus, internal capsule and midbrain developed after drainage of ventricular CSF. Considering the proximity and relationship of thalamic tumors to these structures it appears that the raised pressure as a result of the obstruction in the CSF pathway was in some way protecting these vital organs. In cases of thalamic tumor dilatation of the lateral ventricles could assist in limiting tumor pressure over the surrounding vital structures. Sudden drainage of CSF from the lateral ventricles could result in subtle superior migration of the tumor and secondary stretch over the internal capsule, hypothalamus, and brain stem. As in the cases of suprasellar tumors, in our series of thalamic tumors where our patients worsened following the shunt it was observed that the tumors were of comparatively large size and the ventricular dilatation was more severe. Patients with relatively smaller tumors fared well after the shunt surgery.

LARGE HEMISPHERIC TUMORS

In large hemispheric tumors which result in a significant rise in intracranial pressure, contralaterel ventricular enlargement is frequently seen. In this situation the significance of ventricular enlargement can clearly be observed (Fig. 22.3). The contralateral ventricular enlargement is an attempt to increase the pressure which would prevent herniation of the brain matter across the falx. Such a herniation could result in damage to the midline structures and vessels, an event which could jeopardize life. The significance of the ventricular enlargement of the contralateral side can clearly be observed if one attempts to tap the large ventricle on the contralateral side. This procedure will result in herniation of the brain and events which the natural processes of the brain have continued to avoid.

AN ANALYSIS OF TUMOR-OBSTRUCTIVE HYDROCEPHALUS

Cause of hydrocephalus

In the initial phases, tumor growth is compensated for by subsystem responses of the central nervous system (CNS). The growing tumor distorts the adjacent brain, which is gradually pushed away. This process results in movement of the brain matter into the adjoining subarachnoid space. Patency of the foramina of Magendie and Luschka and free flow of CSF assure an isopressure system within and around the entire CNS so that no single structure is at a greater pressure with regard to any other. Presence of tumor resulting in obstruction to the path of CSF flow is the most accepted and logical explanation of development of hydrocephalus. The concept that the natural response of the brain in the form of enlargement of the ventricles is pathological seems to be inappropriate.

It is seen that in most pathologic states the wisdom of the body swings into action to minimize the damage on any tissue. In cases of injury to the knee, there occurs swelling of the region, resulting in pain and restriction of the movements of the joint. The swelling of the knee is the response of the body and pain and restriction of movement of the knee joint are the symptoms which limit the activity of the knee, thus providing the best opportunity for healing. Isolation of an inflamed appendix by the tightly overlayed omentum is another example to show how nature protects the rest of the abdomen from spreading infection.

In the case of the brain, it is difficult to imagine that nature would commit a major folly. It needs to be re-emphasized that nature has chosen to make the vital centers of the brain stem and hypothalamus in particular more resistant to endogenous or exogenous effects as a part of its survival strategy. The whole science of anesthesia is dependent on the fact that the vital centers in the brain stem are active and kicking when the rest of the sensory and motor areas of the brain are knocked down by anesthetics. It is our assumption, based on a large series of cases, that the hydrocephalus secondary to obstruction in the path of CSF flow by the tumor is a part of nature's defense mechanism. The hydrocephalus accompanying the brain tumor is obviously a hydrodynamic system operative both within and around the CNS because of the patency of the foramen magnum and the foramen of Luschka. We observed that hydrocephalus and increased supratumoral pressure are mechanisms which tend to push the tumor away from the more sensitive areas of the brain. The net effect achieved by the above homeostatic strategy is that the tumor is denied the right to pressurize adjacent centers or blood vessels by being forcibly kept at bay by the CSF push. This was more eloquently observed in cases of posterior fossa vermian and suprasellar lesions. As the tumor increases in size, the supratumoral pressure build-up increases and prevents as much as possible the encroachment of the tumor into the brain stem and the hypothalamus. It is noticed that in the presence of even very large tumors symptoms primarily due to encroachment of the brain stem and hypothalamus or local pressure are late,

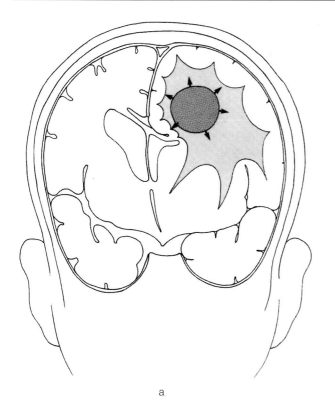

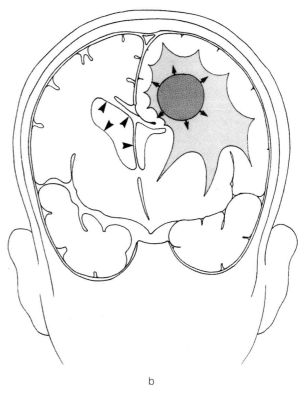

a

b

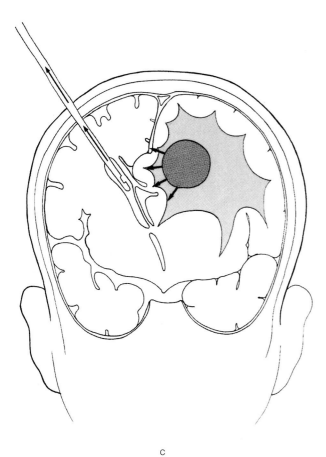

c

Fig. 22.3 **a** Hemispheric tumor with surrounding edema.
Pressure is exerted in all directions by the tumor. **b**
Contralateral ventricular enlargement and rise in pressure
results in an attempt to neutralize the pressure on both sides, at
least to some extent. **c** Cannulation of the contralateral ventricle
and drainage of CSF could result in subfalcine herniation, with
effects on midline structures and vessels.

while symptoms of increased intracranial pressure secondary to hydrocephalus are the principal presenting symptoms. The ventricular enlargement and rise in intracranial pressure correspond to the size of the tumor. The larger the tumor the more severe is the ventricular dilatation and the rise in pressure. This suggests that there is an increasing effort on the part of the body to keep the tumor away from vital structures. Whenever local symptoms arise, the situation is urgent and early treatment should be instituted. The pathways of CSF flow are only rarely completely blocked and alternative channels for CSF outflow are almost always present. In situations where the pathways of CSF flow are completely blocked the ventricular pressure will show an acute rise which could result in transtentorial herniation and other such sequelae. Such a severe rise in intraventricular pressure is rarely seen in the presence of a tumor. In other words, the hydrocephalus per se seldom needs emergency treatment. If symptoms are compelling, decongestive drugs may be used to temporarily tide over the crisis.

Types of tumors and hydrocephalus

It is generally agreed that any tumor which obstructs the pathway of CSF flow will result in hydrocephalus. Large intra-axial brain stem and hypothalamic tumors do not cause hydrocephalus despite the presence in the pathway of flow of CSF. The consensus favors the growth pattern of the tumor responsible for non-development of hydrocephalus. It may be possible that when structures like the hypothalamus and brain stem are already affected the brain needs no additional protective mechanical phenomenon in the form of ventricular enlargement and allows the local growth of the tumor.

Effects of ventricular drainage procedures

The drainage of CSF from the ventricules will result in immediate relief from the symptoms of increased intracranial pressure. However, secondary to the release of supratumoral pressure there may occur subtle movements in the tumor towards the direction of CSF drainage. Such movements in the tumor and in the adjoining brain have been reported to be the cause of reverse tentorial herniations in cases with large posterior fossa tumor. Hemorrhages within the tumor probably secondary to stretch of intra- or paratumoral vessels have also been recorded. Symptomatic impaction of an extramedullary spinal tumor following ventricular CSF drainage shunt surgery has been reported. Such events suggest movements in the tumor. It was observed that following release of lateral ventricular CSF

the initial phase of surgical procedures like dural incisions, cortical manipulation and retraction of the brain become relatively safer. However, as movements of the tumor are towards the brain stem or hypothalamus, surgical dissection of the tumor from these structures could become difficult and dangerous.

Dilatation of the contralateral lateral ventricle in hemispheric tumor could be an attempt to reduce the movements of the brain that may result in subfalcine herniation and anterior cerebral-pericallosal arterial stretch and compromise, and damage to the corpus callosum and medial surface of the hemisphere. An attempt to drain the dilated lateral ventricle of the contralateral side may exaggerate the subfalcine herniation and result in neurological worsening.

TRANSFALCINE APPROACH TO CONTRALATERAL HEMISPHERIC TUMOR

Various approaches to deep-seated tumors have been described. An approach which is direct and shortest, providing a wide exposure, and avoiding the need to traverse or retract vital cerebral cortex, is necessary for successful and safe resection of such a tumor. An interhemispheric fissure transfalcine approach for a contralateral hemispheric tumor in proximity to the falx was found to be most appropriate in four cases (Goel 1995b).

Operative technique

The operative technique is shown in Figures 22.4 and 22.5. A contralateral side craniotomy is performed. The hemisphere is retracted and a wide exposure of the falx is obtained. A window is made in the falx and the lesion is exposed.

Material

Four cases of parafalcine tumors were operated on by a transfalcine approach. All patients were males and their ages ranged from 28 to 50 years. The lesions were situated in the hemisphere in all cases. Two patients had a glioma (anaplastic astrocytoma) in the medial parietal and parieto-occipital region, respectively, one had a choroid plexus papilloma in the region of trigone of the lateral ventricle, and one patient had a deep-seated medial frontal abscess. There was extensive edema surrounding the tumor in all cases. Compression and shift of ipsilateral lateral ventricle was observed in all, while dilatation of the contralateral ventricle was seen in three cases. In case 1 (Fig. 22.6) an

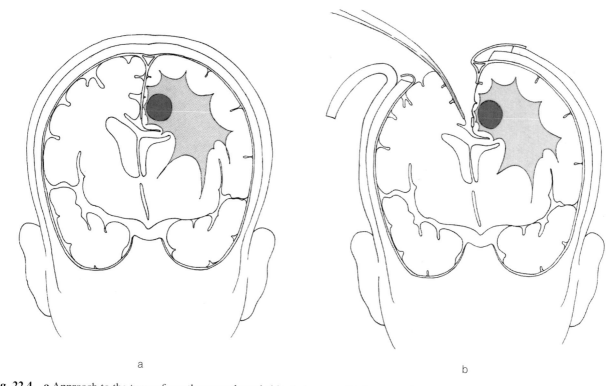

a   b

Fig. 22.4   **a** Approach to the tumor from the contralateral side. A deep parafalcine tumor is seen, with the shaded area depicting extensive edema. The ipsilateral sulci are obliterated and midline structures are displaced. **b** The cerebral cortex has been retracted and a window is made into the falx to expose the lesion on the contralateral side.

ipsilateral posterior parieto-occipital interhemispheric approach was attempted. However, it was difficult to approach the lesion as retraction of the edematous brain resulted in injury to the cortex. The craniotomy was then extended to the right side and a transfalcine approach was successfully performed. In all other cases a contralateral transfalcine approach was chosen as the primary approach.

Case 1

A 50-year-old man was admitted with a 15-day history of headache associated with vomiting and visual obscuration. There was progressive worsening in his behavior and memory. He was markedly disoriented and obeyed only simple commands. Apart from severe papilledema, the rest of the examination was unremarkable. CT of the brain showed a large mixed-density, moderately enhancing tumor, occupying the region of the left temporal horn, trigone and posterior part of the body of the left lateral ventricle. The surrounding white matter was edematous and resulted in obliteration of the ipsilateral sulci. The right lateral ventricle was moderately dilated (Fig. 22.6).

A left-sided posterior parietal craniotomy for an interhemispheric approach along the left side of the falx was carried out. However, on opening the dura the brain was seen to

be markedly edematous and swollen despite the high doses of decongestants. It was observed that retraction of the brain away from the falx could lead to injury to the cortex, bridging veins and sulcal arteries. The craniotomy was then extended to the right side. The brain on the right side was normal in appearance. CSF from the dilated right lateral ventricle and subarachnoid spaces was drained. These maneuvers resulted in further relaxation of the brain on this side. The cortex was retracted away from the falx. A large window was made into the inferior aspect of the falx. The tumor was almost instantly exposed following a shallow cut into the left occipital cortex. A wide and direct exposure of the tumor was possible. A subtotal excision of this grossly malignant and infiltrating tumor was carried out (histopathology: anaplastic astrocytoma). The patient fared well after the operation and the lesion was subjected to radiotherapy.

Cases 2 and 3

The tumors in cases 2 and 3 were located in the medial parietal and trigonal area, respectively. A transfalcine route was selected as the primary approach. The tumor in case 2 was an astrocytoma which was resected subtotally, while the tumor in case 3 was a choroid plexus papilloma and was excised completely. Wide and satisfactory exposure was obtained in these cases. There was no need to drain the lateral ventricle to assist retraction of the non-tumor side of the brain.

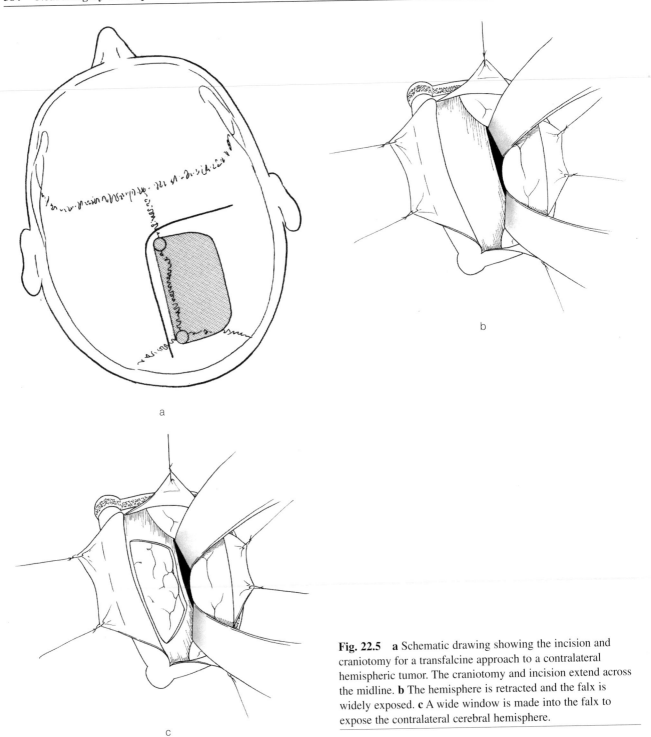

Fig. 22.5 a Schematic drawing showing the incision and craniotomy for a transfalcine approach to a contralateral hemispheric tumor. The craniotomy and incision extend across the midline. **b** The hemisphere is retracted and the falx is widely exposed. **c** A wide window is made into the falx to expose the contralateral cerebral hemisphere.

Case 4

A 28-year-old male patient was admitted with a 2-month history of fever, worsening level of consciousness and progressive right hemiparesis. He was barely moving the limbs on the right side when admitted. There was marked bilateral papilledema. CT scan showed a ring-enhancing left medial frontal lesion with extensive surrounding edema (Fig. 22.7a). The ipsilateral lateral ventricle was markedly compressed and displaced. A transfalcine route was selected. A small cortical incision exposed the subcortical abscess. On incising the wall about 40 ml of thick pus was drained. The wall of the large lesion collapsed and could be removed completely (Fig. 22.7b). The patient showed rapid recovery in his neurological status.

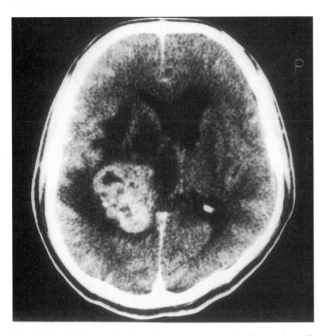

Fig. 22.6 CT scan showing the tumor occupying the region of the trigone of the left lateral ventricle. Extensive surrounding edema is seen. The right lateral ventricle is moderately dilated. (From Goel 1995b, with permission.)

Comments

With the advent of modern anesthetic techniques and decongestive drugs a surgeon seldom confronts a swollen and 'angry' brain. However, in an occasional case with a large tumor and extensive surrounding edema fissural and sulcal approaches are difficult and sometimes impossible. Retraction of the brain to approach a deep-seated lesion may be fraught with dangers of cortical injury and inadequate tumor exposure.

In the described cases an interhemispheric fissure approach from the ipsilateral side is usually considered to be appropriate (Yasargil et al 1986). But under the special conditions of the presented cases the described modified surgical technique was found to be very helpful. It provided a direct approach to the tumor without significantly increasing the distance between surface and lesion compared to the ipsilateral interhemispheric approach. Wide retraction of the brain on the normal side was easily possible. Drainage of CSF from the dilated lateral ventricle (performed in case 1) and subarachnoid cisterns provided additional working space. A large window could be made in the inferior aspect of the falx to approach the tumor. It appears that such an approach, when judiciously employed, can be useful in the occasional case of a deep-seated falcine and parafalcine tumor.

AN ALTERNATIVE SHUNTING PROCEDURE FOR CSF FISTULA

A modified third/fourth ventriculoperitoneal shunt is described (Goel 1993). This procedure was used to deal with postoperative CSF fistulae refractory to treatment by simpler routine measures. The possible indications of the operation are discussed.

Postoperative leakage of CSF from a neurosurgical wound can on occasion become life threatening. Associated wound infections can add to the difficulties. Apart from primary dural repair, CSF leakage is often controlled by simpler measures such as making the site of leak non-dependent and draining CSF by lumbar punctures. Sometimes it is necessary to drain CSF externally or into the peritoneum by inserting a lumbar thecoperitoneal shunt. When the lateral ventricles are dilated, a ventricu-

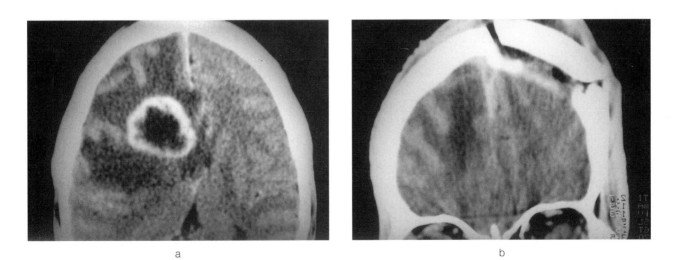

a   b

Fig. 22.7 **a** Contrast-enhanced CT scan showing the large posterior medial frontal ring-enhancing lesion with extensive surrounding edema. (From Goel 1995b, with permission.) **b** Postoperative coronal reconstruction of CT scan shows excision of the abscess through a contralateral craniotomy. (From Goel 1995b, with permission.)

loperitoneal or atrial shunt can sometimes be used. Occasionally, the lumbar area is not available for CSF drainage or lumboperitoneal shunt, for example when the leak is through the wound for dorsolumbar or lumbar surgery and when the lumbar skin is infected. Lateral ventricular drainage shunt may not be possible if the ventricles are small. Faced with such situations, we have drained the third ventricle in three and the fourth ventricle in two patients with a modified shunting procedure, with successful closure of CSF fistula.

The operation

The patient is placed in the prone position and the flank turned to one side (Fig. 22.8). In this position the suboccipital region is available for a midline incision and the lateral aspect of the lower quadrant of the abdomen for the peritoneal surgery. A low suboccipital craniectomy is performed (Fig. 22.9). A V-shaped dural incision is made, the apex being sited at the level of the foramen magnum. If necessary, the occipital sinus is obliterated and divided at the apex of the dural incision. The dural flap is then elevated and kept out of the way. The tonsils are gently separated and retracted so as to open the foramen of Magendie. The ventricular end of the silastic shunt is then introduced blindly but gently along the floor of the fourth ventricle (Fig. 22.10). The dura is closed snugly around the shunt tube. The shunt tubing is then led via a subcutaneous tunnel to the abdomen, where it is inserted into the peritoneal cavity. Scalp and skin sutures are removed on day 8 after surgery and the patient is mobilized once the CSF leak has stopped. In one patient we have inserted a third ventricle to right atrium shunt. Placing the tube in the atrium however, is difficult because of the position of the patient.

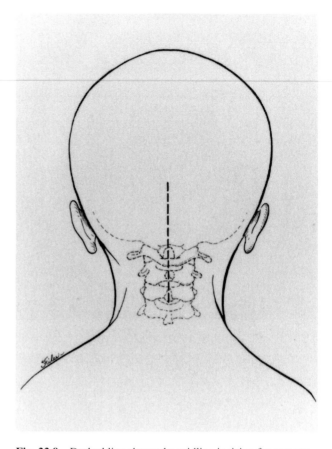

Fig. 22.9   Dashed line shows the midline incision for surgery.

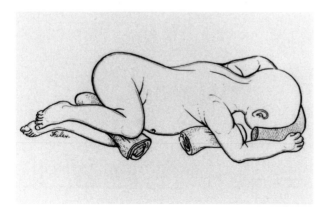

Fig. 22.8   Position of the patient. The head is in the prone position while the trunk is turned into a lateral position. (From Goel & Pandya 1993, with permission.)

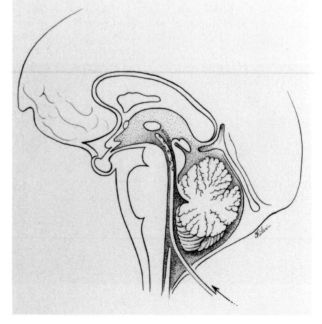

Fig. 22.10   Position of the shunt tube. (From Goel & Pandya 1993, with permission.)

Case 1

A 16-month-old child was brought to us for treatment of paraparesis and incontinence of urine and feces. A lipomeningocele was the cause. At surgery, the spinal cord was released from the intra- and extradural fat. The large dural defect that resulted was meticulously closed using lyophilized dural graft. On the third postoperative day a profuse CSF leak from the wound occurred. The wound was re-explored and a fresh dural repair was carried out. Close approximation of the wound by rotation of the paravertebral muscles and lumbar aponeurosis was performed. The CSF leak continued. CT showed small ventricles. In desperation the third ventricle was drained into the peritoneal cavity as described above. This stopped the leak dramatically. The lumbar, suboccipital and peritoneal wounds healed without incident (Figs. 22.11, 22.12).

Discussion

Most of the CSF is produced by the choroid plexuses in the ventricles of the brain. The common conduit for the bulk of the CSF is the aqueduct of Sylvius. Once the CSF emerges from the fourth ventricle it spreads throughout the subarachnoid spaces. A silastic tube inserted into the aqueduct, or third or fourth ventricle, drains the major portion of the CSF produced away from the subarachnoid space. Such a tube can be drained either into the peritoneal cavity or into the right atrium.

When a CSF leak through a cranial or spinal wound persists despite all the usual measures, the insertion of a shunt as described may prove life saving. The procedure of cannulation of the cerebral aqueduct for relief of obstructive hydrocephalus has been attempted with varying degrees of success in the past. Whilst the operation does not involve making any incision into the neural tissue, the tube travels a very sensitive and delicate path via the fourth ventricle into the aqueduct. Its introduction demands great care. Even so, complications may follow injury to the structures around the aqueduct. A tube placed in the fourth ventricle appears to be safer as possible injury to the brain stem is avoided. Because of the possibility of injury to neural tissue, insertion of this kind of shunt should only be performed when CSF leaks are unmanageable by other methods. Such a situation is rare in present-day neurosurgery. However, in the poorer developing countries, like India, with a relatively high incidence of wound infection, a case of CSF fistula can occasionally lead to a life-threatening situation. Infants and children, who tolerate meningitis and infections poorly, can be salvaged with success by the type of shunt described here.

MENINGOCELE SAC TO PERITONEUM SHUNT

CSF fistula is a dreaded and frequent complication following surgery for varieties of meningocele. Various methods of repair and closure of the dural defect to avoid this problem have been described in the literature. Surgical treatment of failed cases with CSF fistula can be difficult to treat. Persistent CSF leakage can be a source of meningitis in these children, in whom fecal and urinary contamination of the wound is very easily possible. A meningocele sac to

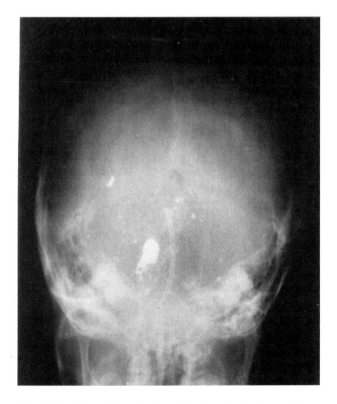

Fig. 22.11 X-ray, Towne's view, showing the location of the tube.

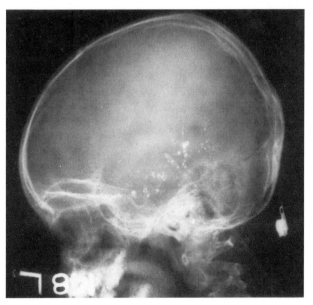

Fig. 22.12 X-ray, lateral view, showing the position of the tube. (From Goel & Pandya 1993, with permission.)

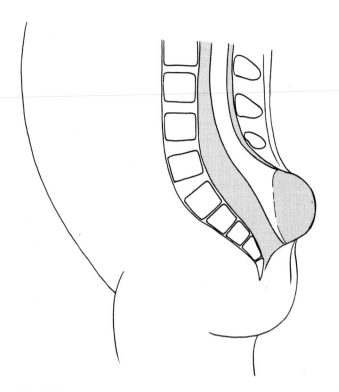

Fig. 22.13 Schematic drawing showing the meningocele sac with tethered cord.

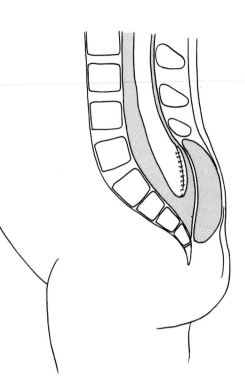

Fig. 22.14 The meningocele sac has been repaired. There is collection of CSF underneath the skin.

peritoneal shunt was found to be an effective and safe method of prevention of CSF fistula in selected cases operated for meningomyelocele (Figs. 22.13–22.15). The method was particularly useful in cases where an initial attempt at repairing the sac had failed. The described shunt procedure can exacerbate symptoms secondary to Arnold–Chiari malformation, which is a common association with these lesions. The procedure was successfully performed in a patient who developed profuse CSF leakage from the wound following detethering of the cord. The tube can be removed at a later date when the wound has completely healed through the abdominal side (Figs. 22.13–22.15).

ROLE OF CEREBRAL EDEMA IN BRAIN PROTECTION

The extent of tumor-reactive cerebral edema varies with the type of tumor. In our experience, the cerebral edema was much greater in more malignant, more vascular and more infective varieties of tumors. Cerebral edema was a reaction to the presence of the tumor. It is possible that the reaction of the brain, in the form of edema, to the presence of the tumor is a protective mechanism of the brain as well. Cerebral edema and the resultant local and generalized rise

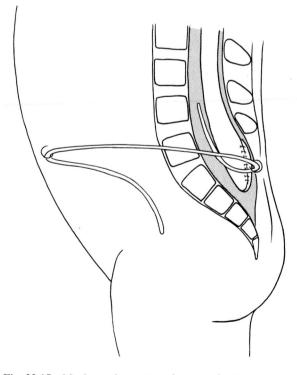

Fig. 22.15 Meningocele sac to peritoneum shunt.

in intracranial pressure could help in limiting the spread of malignant tumor cells and infection. Disproportionately extensive cerebral edema around small abscesses lends some support to the hypothesis. It is possible that circumferential cerebral edema around the tumor could provide support to the delicate and abnormal tumor blood vessels and prevent them from rupturing. The cerebral edema and the resultant rise in intracranial pressure are the cause of the symptoms. On the basis of these observations it appears that unless the symptoms of raised intracranial pressure are crippling, the primary aim of the surgeon should be directed towards the treatment of the pathological lesion and not towards the treatment of cerebral edema. The treatment of cerebral edema should be only in the perioperative phase and aimed towards obtaining a relatively lax brain, which may facilitate safe tumor resection and avoid cortical damage due to retraction and manipulation. Treatment directed to the sole aim of treating the natural brain reaction or cerebral edema and raised intracranial pressure by decongestant drugs and decompressive craniectomies could be disastrous, as is seen in the following cases.

Case 1

A 13-year-old girl presented with a 2-month history of progressive left hemiparesis. She had associated severe bifrontal headache and blurring of vision. When admitted she was drowsy and obeyed only simple commands. There was bilateral marked papilledema. She had grade 3 spastic left hemiparesis. CT scan showed a large hyperdense enhancing right caudate head, body and internal capsule mass (Fig. 22.16). There was moderate surrounding edema and secondary mass effect in the form of effacement of cerebral sulci and displacement of the septum pellucidum to the contralateral side. A large temporoparietal decompressive crainectomy was done. The brain was seen to be tense despite the use of high doses of decongestive drugs. The patient was noted to be drowsy after the surgery and worsened suddenly 8 hours later and died after 2 hours. Postmortem examination of adequately fixed brain showed a large clot in the tumor bed (Fig. 22.17). Histological examination showed that the lesion was anaplastic glioma.

Case 2

A 35-year-old patient was admitted with a 15-day history of severe bifrontal headaches. There was bilateral gross papilledema. There was no focal neurological deficit. MRI showed the patient had a large deep-seated hemispheric tumor (Fig. 22.18). Following decompressive craniectomy the patient suddenly worsened after 45 minutes of surgery and later died within 24 hours. Postmortem examination showed a large intratumoral clot (Fig. 22.19). Histological examination showed that the tumor was glioblastoma multiforme.

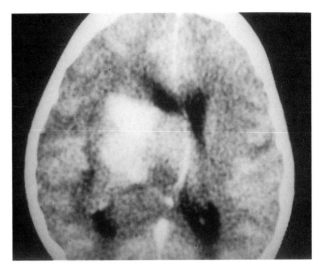

Fig. 22.16   Contrast-enhanced CT scan shows the hyperdense tumor in the region of basal ganglia. Mass effect secondary to the tumor is seen.

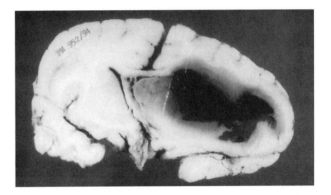

Fig. 22.17   Large intratumoral clot is seen. The clot is extending towards the site of bony decompression.

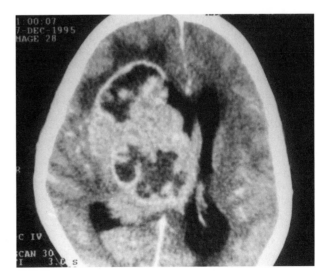

Fig. 22.18   CT scan showing the large hemispheric tumor.

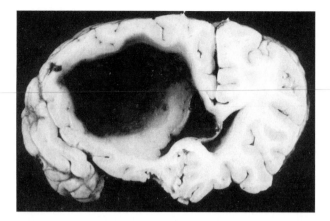

Fig. 22.19 Postmortem photograph showing the intratumoral clot.

Discussion

Subtemporal decompression for deep-seated tumors has been a time-honored procedure advocated to alleviate life and vision-threatening increased intracranial pressure. In present-day neurosurgery, such a treatment is only rarely recommended. The procedure probably resulted in intratumoral bleeding and later death in the reported cases. Our literature search failed to find a report of such a complication.

The popularity of subtemporal decompression surgery for pseudotumor cerebri, 'unresectable' tumors, cerebral contusions and other such conditions has gradually waned with time. With improved anesthesia and quality of decongestive drugs, and improvements in microsurgical and stereotactic surgical techniques, craniectomies are finding less favor with most neurosurgical units. Various authorities have reported favorable results following subtemporal decompression surgery. The additional space provided by subtemporal decompression has been seen to result in an improved buffering effect, reduction of increased intracranial pressure and reduced need of decongestive drugs. Alexander et al (1987) studied the effects of subtemporal decompression and found that the volume increase after subtemporal decompression equals the ventricular volume. Modifications and improvement in the techniques of the decompressive procedure have been described. Hemicraniectomies, complete frontal craniectomies and bilateral massive craniectomies have been advocated. Cooper et al (1979) reported massive edema of the brain occurring under the area of decompression. Later, other authors also reported an increase in brain edema due to compression of blood vessels by the edge of the craniectomy.

In the presented cases such a procedure was adopted as resection of the tumor in proximity to vital neural structures and tracts, in the presence of extensive surrounding edema, was considered to be hazardous. The high incidence of intracranial tuberculomas in India in the age group and sex of the presented patients, their inconsistent radiological features, and excellent response to antituberculous drugs was also a factor that influenced a conservative surgical approach. It was hoped that the decompressive surgery would aid in dissipating the marked increase in intracranial pressure externally.

The exact cause of intratumoral hemorrhage in our patients could not be ascertained. It may be possible that migration of the brain towards the craniectomy resulted in movement in the tumor and traction over its blood vessels. Sudden alteration in the delicately balanced intracranial and intratumoral pressure may have resulted in decompression and bursting of abnormal tumor blood vessels. The relatively large size of the tumor appears to be an important factor that effected the change in intracranial dynamics and caused the resultant hemorrhage. Subtle movements in the tumor following such a procedure could also result in stretch or compressive effects on the vital pathways adjacent to the tumor that could affect their function.

Although no reasonable conclusion can be made on the basis of two reports, the cases are being presented because of their uniqueness and clinical relevance. It appears that further experimental and clinical studies are necessary to evaluate the effects and outcome of decompressive craniectomies. It does appear that cerebral edema and the rise in intracranial pressure were in some way protecting the delicate tumor blood vessels.

REFERENCES

Abraham J, Chandy J 1963 Ventriculo-atrial shunt in the management of posterior fossa tumors: preliminary report. Journal of Neurosurgery 20: 252–253

Albright A L 1982 The value of precraniotomy shunts in children with posterior fossa tumors. Clinical Neurosurgery 30: 278–285

Alexander E, Ball M R, Laster D W 1987 Subtemporal decompression: radiological observations and current surgical experiences. British Journal of Neurosurgery 1: 427–433

Carmel P W 1985 Craniopharyngiomas. In: Wilkins R H, Rengachary S S (eds) Neurosurgery. Mc-Graw Hill, New York, pp 905–916

Cooper P R, Haglet H, Clark W K et al 1979 Enhancement of experimental cerebral edema after decompressive craniectomy: implications for the management of severe head injuries. Neurosurgery 4: 296–300

Cushing H 1931 Experiences with cerebellar astrocytomas: a critical review of seventy six cases. Surgery Gynecology and Obstetrics 51: 129–204

Epstien F, Rajgopalan M 1978 Pediatric posterior fossa tumors: hazards of 'preoperative' shunt. Neurosurgery 3: 348–350

German W J 1961 The gliomas: a follow-up study. Clinical Neurosurgery 7: 1–19

Goel A 1993 Whither preoperative shunts for posterior fossa tumors. British Journal of Neurosurgery 7: 395–399

Goel A 1995a Preoperative shunts in suprasellar tumors. British Journal of Neurosurgery 9: 189–193

Goel A 1995b Transfalcine approach to a contralateral hemispheric tumor. Acta Neurochirurgica 135: 210–212

Goel A, Pandya S K 1993 A shunting procedure for cerebrospinal fluid fistula, employing cannulation of the third and fourth ventricles. British Journal of Neurosurgery 9: 189–193

Ingraham F D, Campbell J B 1941 An apparatus for closed drainage of ventricular system. Annals of Surgery 114: 1096–1098

Pitts L H, Wilson C B, Dedo H H et al 1975 Pneumocephalus following ventriculoperitoneal shunt: case report. Journal of Neurosurgery 43: 631–633

Vaquero J, Cabezudo J M, DeSola R G et al 1981 Intratumoral hemorrhage in posterior fossa tumors after ventricular drainage. Report of two cases. Journal of Neurosurgery 54: 406–408

Yasargil M G, Cravens G F, Roth P 1986 Surgical approaches to 'inaccessible' brain tumors. Clinical Neurosurgery 34: 42–110

Bone defects should preferably be reconstructed in the following situations:

1. Larger defects over the tegmen tympani and orbital roof should preferably be replaced with bone as the dura in this region is relatively thin and the region is deprived of large basal CSF cisterns; consequently initially brain pulsations can be transmitted and later the brain can herniate into these spaces.
2. Support for brain tissue may be necessary where large bone defects are created following the operation.
3. Reconstruction of the bone is also carried out to support the dura and help in the provision of watertight sealing of the base and avoiding formation of CSF fistulae.
4. Protection of the brain from future injury and restoration of a reasonable appearance and quality of life are other important objectives.

The size of the defect and its site, extent of resection of the associated structures, history of previous operative procedures, and endovascular and radiation treatment are important variables that determine the appropriate reconstructive procedure. Various methods of reconstruction of basal bone have been described. Reconstruction of bone defects in the cranial base should preferably be done with the help of bone. In sterile fields free small or large bone pieces can be used for this purpose. Ribs, iliac crest and scapular grafts have been successfully used. Acrylic and metal plates can also be used in such a situation. However, in potentially infective fields which are more frequently encountered after a skull base operation, use of a bone flap based on a vascularized pedicle is recommended.

Vascularized osteomyoplastic flap (Goel 1994a)

Various experimental studies have been conducted on the evolution of temporalis osteomuscular flaps compared with calvarial free bone grafts (Antonyshyn et al 1986, Combelles & Zadeh 1984, Fasano et al 1987). The studies confirmed that vascularized bone flaps remain viable and are characterized by normal evolution, while free bone grafts show typical signs of necrosis and resorption. Such vascularized bone flaps based on a muscle pedicle have been used in cosmetic facial surgery and mandibular, maxillary and palatal reconstruction and mastoid cavity obliteration (Bite et al 1987, Choung et al 1991).

We performed skull base reconstruction using split or full-thickness cranial bone pedicled on muscle flaps. Temporalis muscle, being in close proximity to the skull base and also the ease with which it could be rotated in various directions, was used effectively for such an osteomyoplastic flap skull base reconstruction (Figs. 23.1, 23.2).

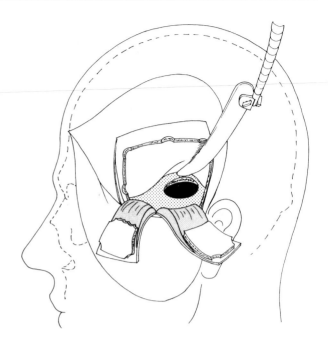

Fig. 23.1 Bone defect in the middle cranial fossa base on retracting the temporal brain. The temporal bone is split into two, each piece being placed on temporalis muscle pedicle.

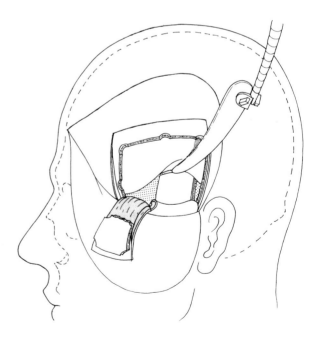

Fig. 23.2 The posterior piece of the temporal bone flap is rotated to fill the defect. This forms the osteomyoplastic flap. The anterior piece of the temporal bone flap is replaced in the convexity.

The temporalis muscle has an extensive blood supply to the calvarium through multiple perforators. Elevation of the bone flap with wide attachment to the muscle pedicle results in a well-vascularized flap. Vascularized bone flap can also be based on muscles of the nape of the neck. Judicious use of split cranial grafts can fill the resulting defects in the skull. Osteomyoplastic flaps can be used for reconstruction of middle fossa and petrous bone defects with relative ease. The fascial layers covering the temporalis muscle can be used to seal the defects in the basal dura while the muscle and bone occupy the area of bone defect. Unlike pericranial and galeal flaps which can be raised either before or after the surgical resection, osteomyoplastic flaps, on most occasions, have to be planned and fashioned in the exposure stage of the operation. The incisions and dissection in the muscle and fascial planes are modified to avoid transection of blood supply, which could be crucial to sustain the bone flap.

Case 1

A 12-year-old boy had suffered three episodes of pyogenic meningitis, the last attack being 3 months before admission to our unit. At the age of 3 years he had suffered a fall from a height of about 8 m following which he was unconscious for 2 days and subsequently recovered. Following the injury he had diminished hearing in the left ear. There was no history suggestive of CSF fistula. On examination, apart from grossly affected hearing in the left ear he had no neurological deficit. X-rays of the skull and computed tomography (CT) showed a large defect in the left temporal squamous and petrous bone. There was a hypodense area in the brain around the left petrous bone suggestive of encephalomalacia and an ipsilateral enlargement of the lateral ventricle. The petrous bone was invaded by soft tissue. Small air spaces could be seen connecting the external ear canal with the brain and Eustachian tube (Fig. 23.3a, b). During surgery a large dural defect was encountered in the middle fossa base. There was evidence of herniation of brain matter through the bone defect in the tegmen

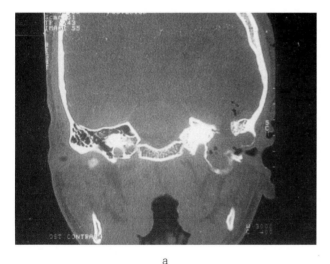

a

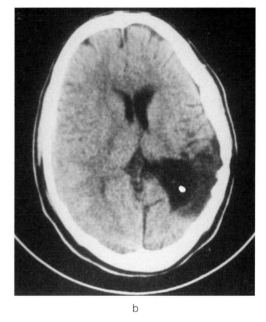

b

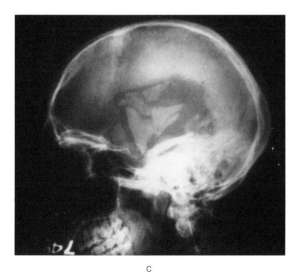

c

Fig. 23.3 **a** Bone window of the CT scan showing a bone defect in the tegmen. Soft tissue shadow in the petrous bone is seen. Also note air spaces in the external ear canal, petrous bone and intracranially. (From Goel 1994a, with permission.) **b** A plain CT scan shows encephalomalacia of the parietotemporal brain and ipsilateral enlargement of the lateral ventricle. (From Goel 1994a, with permission.) **c** Postoperative skull X-ray showing the large temporal squamous bone flap (seen end on) over the petrous bone. Bone pieces fill the bone defect created. No evidence of intracranial air is seen. (From Goel 1994a, with permission.)

tympani region into the petrous bone. The herniated brain was continuous with a glistening tumor occupying the petrous bone (histopathology: epidermoid). The tumor and the brain matter that had herniated into the petrous bone were carefully removed. The middle ear structures were completely destroyed by the mass, which occupied a large part of the mastoid antrum, middle ear and extended into the Eustachian tube. There was some granulation tissue suggesting chronic infection in the region. The dilated temporal horn of the lateral ventricle was widely opened in the process.

The temporalis muscle, with its fascia and part of the squamous bone, was rotated to fill up the defect in the base. The dural defect was repaired with the temporalis fascia which remained attached to the temporalis muscle, thus retaining its vascularity. Smaller empty spaces were packed with free fat grafts taken from the thigh. The defect created in the temporal squamous bone was reconstructed with a split parietal bone flap and by bone debris. Follow-up X-ray after 6 months of surgery (Fig. 23.3c) showed that the bone flap had been well accepted. No intracranial air was seen. The patient showed no clinical evidence of persisting CSF fistula when assessed 3 years after surgery.

Pericranium-based bone flaps (Goel 1994b)

Pericranial and galeal flaps have been described for reconstruction of anterior cranial base and craniofacial deformities. The pericranium comprises an outer layer of loose aereolar tissue and an inner layer of osteoblasts, and contains an extensive vascular network. The pericranium derives blood supply anteriorly from the supratrochlear and supraorbital arteries and laterally from the superficial temporal arteries. Pericranial layer pedicled flaps can be based on either of these vessels, and accordingly rotated anteriorly or laterally. The pericranium can sustain the calvarial flap by means of multiple small, vertical perforators. Studies have shown that calvarial flaps can safely be pedicled on the pericranial layer or galeopericranial layer (Casanova et al 1986, Cutting et al 1984, Price et al 1988, Snyderman et al 1990, Watson Jones 1993). Bone flaps of the calvarium can be either of full thickness or only of the outer table. A split-thickness osteogaleopericranial flap as shown in Figures 23.4 and 23.5 can be used to reconstruct the anterior cranial fossa base. Easy availability, rotational capability, long length and close proximity to the operative area of such vascularized flaps make them ideally suited for skull base reconstruction. The bone piece can be pedicled on a large base of pericranium and can be additionally nourished by the galeal flaps. Whenever necessary, the bone flap can be turned upside down so that the bone surface is not directly exposed to the paranasal sinuses. The flap can even be sandwiched between the pericranial layers. In cases with extensive defects, an extended subgaleal fascia–pericranial

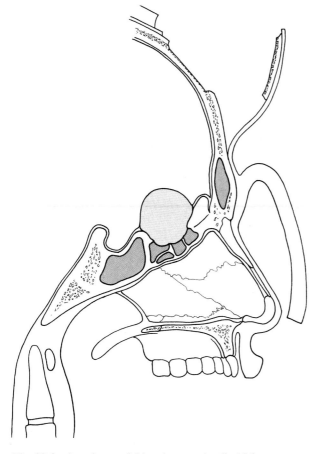

Fig. 23.4 Anterior cranial basal tumor. A split-thickness calvarial graft pedicled on the galeopericranial layer is taken.

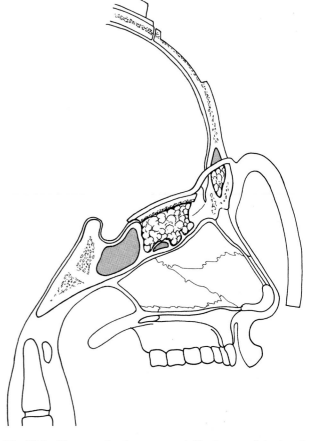

Fig. 23.5 The tumor has been resected. The bone graft is placed in the resultant basal defect. Fat occupies the opened sinuses.

Reconstruction of the skull base

temporalis flap can first be placed in the region of the defect (Goel & Gahankari 1995), over which the described bone flap can be placed. Reconstruction can thus be with multiple layers of vascularized tissue. The bone piece can be fractured into two or more pieces, retaining its attachment to the pericranium so that its contour can be adjusted to suit the local environment. Such vascularized flaps are more resistant to infection, tolerate radiation therapy better, are mechanically stronger, contract less and survive better in a poorly vascularized bed when compared to free bone grafts. It is presumed that such flaps would be ideal while treating basal encephaloceles.

Case 1

A 28-year-old male patient was operated upon for a massive olfactory groove meningioma (Fig. 23.6a). The tumor invaded the ethmoid sinuses extensively (Fig. 23.6b). Difficulties in basal reconstruction were anticipated and the described bone flap was planned. A bicoronal scalp flap was reflected anteriorly in the subgaleal plane, leaving the pericranium attached to the bone. A small part of the outer table of the frontal bone, at the posterior end of the proposed craniotomy, measuring about 4 × 4 cm, was split with the help of an oscillating saw, chisel and hammer, and was fractured anteriorly. The entire pericranium of

the proposed bifrontal craniotomy was cut and reflected anteriorly along with the piece of the outer table of calvarial bone (Figure 23.6c).

A bifrontal basal craniotomy was performed. The intracranial and ethmoid sinus tumor was excised along with the involved basal dura and bone. The cranial cavity was now communicating with the paranasal sinuses through a wide defect. The large anterior cranial fossa floor defect and exposed mucosa-denuded sinuses were first packed with fat and then covered with a wide-based and long-pedicled osteopericranial flap. A strip of galea based on the left supraorbital vessels was then dissected from the scalp flap and placed over the pericranial flap for provision of additional blood supply to the flap and was also used to reconstruct the dural defect at the base. The wound healed without incident and the flap was well accepted when the patient was seen 6 months later.

Long vascular pedicle composite cranial flap (Goel 1995a)

The flap described is a split or full-thickness cranial bone flap based on the pericranial layer which receives its vascular nourishment from the temporalis muscle and its overlying fascial layers. Subgaleal elevation of the scalp is

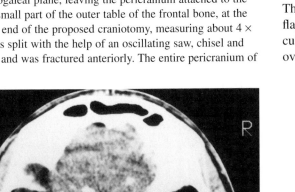

a

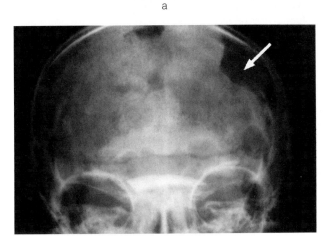

c

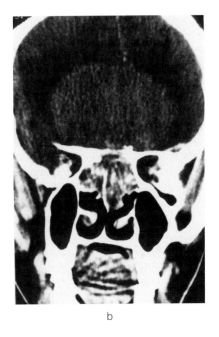

b

Fig. 23.6   a CT showing the large olfactory groove meningioma. (From Goel 1994b, with permission.) **b** Note the involvement of the ethmoid sinuses by the tumor. (From Goel 1994b, with permission.) **c** Postoperative skull X-ray shows that the bone flap occupies the region of resected tumor. Arrowhead shows the site from where the partial-thickness split cranial graft was taken. (From Goel 1994b, with permission.)

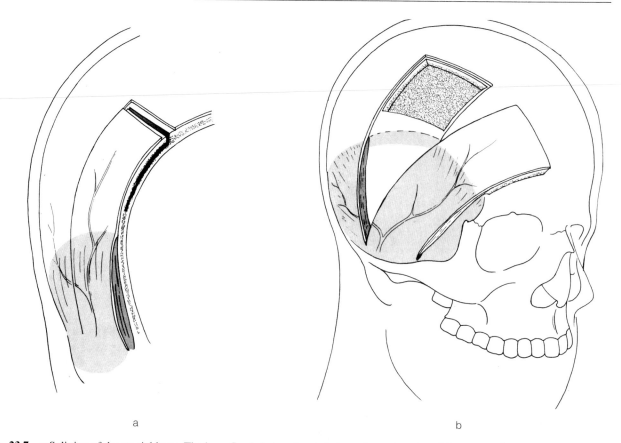

a   b

Fig. 23.7   **a** Splitting of the cranial bone. The bone flap is being elevated along the pericranium. The temporalis muscle and its fascial envelope form the pedicle of the flap. **b** Drawing shows how the described flap will be harvested and rotated towards the site of bone defect. The temporalis muscle has been split vertically.

carried out. The temporalis muscle with its overlying fascial layers and the pericranial layer is retained with the skull. The outer table of the skull bone is split as shown in Figure 23.7a, preserving the overlying pericranium. A part of the temporalis muscle (and fascial layers) along with the pericranium is elevated and rotated as required (Fig. 23.7b). The superficial fascial layer over the temporalis muscle is a part of the pericranial aponeurosis, whilst the deep temporal fascial layer completely invests the superficial aspect of the temporalis muscle. The temporalis muscle and its fascial envelope and the pericranium receive their blood supply from the anterior, middle and posterior deep temporal and superficial temporal arteries. Subperiosteal elevation of the temporalis muscle along with the fascial layers preserves the integrity of all the major vascular supply. The split or full-thickness cranial bone based on the pericranial layer and the temporalis musculofascial layer as described, results in a viable flap with abundance of vascular supply. Vertical splitting of the temporalis muscle into half or one-third would still preserve at least one or two of the main feeding vessels. This splitting would not adversely affect circulation to the flap and may help in preservation of the function of the tempo-

ralis muscle. The skull bone is thicker superior to the temporal line which marks the attachment of the temporalis muscle. Splitting of the skull bone is easier in the paramedian parietal bone due to the well-formed diploic channels. The split-thickness bone can be broken into pieces and can be suitably contoured, preserving the attachment of the pericranium. The long length, local availability and maneuverability of the flap make it versatile, with great potential for reconstruction of skull convexity and basal defects. The other advantages of such a flap include harvesting of grafts of adequate size, ease of access within the same operative field, and no or minimal postoperative morbidity and discomfort for the patient. The described flap can be used particularly to reconstruct cranial defects where there is poor local nourishment and potentially infective fields and areas which are cosmetically crucial.

Case 1

A 12-year-old boy underwent nephrectomy for a Wilm's tumor. He developed a swelling on the forehead considered to be a solitary metastasis from the kidney tumor. The swelling was treated by local irradiation, but local pain forced neurosurgical treatment. CT showed the bony lesion in the frontal midline over the forehead. Radiographs showed a sun-ray appearance of the lesion (Fig. 23.8a, b). The tumor was resected piecemeal with the help of a chisel and hammer and a micro-drill. After the entire tumor had been resected a large boney defect had been created. There was poor vascularity of the area secondary to local irradiation and it was considered that a free flap would not be suitable for the large defect. A vascularized pedicle temporalis musculofascial full-thickness bone flap was turned from the posterior frontoparietal region and placed over the bone defect and sutured in place. Splitting of the flap was not possible due to the thin skull bone in this child. Histological examination showed that the lesion was a benign fibrous dysplasia. The forehead contour was acceptable when the child was seen 6 months after the operation (Fig. 23.8c).

Case 2

A 32-year-old man was admitted with a complaint of frontal headache and a swelling on the right side of the forehead for 5 years. He also complained of diplopia and decreased vision in the right eye for 3 years. He had a well-circumscribed 6 × 6 cm bony swelling over the right supraorbital region. CT and magnetic resonance imaging (MRI) showed a right frontal extracerebral enhancing lesion extending into the ethmoid sinus. Thickening of the bone was noted (Fig. 23.9a, b). A transcranial biopsy by the otolaryngology unit confirmed that the lesion was a meningioma. Four weeks after the first procedure, the lesion was excised by the transcranial route. The pericranium was thickened and the region of the swelling was soft and friable bone. The bone swelling and the thickened pericranium were excised until normal areas were seen. The dura underneath the swelling was tumor ridden and was excised with intradural tumor. Tumor extension into the ethmoid sinus was removed en masse. The dural defect was covered by a pericranial graft. The bone defect was covered by a split-thickness posterior frontal flap with a vascularized pedicle based on the pericranium and temporalis muscle. The ethmoid sinus was packed with fat taken from the abdominal wall. The wounds healed well. When the patient was seen 4 months after the surgery the flap was well accepted (Fig. 23.9c).

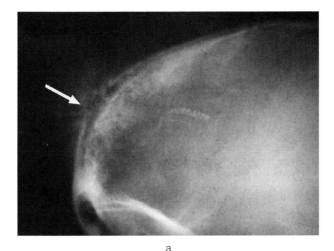

a

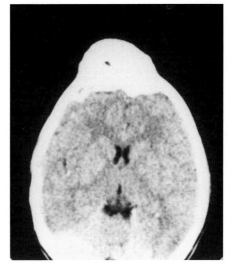

b

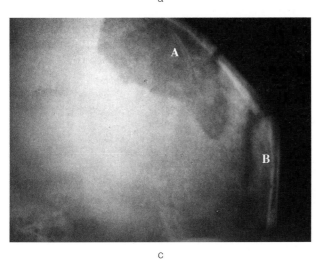

c

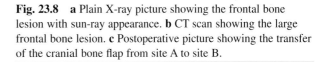

Fig. 23.8 **a** Plain X-ray picture showing the frontal bone lesion with sun-ray appearance. **b** CT scan showing the large frontal bone lesion. **c** Postoperative picture showing the transfer of the cranial bone flap from site A to site B.

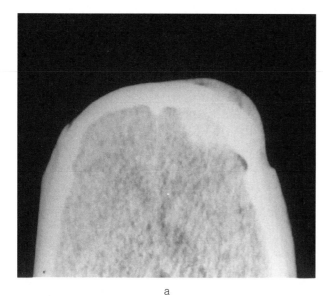

a

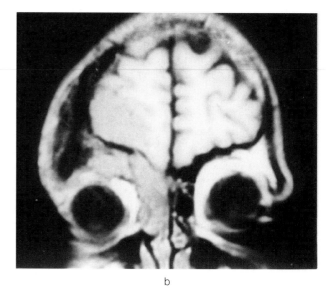

b

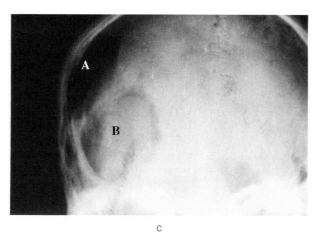

c

Fig. 23.9 **a** CT scan showing the extracerebral enhancing meningioma in the frontal region with hyperostotic bone changes. **b** MRI shows the frontal lesion and its extension into the ethmoid sinus. **c** Radiograph, with A suggesting the donor site where the cranial bone was slit and B showing the receptor area. (From Goel 1995a, with permission.)

Use of bone dust and debris

With the use of modern craniotomes for making burr holes, a large amount of bone dust can be obtained. Figure 23.10 shows the amount of bone dust obtained after drilling one burr hole. The bone dust can be flattened and placed in the form of a sheet over the site of defect. Small bone chips and bone debris which are generally available during a craniotomy can be placed interspersed in the bone dust. This forms a template over which new bone and fibrous tissue are laid and a firm, strong and resistant barrier is formed.

Reconstruction of skull base with free bone graft

Whenever possible bone defects should be filled with a

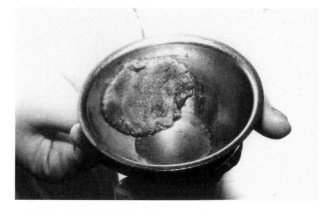

Fig. 23.10 The bone dust obtained after drilling one burr hole has been collected in a bowl and spread into a sheet.

vascularized pedicle bone flap. However, such a vascularized bone flap is sometimes not available and in this situation a free bone graft may be required. A free bone graft should not be directly exposed to the paranasal sinuses or mucosal surfaces. Whenever such a free bone graft is placed in the skull base, it should be as small as possible and care should be taken that it is covered on both sides with vascularized and viable soft tissue. Such a 'sandwich' free bone graft can be placed between muscle and fascial–pericranial layers. Postoperative collection of hematoma around the bone graft should also be avoided and whenever necessary external drains can be placed. Tenting scalp stitches can be used (Goel 1994c) whenever possible and indicated.

Suturing of bone pieces

Suturing of the small bone pieces, like those obtained after zygomatic and orbital osteotomy, should preferably be carried out with thin wires or unbraided silk or nylon stitches. As no significant movements are expected in the basal cranial bones use of miniplates, screws, and excessive volume of metal can be avoided.

Placement of soft tissue in place of bone, although not consistent with generally taught principles of reconstruction, can form a firm barrier of fibrous tissue and serve the purpose in cases of basal bone defects. Rotation of a vascularized pedicle muscle, pericranial or fascia flap or free fat graft or muscle can be performed to occupy the area of bone defect and empty spaces (Goel 1994c, Goel 1994d).

Subgaleal preservation of bone flaps
(Goel 1995c)

Convexity and basal bone flaps can be preserved in some rare situations like brain swelling, potentially infective operative fields and other such conditions and can be replaced to the original site after a period of time. Various techniques of preservation of bone flaps have been described, both inside and outside the body. The flaps have been more frequently and successfully stored in the subcutaneous plane of the abdominal wall or in the thigh (Fig. 23.11). External storage methods include deep freezing, autoclaving it while replacing, storing after radiation treatment and using antibiotic solutions.

An alternative method of preservation of the skull bone flap in the subgaleal space was found to be effective. The subgaleal plane adjacent to the site of operation is exposed widely using blunt dissection. The bone flap is placed in this plane, taking care that the curvature of the bone flap does not excessively elevate the scalp or cause tension over the scalp edges. In cases where larger subgaleal bone flaps are placed the curvature may necessitate fracturing of the bone flap in two or more pieces. The relative avascularity of the subgaleal plane helps in limiting the rate of reabsorption of the bone. There was no significant bone resorption in any of the patients in our series of 13 cases during the period of observation, which varied from 2 to 24 months. The subgaleal space can be easily exposed widely, providing a large area for bone placement. Such a

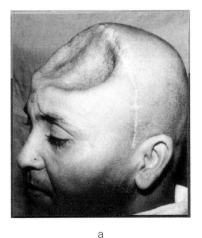

a

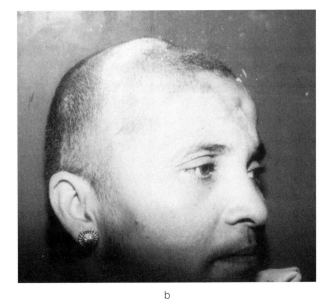

b

Fig. 23.11 **a** Profile of the patient with large anterior skull base defect. The bone flap was placed in the subcutaneous fat layer of the abdomen. **b** After 18 months the bone flap was replaced into the area of the defect resulting in satisfactory cosmesis.

large and avascular space is not available elsewhere in the body. Frequently the curvature of the bone flap matches that of the adjacent bone, which assists in the ease of placement. The flap is placed and replaced to the original site in one operative field. As no additional incision is necessary, the procedure is quick to perform. Whenever, such bone preservation is not anticipated the abdomen or thigh is not shaved or adequately prepared. Such maneuvers at the termination of a surgical procedure may not be satisfactorily performed, adding to the risk of infection. None of the patients in the presented series complained of any discomfort due to the flap placement.

Use of synthetic material in skull base bone reconstruction

Synthetic material is rarely required and advocated to reconstruct basal bone. Issues of biocompatibility, corrosion characteristics and metallurgic properties of the implant, hardness and malleability and suitability of the host area to adjust to the foreign intrusion and various other factors have to be adequately analyzed prior to selection of such material. Various substances including acrylic casts, plastics, glass-ionomer cement, silicone bars, proline mesh, stainless steel and titanium miniplates, screws and wires have been used. Such material is presently sometimes used whilst reconstructing cosmetically sensitive areas like orbital rim, zygomatic arch and for facial re-animation. Patients with large and complex bone defects sometimes present with major functional and esthetic disability. Adequate reconstruction is necessary and important to restore them to their accustomed way of life.

RECONSTRUCTION OF THE DURAL AND SOFT TISSUE DEFECTS

Dural closure

It is frequently not possible to perform a water tight dural closure in the base. Sometimes it is necessary to resect the basal dura after a tumor resection. Large spaces also need to be filled after tumor, bone and soft tissue resection.

Fat and free muscle as a packing material

Small and large pieces of fat have been effectively used for this purpose. The fat globules become vascularized early from the surrounding tissues. Whenever free muscle is being used as a packing material, it should be ground into small pieces so that these pieces can become vascularized from the surrounding tissues. If large pieces of muscle are

placed, it becomes vascularized from the periphery and the central portions of the tissue can become necrotic. Such a necrosed tissue can be absorbed or even pose a problem of infection. A free tissue should never be placed over a free tissue as this procedure can lead to ischemic necrosis of the tissue most distant from the vascularized structures.

Lyophilized dura and fascia lata

These dural substitutes have been used extensively and successfully for basal reconstruction. However, whenever possible a live and vascularized pedicle fascial material may be used to obtain a compact closure.

Use of pericranial and galeal flaps

Pericranial and galeal flaps have been extensively used for reconstruction of basal defects. Their use is more effectively possible for reconstruction of bone and dural defects in the anterior cranial base. The pericranium contains an extensive vascular network and forms an effective flap. It comprises an outer layer of loose aereolar tissue and an inner layer of osteoblasts and derives blood supply anteriorly from the supratrochlear and supraorbital arteries and laterally from the superficial temporal arteries. Pericranial layer pedicled flaps can be based on either of these vessels, and accordingly rotated anteriorly or laterally. The pericranium is thin in the region of frontal bosses and over the region of parietal convexity and can be torn easily if insufficient care is taken while harvesting the flap.

Use of rotation of muscle flap

Temporalis muscle can be effectively rotated to cover middle fossa defects. Sternocleidomastoid and other muscles of the nape of the neck can be rotated superiorly to cover defects in posterior cranial basal defects.

Extended vascularized temporalis muscle-fascia flap (Goel 1994c)

The deep layer of the temporalis fascia is everted partially over the temporalis muscle, preserving its vascularity. A composite flap comprising temporalis muscle and its fascia attached along its superior border is rotated for reconstruction of postoperative defects in the middle cranial fossa floor and mastoidectomy cavities (Fig. 23.14c). Partial eversion of the temporalis fascia over the muscle increases the length of the flap while retaining its vascular pedicle. The long-length vascularized pedicle flap can be used to cover defects, may be folded for bulk and may be used to carry blood supply to poorly vascularized recipient sites. Such a flap can be effectively used to line the middle cranial fossa floor and mastoidectomy defects. Similar flaps using the thinner superficial layer of temporalis fascia have been used in craniofacial reconstruction (Casanova et al 1986), filling up post-traumatic defects in the anterior cranial fossa and for facial reanimation (Mathog & Ragab, 1985, Renner et al 1984). As discussed above, the superficial temporal fascial layer is part of the pericranial aponeurosis whilst the deep temporal fascial layer invests the superficial aspects of the temporalis muscle down to the zygomatic arch. These fascial layers have a separate arterial and venous supply and have been used as a homograft, a rotation flap or free microvascular flap. The deep temporalis fascia is separated from the superficial fascia by a plane of loose aereolar tissue (subgaleal fascia – discussed later). The temporalis muscle and the deep layer of the fascia receive their blood supply from the anterior, middle and posterior deep temporal arteries. These vessels run between the muscle and the periosteum, and subperiosteal elevation of this fan-shaped muscle results in a viable muscle flap. The deep layer of the temporalis fascia is nourished by multiple small branches which traverse through the muscle. Partial eversion of the deep layer of fascia with an attempt to preserve small vascular connections can result in a long vascularized flap.

Fat and free muscle have been effectively used as a packing material of mastoidectomy defects. However, in some cases, particularly where there is infection in the receptor area, vascularized pedicle graft may be necessary. Temporalis muscle can be easily rotated to cover the mastoid defects. However, the length of the muscle is not sufficient for it to be used to pack large mastoid bone defects. Also, often the thickness of the muscle restricts its rotation and laying on the middle fossa base. Rotation of muscle flap from the neck or provision of a distant muscle flap (viz., rectus abdominis) with microvascular anastomosis can be used in such a situation. However, an extended temporalis muscle-fascia flap provides a simple, easily maneuverable and locally available alternative. A similar flap can also be used for reconstruction of large defects in the middle cranial fossa base.

Case 1

Radical resection of a massive recurrent petrous bone cholesteatoma was carried out in a 60-year-old patient. A large part of the petrous bone, including the condyle of the occipital bone, was destroyed by the tumor. The nerves in the internal auditory meatus were involved by the cholesteatoma and were sacrificed. The dural defect in the region of the internal auditory canal was sutured with absorbable sutures. The external ear canal was left open after meatoplasty to provide for drainage of

cholesteatoma. The large mastoid defect was packed with a free fat graft taken from the abdominal wall. On the third postoperative day, the patient developed profuse CSF leak from the ear. A lumbar thecoperitoneal shunt was performed. However, the CSF leak continued. Meanwhile, there was pus discharge from the mastoid wound and meningitis developed. A persistent CSF leak in an infected wound was a threat to life. The wound was reopened and the free graft was removed. The CSF fistula site at the internal auditory meatus was identified. Attempted resuturing of the defect failed as the dura was very fragile in the region. There was no alternative but to provide a vascularized pedicle flap with which to pack the mastoid defect. An attempt was made to rotate the temporalis muscle into the receptor area, but the length of the muscle was insufficient. The deep temporalis fascia was everted partially over the muscle, and the muscle with the fascia attached along its superior border was rotated into the region, thus providing the crucial extra length of vascularized graft (Fig. 23.14c). The fascia was stabilized in the region by a stay suture. Adequate antibiotic cover was provided. The CSF leak stopped and the wound healed without incident.

Extended subgaleal fascia–pericranial temporalis flap (Goel & Gahankari 1995)

A long pericranial flap can be used to line an anterior skull base defect. The temporalis muscle is rotated along the pericranial flap and forms the vascular pedicle of the flap. Subgaleal fascia is preserved to enhance the vascularity of this long flap. Subgaleal fascia – known previously as the 'loose aereolar tissue layer' of the scalp and believed to be a relatively avascular zone – has now been shown to have an independent and extensive blood supply entering it at the base of the cranial vault circumferentially. Casanova et al (1985) called the same layer the innominate fascia. It is a thin but well-defined trilaminar fibrous structure and a discretely separable layer. The superficial temporal artery and its branches which supply the galea also give off minute but many branches (Tremolada et al 1994) to the subgaleal fascia, which is closely approximated to the pericranial layer. The blood supply to the subgaleal fascia is also enhanced by vascular connections with branches of the deep temporal arteries which supply the temporalis muscle and its fascial coverings. The pericranial layer and subgaleal fascia are continuous laterally with the superficial layer of the temporalis muscle. The pericranial layer is supplied by the perforating branches of the superficial temporal artery which traverse the subgaleal fascia and those of deep temporal arteries which traverse through the temporalis muscle and its fascial envelope. There are also a few vascular channels connecting the pericranium with the meningeal vessels (Abul Hassan et al 1986, Chazen & Nathan 1974, Marty et al 1986, Price et al 1988). Preservation of the subgaleal fascia and subperiosteal elevation of the temporalis muscle along with the fascial layers maintain the integrity of the major vascular supply to the pericranial layer. It is presumed that such a twin source of vascular supply may sustain a long length of pericranial flap. Although laterally based pericranial flaps are described for covering anterior central skull base defects, successful use of such a flap taken beyond the midline has not been reported (Fig. 23.12). The rotation of the pericranial flap along with the temporalis muscle and its fascial layers forms a viable flap. While elevating the pericranial flap some of the subgaleal fascia is almost always included. A specific attempt to preserve this layer by conscious and careful dissection from the galea in an attempt to preserve additional vascular supply to the pericranial layer may be critically important in long pericranial flaps as described. Although the temporalis muscle can be used in its entirety, vertical splitting of the temporalis muscle into half or one-third would preserve at least one or two of the main feeding vessels.

The described flap can sometimes be used to reconstruct cranial defects where there is poor local nourishment and in potentially infective fields. Relative ease of harvesting and the ability to alter the arc of rotation of this flap can be effectively used.

Case 1

A 45-year-old man, a known diabetic and hypertensive, was operated by a frontal basal approach for a massive sellar and parasellar tumor. A bicoronal scalp flap was taken which was followed by a bifrontal basal craniotomy. The cribriform plate and a part of the planum sphenoidale were removed during the exposure. A subtotal resection of the tumor was achieved. During the operation rents were created in the basal dural inadvertently. Rotation of the anteriorly based pericranial flap to the base was not possible as this layer was torn in several places during the eversion. A layer of galea from the scalp was rotated to the base for reconstruction. Fat was taken from the abdominal wall and stuffed into the exposed sinuses. Frontobasal ducts were carefully packed. A lumbar thecoperitoneal shunt was performed to prevent CSF leakage.

The patient, however, developed severe meningitis. Purulent discharge was noted from the nose. On the 10th postoperative day, following a fit, he became severely drowsy. CT scan showed that there was a large amount of intracranial air and subdural fluid collection. He also developed pneumonia for which tracheostomy was done.

Reconstruction of the persistent anterior cranial base defect was planned. His toxic state and poor general condition did not permit any elaborate reconstructive procedure, such as the use

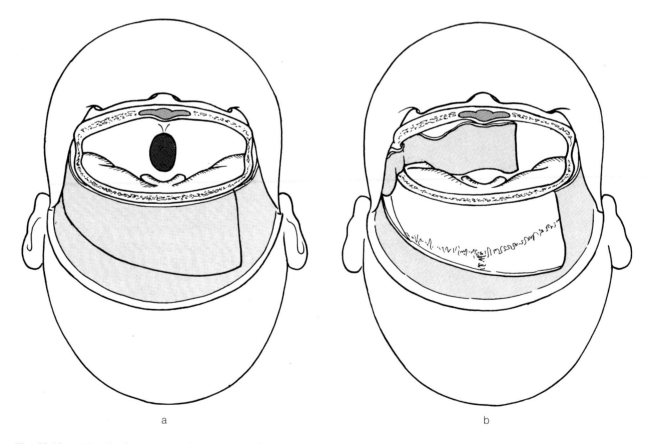

a

b

Fig. 23.12   a The site from where a long subgaleal fascia pericranial flap will be harvested. **b** After rotation of the long subgaleal fascia–pericranial flap it adequately covers the site of the anterior cranial floor defect.

of a distant flap with microvascular anastomosis. The scalp wound was reopened. The absence of galea and pericranial layer from the scalp flap, and the desperate need for a vascular flap, forced us to use the described flap.

The scalp posterior to the bicoronal incision was everted, preserving the subgaleal fascia over the pericranial layer. A long length of the subgaleal fascia–pericranial flap could be obtained and was rotated along with the entire temporalis muscle (Fig. 23.13). The length and size of the flap measuring 18 × 7 cm even permitted double breasting of the flap at the site of dural defect. The flap took well and the patient rapidly improved.

Muscle–fascia flap

The temporalis muscle along with its fascial coverings can be rotated along with the pericranium to form a long flap. The fascial cover of the temporalis muscle can be everted as shown in Figures 14a, b to form a thick peripheral flap.

MULTILAYERED BASAL RECONSTRUCTION (Goel 1996)

Multilayer reconstruction of middle fossa base

Frequently there are large dead spaces that need to be filled after basal bone, soft tissue and tumor resection. Such spaces can be a site for collection of hematoma or CSF loculation. Both these events may enhance the possibilities of infection and CSF fistulae. Use of multiple layers of vascularized tissue for reconstruction not only provides a compact sealing of the defect, but by virtue of its volume helps in reducing the dead space. Two methods of multilayer reconstruction of the middle cranial basal defects are shown in Figure 23.14. The procedure involves use of an osteomyoplastic flap which was placed over one of the two described types of temporalis muscle–fascia flap.

As mentioned earlier, the superficial fascial layer covering the temporalis muscle is a part of the pericranial aponeurosis. Over the temporalis muscle it is relatively thin. The temporalis muscle and its two fascial coverings receive their blood supply from the anterior, middle and posterior deep temporal and superficial temporal arteries. The pericranium receives its blood supply circumferentially. On the lateral aspect its chief source of vascular nourishment is through the vessels feeding the superficial layer of the temporalis muscle. The deep temporal arteries traverse through the muscle and supply the two fascial layers from their deep surface, while the superficial temporal artery supplies these layers in a reverse direction from superficial to deep layer. Elevation of the pericranial layer along with the temporalis muscle and fascial layers as shown in Figure 23.28a, b, results in a long viable flap with

abundance of vascular supply. In situations where this flaps is sufficiently thick it can be used as the *primary* flap. Whenever the pericranial part of the flap is not very thick, or for some reason cannot be harvested, a muscle–fascia flap (described earlier) can be rotated. In this method, partial eversion of the superficial and the deep layers of the temporalis fascia by cutting these two layers just above the zygomatic arch (Fig. 23.14b–d) is performed. The peripheral part of the flap now has three fascial layers comprising pericranium and superficial and deep layers of temporalis fascia. This makes the distal end of the flap relatively thick. The proximal end of the flap is formed by the full thickness of the muscle. The result is a long and thick flap. Vertical splitting of the temporalis muscle into half or one-third would still preserve at least one or two of the main feeding vessels. This splitting would not adversely affect circulation to the flap. The anterior or posterior part of the split temporalis muscle can be used to harvest a vascularized pedicle osteomyoplastic flap (Fig. 23.14a–d). This forms the *secondary* flap. Split or full-thickness bone can be used. The bone piece can be fractured into two or more pieces, retaining its attachment to the muscle so that its contour can be adjusted to suit the local environment. The *primary* flap consisting of either of the two types of muscle–fascial flap is first placed over the site of middle fossa bone defect (Fig. 23.14e) over which the *secondary* osteomyoplastic flap is placed (Fig. 23.14f). This forms a compact and multilayered construct of vascularized pedicle flaps. Whenever it is felt that bone replacement over the site of the defect is not essential only soft tissue flaps may be used. The temporal bone defect resulting from

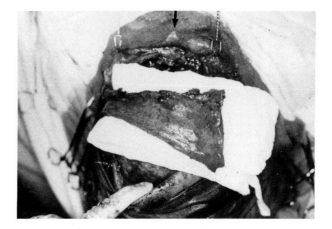

Fig. 23.13 Intraoperative photograph showing the extended subgaleal fascia–pericranial temporalis flap placed over the surgical mop. The exposure is basal frontal. Anteriorly the scalp flap is everted by hooks. Posteriorly the surgeon's index finger is retracting the scalp flap, exposing the cranial bone from where the flap is raised. Arrow indicates the midline. (From Goel & Gahankari 1995, with permission.)

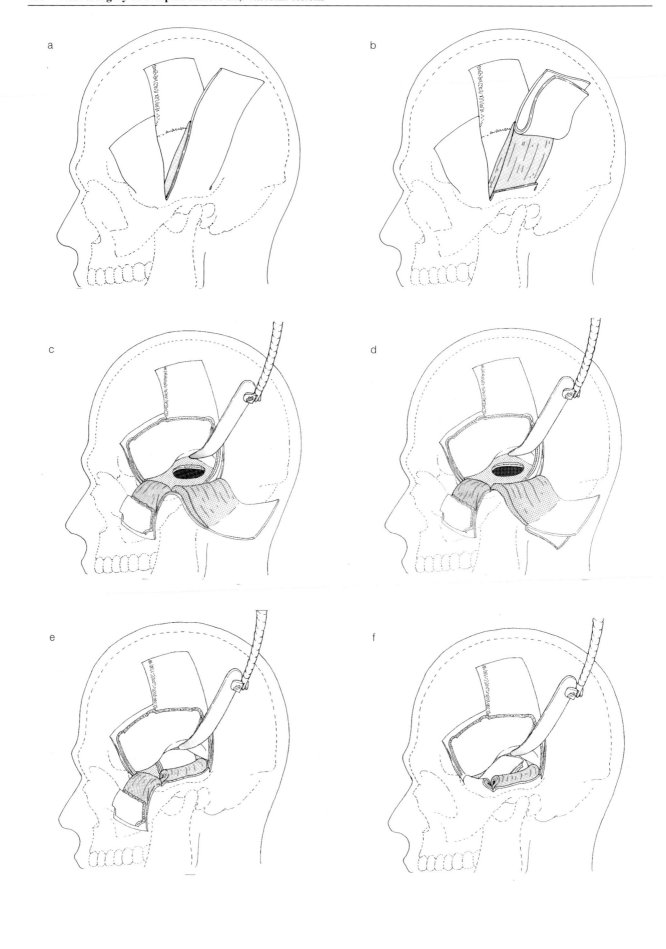

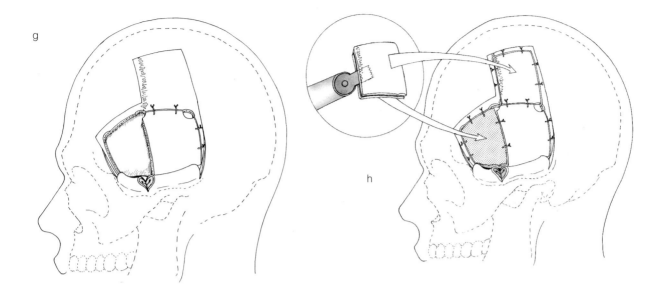

Fig. 23.14 Multilayered vascularized flap. **a** Fashioning of the flap. The temporalis muscle is split into two parts. The anterior part is used to harvest an osteomyoplastic flap (secondary flap) while in the posterior part the temporalis muscle and its fascial envelope are elevated along with the pericranial layer of the parietal bone (primary flap). This forms a long vascularized pedicled temporalis muscle–pericranial flap (primary flap). **b** The deep and superficial fascial layers of the temporalis muscle are cut at the inferior aspect and rotated superiorly towards the pericranial layer. This procedure makes the distal segment of the vascularized flap relatively thick (primary flap). **c** Craniectomy. The temporal brain is retracted to expose the middle cranial fossa bone defect. The anterior half of the flap is an osteomyoplastic flap (secondary flap), while the posterior half of the flap is a long temporalis muscle–fascia–pericranial flap (primary flap). **d** The primary flap is a thick muscle fascia flap. **e** The primary flap (which can be as described in Figure 23.13a or b) is rotated first towards the middle fossa floor defect. **f** The secondary osteomyoplastic flap is then rotated so that it lies on the previously laid primary flap. This results in the formation of multilayer construct with vascularized pedicle flaps. **g** The posterior half of the free squamous temporal bone is replaced at its original site after the basal reconstruction. The anterior half of the temporal bone defect remains. **h** Parietal bone flap (from where the pericranium is harvested) is elevated and split into two halves. The temporal bone defect is reconstructed with the inner table of the bone flap (as shown in the insert) and sutured in situ.

basal rotation can be reconstructed with split cranial bone flaps as shown in Figures 23.14g, h.

In most cases of middle fossa defects a simpler method of reconstruction may suffice. However, in an occasional case with a complex defect, information about the feasibility of the described method of reconstruction may be a useful adjunct. The multilayered reconstruction, as discussed, could be performed as a radical measure in situations where problems of CSF fistula or those related to herniation of brain matter are anticipated, or where earlier attempts at reconstruction have failed. Such a multilayered flap fashioned entirely with vascularized pedicles, by virtue of its bulk and long length, can be used to cover bone defects, may be folded for bulk and may be used to carry blood supply to poorly vascularized recipient sites. In an occasional case of CSF otorrhoea, such an elaborate reconstruction could be a life-saving operation.

Case 1

A 4-year-old boy was noticed to have a small swelling in the external ear canal for 6 months. For 3 months there was an associated intermittent clear fluid discharge from the ear. There

was no evidence of meningitis. The child was otherwise active and playful. He had a mild right infranuclear facial paresis and conductive deafness in the right ear. The swelling in the external auditory meatus was soft and compressible in nature (Fig. 23.15a). Examination of the fluid discharge from the ear was consistent with CSF. CT scanning (Fig. 23.15b) and MRI (Fig. 23.15c) revealed a large defect in the floor of the middle cranial fossa and the tegmen tympani through which a temporal brain herniation was seen extending into the infratemporal fossa, middle ear, external ear canal and parapharyngeal region. The various issues involved in surgical treatment were analyzed and a multilayered flap was planned. The necrotic herniated brain was resected and the large basal dural and bone defect was identified. The bone covering the petrous carotid artery and the Eustachian tube was eroded and these structures were exposed on removal of the brain matter. The greater and lesser petrosal nerves were not identified during surgery. The middle ear cavity was completely occupied by the herniated brain tissue. The herniated brain was resected. The tympanic segment of the facial nerve was denuded of bone. Direct pressure of the brain over this segment of the nerve appeared to be the cause of his facial nerve weakness. After resection of the herniated brain tissue the middle ear cavity and the Eustachian tube, external ear canal and the intracranial cavity communicated freely. The multilayer reconstruction is shown in the Figure 23.14. A 3 ×

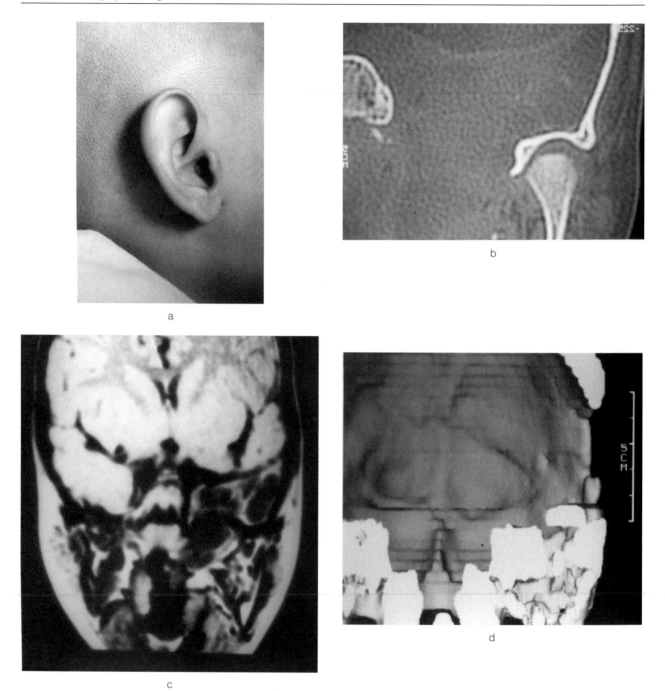

Fig. 23.15 **a** A small swelling is seen in the external ear canal. The photograph does not clearly show the leaking CSF. (From Goel 1996, with permission.) **b** CT scan showing the large defect in the floor of the middle cranial fossa. (From Goel 1996, with permission.) **c** MRI showing the herniation of a multicystic temporal lobe into the infratemporal fossa. (From Goel 1996, with permission.) **d** Postoperative three-dimensional CT scan shows the large defect in the petrous bone roofed almost completely by the rotated bone flap. (From Goel 1996, with permission.)

3 cm portion of full-thickness temporal squamous bone was retained with the anterior half of the split temporalis muscle. A small defect in the skin of the external ear canal was left unrepaired. The patient had no further CSF otorrhoea. At 14 months follow-up the child was asymptomatic. His facial paresis completely recovered. He was deaf in the right ear. A

three-dimensional CT scan showed that the large middle fossa and petrous bone defect was almost completely covered with the bone flap (Fig. 23.15d).

Another patient with a large defect in the floor of the middle cranial fossa as a result of a large epidermal cyst was treated with multilayer reconstruction (Fig. 23.16).

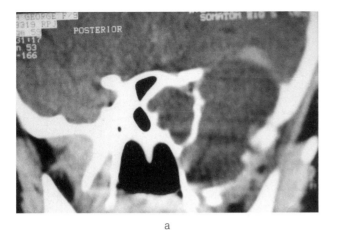

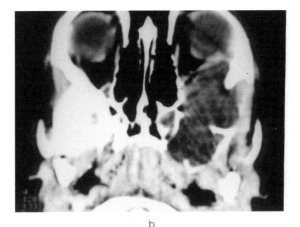

a

b

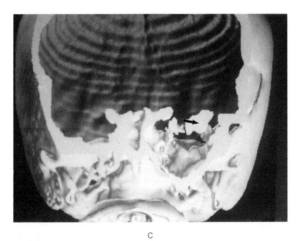

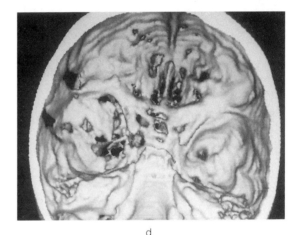

c

d

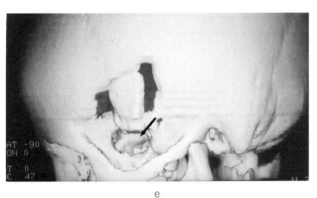

e

Fig. 23.16 **a** CT scan showing a large defect in the middle fossa floor as a result of a large epidermal cyst. **b** Axial cut showing the extent of the cyst and the bone defect. **c** Three-dimensional scan, the arrow showing the rotated temporal bone flap in a multilayer construct. **d** Arrow shows the middle fossa defect covered by temporal squamous bone flap. **e** Arrow shows the basally displaced temporal squamous bone flap.

Multilayer reconstruction of the anterior cranial fossa floor (Goel, 1994d)

Multiple combinations of flaps can be used to cover anterior cranial basal defects. Two multilayer flaps are shown in Figures 23.17 and 23.18. The flaps may comprise only soft tissues (Fig. 23.17) or may include a bone piece (Fig. 23.18).

A bicoronal incision is made and scalp flaps are reflect-ed both anteriorly and posteriorly in the subgaleal plane. The pericranium over the frontal bosses is relatively thin and harvesting an intact pericranial flap could be difficult. Whenever such an elevation is possible the frontal pericranium can be rotated over the defect in the anterior cranial base. Everting the posterior part of the scalp results in a wide exposure of the pericranium over the parietal or even occipital region. Harvesting a long pericranial flap based on the temporalis muscle and its fascial cover from both

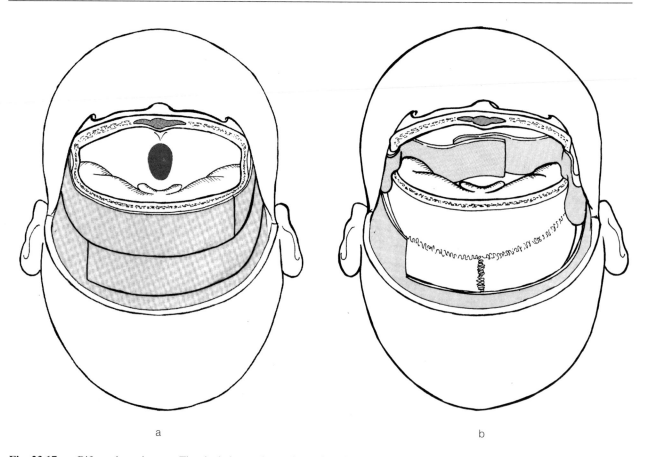

a   b

Fig. 23.17 **a** Bifrontal craniotomy. The shaded area shows the pericranial cover of the skull bone. The transverse lines show the sites of pericranial layer incision for the purpose of harvesting the flaps. **b** The two pericranial flaps from both sides are harvested and rotated along with the temporalis muscle towards the defect in the anterior skull base, one over the other, forming a multilayer reconstruction.

sides and rotating them over the anterior cranial fossa defect can result in a multilayer closure. The long length of the flaps can be useful in placing the flaps loosely or even double-breasting it over the defect.

Whenever it is felt that addition of bone is necessary for adequate reconstruction, a vascularized pericranial-based bone flap as described earlier can be used. The split or full-thickness bone flap can also be pedicled on a laterally based pericranial flap. A long pericranial flap is harvested from the contralateral side as shown in Figures 23.17 and 23.18. Both these pericranial flaps (one containing bone piece) are then rotated along with the temporalis muscle and its fascial coverings. On both sides the temporalis muscle can be split vertically to retain its function. On one side the anterior portion of the split muscle is used as the base of the pericranial flap over the anterior parietal region, while on the other side the posterior portion of the split muscle forms the base of the pericranial flap over the posterior parietal region. A specific attempt is made to pre-serve the subgaleal fascia to enhance the vascularity of the designed flaps. Both these flaps are rotated anteriorly and laid down one over the other in the region of the defect in the base. The vascularized pedicle bone flap is placed superior to these flaps so as to avoid direct exposure of the bone to the paranasal sinuses.

Case 1

A 10-year-old girl complained of a blocked nose for 6 months. She had a nasal twang to her speech, and had oral breathing. On examination she was noticed to have temporal field defects in both eyes. CT scan showed a massive bony tumor occupying the nasopharynx, sphenoid and posterior ethmoid sinuses which displaced the anterior cranial fossa floor, including the sella, planum sphenoidale superiorly sella, and stretched the optic nerves laterally (Fig. 23.19). A transcranial basal frontal approach was considered safe and suitable for surgical resection of the tumor. The basal bone was destroyed by the tumor and some bone had to be resected to obtain the exposure. These problems were anticipated prior to surgery and a multiple-layer flap as described was harvested at the time of the exposure.

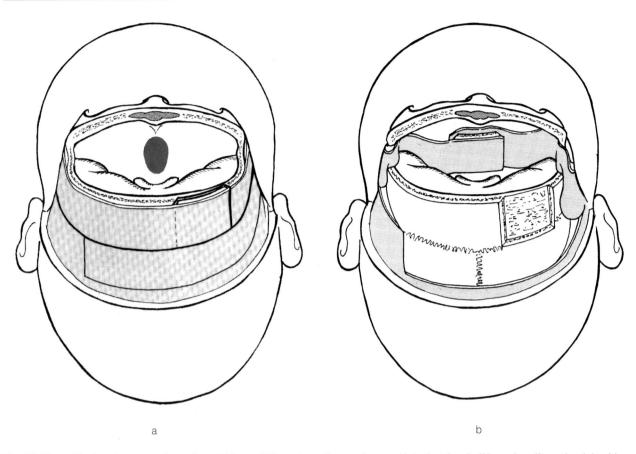

Fig. 23.18   a The incisions over the pericranial layer. Bifrontal craniotomy is seen. Note that the skull bone is split on the right side so that it can be rotated along with the pericranium to form a vascularized pedicled bone flap. **b** Anterior cranial basal multilayer reconstruction.

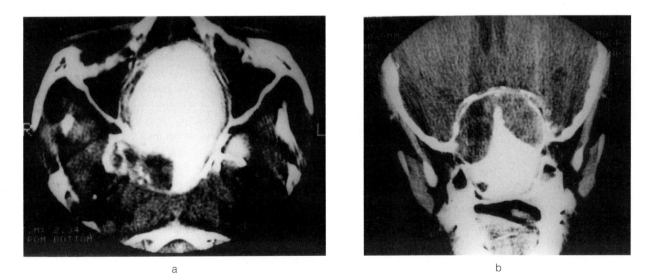

Fig. 23.19   a CT scan showed a massive bony tumor occupying the nasopharynx, sphenoid and posterior ethmoid sinuses, which displaced the anterior cranial fossa floor including the sella, planum sphenoidale superiorly sella, and stretched the optic nerves laterally. Multilayer reconstruction was used to repair the skull defect after tumor excision. **b** Axial view of the CT scan showing the large bony tumor.

Use of outer layer of dura as a pedicled flap (Goel 1995b)

Cranial dura is formed by two layers: the outer endosteal layer and the inner meningeal layer. These layers are well defined and 'separable' by manual dissection, particularly in younger individuals. The dura is supplied by multiple small and medium-sized arteries circumferentially. The meningeal blood vessels are largely located in the endosteal layer. When preserved intact the outer endosteal layer can be rotated and used to cover defects in the proximity. The principal advantage of using such a material is that it may be used as a vascularized pedicle flap or a free graft (Fig. 23.20). The consistency and quality of the material match with that of adjacent dura. Local availability and ease of rotation of this flap are the other advantages. Despite the limitations in using this flap due to technical difficulties in separating the layers, it can come in useful in an occasional patient.

Case 1

A 35-year-old man was operated on for a large petroclival chordoma. A Gigli's guide was passed between two burr holes during the procedure of temporal craniotomy. Accidentally, the guide passed between the two dura layers, giving the impression, when observed from the distal burr hole, that it had pierced the dura. After readjustment of the guide the craniotomy was completed. It was observed that the guide had widely separated the dural layers. The layers were gently peeled further. A large additional layer of dura that resulted was used to partially cover mastoid air cells which had been packed earlier with bone wax (Fig. 23.20).

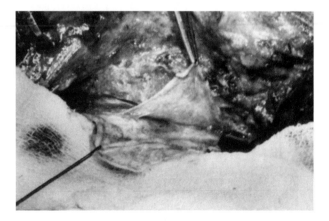

Fig. 23.20 Operative picture showing the two slit dural layers. The layer held by a stay suture is the cerebral layer, while that held by forceps is the endosteal layer. The endosteal layer was rotated to cover the mastoid air cells. (From Goel 1995b, with permission.)

Lumbar drainage of CSF

Many groups prefer lumbar drainage of CSF following skull basal surgical procedure. Such a procedure is seldom required. In the event of postoperative CSF fistula lumbar drainage of CSF may be performed only if basal reconstruction has been elaborate. The potential for ascending infections following lumbar drainage should be kept in mind while performing this procedure. In cases where basal reconstruction is not considered to be adequate it is preferable to consolidate the reconstruction by re-exploration of the entire wound rather than resorting to lumbar drainage.

Tenting scalp stitches (Goel 1992)

Postoperative collections underneath the scalp are common, although are usually no more than a nuisance to the surgeon and the patient. However, sometimes these collections can be a source of secondary complications such as wound breakdown and infection. Such complications are particularly relevant after a long skull base operation. The problem can occur after an osteoplastic craniotomy when the collection develops between the galea and the pericranium, or following free bone flap exposure in which case the collection is between the pericranial layer and the bone flap. Suction drains and tight head dressings are frequently used at the time of closure to avoid this problem. Occasionally, there is a need to drain the collection and approximate the scalp layers by a large bore needle, and sometimes lumbar drainage of CSF may be necessary. Suction or gravity drains often become clogged, or only approximate the layers of the scalp in a limited area. They cannot be used for long periods because of the risk of infection. Tight head dressings loosen over a period of time, can be a source of discomfort to the patient, and occasionally compromise the blood supply of the skin flap.

'Tenting' sutures of the dura are routine after every craniotomy. These stitches help to prevent the occurrence and expansion of extradural collections. The stitches shown in Figures 23.21 and 23.22 are similar in principle and action for the scalp. This is a simple and non-time-consuming technique. The sutures help to seal surgically created space between the layers of the scalp and act as internal compression. The closer approximation of the scalp to the bone improves the vascularity of the bone by providing an additional pathway for the blood supply in the initial postoperative phase.

Technique

After adequate hemostasis when the scalp is reflected back for closure, three to four (or more) sutures are placed between the galea and pericranium as shown in

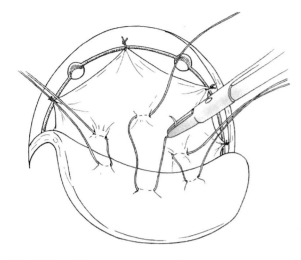

Fig. 23.21   Galea to pericranium stitches.

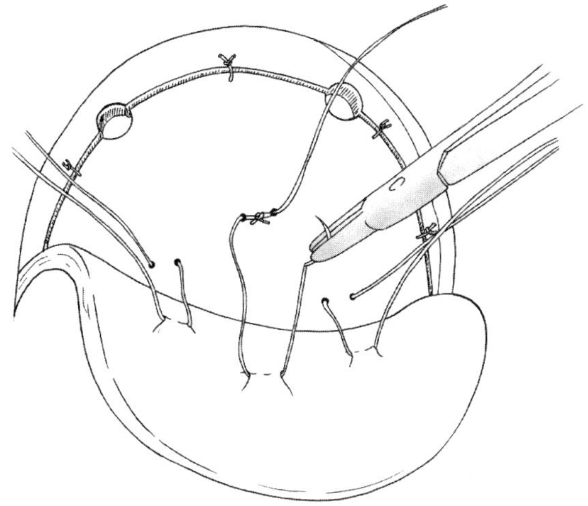

Fig. 23.22   Galea–pericranial layer bone flap stitches. Note that the dural tenting sutures have already been placed and tied in the central bone holes.

Figure 23.21. The site of the sutures is carefully judged so that the scalp wound can approximate closely. It is usually easier to place the sutures at a distance of about 5 cm from the scalp incision. The greater the number of sutures placed, the more compact is the closure of the layers. It is easier to tie knots after all the sutures have traversed the layers. In the case of a free bone flap, the pericranial layer is sutured to the bone after drilling holes in the bone. The holes used for 'tenting' the dura in the center of the bone flap can be used for this purpose (Fig. 23.22).

REFERENCES

Abul Hassan H S, von Drasek Ascher G, Acland R D 1986 Surgical anatomy and blood supply of the fascial layers of the temporal region. Plastic and Reconstructive Surgery 77: 17–28

Antonyshyn O, Cocleugh R F, Hurst L N et al 1986 The temporalis myo-osseous flap: an experimental study. Plastic and Reconstructive Surgery 77(3): 406–415

Bite U, Jackson I T, Wahner H W et al 1987 Vascularized skull bone grafts in craniofacial surgery. Annals of Plastic Surgery 19(1): 3–15

Casanova R, Cavalcante D, Grotting J C et al 1985 Anatomic basis for vascularized outer-table calvarial bone flaps. Plastic and Reconstructive Surgery 78: 300–308

Chazen D, Nathan H 1974 Anatomical observations on the subgaleotic fascia of the scalp. Acta Anatomica 87: 427–431

Choung P H, Nam I W, Kim K S 1991 Vascularized cranial bone grafts for mandibular and maxillary reconstruction: the parietal osteofascial flap. Journal of Craniomaxillofacial Surgery 19: 235–242

Combelles R, Zadeh J 1984 Temporalis osteomuscular flap: anatomical study and experimental and surgical technique. Revenue de Stomatologie et de Chirurgie Maxillofaciale 85: 351–354

Cutting C B, McCarthy J G, Berenstein A 1984 Blood supply of the upper craniofacial skeleton: the search for composite calvarial bone flaps. Plastic and Reconstructive Surgery 74: 603–610

Fasano D, Menoni V, Riberti C et al 1987 The temporalis osteomuscular flap versus the free calvarial bone graft: an experimental study in growing rabbit. Journal of Craniomaxillofacial Surgery 15(6): 332–341

Goel A 1992 'Tenting' stitches for the scalp. British Journal of Neurosurgery 6: 357–358

Goel A 1994a Vascularized osteomyoplastic flap for skull base reconstruction. British Journal of Neurosurgery 8: 79–82

Goel A 1994b Vascularized bone flap for skull base reconstruction. Acta Neurochirurgica 128: 166–168

Goel A 1994c Extended temporalis muscle–fascia flap. British Journal of Neurosurgery 8: 731–733

Goel A 1994d Multilayered vascularized pedicle reconstruction of the anterior cranial fossa floor. Paper presented in the fifth advanced course in head and neck cancer surgery, organized by the Singapore Society for Head and Neck cancer surgery, 21–23 November

Goel A 1995a Long vascular pedicle composite cranial flap. British Journal of Neurosurgery 9: 667–670

Goel A 1995b Use of outer layer of dura as a pedicled flap. Surgical Neurology 44: 92–93

Goel A 1995c Subgaleal preservation of the calvarial bone flap. Surgical Neurology 44: 181–183

Goel A 1996 Multilayered vascularized pedicle reconstruction of the middle fossa floor. Acta Neurochirurgica (Wien) 138: 584–589

Goel A, Gahankari D 1995 Extended subgaleal
fascia–pericranial temporalis flap for skull base
reconstruction. Acta Neurochirurgica (Wien) 135: 203–205

Marty F, Montandon D, Guniener R, Zbrodowski A (1986)
Subcutaneous tissue in the scalp: anatomical, physiological
and clinical study. Annals of Plastic Surgery 16: 368–376

Mathog R H, Ragab M A 1985 Temporalis muscle–galea flap in
facial reanimation. Archives of Otolaryngology. 111:
168–173

Price J C, Loury M, Carson et al 1988 The pericranial flap for
reconstruction of anterior skull base defects. Laryngoscope
98: 1159–1164

Renner G, Davis W E, Templer J 1984 Temporalis pericranial
muscle flap for reconstruction of the lateral face and head.
Laryngoscope 94: 1418–1422

Snyderman C H, Janecka I P, Sekhar L N et al 1990 Anterior
cranial base reconstruction: role of galeal and pericranial
flaps. Laryngoscope 100: 607–614

Tremolada C, Candiani P, Signorini M et al (1994) The surgical
anatomy of the subcutaneous fascial system of the scalp.
Annals of Plastic Surgery 32: 8–14

Watson Jones R 1993 The repair of the skull defects by a new
pedicle bone-graft operation. British Medical Journal 1: 780

Computers in neurosurgery

Hiroshi Okudera   Shigeaki Kobayashi   Kazuhiro Hongo

GENERAL CONSIDERATIONS

Innovations and progress in computer technology have had a remarkable influence in neurosurgical practice. Some techniques using computer technology improvised and developed by us are discussed in this section.

Intraoperative computed tomography scanner system

Planning an approach and intraoperative strategy only on the basis of topographic measurements taken from the preoperative computed tomography (CT) scan can sometimes be inadequate. This is because the structural shift of the lesion (Okudera et al 1994c) and the brain matter may occur during the surgery secondary to manipulation, brain edema or hemorrhage. We have developed a CT scanner

system for use in the operating room (Fig. 24.1). The prototype consists of a CT scanner system (TCT-300), Toshiba, Tokyo), operating table with a digital connector (MST-7100B, Mizuho, Tokyo) and a modified head fixation system (Okudera et al 1992) (Fig. 24.2).

For feasibility of use of CT scanner in the operating room various technical problems have to be overcome. The gantry of the CT scanner system is mobilized by a gantry carrier (Okudera et al 1991c). The scanner gantry can be moved within a range of 10 m (Fig. 24.3). Such a range of mobility is usually sufficient for actual use in the operating room. The gantry can move in any direction like an ordinary mobile X-ray unit.

We have designed a special digitally controlled operating table (Okudera et al 1990b). A digital-control power unit and an encoder system are installed in the operating table so that table motion can be controlled directly from the computer of the CT. The digital operating table provides

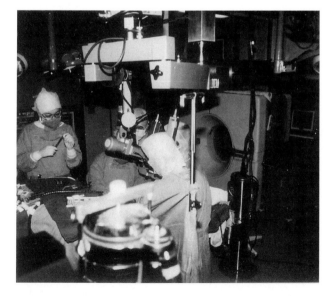

Fig. 24.1 Mobile CT scanner gantry of the operating CT scanner system in the Sugita operating theater.

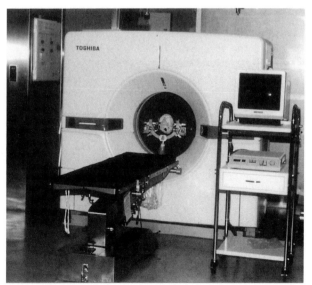

Fig. 24.2 Mobile CT scanner gantry of the operating CT scanner. Drawing shows a modified head fixation system.

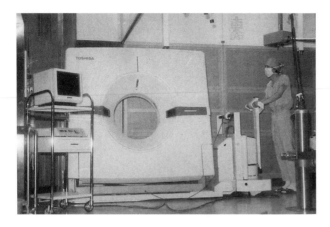

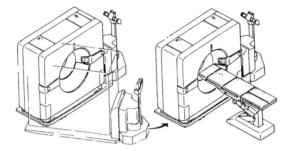

Fig. 24.3 The gantry of the CT scanner system being mobilized by a gantry carrier.

accurate motion entirely comparable to an ordinary scanner bed. An accuracy test using the CT scanner with mobile gantry and digitally controlled operating table was performed in the laboratory and yielded a similar degree of error when compared to the ordinary CT scanner with a scanner bed. Some authors have reported trials of intraoperative CT scanning and its clinical applications (Shalit et

al 1979, 1982, Lunsford et al 1984). These attempts are limited to a patient placed on the ordinary scanner bed. Because of the limited movement of the scanner bed and inability for suitable positioning of the patient during surgery, their systems cannot be conveniently applied during neurosurgical procedures. In the operating CT scanner system, combination of mobile gantry and digital operating table allows scanning of the patient in any head position (Okudera et al 1991a).

USES OF INTRAOPERATIVE CT SCANNING IN NEUROSURGERY

The operating room CT scanning system provides several advantages during surgery. Intraoperative CT (IOCT) scanning is useful in location of deep-seated paraventricular lesions. IOCT images can demonstrate structural shifts of the brain (Okudera et al 1994c). CT-guided transsphenoidal surgery for pituitary tumours can be a useful and safer modality of treatment (Okudera et al 1993a) (Fig. 24.4). The tumor can be identified easily after contrast administration and thus residual tumor can be detectable intraoperatively. Contrast-enhanced IOCT scan can demonstrate major cerebral arteries in the basal cistern. One can demonstrate intraoperative complications such as hemorrhage, pneumocephalus and can reliably show the radicality of tumor resection. IOCT is also helpful during skull base surgery (Okudera et al 1994c). Stereotactic procedures using the operating CT scanner are beneficial in various ways (Okudera et al 1990c). It permits carrying out the entire procedure in a sterile operating room. Craniotomy or any other surgical procedure can be performed as necessary. A CT scan can be done during or immediately after surgery in the operating room. In our practice immediate postoperative

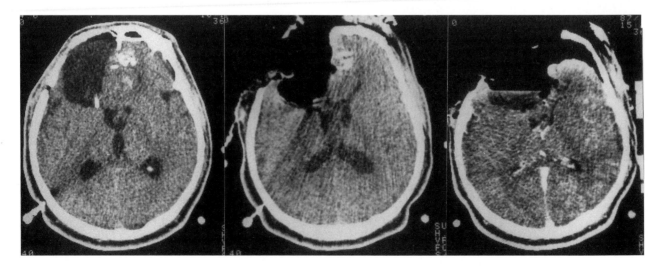

Fig. 24.4 Intraoperative serial CT scanning showing structural shifts.

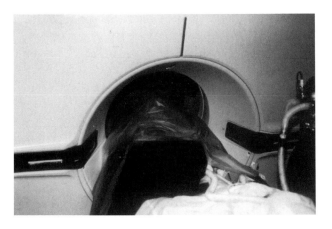

Fig. 24.5   Intraoperative CT scanning being performed.

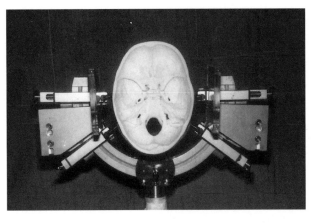

Fig. 24.6   Radiolucent version of Sugita head frame and fixation.

CT scanning is now a routine for all neurosurgical cases (Fig. 24.5) (Harada et al 1991).

RADIOLUCENT SUGITA HEAD FRAME AND FIXATION

Intraoperative radiological diagnostic methods such as digital subtraction angiography (DSA) and CT have been recently introduced. For satisfactory conduct of these investigations, it has become necessary to have a radiolucent head fixation system. Following the introduction of a CT scanner in our operating room, we have modified the Sugita head fixation (Sugita et al 1978). Initially, we modified the head holder and pins of the Sugita head fixation using an 'L'-shaped head pin held by a supporting device which is applied to the head holder. Recently, we developed a novel head fixation system for IOCT scanning (Fig. 24.6). The system is a new version of the Sugita multipur-pose head frame and is made up of two kinds of advanced engineering material: carbon fiber-reinforced plastic for head holder and frames, and polyamide-imide polymer for joints, screws and head pins (Fig. 24.7). Clinical tests including autoclaving and sterilization were performed and revealed that the material had sufficient strength for clinical use. This fixation system enables us to increase the efficacy of IOCT scanning during open-field neurosurgery.

The radiolucent multipurpose head frame, which has been developed for intraoperative CT scanning, can also be used for intraoperative angiography (Okudera et al 1994a). All parts of the radiolucent multipurpose head frame were designed to have interchangeability with that of the ordinary metallic Sugita system. Therefore, one can use the metallic accessories of the ordinary multipurpose head frame, such as the sliding base of the self-retaining retractor and the hand rest, together with the radiolucent frame as needed.

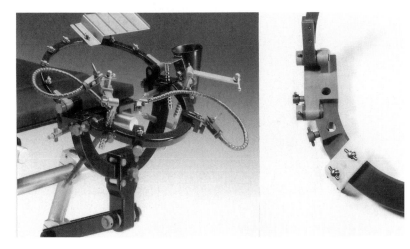

Fig. 24.7   The radiolucent Sugita head fixation frame is designed to maintain interchangeability with that of the original metallic Sugita system. Malleable retractors and other instruments can be used on this system.

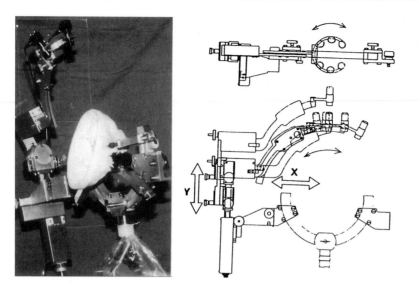

Fig. 24.8   Intraoperative stereotactic guide system in Shinshsu University.

INTRAOPERATIVE NAVIGATION

Intraoperative navigation is one of the promising neurosurgical techniques. Based on the ordinary stereotactic methodology, several navigation methods have been developed using ultrasound (Roberts et al 1986), mechanical arm with potentiometer (Watanabe et al 1987) and magnetic field (Kato et al 1991). We have developed a three-dimensional (3-D) stereotactic guide system concurrently with the operating CT scanner system (Okudera et al 1990a). The Shinshu system has been developed to target a point in the IOCT images directly onto the actual operative field by the intersection of laser pointers (Fig. 24.8). A laser guide arm with twin laser pointers was developed for the system (Okudera et al 1991b). The current version of the laser guide system yields similar accuracy to the ordinary CT stereotactic systems (Okudera 1993). As a navigation method, we used Neuronavigator (Watanabe et al 1987) (Mizuho, Tokyo) using exclusively designed attachment device for the Sugita head fixation system (Singh et al 1994) (Fig. 24.9).

COMPUTER-ASSISTED IMAGING TECHNOLOGY IN NEUROSURGERY

High-definition television system

The stereoscopic biocular operating microscope with a beam splitter is an essential microsurgical tool. We have used a triple binocular microscope in our operating theater (Sugita & Tsugane 1976) (Fig. 24.10). Based on the Sugita stereoscopic microscope system, the first-generation

stereoscopic recording was carried out using an ordinary NTSC (National Television System Committee) video system (Sugita et al 1985).

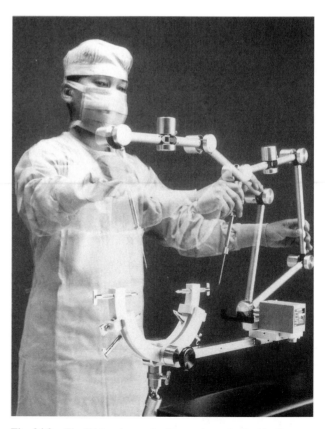

Fig. 24.9   The Watanabe navigation system attached to the Sugita head frame.

Visual documentation using a television and video system plays a significant role in modern neurosurgery. It is especially useful for the education of medical students, training of residents and recording medical conferences. In the documentation of microsurgery and endoscopic surgery, a video system is essential.

Recently, several high-definition television (HDTV) systems have been developed. The Hivision system is a completed HDTV system supporting high-quality pictures, which are comparable to 35 mm movie film, produced by 1125 scanning lines (Fujio 1985). It has been developed to replace the ordinary NTSC video system and realizes distinctive high-quality imaging. In the medical field in general, it provides superior quality images for recording surgical procedures under the microscope and endoscope. We first introduced the Hivision system to the medical field for relaying and recording neurosurgical procedures under the operating microscope (Okudera et al 1990d). Stereoscopic recording and presentation were realized using two sets of Hivision camera and Hivision recorder (Okudera et al 1993b) (Fig. 24.11). Recently we used a 3-D Hivision system for microneurosurgical documentation based on the Wide Vision Telepresence system (Okudera et al 1993b). The system enables us to realize 3-D medical documentation using one Hivision camera and one Hivision monitor. As in the traditional stereoscopic method of angiography, the system provides excellent 3-D microneurosurgical images and printed matter on one screen without the need for any optical devices.

A 3-D attachment device exclusively for the stereoscopic operating microscope has been developed. The device connects to the split right and left beam outputs of the stereoscopic operating microscope. It conducts two images from right and left outputs to one visual field individually. Because the Hivision system has a 9×16 image field, bilateral images can be recorded simultaneously in one Hivision image (Fig. 24.12). Using a traditional parallel stereoscopic viewer, the recorded Hivision images provide 3-D documentation of microneurosurgical practice on a monitor, on screen using a video projector and on printed matter. We introduced the 3-D Hivision system in cadaveric microneurosurgical hands-on workshops (Okudera et al 1996). The system was found to be a useful means of exact communication between the instructor and the participants and avoided congestion on the instructor's table. The entire proceeding could be recorded three-dimensionally for later use and educational purposes.

Computer-assisted infrared imaging

Brain temperature has been an important monitoring factor of cerebral blood flow and brain metabolism. We have introduced a high-resolution infrared (IR) video camera, developed for thermography applicable during microneurosurgery. Thermography is a well-established method for measuring the surface temperature of human organs. With the progress in electronic technology, a small-sized and lightweight thermographic camera is commercially available. It allows one to obtain not only static images but also real-time motion images. Intraoperative IR imaging during open neurosurgery was first performed in the surgical resection of a cerebral arteriovenous malformation (AVM) (Okudera et al 1995) (Fig. 24.13). For this purpose, a real-time mode IR camera was installed to the Sugita operating microscope using an exclusively developed

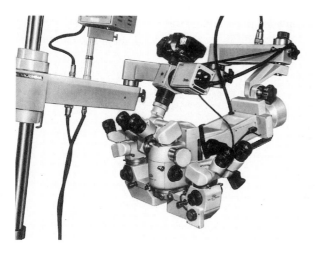

Fig. 24.10 The Sugita triple binocular microscope used in our operation room.

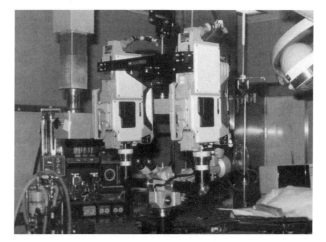

Fig. 24.11 3-D Hivision system based on the Wide vision Telepresence system using one camera and one monitor.

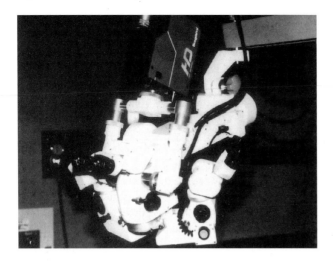

Fig. 24.12   Hivision camera system attached to the Sugita microscope.

attachment device. The camera demonstrated intraoperative regional and functional IR images. Changes of surface temperature of the cortical draining vein and surrounding cortical surface were observed intraoperatively before and after occlusion of the main feeder. Intraoperative functional thermography using cold physiological saline solution demonstrated change in heat clearance of the draining vein after complete obliteration of the feeder. Nowadays, we use a new digital mode IR camera with an operating microscope and obtain IR images during cerebrovascular surgery (Okudera & Kobayashi 1995). The new IR camera has a two-dimensional electronic IR sensor and Starling cooling unit. The system is developed for medical use. It realizes high-speed (60 image frames per second) and high resolutional digital IR imaging. Intraoperative surface IR imaging provides limited information within a few millimeters depth from the surface. However, it provides further objective information of the circulatory changes during surgery of cerebrovascular lesions as well as

helping in performing a minimal invasive resection of lesions. Intraoperative IR imaging realizes a non-contact and non-invasive real-time monitoring technique without the use of contrast materials.

Digital angiotomosynthesis

Digital tomosynthesis is the computer-assisted technique of reconstructing a tomogram of an object at any desired depth using a set of tomographic projection images taken from movement of the equipment (Sone et al 1991). In neurosurgical practice, conventional angiography is indispensable for evaluating complex cerebrovascular lesions even in the era of CT and MRI. The application of digital tomosynthesis to cerebral angiography provides several advantages over conventional angiography (Shigeta et al 1994). The digital tomographic image reveals fine details of the vascular lesion such as giant aneurysms and arteriovenous malformations.

Surgical simulation and computer graphics

At surgery for an intracranial mass lesion, the neurosurgeon often wishes to know the 3-D shape of the lesion and its topographical relationship to the surrounding anatomical structures. For surgical simulation of mass lesions we designed a simple 3-D display model based on off-line CT data (Okudera et al 1984). We have developed a computer-assisted geometric design of cerebral aneurysms for surgical simulation (Koyama et al 1995). The technique is based on the approximation power of the parametric spline function, which achieves interpolation and surface fitting of the geographical information of the intracranial arteries obtained by conventional angiography (Fig. 24.14). Computer graphic transformations including rotation, scaling and shifting make it possible to obtain the surgical

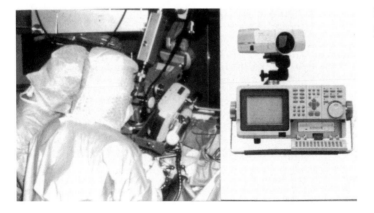

Fig. 24.13   Intraoperative real-time IR imaging system.

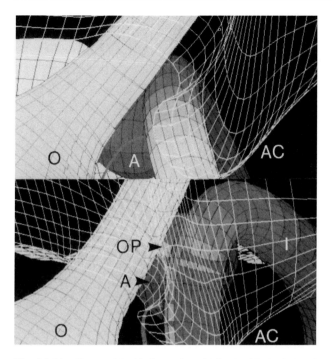

Fig. 24.14 Geographical information obtained with the help of computer graphics. Carotid cave aneurysm is seen (A) in relationship to the internal carotid artery (I), anterior clinoid process (AC), optic nerve (O) and ophthalmic artery (OP).

simulation of complex cerebral aneurysms such as basilar aneurysms and carotid cave aneurysms (Koyama et al 1996).

COMPUTER COMMUNICATION IN NEUROSURGERY

The personal computer is well established and widespread among medical doctors. In neurosurgery, the microcomputer has been applied to manage medical information such as patients' personal data, surgical data and follow-up (Manaka 1984). Recently, personal computer communication has become an important and basic tool in medical communication. It is useful in management of closed medical meetings (Okudera et al 1990) and wide-area computer networks (Bailes 1994).

REFERENCES

Bailes J E 1994 Neurolink: a neurosurgical wide-area computer network. Neurosurgery 35: 732–736

Fujio T 1985 High-definition television systems. Proceedings of the IEEE 73: 646–655

Harada T, Okudera H, Kobayashi S et al 1991 Computerized tomography immediately after surgery in the neurosurgical operating theater. Neurological Surgery 19: 415–419

Kato A, Yoshimine T, Hayakawa T 1991 A frameless, armless navigational system for computer-assisted surgery. Journal of Neurosurgery 74: 845–849

Koyama T, Okudera H, Kobayashi S 1995 Computer-assisted geometric design of cerebral aneurysm. Neurosurgery 36: 541–547

Koyama T, Gibo H, Okudera H et al 1996 Clinical implication of computer-assisted surgical design in a carotid cave aneurysm. Journal of Clinical Neurosciences 3: 363–365

Lunsford L D, Parrish R, Albright L 1984 Intraoperative imaging with a therapeutic computed tomographic scanner. Neurosurgery 15: 559–561

Manaka S 1984 Development and application of computerized database for neurosurgery. Neurological Surgery (Tokyo) 12: 889–898 (in Japanese)

Okudera H 1993 Development of stereotactic guide system for open neurosurgery. Shinshu Medical Journal 41: 571–578 (in Japanese)

Okudera H, Kobayashi S 1995 Clinical implications of intraoperative infrared imaging in cerebrovascular surgery: state of the art. Advances in Clinical Neurosciences 5: 469–473

Okudera H, Kobayashi S, Sugita K 1984 A simple three-dimensional display model based on recorded CT scan films for surgical reference. Technical note. Acta Neurochirurgica (Wien) 71: 47–53

Okudera H, Kobayashi S, Sugita K 1990a Three-dimensional neurosurgical guide system based on intraoperative computerized tomography. Progress in Clinical Neurosciences 6: 17–23

Okudera H, Kobayashi S, Sugita K 1990b Digitally controlled neurosurgical operating table. Technical note. Neurologia Medicochirurgica (Tokyo) 30: 201–203

Okudera H, Kobayashi S, Tanizaki Y 1990c Operating computed tomography (CT) scanner system for stereotactic surgery in the operating room. Stereotactic and Functional Neurosurgery 54–55: 418–419

Okudera H, Kobayashi S, Takemae T 1990d Stereoscopic HDTV (high definition TV) projection system for use with the operating microscope. In: Sugita K, Shibuya M (eds) Intracranial aneurysms and arteriovenous malformations. Nagoya University COOP Press, Nagoya, pp 413–414

Okudera H, Kobayashi S, Sugita K 1991a Development of the operating computerized tomographic scanner system for neurosurgery. Acta Neurochirurgica (Wien) 111: 61–63

Okudera H, Kobayashi S, Sugita K 1991b Computer-assisted three-dimensional surgical guide system using a laser guide arm based on intraoperative computerized tomography, in Brock M, Banerji A K, Sambasivan M (eds) Modern Neurosurgery 2. San Jose Press, Trivandrum, pp 471–477

Okudera H, Kobayashi S, Sugita K 1991c Technical note. Mobile CT scanner gantry for use in the operating room. American Journal of Neuroradiology 12: 131–132

Okudera H, Kobayashi S, Sugita K 1992 Modified head fixation system for intraoperative CT scanning. Technical Note. Neurologia Medicochirurgica (Tokyo) 31: 38–39

Okudera H, Kobayashi K, Takemae T 1993a Intraoperative CT scanning during transsphenoidal surgery. Technical note. Neurosurgery 32: 1041–1043

Okudera H, Kobayashi S, Kyoshima K 1993b Three-dimensional Hi-Vision system for microneurosurgical documentation based on wide-vision telepresence system using one camera and one monitor. Neurologia Medicochirurgica (Tokyo) 33: 719–721

Okudera H, Tokushige K, Kobayashi S 1994a Intraoperative angiography using a radiolucent multipurpose head frame for intraoperative CT scanning: a case with basilar bifurcation aneurysm. Japanese Journal of Neurosurgery (Tokyo) 3: 159–161

Okudera H, Kobayashi S, Toriyama T 1994b Intraoperative regional and functional thermography during resection of cerebral arteriovenous malformation. Neurosurgery 34: 1065–1067

Okudera H, Kyoshima K, Kobayashi S 1994c Intraoperative CT scan findings during resection of glial tumours. Neurological Research 16: 265–267

Okudera H, Kobayashi S, Takemae T 1994d Intraoperative CT scanning during skull base surgery. In: Samii M (ed) Skull base surgery. Karger, Basel, pp 26–28

Okudera H, Goel A, Kyoshima K et al (in press) Cadaveric hands-on workshop using three-dimensional high definition television system. Skull Base Surgery 6: 191–192

Roberts D W, Strihbehn J W, Hatch J F 1986 A frameless stereotactic integration of computerized tomographic imaging and the operating microscope. Journal of Neurosurgery 65: 545–549

Shalit M N, Israeli Y, Matz S et al 1979 Intraoperative computerized axial tomography. Surgical Neurology 11: 382–384

Shalit M N, Israeli Y, Matz S et al 1982 Experience with intraoperative CT scanning in brain tumors. Surgical Neurology 17: 376–382

Shigeta H, Sone S, Kasuga T 1994 Digital angiotomosynthesis for preoperative evaluation of cerebral arteriovenous malformations and giant aneurysms. American Journal of Neuroradiology 15: 543–549

Singh A K, Okudera H, Kobayashi S 1994 Newly developed attachment device of the multipurpose head frame for Neuronavigator. Acta Neurochirurgica (Wien) 129: 97–99

Sone S, Kasuga T, Sakai F 1991 Development of a high-resolution digital tomosynthesis system and its clinical application. Radiographics 11: 807–822

Sugita K, Tsugane R 1976 Triplescope for neurosurgery (Nagashima II). In: Koos W T, Bock F W, Spetzler R F (eds) Clinical microneurosurgery. Thieme, Stuttgart, pp 5–6

Sugita K, Hirota T, Mizutani T 1978 A newly designed multipurpose micro neurosurgical head frame. Technical note. Journal of Neurosurgery 48: 656–657

Sugita K, Ohohigashi Y, Kobayashi S 1985 Stereoscopic television system for use with the operating microscope. Technical note. Journal of Neurosurgery 62: 610–611

Watanabe E, Watanabe T, Manaka S 1987 Three-dimensional digitizer (neuronavigator): new equipment of computed tomography-guided stereotaxic surgery. Surgical Neurology 27: 543–547

Image-guided Neurosurgery: Applications in Skull Base Surgery
Prem Pillay

Image-guided neurosurgery refers to the technological advances in computer science, particularly 3-D graphics and frameless neuronavigation, improved optical imaging systems such as video endoscopy and computer-guided radiosurgery, which have over the last decade created a paradigm shift in neurosurgery.

Frameless Stereotaxis in Skull Base Surgery: In frameless stereotaxis, intraoperative neuronavigation can be carried out without the requirement of frame fixation prior to surgery. The advantage of this system is that there is no frame to interfere with patient positioning and access to any area of the cranium and skull base. At the same time, using a pointer or 'wand' in the Viewing Wand system, for example, the neurosurgeon is able to define any point in the operative field in terms of a cross-hair on axial, sagittal and coronal MRI or CT scans. A 3-D reconstruction of the tumor and adjacent important anatomical structures such as the carotid artery, cranial nerves, optic nerve and brain stem can be created to provide feedback to the surgeon during the operation. Another use is to guide the placement of a craniotomy, optimize and minimize the skull opening, navigate precisely to the target lesion, avoid critical structures, and maximize tumor removal. The latest frameless

system is called the stereotactic microscope (MKM microscope, Zeiss). Preoperative MRI and CT images of the skull base lesion are input into a computer workstation where processing takes place. Fiducial markers placed on the patient's scalp are registered on the operating table with a class I laser built into the microscope to define the stereotactic volume. Intraoperative navigation can now take place guided by a cross-hair and head-up navigational display within the viewing field of microscope. A 3–D video monitoring system can be used in conjunction with the stereotactic microscope. It is conceivable that with improved developments in monitor resolution in the near future it will be unnecessary for the neurosurgeon to look through the eyepieces of the microscope.

In our clinical research on the use of frameless stereotaxis in skull base surgery at our Brain Center, we have used these systems on approximately 176 patients with skull base tumors, including pituitary tumors, acoustic neurinomas, skull base meningiomas and various other tumors including clivus chordomas, orbital lymphoma and melanoma, esthesioneuroblastomas, and foramen magnum meningiomas. We found that neuronavigational techniques were particularly useful in planning appropriate approaches in these tumors and in defining critical structures where normal anatomy was grossly distorted by large tumors. In skull base tumors encasing the carotid artery, for instance, it was useful to know the distance and trajectory to the carotid artery while in the process of removing the tumor. In large acoustic neurinomas, the initial phase of debulking the tumor with an ultrasonic cavitron could take place by knowing the distance to the brain stem, followed by complete tumor excision. In the middle fossa approach to smaller acoustic neurinomas, drilling through the petrous bone with preservation of the cochlear function and precisely locating the tumor could be easily accomplished with image-guided frameless stereotaxis. In small pituitary microadenomas, accurate intraoperative location was carried out using the Viewing Wand system linked to an endoscope.

Video Endoscopic Skull Base Surgery: Since 1993, we have been exploring the use of endoscopes in the skull base. We started with endoscopic cadaveric dissections to define approaches and surgical endoscopic anatomy. This was followed by developing transnasal, transethmoidal as well as transnasal transsphenoidal endoscopic approaches to the sellar, suprasellar, clival and cavernous sinus regions. The most useful approach has been the transnasal transsphenoidal endoscopic procedure for resection of pituitary tumors. Only a small unilateral incision, approximately 8 mm in length, is required to create a submucoperichondrial tunnel with minimal displacement of the septal cartilage to reach the sphenoid. 4 mm rigid endoscopes are used with 0°, 30°, 70° and 120° of view. A three-chip color video camera is attached to the end of the endoscope and the surgeon operates from the view on a 21-inch high-resolution color monitor. Once the sphenoid sinus is entered an excellent panoramic view is obtained of the carotid arteries, the optic nerve and chiasm in their natural bony coverings and their relationship to the sella. Image-guided frameless stereotaxis is used to determine the site of intrasellar exposure for a small microadenoma in conjunction with the endoscope. In large pituitary macroadenomas, a 2 mm endoscope can be introduced into the pituitary fossa visualized with the microscope. The difference between tumor invasion and mere displacement of the cavernous sinus can be determined. The risk of carotid artery injury can be reduced. We have found that excellent tumor removal can be obtained even in large suprasellar tumors. We have carried out video endoscopic resection in 106 pituitary tumors and in 12 other skull base lesions including craniopharyngiomas, lymphoma, rhabdomyosarcoma and giant cell tumor of the bone. Video endoscopy is an important addition to the armamentarium of the skull base surgeon.

Combined Microsurgery and Radiosurgery for Skull Base Tumors: Radiosurgery refers to image-guided computer-planned and guided, focused radiation beams to ablate an intracranial target. The gamma knife is the 'gold' standard but LINAC systems are also in use. A large

volume of experience has been accumulated in applying radiosurgery to the treatment of skull base lesions, including cavernous sinus meningiomas, petroclival meningiomas, acoustic neurinomas and pituitary tumors. Most of these patients were deemed unfit for open surgery or had recurrent or residual tumors after attempts at radical surgery. A new and emerging concept that we are developing in skull base surgery is that of preplanned combined microsurgery and radiosurgery (CMR). This is particularly useful in large tumors involving either one or both cavernous sinuses, or in larger acoustic neurinomas. An important issue in radical skull base surgery is when dealing with benign tumors such as a meningioma of the middle fossa that has infiltrated the cavernous sinus radiologically but has not caused the patient any or at most mild cranial neuropathy, whether the degree of postoperative neuropathy is justified in attempting to 'cure' the patient of his tumor. In some patients this surgical complication is permanent. There are now several reports that cavernous sinus meningiomas infiltrate the cranial nerve sheaths and even the carotid artery. Certainly, in these patients, radical surgery will not offer a long-term cure. We are currently treating these larger tumors with radical image-guided microsurgery of these parts of the tumor which can be accessed with low morbidity and deliberately leaving and shaping the intracavernous tumor for optimal treatment with the gamma knife The functional results for the patient have been excellent but clearly a long-term study will have to be carried out in several institutions, including randomizing patients to either radical microsurgery or CMR, to determine its role.

Conclusions: There are several new areas to explore in the skull base surgery of the future. Telesurgery, robotics, virtual reality and even the Internet, all of which are image dependent, will impact on our practice. It is prudent for us to be aware of these advances and incorporate them into our repertoire of skills for the benefit of our patients.

References

Pillay P K 1995a The stereotactic microscope. In: Gildenberg P, Taskar R (eds) Textbook of stereotactic and functional neurosurgery. McGraw-Hill, New York (in press)

Pillay P K 1995b Stereotactic techniques. In: Andrews R (ed) Intraoperative neuroprotection. Williams & Wilkins, Baltimore, pp 395–422

Pillay P K, Sethi D S Endoscopic skull base surgery. Skull Base Surgery (in press)

Sethi D S, Pillay P K 1995a Endoscopic anatomy of the sphenoid sinus and sella turcica. Journal of Laryngology and Otology 109: 951–955

Sethi D S, Pillay P K 1995b Endoscopic management of lesions of the sella turcica. Journal of Laryngology and Otology 109: 956–962

Computed Tomography-guided Stereotactic Management of Brain Stem Masses
Vedantam Rajshekhar

Introduction: Management of intrinsic brain stem masses is rapidly evolving and is also the subject of much recent debate and discussion. Contributory to the change in the existing conservative approach to these masses, located in undoubtedly the most vital of intracranial structures, have been the remarkable advances in imaging the brain stem and surgical techniques, and evolution of protocols for monitoring the function of nervous structures within the brain stem. Image-guided, both CT and MRI, stereotactic techniques are one of those technical advances which enable a surgeon to access pathology in the brain stem with relative safety.

Historic Perspective: Ablative stereotactic procedures involving the spinothalamic tract in the midbrain (stereotactic mesencephalotomy) were performed by Spiegel and Wycis as far back as 1947 (Wycis & Spiegel 1962). Several others have performed this surgery for pain using pneumoencephalograms or positive-contrast ventriculography to guide the placement of the lesion. None of the conventional imaging techniques, however, afforded visualization of lesions within the brain stem for biopsy or aspiration and therefore morphological stereotactic surgery of the brain stem gained widespread acceptability only with the advent of stereotactic systems compatible with CT. Several reports of CT-guided stereotactic surgery on the brain stem since the mid-1980s are testimony to its increasing application in the management of brain stem masses (Abernathy et al 1989, Coffey & Lunsford 1985, Hood et al 1986, Hood & McKeever 1989, Kratimenos & Thomas 1993, Rajshekhar & Chandy 1994, 1995).

Stereotactic Access to the Brain Stem: The brain stem can be approached stereotactically through two routes (Hood et al 1986). In both approaches the basic principle is to violate only one pial plane, that is, the one closest to the cranial entry point. A second plane such as at the base of the brain should not be breached as the pial vessels in the basal cisterns and also those on the ventral surface of the brain stem can be damaged by the probe. Thus in both approaches the corridor of access remains within the brain parenchyma as far as possible. The surgery can be performed under local anesthesia in most cooperative adults.

Transfrontal Route: With the patient in the supine position, a cranial entry point just anterior or posterior to the coronal suture and about 3 cm lateral to the midline is chosen. A right frontal entry is generally preferred for all masses which are not lateralized to the left of the midline. Through a twist-drill craniostomy or a burr hole at this site, a stereotactic probe can be directed through the entire vertical extent of the brain stem. The probe track passes through the cerebral white matter, body of the lateral ventricle (depending on its size and therefore lateral extent) and then through the thalamus to reach the mesencephalon. If the cranial entry point is too far anterior, the probe will perforate the ventral surface of the brain, and too far posterior or lateral entry may result in entry into the dorsal surface of the tentorium at its hiatus. Thus the cranial entry is chosen to direct the stereotactic probe through the brain parenchyma as it passes through the tentorial hiatus and avoiding the edges of the tentorium.

Transcerebellar Route: With the patient in the prone position, a cranial entry point is chosen below the level of the transverse sinus and at an appropriate distance lateral to the midline to enable access to the pons through the middle cerebellar peduncle. The limitation of this approach is that it cannot be employed for masses in the midbrain and medulla.

Indications: Stereotactic surgery for a brain stem mass is mandated in two principal situations:

Histological Verification: This is by far the commonest indication for stereotactic exploration of the brain stem. Even the best available imaging modality (gadolinium-enhanced MRI) can on occasion be misleading with respect to pathology of a mass and even its exact location (extrinsic versus intrinsic). Hence histological verification of an intrinsic brain stem mass would ideally be necessary to direct a rational management plan in most instances. There is a great deal of controversy regarding the need to obtain a biopsy in children with diffuse brain stem gliomas. Some surgeons are comfortable with prescribing radiation therapy to these patients, without a biopsy diagnosis, on the basis of a typical clinical and MRI picture of a diffuse hypointense mass on T1-weighted images and a hyperintense mass on T2-weighted images (Albright et al 1989). Everyone is, however, agreed on the need to verify the histology of all focal and enhancing brain stem lesions and a brain stem mass in any patient with atypical clinical or MRI features (Albright et al 1989, Rajshekhar & Chandy 1995).

Aspiration of Cysts and Hematomas: Tumors cysts, abscesses (pyogenic and tuberculous) and hematomas within the brain stem can safely be evacuated using stereotactic methods (Hood & McKeever 1989, Kratimenos & Thomas 1993, Rajshekhar & Chandy 1994, Rajshekhar & Chandy 1995). In addition, radioisotopes have been instilled into glioma cavities after aspirating their contents (Hood & McKeever 1989).

Results and Benefits of Stereotactic Surgery: The yield from stereotactic biopsies of brain stem masses is very high, with reported positive biopsy rates from 94% to 100% (Abernathy et al 1989, Coffey & Lunsford 1985, Hood et al 1986, Hood & McKeever 1989, Kratimenos & Thomas 1993, Rajshekhar & Chandy 1995). More significant is the fact that an unexpected diagnosis emerged from the biopsy in 15–50% of instances (Kratimenos & Thomas 1993, Rajshekhar & Chandy 1995). In our series gathered over a period of 8 years, 103 patients with brain stem masses underwent 105 stereotactic procedures and a benign lesion was disclosed in 11/103 (10.6%) of those who had been diagnosed to have a malignant mass on their images (CT or MRI). While analyzing the benefits of the procedure in our patients we found that such a misdiagnosis was most likely to occur in patients with focal masses (<2 cm or restricted to one brain stem segment) and those with enhancing masses on CT, both focal and diffuse (Rajshekhar & Chandy 1995). Benign lesions which could mimic gliomas include demyelination, encephalitis, inflammatory granulomas, pyogenic abscesses, metastasis, lymphomas and occasionally masses adjacent to the brain stem such as cystic trigeminal schwannomas, epidermoids and prepontine neuroepithelial cysts (Abernathy et al 1989, Hood et al 1986, Kratimenos & Thomas 1993, Rajshekhar & Chandy 1995). Stereotactic biopsy avoids the obvious hazards of identifying a benign mass as a malignant tumor and empiric radiation therapy. In patients with brain stem tuberculomas, most often a stereotactic biopsy only excludes a neoplastic process and a definitive diagnosis of a tuberculoma can be made only in about 20% of cases (Rajshekhar & Chandy 1993, 1995).

The other major benefit that can accrue from stereotactic procedures for brain stem masses is the rapid amelioration of neurological symptoms in patients with cystic masses (Rajshekhar & Chandy 1993). Moreover, in the case of abscesses the causative organism can be identified and its antibiotic sensitivity pattern determined (Rajshekhar & Chandy 1994, 1995). The incidence of such cystic masses in our series was about 7%. We concluded that overall about 18% of patients benefited from the stereotactic procedure from a change in the projected management before the procedure and/or improvement in their neurological status following aspiration of cystic lesion (Rajshekhar & Chandy 1995).

We are not convinced that there is a correlation between the histological grade of a glioma determined from a stereotactic biopsy and the outcome (Rajshekhar & Chandy 1995). But others have shown that patients with low-grade brain stem glioma diagnosed on a stereotactic biopsy may have a better outcome than those with a biopsy diagnosis of a high-grade or malignant glioma (Hood et al 1986, Kratimenos & Thomas 1993).

Complications: The major complications of stereotactic procedures on the brain stem are those common to these procedures in general, namely hemorrhage along the probe track or at the biopsy site, and those specific to the brain stem. The latter category of complications can result from any technical error or shift of a firm mass away from the blunt stereotactic probe and damage to the surrounding normal brain stem structures. Occasionally, swelling of a mass may follow the procedure leading to an increase in existing neurological deficits. Another procedure-related complication noted by us has been the delay (24–48 hours) in awakening of four children with diffuse brain stem gliomas who underwent a stereotactic biopsy under general anesthesia (Rajshekhar & Chandy 1995). There has been no procedure-related mortality in our series of 103 patients; one patient developed permanent morbidity and six others had transient morbidity (including the four children with delayed awakening) which resolved within a week.

Conclusions: Our present policy is to verify isolated brain stem masses histologically in virtually every patient. This is mandatory for any focal or enhancing mass (focal or diffuse) and less so for children with diffuse non-enhancing masses on CT, provided gadolinium-enhanced MRI does not reveal any enhancement and the history and findings are typical for a brain stem glioma. But whenever there is the slightest doubt we tend to err on the side of obtaining a biopsy diagnosis. Patients with dorsally exophytic brain stem masses and those at the cervicomedullary junction (which are difficult to image on the CT and hence target) are generally subjected to open surgical exploration. We believe that it is prudent to obtain a stereotactic biopsy for any focal brain stem mass in which radical surgical excision is being contemplated (Rajshekhar & Chandy 1995). Identification of a malignant mass on the biopsy may alter the decision to go ahead with radical surgery as it is now well known that such surgery does not improve the survival of patients with malignant focal tumors of the brain stem.

References

Abernathy C D, Camacho A, Kelly P J 1989 Stereotaxic suboccipital transcerebellar biopsy of pontine mass lesions. Journal of Neurosurgery 70: 195–200

Albright A L, Packer R J, Zimmerman R et al 1989 Magnetic resonance scans should replace biopsies for the diagnosis of diffuse brain stem gliomas: a report from the Children's Cancer. Neurosurgery 70: 195–200

Coffey R J, Lunsford L D 1985 Stereotactic surgery for mass lesions of the midbrain and pons. Neurosurgery 17: 12–18

Hood T W, McKeever P E 1989 Stereotactic managment of cystic gliomas of the brain stem. Neurosurgery 24: 373–378

Hood T W, Gewbarski S S, McKeever P E et al 1986 Stereotaxic biopsy of intrinsic lesions of the brain stem. Journal of Neurosurgery 65: 172–176

426   Neurosurgery of complex tumors and vascular lesions

Kratimenos G P, Thomas D G T 1993 The role of image-directed biopsy in the diagnosis and management of brainstem lesions. British Journal of Neurosurgery 7: 155–164

Rajshekhar V, Chandy M J 1993 CT guided stereotactic managment of intracranial tuberculomas. British Journal of Neurosurgery 7: 619–624

Rajshekhar V, Chandy M J 1994 Successful stereotactic management of a large cardiogenic brain stem abscess. Neurosurgery 34: 368–371

Rajshekhar V, Chandy M J 1995 Computerized tomography-guided stereotactic surgery for brainstem masses: a risk-benefit analysis in 71 patients. Journal of Neurosurgery 82: 976–981

Wycis H T, Spiegel E A 1962 Long-range results in the treatment of intractable pain by stereotactic midbrain surgery. Journal of Neurosurgery 19: 101–107

Neuronavigator
Eiju Watanabe

Neuronavigator was first developed in 1987 by Watanabe et al (1987). Since then, more than 10 navigation systems have been invented with a similar underlying idea. The navigation system translates the location in the surgical field into the preoperative CT/MRI image. The Neuronavigator consists of a personal computer, a multi-joint sensing arm and an image scanner (Fig. 24.15). The 3-D coordinates of the arm tip are monitored by the computer and automatically translated into CT or MRI coordinates and finally displayed with a cursor on the CT or MRI images on the computer screen (Fig. 24.16) (Watanabe et al 1987, Watanabe et al 1991, 1992, Watanabe & Kosugi 1993). The navigator is one of the stereotactic operation systems; however, it has several differences from the conventional CT/MRI-guided stereotactic frames. The most fundamental difference is the direction of the conversion of spatial information. In the conventional system, the CT/MRI coordinates of lesion are measured and translated into a patient's coordinates. The surgeon then sets the frame parameters corresponding to the patient coordinates to reach the lesion. With the navigator, we first place the arm tip on the patient's head to obtain the patient's coordinates. The computer automatically indicates the location in the corresponding CT/MRI image. In short, in the stereotactic system, the spatial information is translated from CT/MRI coordinates into patient's coordinates, whereas in the navigator system, the information is translated from a patient's coordinates into CT/MRI coordinates. When we target one particular point in the cranium as in needle biopsy, the former method is reasonable. But when we want to monitor our direction of approach or monitor our location, the navigator's method is more comfortable. It is similar to the flow of information in a surgeon's own thinking process during surgery, in approaching the intracranial target.

The overall accuracy of the Neuronavigator is about 2.5 mm (Watanabe et al 1991). Because we use nasion and tragi as fiducials, the accuracy becomes better when the target lies nearer to the skull base. We must be careful of the fact that the brain tissue deviates when considerable amounts of CSF or tumor tissue are removed. In a practical sense, however, it is often recognized that just opening the dura mater does not cause significant deviation of the tissue. As far as we use the preoperative CT/MRI images in navigation, this problem cannot be avoided. The easiest way to overcome this problem is to achieve orientation at the earlier phase of the surgery. The fundamental solution to this problem would be a real-time image-updating technique such as intraoperative CT or MRI.

As for future applications, the use of Neuronavigator to translate the information of functional mapping into the surgical field is promising (Sakai et al 1995). Magnetoencephalography is one of the effective alternatives to localize the somatosensory cortex of the individual brain. When this information is superimposed onto the individual magnetic resonance image, the navigator can indicate accurately the somatosensory cortex or central sulcus on the actual brain surface of the patient during the operation. Using this type of guidance we could easily achieve lower postoperative morbidity in a shorter operation time.

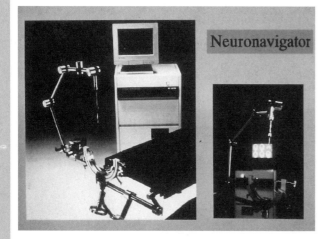

Fig. 24.15   The Neuronavigator consists of a personal computer, a multi-joint sensing arm and an image scanner.

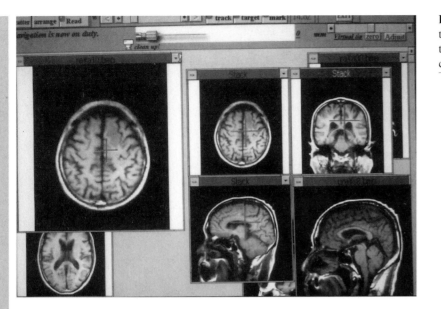

Fig. 24.16   Computer display. Location of the arm tip is calibrated and displayed on the corresponding CT/MRI slice with the cross-hair cursor.

References

Sakai K, Watanabe E, Onodera Y et al 1995 Functional mapping of the human somatosensory cortex with echo-planar MRI. Magnetic Resonance Medicine 33: 736–743

Watanabe E, Watanabe T, Manaka S et al 1987 Three dimensional digitizer (Neuronavigator): new equipment for computerized tomography-guided stereotactic surgery. Surgical Neurology 27: 543–547

Watanabe E, Mayanagi Y, Kosugi Y et al 1991 Open surgery assisted by the neuronavigator, a stereotactic articulated, sensitive arm. Neurosurgery 28: 792–800

Watanabe E, Mayanagi Y, Takakura K 1992 Stereotactic guidance of TCD probe using a computer assisted frameless stereotactic guiding system (Neuronavigator). Recent Advances in Neurosonology 481–486

Watanabe E, Kosugi Y 1993 Intraoperative neuronavigator system in neurosurgery and computer surgery. in Fujino T (ed) Simulation and computer-aided surgery. Wiley, Chichester, pp 157–162

Index